Chronic Illness

THE JONES AND BARTLETT SERIES IN NURSING

THIRD EDITION

Chronic Illness

Impact and Interventions

Ilene Morof Lubkin, RN, MS, CGNP

Professor Emeritus
California State University
Hayward, California

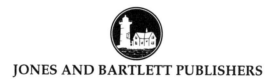

JONES AND BARTLETT PUBLISHERS

Sudbury, Massachusetts

Boston   London   Singapore

Editorial, Sales, and Customer Service Offices
Jones and Bartlett Publishers
40 Tall Pine Drive
Sudbury, MA 01776
508-443-5000
800-832-0034

Jones and Bartlett Publishers International
Barb House, Barb Mews
London W6 7PA
UK

Library of Congress Cataloging-in-Publication Data

Lubkin, Ilene Morof
    Chronic illness : impact and interventions / Ilene Morof Lubkin—3rd ed.
       p.   cm. — (Jones and Bartlett series in nursing)
    Includes bibliographical references and index.
    ISBN 0-86720-712-4
    1. Chronic diseases—Psychological aspects. 2. Chronically ill—Family
relationships. 3. Nurse and patient. I. Title. II. Series.
    [DNLM 1. Chronic Disease—psychology. 2. Professional-Patient
Relations. 3. Professional–Family Relations.   W 62 L929c 1995]
RC108.L83   1995
616–dc20
DNLM/DLC
for Library of Congress   94-37265
                                                CIP

Acquisitions Editor: Jan Wall
Production Editor: Mary Cervantes Sanger
Manufacturing Buyer: Dana L. Cerrito
Editorial Production Service: Ocean Publication Services
Typesetting: Modern Graphics, Inc.
Cover Design: Hannus Design Associates
Printing and Binding: Hamilton Printing Company
Cover Printing: John P. Pow Company

Printed in the United States of America
98 97 96   10 9 8 7 6 5 4 3

CONTENTS

FOREWORD

The medical arts and sciences have had their finest moments in the address of acute diseases. Modern surgery, technology, and antibiotics have transformed the roster of major killers that ruled for centuries, so at the end of this millennium we find ourselves with markedly fewer acute problems. The extraordinary atrophy of the hospital as the center of medical enterprise is vivid testimony to the shift from acute to chronic conditions.

It is clear that this epochal transition finds a lack of adequate conceptual framework from which policy and practice can derive. Biology, sociology, economics, and civics are ill equipped to confront the new reality. The major effort now directed to health care reform is, to a large degree, due to the inability of prior structures to deal with the present situation.

Fee-for-service medicine was an appropriate administrative arrangement for acute problems. The transaction was simple, direct, and time insensitive. Unfortunately, the conditions that create our current morbidity and mortality are not susceptible to cure. We palliate rather than cure heart attacks, stroke, diabetes, arthritis, emphysema, and Alzheimer's disease, among others. We spend huge amounts of effort and money on a curative philosophy and practice when cure does not pertain. Unfortunately, disease prevention, health promotion, and restorative efforts languish because they lack glamour, prestige, and payment incentives.

Chronic illness also brings with it the concept of team management. Whereas acute problems usually lend themselves to a simple paternalistic entrepreneurial contract, the degenerative conditions that now predominate demand a diverse therapeutic perspective and competence. This team, when truly functional, is able to initiate and sustain treatment protocols that no single health professional can possibly provide. As a result, the patient becomes the beneficiary of biologic, psychologic, and social knowledge. However, the shaping of team structure and function is still in its infancy. Health professionals need to become comfortable with the concept of the patient and family being the center of the team. Experimentation is mandatory to find out what works and what does not and, importantly, how much it will cost.

A principal element underlying the entire paradigm shift involves the participation of time. Until now, time was undervalued as a participating agency in the course of our affairs. Until now, life was analyzed largely as a set of episodic unconnected events rather than as a series of interconnected and time-dependent processes. Adding a time dimension increases the complexity of our understanding immeasurably.

We are fortunate that as time is increasingly being identified as a major contributing agency to this human condition, outcomes assessment technology is also emerging. This technology encompasses the time variable and greatly enriches our understanding of the area under the curve rather than at a group of isolated points in time. Further, outcomes technology shifts the emphasis from the analysis of what happens to the individual at a single moment, to how the individual and community perceive the outcome of a group of variables over time. The individual at risk is described, not just as a passive partner in an isolated event, but as an active participant who both shapes and is shaped by the environment. Such a shift in emphasis is equivalent to the evolution of physics from the time-insensitive Newtonian era of mechanics to the expanded era of quantum principles that encompasses uncertainty and complexity.

I have experienced innumerable intense patient–physician encounters in which the proposed approach or solution of today melts into tomorrow's new realities. The reality of time ensures modesty.

This revised edition of *Chronic Illness: Impact and Interventions* explores the emerging awareness. It emphasizes time courses, trajectories, developmental process, life quality, and the embeddedness of the individual and the caregiver in a social fabric. No one can pretend that this approach is neat and tidy, but at least it has relevancy in the present circumstance.

To apply the old model to the current situation is naive at best. More accurately, it is stupid, wasteful, and dangerous for our society. The application of solutions from our parents' era to our children's problems won't work. As we enlarge our vision to incorporate time-dependent complexities, we place ourselves in consonance with the universal law. This volume takes us into the richness of human illness over time. It displays the problems and challenges; it notes progress made and areas of lack. It provides a framework for eager address of a critical societal issue of our time.

Walter M. Bortz, II, M.D.
Physician, Palo Alto Medical Foundation;
Clinical Associate of Medicine,
Stanford Medical Center

PREFACE

As I complete work on this third edition, I reflect on the origin of this book and the frustration I felt over the lack of an adequate text that dealt with how chronic illness impacted on individuals. Then, as now, I had no need to create a text that dealt with disease process or management, subjects that are well covered in numerous other sources.

Originally, the experience and themes that proved meaningful to nursing students guided the selection of the text's content. This material continues to be of value and has been updated. Much of the new content grows out of the turmoil that exists in today's ongoing debate over the direction that health care will take. Most individuals agree that change is necessary.

Since the book was first published, much has changed in the provision of health care, even though a great deal remains the same. Our health care system continues to focus on acute care, although there are fewer acute conditions. Health care in the United States is of the highest quality, yet because of escalating costs and the lack of or inadequate insurance, more and more individuals find they are unable to avail themselves of this care. Technology has burgeoned, providing us with many new and exciting methods of diagnosis and treatment; however, we have no solutions to the problems and complications of conditions that are chronic in nature: cardiac illnesses, strokes, long-term prob-lems of prematures, mental deterioration, diabetes, AIDS, and so forth.

This text continues to focus on the many factors and issues that influence clients and families who are dealing with chronic conditions and who see their disorders as entailing more than physiological and psychological pathology. These individuals deal not only with their diseases but with managing their lives on a day-to-day basis from sociological, psychological, ethical, organizational, and financial perspectives. Most health professionals, on the other hand, continue to think of illness as acute and episodic in nature rather than as conditions that have a long-term impact on their clients.

The publication of a third edition provides an opportunity both to update and to add additional content that seems appropriate. To this end, chapters on growth and development, social isolation, nursing case management, nursing ethics, and social/health policy have been added. The Appendix has also been updated. Content on nursing diagnosis comes from Taxonomy I (1987) and *NANDA Nursing Diagnosis: Definitions and Classification* (1994), published by the North American Nursing Diagnosis Association.

As in previous editions, the text presents a cohesive whole by developing the interrelationship of topics throughout. However, each chapter stands alone, providing information and help in the area discussed. It is hoped that the content herein will expand health professionals' knowledge of chronicity so they can better help their clients take on the responsibilities of self-care management while providing more sensitive care. Only by understanding the topics addressed from the perspective of chronicity can one develop a thorough appreciation of the long-term impact of chronic diseases and the many challenges facing health care today.

Acknowledgments

I wish to acknowledge the many people who supported and encouraged me in the creation of this edition: my publisher for having enough faith in the book to want another edition; my attorney, Alan Freeland, for his excellent legal advice; and the reviewers who went over both new and greatly revised chapters. I also want to give thanks to those contributors who worked with me on the first two editions but were unable to do so for this edition: Brenda Bailey, R.N., D.N.Sc.; Marie-Luise Friedemann, R.N., Ph.D.; Eileen Jackson, R.N., Ph.D.; Terry Neifing, M.S.W., L.C.S.W.; Margene Nordstrom, R.N., D.N.Sc.; Barbara Scheffer, R.N., Ph.D.; and Anne Shanck, R.N., M.S., M.A. Their work was greatly appreciated. And thanks must be given to those contributors who made time to modify their chapters and to those who either wrote new material or updated and modified prior content.

A special thanks to my many friends, family, and colleagues who are always there for me when I undertake a major writing project and who see that I have nonwriting outlets so I don't become isolated with my computer.

CONTRIBUTORS

Ilene Lubkin, RN, MS, CGNP
Professor Emeritus
Department of Nursing
California State University, Hayward
Hayward, California

Diana Biordi, RN, PhD
Associate Professor
Assistant Dean, Research and
 Graduate Affairs
School of Nursing
Kent State University
Kent, Ohio

Dorothy Blevins, RN, MSN
Associate Professor
School of Nursing
Kent State University
Kent, Ohio

Audrey Bopp, RN, MSN
Chair
Health Occupations Education
 Department
Front Range Community College
 —Larimer Campus
Ft. Collins, Colorado

Karna Bramble, RN, PhD, CGNP
Associate Professor of Nursing
California State University, Long Beach
Nurse Practitioner
Veterans' Administration Hospital
Long Beach, California

Margaret Burns, RN, DNSc
Associate Professor
School of Nursing
Loma Linda University
Loma Linda, California

Deborah H. Burton, PhD, RN
Associate Chief Nurse
Department of Veterans Affairs
 Medical Center
Portland, Oregon
Adjunct Assistant Professor
University of Portland School of Nursing

Mary Curtin, RN, MS, CANP
Nurse Practitioner
Coalinga Health Center
Coalinga, California

Elizabeth Dixon, RN, PhD
Professor
School of Nursing
Mankato State University
Mankato, Minnesota

Christine Elnitsky, RN, BSN, MSc
Graduate Research Assistant
Old Dominion University
Norfolk, Virginia

Sheila Ostrow Flodberg, RN, MS, CGNP
Nurse Practitioner
Developmentally Disabled Mentally Retarded
Utah State Developmental Center
American Fork, Utah

Barbara A. Harris, MS, RN, PhDc
University of Illinois at Chicago
Chicago, Illinois

Elizabeth Johnston-Taylor, RN, PhD
Post-Doctoral Fellow
University of California, Los Angeles
Los Angeles, California

Patricia S. Jones, RN, PhD
Professor
School of Nursing
Loma Linda University
Loma Linda, California

Arlene Miller Kahn, RN, EdD
Professor and Chair
Department of Nursing
California State University, Hayward
Hayward, California

Katheliene Kohler, RN, MS, CANP
Support Services Manager
Kaiser Permanente Medical Center
Martinez, California

Karen Thornbury Labuhn, RN, PhD
Senior Research Associate
Center for Health & Research
Kaiser Permanente North West Region
Portland, Oregon

Pamala D. Larsen, RN, PhD, CRRN
Associate Professor
School of Nursing
College of Health and Human Sciences
University of Northern Colorado
Greeley, Colorado

Carolyn Lewis, PhD, RN
Program Services Manager
American Nurses Credentialing Center
Washington, D.C.

Patricia Ryan Lewis, RN, PhD
Assistant Professor and Associate Chair
School of Nursing
Northern Illinois University
DeKalb, Illinois

Beverly J. McElmurry, RN, EdD, FAAN
Professor and Associate Dean
Office for International Studies
College of Nursing
University of Illinois at Chicago
Chicago, Illinois

Cathy Michaels, RN, PhD
Clinical Director, Research
Professional Nurse Case Manager
Carondolet St. Mary's
Tucson, Arizona

Susan J. Misner, MS, RN
Research Specialist
Department of Public Health
College of Nursing
University of Illinois at Chicago
Chicago, Illinois

Geri Budesheim Neuberger, RN, EdD
Associate Professor
School of Nursing
College of Health Sciences
University of Kansas
Kansas City, Kansas

Linda L. Olson, MS, RN, PhDc
University of Illinois at Chicago
Chicago, Illinois

Judith Papenhausen, RN, PhDc
Associate Chairperson and Professor
Department of Nursing
California State University, Los Angeles
Los Angeles, California

Mary Elizabeth Payne, RN, PhDc
Director of Nursing
Dial-A-Nurse
L. W. Consulting Services, Inc.
Naples, Florida

Diane Peters, RN, PhD
Associate Professor
College of Health and Human Science
School of Nursing
University of Northern Colorado
Greeley, Colorado

Timothy A. Philipp, RN, PhD
Consultant
T. A. Philipp and Associates
Chicago, Illinois

Coleen Saylor, RN, PhD
Professor
School of Nursing
San Jose State University
San Jose, California

Mary Therese Schweikert-Stary, MA
Advisor, Student Life Programs
California State University, Hayward
Hayward, California

Nancy E. White, RN, PhD
Associate Professor
College of Health and Human Sciences
School of Nursing
University of Northern Colorado
Greeley, Colorado

Cynthia Thorne Woods, RN, PhD
Assistant Professor
School of Nursing
College of Health Sciences
University of Kansas
Kansas City, Kansas

PART I

Impact of the Disease

CHAPTER 1

What Is Chronicity?

Mary Curtin • Ilene Lubkin

Introduction

Chronic illness constitutes our nation's number-one medical malady, demanding that medical and social leadership construct new visions and goals. Comprehensive planning is needed to prevent events that might lead to the initial long-term illness, as well as to deter the worsening of existing disabilities. Research efforts expand their probe of causes and eradication of illnesses that become chronic states. Policy changes lead to legislation that attempts to keep pace with the burdens of chronicity—especially the social, medical, and economic costs. Increasingly, partnerships of those who require services with those who provide services are making past delivery systems obsolete and opening opportunities for the redefinition of roles, activities, and goals.

Chronic illnesses take many forms. They can occur suddenly or through an insidious process; they can have episodic flare-ups or exacerbations or remain in remission with an absence of symptoms for long periods of time. Maintaining a degree of wellness or keeping symptoms in remission can be a juggling act of balancing treatment and regimens. For example, heart failure makes one person a bedridden invalid, although another with a similar degree of failure attains a satisfactory social life through the understanding support of others and knowledgeable manipulation of cardiac medication.

Historical Perspective

Human beings throughout history have recognized the presence of illness and attempted to repair or minimize disease. Evidence of early healing attempts is shown in a Sumerian tablet (approximately 2100 B.C.) that deals primarily with poultices. The "Treatise of Medical Diagnosis and Prognosis" (Mesopotamian tablets possibly from 1600 B.C.) lists diseases and outcomes based on a variety of signs (Majno, 1975). Interventions that combined medical means and mysticism were often used to treat the tangible and intangible aspects of disease. In the 1600s, secondary to traditional interpretation of cause and effect, health authorities ventilated city alleys and legislated the storage of manure in an effort to do battle against bad odors and humors, thought to be the source of the plague (Cipolla, 1992).

Beginning in the 19th century, after discoveries in disease causation and process, people began to apply scientific methodologies to health care. Health fields, such as medicine and nursing, now deal with an increasing variety of health events that move from acute to chronic, as well as with the iatrogenic effects of successful and wide-ranging interventions. Current health workers face the prospect that in the next quarter of a century there will be clients with health conditions as yet unknown who will require health care by means not yet comprehensible. Looking at the coming century, politicians and scientists will need to balance anticipated longer life spans with the economic, societal, and environmental resources needed to maintain lengthened years (Lowenstein, 1992).

Factors Influencing Increasing Chronicity

The course of any disease follows some kind of general trend or trajectory (see Chapter 3, on illness trajectory) depending on the specific entity diagnosed, its severity and rate of progression, and the psychological makeup and expectations of the person. In the past, trajectories tended to be fairly predictable, but the advent of new technology, such as donor and mechanical organ transplants, has dramatically altered such courses. The presence of multiple disease entities further changes the trajectory, making projecting outcomes difficult for physicians and other health professionals, as well as making future planning uncertain for the client and the family.

Developments in the fields of bacteriology, immunology, public health, and pharmacology have resulted in a precipitous drop in mortality from communicable and other acute diseases. Since the 1970s, however, there has been an emergence of newly identified illnesses and syndromes. For example, an outbreak of *E. coli* in commercial hamburger meat caused a serious outbreak and four deaths. The virulence of this organism and the potential impact on public health expanded regulatory and surveillance activities to include this once little regarded pathogen (CDC, 1993).

Decreased mortality from acute illness has led to lengthened life spans and, incidentally, greater vulnerability to accident and disease events that can accumulate as chronic conditions. Medical success has also contributed, in part, to the unprecedented growth of chronic illness. For instance, biotechnology and nuclear medicine bring about life-saving and life-sustaining interrelationships with machines.

Given these factors, it becomes apparent that the prevalence of chronic disease is increasing dramatically. For instance, pharmacotherapy has changed the character of the AIDS epidemic from an acute terminal illness to a chronic one. HIV infection itself will increasingly require chronicity management (Fee & Fox, 1992). The World Health Organization (WHO) estimates that between 8 and 10 million persons worldwide have been infected. While the world case total of AIDS has risen, there has been a decrease of diagnosed cases in the United States. As is characteristic of any early chronic health problem, future AIDS cases will reflect the current HIV infection rates (WHO, 1992).

Human behavior is a major factor determining health. For instance, it is projected worldwide that the effects of smoking tobacco will cause chronic illnesses that will lead to 10 million deaths yearly. Controlling such disorders as hepatitis B infections, hypertension, and elevated blood cholesterol will greatly lower global chronic disease rates (Peto, 1992). Chronic disabilities are disproportionately found among minorities, the lower socioeconomic populations, and the elderly. In addition, about one in every seven persons of all ages has a disabling condition that limits life activities (Institute of Medicine, 1991).

Chronic illness can begin with a seemingly insignificant acute condition that is only partially resolved. Although the outcome may be free of profound disability or death, the accumulation of events can lead to a drastically altered lifestyle. The case history of Mr. W. demonstrates such an occurrence.

Perceptions of Chronic Illness

Health professionals can view chronicity positively, as a state that can continue to contribute to the potential growth of an individual, family, or society, or negatively, as a state of failure to recover completely. Some of this negativity flows from the fact that a majority of health workers participate in the client's care only at the worst times, since most health care settings provide episodic care based on the worsening or exacerbation of symptoms. With this piecemeal exposure, the disease entity reinforces the attitude

CASE STUDY

A Case of Progressive Dermatitis

While looking after his small herd of cattle, Mr. W., aged 52, wore boots that were higher than his sock length, producing chafing in both calves. One area became increasingly inflamed and then infected. He self-medicated for a week with veterinary penicillin ointment on hand for use with cattle. By the time he went to his physician, the formerly reddened area had progressed into cellulitis with draining lesions from foot to midthigh. Two medications were tried without improvement.

After two weeks, a dermatology consultation led to hospitalization and orders for bedrest, daily leg soaks, diet restrictions, and further medication changes. Several months later he had still not healed. Social contacts were reduced; he sold the cattle herd because he was unable to work regularly. Reemployment as a yard foreman required job modification due to exacerbation of the leg lesions with activity. When not at work, Mr. W. kept his legs elevated and wrapped with ace bandages. At age 58 he retired because of chronic leg debility.

---

that extended life may indeed offer only increasing disability, pain, and deterioration. To counteract negativity of this kind, the health professional must strive to keep the client's entire life pattern in focus.

Statistics, which are an invaluable aid for appreciating the scope of a particular disease condition through analysis of characteristics, impact, prevalence, costs, and so on, also influence attitudes about chronic conditions. From a positive dimension, statistics provide information that demonstrates probable cause and effect of a disease process, as well as the impact of preventive measures. For example, chronic obstructive pulmonary disease (COPD) mortality is second only to that of coronary heart disease; morbidity from this one disorder is about 10 to 15 percent of all adults over 55 years of age (Department of Commerce, 1992). The number of individuals with COPD is expected to slow following the decline of tobacco use. Because COPD evolves from a long period of destruction before symptoms are noted, statistics do not, as yet, reflect the degree of tobacco cessation. However, 80 to 90 percent of people with early COPD have stopped smoking cigarettes, and this is expected to lead to a decrease in severe COPD cases in the future (Ries, 1993).

In spite of findings like these, statistics tend to reinforce negative attitudes about chronic diseases. For instance, information about the decline of heart disease in the United States describes the disease's characteristics in terms of physical disability, economic costs, and death rates. Seldom are reemployment rates provided for comparison to rates demonstrating individuals' dependency on society. Additionally, researchers looking into the impact of chronic disease have been hampered by measures of health status emphasizing performance of activities of daily living (ADLs) rather than a full range of employment and social activities (Lubeck & Yelin, 1988). To investigate these broader approaches, a telephone survey posed questions based on the inherent value of activities, past and present, to evaluate the indirect costs of limitation. Among respondents over the age of 40 with at least one limitation, it was found that work was less important than maintaining the capacity for social contacts and performing personal activities such as shopping and home endeavors. Although these findings emphasize the importance of ADLs, it was conjectured that a younger population would possibly find employment capability of significant importance (Lubeck & Yelin, 1988).

Acute illnesses generally have a sudden, dynamic onset, with signs and symptoms usually related to the disease process itself. Acute illness ends shortly either with complete recovery and resumption of prior activities or with death. Acute illness may be compared to an unexpected visitor who leaves one's house after a short-term stay.

Chronic illness, on the other hand, announces plans to visit for an indefinite stay and gradually becomes part of the household. Although this "guest" is a welcome alternative to death, the illness provides a mixed blessing to the host household and to society at large. In addition, the illness frequently becomes the person's identity. For example, an individual having leukemia, even in remission after chemotherapy, acquires the label "that person with leukemia" (see Chapter 5, on stigma).

Difficulty in Defining Chronicity

Answering the question of what chronicity is becomes very complex. Many individuals have attempted to present an all-encompassing yet clear definition of chronic illness (see Table 1-1). It is interesting to note that there are no nursing definitions. The characteristics of chronic diseases were identified by the Commission on Chronic Illness as all impairments or deviations from normal that include one or more of the following: permanency; residual disability; nonpathological alteration; required rehabilitation; or a long period of supervision, observation, and care (Roberts, 1954). The National Conference on Care of the Long-Term Patient added a further time dimension to these characteristics: chronic disease or impairment necessitating acute hospitalization exceeding 30 days, or medical supervision and rehabilitation of 3 months or longer in another caretaking setting (Roberts, 1954). Many conditions, such as birth defects and postinjury and postsurgical states, are included within the umbrella-like classification of chronic illness under the terms these two agencies present.

Determining a definition for chronic disease is more difficult when one attempts to establish the origin of a specific condition. Many chronic diseases have multiple factors that can take many years to accumulate sufficiently to produce frank symptoms. Do we say that bowel cancer that manifests itself at the age of 50 originated when the first mutant cell divided 30 years earlier? Or was it the result of a particular diet or life-style? Or can we say it started at the time of biopsy? Like life itself, the time of origin is debatable. For chronic disease, origin is highly critical in seeking measures that may prevent or ameliorate the eventual disease.

The extent and direction of chronic illness further complicate attempts to provide a firm definition. A measurable quantity of disability from chronic illness depends not only on the kind of condition and its severity but also on the implications it holds for the person. A teenager may require greater adjustment to the restrictions necessitated by a bone cancer than an individual who is past the age of 60. The degree of disability and altered life-style, part of a traditional definition, may relate as much to the client's views of the impact of the disease on self as to the specific disease.

Long-term and iatrogenic effects of some treatment methods may constitute chronic conditions eligible for definition as chronic illness. This situation is well represented by the necessary changes in life patterns required of clients on hemodialysis. Lifesaving procedures can create other problems. Abdominal radiation that arrested metastatic intestinal cancer when an individual was age 30 can contribute to a malabsorption problem several years later, so that almost continuous diarrhea may force the now cachectic and exhausted person to stay close to toilet facilities. Fortunately, these are extreme examples of life-style changes provoked by treatment procedures.

Chronic illness, by its very nature, is never completely cured or prevented. The inevitable breakdown of cultural, economic, emotional, and social factors all affect body integrity. Biologically, the human body wears out unevenly. Medical advances cause older persons to need a progressively wider variety of specialized services for increasingly complicated bodily conditions. In the words of Emanuel (1982), "Life is the accumulation of chronic illness beneath the load of which we eventually succumb."

So we are left with the problem of defining chronicity. All of us, depending on our own state and perspective, may define it differently, but a more comprehensive and flexible definition is needed. The primary author offers the following in the hope of meeting these conditions:

Chronic illness is the irreversible presence, accumulation, or latency of disease states or

TABLE 1-1. Definitions of chronic illness

Author	Definitions	Advantages	Disadvantages
Commission of Chronic Diseases (1949)	All impairments or deviations from normal that have the following characteristics: permanency, residual disability caused by nonreversible pathological alteration, require rehabilitation, and may require a long period of supervision, observation, or care	Concise Generally applicable	Patriarchal Medicine-based interventions Not flexible Unilateral approach
National Conference on Care of the Long-Term Patient (1954)	Requires a continuous or prolonged period of care, at least 30 acute hospital days, or 3 months of medical supervision and/or rehabilitation in a different setting [summarized]	Gives definite time dimension	Primarily based on hospital settings How much intervention emphasizes shortening hospital stay and preventing exacerbations
Abram (1972)	Any impairment of bodily function over a period of time requiring general adaptation [summarized]	Behaviorally oriented Concise	Too brief
Feldman (1974)	Ongoing medical condition with spectrum of social, economic, and behavioral complications that require meaningful and continuous personal and professional involvement [summarized]	Directs attention to context of all human involvement Provides sound basis for intervention by all disciplines	Complex More cognizant of caretaker's than client's role
Buergin et al. (1979)	Symptoms and signs caused by a disease within a variable period of time that runs a long course and from which recovery is only partial	Concise Traditional	Disease-oriented
Cluff (1981)	A condition not cured by medical intervention requiring periodic monitoring and supportive care to reduce the degree of illness, maximize the person's functioning and responsibility for self-care [summarized]	Puts person with chronic illness into a major self-care role Flexible Includes other disciplines subtly Defines role of medical intervention	Somewhat medically oriented
Mazzuca (1982)	A condition requiring a high level of self-responsibility for successful day-to-day management [summarized]	Acknowledges role of self-help Futuristic	Too brief
Verbrugge (1982)	A degenerative illness	—	Too simplistic
Bachrach (1992)	Refers to individuals who suffer major mental illness experiences resulting in severe disabilities for long period, or lifetime	Homogenization of the diverse for facilitation of policy development and service planning	Mental health oriented Application of term may suggest hopelessness and invite stigma

impairments that involve the total human environment for supportive care and self-care, maintenance of function, and prevention of further disability.

Impact of Chronic Illness

Confirmation of a chronic condition tends to affect social, psychological, physical, and economic aspects of a person's life, often in a cyclic manner. The impact of physical disability changes the psychological status, which impinges on economic capability, and so on. Each area acts as its own stressor. Problems inevitably faced include intrafamily and sexual stresses, social isolation, independence versus dependence conflicts, enforced self-image insults and modifications, economic pressures, and the threat of death (Levy, 1979). The way an individual responds to diagnosis and then copes with chronicity usually relates to prior experiences with crises and accumulated strengths and weaknesses (Feldman, 1974).

The case history of J. O. illustrates the impact of progressive disability on the individual, the family, and the community, and the interrelatedness of aspects of this illness on one client's life. J. O. initially denied the presence of a physical problem. When confronted by the diagnosis, he heard threats to his marriage and the prediction of his impending death. He responded by sequestering himself and his family as he grappled with his newly acquired sick role and changed image. For the first time as an adult, he became dependent on others to fulfill his needs.

Self-imposed isolation led to jealousy, perceived loss, hopelessness, powerlessness, and finally depression. Family and friends were then unable to maintain the degree of support sufficient to confirm his own esteem and worthiness. The threat of suicide led to potent crisis intervention and interruption of that overwhelming cycle. He grieved for his lost premorbid potential and independence and finally concluded, "I'll live with it." This successful accommodation of different levels of normality allows J. O. to face and participate in day-to-day problem solving. He finds that life holds value (Strauss, 1975).

Issues of Quality and Quantity of Life

Adapting successfully to chronic illness includes a conception that the quality of life is worth the struggle. Illness is only one of innumerable factors that influence the totality of a perceived life scheme that impacts a person's quality of life. The same medical condition may be tolerable to one person and overwhelmingly intolerable to another. Quality-of-life goals may be the standard for measuring the performance of health care (Institute of Medicine, 1991). Quality specifies the functional capacity and independence of the affected person and also provides a means for evaluating achievement of the person's goals. The characteristics of the illness, age of the individual, degree of collective disability, and extent of medical intervention required to maintain a condition all have implications for individual and community decision making (see Chapter 9, on quality of life).

Professional caregivers face changing dilemmas as medical technology creates new methods to preserve and prolong life. The medical community has long confronted the question of who receives which life-giving measure and who should finance treatment. With the advent of multiple complex treatment modalities and mechanical organ transplants, broad-based planning must establish the guidelines for designating recipients. Even the process of dying and the moment of death itself can be controlled by machinery that dictates bodily functioning. The Patient Self-Determination Act of 1990 has changed the responsibilities of medical staffs from decision makers to educators and facilators. Clients are now placed in the collaborative role of making early end-of-life decisions in documents called advanced directives (Meyer, 1993). (See Table 19–4 in Chapter 19, on nursing ethics.)

Assisted suicide and euthanasia are issues with implications outside traditional medical arenas. At present there exists a vacillating medical/legal acceptance of self-directed timing of death. Of critical importance to society is seeking an answer to the question, When is a client's request for cessation of treatment death with dignity, and when is it suicide?

CASE STUDY

Interrelated Problems of Chronic Illness

Seven years ago, J. O., then a 30-year-old, was surprised by a sudden inability to control his hand grip. Tools fell unaccountably, and he noticed a numbness of his hands and a gradual inability to identify hand-held objects. For several months he attributed the lack of sensation to other causes until intermittent double vision led him to a family physician, who diagnosed multiple sclerosis. The doctor provided J. O. with what he saw as a dismal description of progressive deterioration. He also alarmed J. O. with the statement that "90 percent of marriages end in divorce by the fifth year." Recurrent, progressive symptoms led to J. O.'s decision to leave his job and remain at home.

Friends and associates who visited were confused and apprehensive when looking at this robust-appearing man who had been so physically strong. They often talked all around the subject of his health, preferring to keep communication light. He did not benefit from these visits. He felt tired, defeated, and resentful and experienced pain from muscle spasms. He also was suspicious of his associates' intentions toward his wife. He rebuffed offers of activities that once were pleasurable and maintained an uncivil attitude toward all. Rarely did he leave the house for fear of being trapped in a situation in which his awkward ambulation or appearance in a wheelchair would cause him to seem foolish or pitiable.

J. O.'s marriage was under stress. He felt that his wife deserved a more sexually capable mate and their young children a more involved parent. The children knew their father was ill and that his legs wouldn't work, but they did not understand his frequent irritability. They seemed to take particular delight in adapting or mimicking his dysfunctional mannerisms. He considered suicide to hasten the ultimate outcome. This threatened action necessitated a psychiatric consult and treatment and later referral to vocational rehabilitation.

J. O. and his family now balance what they want from life with what they must concede. He works from home as a telephone research surveyor. His wife has taken a full-time position nearby. They coordinate child care with a flexible child care service. Monthly visits to a neurologist provide a consistent medical regimen and support, some pain relief, and increased optimism about the disease progression and remissions. Family and friends continue to visit occasionally, and some invite J. O. out to their homes or to various community events. He now feels more relaxed in public places that afford accessibility to him, and he looks upon his wheelchair as a good friend that provides comfort and safety. Conversation frequently turns to hopeful talk about a new medication or cure, or at least to lengthy remission. General plans include events several years in the future.

J. O. says, "This is not a pleasant thing to have but I've got it and I'm going to live with it." The couple seem to agree that life is more complex and uncertain. His wife describes his efforts: "Every day you get up to work is a struggle and a challenge for the day." Communication is more open than ever before. They have developed a rather global outlook on the course of life's events for themselves and those around them.

Impact on the Client

An individual is destined to age, progressing toward senescence. Age and life stages influence the types of problems and consequences impacting the person having a chronic condition. In spite of the disability, the individual must accomplish developmental tasks allowing psychological and cognitive transition from one stage to the next. Each age group—child, adolescent, middle-aged, and old—demonstrates particular characteristics (see Chapter 2, on growth and development).

Infancy through Adolescence Chronic illness has replaced acute illness as the leading health concern for children. Jackson and Vessey (1992) estimate that between 10 and 20 percent of the pediatric population have a chronic condition. A survey of over 17,000 households in 1988 for child health concerns elicited estimated findings that 31 percent of children under 18 years of age have one or more chronic conditions. While only 2 percent of these children experience multiple and severe chronic conditions, this group requires a significant level of physician, hospital, and medication intervention (Newacheck & Taylor, 1992). From infancy to 18 years of age, the four most prevalent chronic conditions are hay fever, chronic sinusitis, chronic bronchitis, and asthma (National Health Survey, 1993).

Stein (1989), who prefers the term "serious ongoing physical health conditions" to the term "chronic illness," sees either designation as a framework for thinking about the health need spectrum of morbid youngsters. Childhood chronic illness poses several considerations for long-term health planning and delivery. The potential disabilities of this population will persist in terms of actual economic burden as well as social and psychological demands on family and community. Because of the unique period of childhood, growth and development needs require sequence of care different from their age groups (see Chapter 2, on growth and development).

Parents face a balancing act of managing the normal requirements of growth and development with the complications posed by the illness. The two sets of opposing forces include

The child's need to socialize and explore versus health risks and consequences.

The child's need for appropriate limits versus the desire to "make up" for the illness.

The needs of other family members versus time and financial resources consumed by the illness.

The child's natural process of becoming independent versus the need for increased supervision.

The natural experimentation of childhood versus the limitations of the illness and physical vulnerabilities.

The role of spouse versus the role of parent.

Parents as medical monitors, service seekers, and medication givers versus the advice of professionals.

The need for the child to become responsible versus extra attention and reduced expectations that come with being sick.[1]

Case management may help define levels of care needed. Families generally need assistance with medical and nursing services, respite and day care, education, life planning, financial and legal services, speech therapy, transportation, recreational activities, and advocacy causes (Marcenko & Smith, 1992). Currently, child health policies promote access to primary care for acute and preventive health care needs. The "noncategorical approach to illness" points out the commonalities of children with chronic conditions and healthy youngsters (Kelley et al., 1991).

Siblings play multiple roles in actively shaping one another's lives and preparing each other for adult life. They experience a gamut of emotional reactions to having a "different" brother or sister; often their lives reflect the routines made necessary by the affected child's illness or disability. In a review of studies on siblings, it was found that a child's disability or illness was not likely to have a detrimental effect on the sibling's psychological adjustment (Lobato, 1990). Further studies are suggested to see if there are positive effects that a child's disabilities have on all family members (Cadman et al., 1991). Because of the multi-impacted timing of a child's long-term illness on family members, health providers have an ongoing role in the assessment of the total family's psychosocial well-being.

The adolescent who has a chronic illness faces a dual role of normal adult development and acceptance of a life with limitation. A major task confronting an adolescent is the necessity to grow into a life of what is and can be rather than one of what might have been. Stein (1989) identified eight social experiences that are important for the transition from childhood to adulthood:

[1] From "Parenting the Child with Chronic Illness, a Balancing Act" developed by the Community Resource Committee of the Infant-Toddler Interagency Collaboration Project of San Diego and Imperial counties.

1. Shifts in social relations from parents to self to peers
2. Functioning in the peer culture through assimilation of information and peer culture
3. Taking responsibility for one's own affairs, including obtaining income and controlling how it is spent
4. Learning adult behaviors appropriate for adult responsibility and activities
5. Developing skills in social relations, including ease with language and participation encounters
6. Self-regulation for routine obligations such as employment and travel
7. Tolerance for departures from autonomous adult behavior, especially in an entry-level work role
8. Appearance, dress, and manner appropriate to blend in with peers

In consideration of the above normal adolescent socialization steps, opportunities to involve the chronically ill adolescent in all areas is vital to adjustment and fulfillment as an adult. In the case study of M. T., her motivation to progress from child to adult, regardless of the regimens imposed by cystic fibrosis, is clearly apparent.

Young to Middle-Aged Adults The young to middle years are typically a time of high activity and productivity. Individuals launch careers and marriages, begin and raise families, experience changes in status, and prepare for retirement. According to 1989 data, chronic sinusitis and deformities or orthopedic impairments were the most prevalent chronic illnesses among young to middle-aged adults (National Health Survey, 1993). Increasingly, the results of research into the causes of illness and debility in the elderly demonstrate the effects of life-style behaviors and habits in the early and mid-life years. Of current alarm is the observation that of the 14 million individuals worldwide who are HIV infected, 50 percent acquired the virus between the ages of 15 and 24. In the United States, AIDS accounted for 16.5 percent of all 1990 deaths in men and 4.8 percent in women aged 25 to 44 (Hein, 1993).

The presence of a chronic condition can complicate the conception and completion of goals and dreams. At a time when creative energy is generally directed outward, the individual may need to utilize most inner resources to cope with the condition. The case history of T.Y. discusses the impact of an uncertain illness during a time of usual high energy and career accomplishment. Cohen (1993) researched the effects on family life of children living under conditions of sustained uncertainty. Applicable to T.Y. and other persons suffering from a baffling illness is the appreciation for sustained uncertainty as a unique phenomenon at a time when society expects absolutes in disease source, progress, and termination.

Older Adults The greatest proportion of chronic illness affects the older population. Diagnoses of chronic illness are frequently multiple. To the older chronically ill person, longer life expectancy means periods of disability, vulnerability to other health problems, financial expense, and increasing care concerns.

Demographics from 1991 show a preponderance of older women over older men in North America. At age 65 and over, there are 1,000 women to every 674 men. Over age 75, the proportion increases to 1,000 women to 548 men (Department of Commerce, 1992). Chronic conditions with the highest prevalence for persons 45 to 75 and over are arthritis and hypertension. Hearing impairments and heart conditions follow in prevalence for ages 65 and over (Department of Commerce, 1992). The older woman who is alone must meet the normal challenges of financing and running a household. Her support system often depends on the presence of children and friends and their ability to help. This woman tends to be less assertive and less well educated than younger single women; cohort differences exist in the changing role of women and their dependence.

In general, society views both the aged and chronically ill negatively. There is a tendency to look at age and disability in terms of their effect on the national pocketbook. Indeed, persons aged 65 and older accounted for one-third of the 1988 health care costs (Binstock & Post, 1991).

CASE STUDY

Impact on the Client and Family

M. T. was the second-born and seemed normal until repeated upper respiratory infections and consistent lack of weight gain necessitated a referral to a regional medical center when she was 14 months old. Cystic fibrosis was diagnosed through a positive sweat test. The diagnosis could not have come at a worse time. The mother was in her second trimester of pregnancy, and the family's finances already were not covering assorted medical expenses.

M. T.'s parents learned to perform the postural drainage and percussion exercises required several times daily to keep M. T.'s lungs functioning. With urging, they attended group meetings at the center. Inherent in these meetings were shared experiences and emotional support. After two meetings the father stopped attending: "I wasn't getting anything from them. My wife became the expert and ran the meeting. Even the therapists had a hard time talking."

As M. T. grew older, the mother became obsessed with the home regimen and perceived need to keep M. T. away from disease-causing people or things. People were not invited to the home, and M. T. did not go into crowds. The father gradually assumed a background role in family decision making in regard to M. T.'s illness. His concern for his wife's preoccupation led him to suggest that she consult a psychiatrist. She of course refused. When the public health nurse, visiting for Crippled Children's Services, suggested mental health counseling to the mother, she was told to mind her own business: "I'm not crazy."

The older sibling, a girl five years M. T.'s senior, had always been expected to conform to the demands her sister's illness placed on the household. She was a serious child, close to her father, and

until she was 16 was the major caregiver to the youngest girl. She eloped at that time. The youngest girl, who proved to be free of cystic fibrosis after delivery, varied between overdependence and stubborn independence. Although close to M. T. in age, she generally kept an emotional distance. The siblings chose not to entertain their friends around M. T. and centered their activities out of the home.

By the time M. T. reached school age she needed to rise an hour and a half earlier than her sisters to allow for the first pulmonary exercise program. Dietary requirements and occasional added postural drainage at noontime necessitated that the mother transport M. T. home and back to school daily. After school, a pulmonary session was followed by homework, a rest period, and dinner. M. T. had an early bedtime. She slept nightly in a mist tent.

Regardless of the restrictive circumstances, M. T. developed into a bright, energetic child who was outgoing and well liked. Friends did not visit often because of the home routine and the unpleasant but necessary production of sputum. Until she was 10 years of age, M. T. followed her mother's directions without argument.

During the fifth grade, illness forced M. T. to miss a lot of school. All her spare time had to be spent studying. One day she told her mother she was joining the Girl Scouts "to have some fun with my friends." The mother pointed out that group activities would expose her to fatigue, germs, and a change of routine, but the child was adamant. From that time on, regardless of her mother's wishes, M. T. continued to direct her own life.

Future population projections imply growth in both the amount and percentage of health care dollars for future older care (see Chapter 22, on financial impact). Unlike children, the investment for older adults brings limited promise of return.

The old who are chronically ill also carry a double yoke of undesirability when they become

inpatients because they are often less rewarding to care for in terms of recovery, reduction of disease states, and economics. The national policy outcome of a prospective payment system, introduced in 1983, and its impact on health care provisions for older Americans reveal a care gap of crisis proportions in the community-based long-term care system, especially regarding ac-

CASE STUDY
Tired of Chronic Fatigue Syndrome

Once supervising the serving of 300 meals nightly in a chic restaurant, 33-year-old T. Y. now measures a "good day" if she can prepare two meals of natural foods for herself. A "bad day" is when her symptoms occur all at once and she ends up staying in bed all day.

A case of "flu" became chronic over three months. A variety of diagnoses led to multiple, and unsuccessful, treatments. She was finally diagnosed as having chronic fatigue syndrome (CFS) and given orders to take multivitamins and to rest. Expecting at most a six-month recovery period, she hired someone to manage the restaurant and returned to her parents' home for recuperation. About the diagnosis she says, "It was devastating, but I was glad the problem was not life threatening."

Two and a half years later she lives in the dark, avoiding sudden increases in light. Even the light caused by opening the refrigerator door can set off a crushing headache with blurred vision and green "zig zags" in her visual field. Reading and watching television are out of the question. She also experiences multiple symptoms of arm, stomach, and foot pain, as well as the omnipresent fatigue. She admits to now being "sort of anti-drug, anti-doctor." She has told doctors she doesn't want more medicine, just answers.

She has turned to friends and other sufferers of CFS for suggestions and answers. Natural foods, especially raw juices, seem to give her strength and relieve her stomach symptoms. Her social life is nonexistent. Visitors are welcome, but prove tiring. With the best of intentions many of them bring recommendations for specialists to try, medications to take, or the gentle admonition to "just get out and be with people." She has not driven in two years. She says, "I'm almost convinced that this virus is in my body and is going to stay there no matter what. But I have a strong feeling that my dietary approach will be the answer to clearing it out. I really thought I'd just get over this, but that was a long time ago."

---

cess to nonmedical services (Estes et al., 1993). Bortz (1990) reviewed records of 97 geriatric patients who died in 1987 and found that more than half of them had little dysfunction that year regardless of actual age. Another study found that disability rates, not the number of diseases, escalated with increasing age at death. The common theme characterizing both of these studies is that functionality, not age, is important in establishing guidelines for end-of-life care. Bortz (1988) places prevention strategies, functional assessment, and rehabilitation therapy ahead of cure allocations. At this time of increasing financial concerns and rationing of dollars, health care workers must put into ethical perspective issues of age and function and quality of life for economic decision making (Binstock & Post, 1991).

Even though an older person may have been independent just before a crisis, other persons' caution and reluctance to relinquish the helping role may negate return to an independent state. The case study on A. C. and her loss of independence demonstrates just such a situation.

Sociocultural Impact

To date, society defines illness and debility largely with a disease-specific focus. This acute illness model places chronically ill individuals at a disadvantage. Rather than seeking cure of disease, the chronically ill person needs to be considered not as incurable but as modified. Such a perspective leads to maximization of well-being, creativity, and productivity. However, society often sees the disabled as nonproductive. Interestingly enough, the artist Joe Dauley found that the effects of Parkinson's disease increased his marketability. The hand tremors he developed caused his painting style to change from realistic to impressionistic, featuring a renaissance of color and subjects. His patrons are numerous and generous. He says that, oddly enough, Parkinson's has been a boon; he's a much better painter (Dowling & Hollister, 1993).

Hamera and Shontz (1978) studied clients', families', and nurses' attitudes toward positive and negative aspects of chronic illness. They

CASE STUDY
Losing Independence

A. C., a 72-year-old retired businesswoman and widow of six years, was healthy except for a history of peptic ulcer and cataract of the left eye. She stumbled and fell, sustaining a fractured femur that was pinned without complication. She was transferred from the acute care facility to a convalescent hospital for continued physical therapy and recovery. During a transfer from her wheelchair to the toilet, she fell without sustaining injury. However, her self-confidence was shattered. Subsequently, two nursing assistants helped her with ambulation and transfers. Her daughter, who lived out of town, noted this increase in aid and advised her mother to stay at the hospital until she could take care of herself as before.

A bladder infection caused problems with urinary continence. A. C. began to exhibit confusion and made several attempts to get out of bed at night without alerting the staff. After retrieving her from the floor twice, they applied restraints at night to prevent further falls. A representative from a home health agency attempted to arrange discharge and visitation schedules. A. C. expressed fear about being at home alone. Family and staff now assumed most of her daily living tasks and business transactions. Alternative living situations were considered. Her wish to return to her own home is very uncertain.

found that subjects who had close contact to the illness had a more positive perspective than those who were less close. One may take some liberty with this conclusion by casting society in the role of an outsider who emphasizes negative aspects of chronic illness because of perceived dismal outcomes.

Recently, nationally recognized political figures have stepped forward to make statements as active persons who coincidentally have disabling or terminal illnesses. Their conditions include alcoholism, cancer, and neurological and coronary diseases. These persons' courage and farsightedness encourage a more objective and closer appraisal of legislation and funding by lawmakers.

Use of Health Services   Traditionally, chronic disease has been that condition left after incomplete resolution of acute disease. As a result of the gradual evolution of chronic disease in this manner, acute modalities have been the management approaches used. The physical design of hospitals well defines this mode, given that they are planned for efficient disposition of diagnosis, treatment, and care.

The great uncertainty clouding the future of an individual's life may not be caused by the demands of his or her condition but by the intricacies of the medical system. Dealing with various services or providers can be difficult for people who lack knowledge or energy. Physicians' offices tend to reflect efforts to maintain efficiency and control of the clients' behaviors. Health personnel often do not recognize that a general conversation can elicit the extent to which a person is affected and the adaptation required for lengthy disability. The need for professionals to see chronic illness as more than pathology is essential for providing optimal support and interventions.

Utilization of services varies by sex and age. Both the elderly (65 years of age and older) and women use health services more than younger populations or men (Department of Commerce, 1992). Women who attend prenatal and well-baby care programs are more exposed to the importance of prevention and health promotion, which may partly account for their increased utilization of these services. The existence and extent of health inequities, such as education, income, and marital status factors, have been better documented than have the reasons that explain why these inequalities continue. In his extensive critical review of the relationship between socioeconomic status and health,

Feinstein (1993) concludes that individuals of lower-income and lower-status employment do less well in the health care system. Additionally, materialistic and behavioral factors contribute to the inequalities.

Society's laws have supported illness and disability as acute processes that shape and dominate the environment of the client's life. The nursing home industry well illustrates this perspective. Although striving to make the most of remaining health and ability, these facilities offer a pervasive illness model with stark walls and white uniforms of caretakers serving as a daily reminder of the need for intensive care. Health workers need to appreciate how the environments they work in may influence attitudes toward chronic illness and the chronically ill.

Recent inroads in chronic care management are redefining environments and services. Many nursing homes have decor that stimulates and helps orient their residents. Also for the residents, greater accessibility to the community encourages fuller life experiences and expectations. Increasingly, medical centers are providing transportation units for easier access to doctors' offices or other required appointments. As primary care refocuses on the needs of the individual, some physicians or other members of the health team are making house calls to evaluate medical status. Access goes hand in hand with availability.

Rehabilitation Medical rehabilitation has been described as the third phase of medical care, the first and second being prevention and cure *(Directory of Medical Rehabilitation Programs,* 1990). Rehabilitation for the chronically ill can play a major role in restoring or maintaining function. As with acute illness, planning and implementation of restorative methods must soon follow diagnosis. Critical functions, such as hand flexibility and bladder continence, must be assessed for competency. Efforts should address those areas that potentially lessen independence. In response to heavy financial burdens, public policy and health planning tend to deny the accessibility of physical and sociopsychological rehabilitation to the chronically ill (see Chapter 24, on rehabilitation).

Cultural View of Illness Illness belief systems form the cultural milieu that defines caregivers' and individuals' attitudes toward illness. Conceptions about the source of illness and required treatment affect the types of therapy the caregiver offers as well as the outcome the client expects. As Hispanics are the single largest, and also the youngest, minority group in the United States, approaches to health care for them are of concern for effective planning that is culturally appropriate. Cited during a workshop on Hispanic and Latino health was the fatalistic expectation that life offers suffering and death. Preventive health is a new idea to many persons (Branch & Malik, 1993). As different ethnic groups have different health conditions and needs, specific and individual guidelines must be designed in planning strategies (CDC, 1992).

Political Impact

Ideally life is active, full, and lengthy and terminates in a speedy decline and death. However, the largest contributors to national morbidity concerns and policies have been the disease states of atherosclerosis and lung cancer and automobile accidents. All cause long-term conditions, and all lead to life-style behaviors that are modified.

National policies and financing for prevention of early-onset morbidity could be cost-effective. With the current debate on health care reform, including health promotion measures, legislative actions may affect the life span characteristics of our national population more than at any time before. As the total population ages, interventions must be directed to decreasing the source and amount of disability. For example, osteoarthritis, once thought to be the plight of aging persons, is now recognized to be a multifactorial product of body use and abuse, obesity, and sedentary life-style, among other factors (Fries, 1989). Answers lie in using known risk factors. However, life expectancy limits are debatable. Current life expectancy in the United States is 75.5 years (Connell, 1993)—an all time high. If life expectancy continues to increase, the proportion of persons dying at the oldest ages will also increase (Guralnick et al., 1991).

Financial Cost

Illness is expensive. During fiscal year 1989, the total reported expenditure for chronic disease control activities in the United States was over $245 million (CDC, 1991a), with costs escalating for care of the elderly. Seventy-one percent of all deaths occur among people aged 65 and older. Twenty-eight percent of all Medicare costs were incurred by 6 percent of those covered who died within the next 12 months (Guralnick et al., 1991). As the economic impact of chronic illness causes legislative turmoil on a national level, community impact and family desperation continue on the local level. Families are characterized by reduction of income and benefits, change to poorer housing, marital instability, and decreased opportunities to educate their children.

Interventions

Interventions on behalf of the chronically ill require responsible management by health providers and responsible achievement by the involved individual. Intervention occurs after an illness is diagnosed or when prevention of further disability is necessary. Proactive intervention is a growing strategy, with areas known to cause chronic illness as well as areas of high risk for each illness. Temple and Burkitt (1993) describe this activity as "moving from a rearguard action to a grand offensive." An area where proactive intervention would be effective is referral for present or potential mental health disorders. Yet parents who reported behavioral problems exhibited by their chronically ill children made little use of mental health services for this high-risk population (Gortmaker et al., 1990). In addition, children with "serious" chronic disorders tended to have more behavioral and emotional problems than those with "minor" chronic disorders. At highest risk for both problems were children with serious disorders involving the central nervous system (Weiland et al., 1992). Comprehensive interventions should include ongoing assessment of need based on knowledge of the individual's disease course and vulnerability to inherent risks.

Coming to Terms with Chronicity

Successful management of chronic illness requires a high level of client or family responsibility. The individual's attitudes toward a specific therapy can have profound effects on outcome. A very personal problem the client must confront is determining the treatment that offers the wished-for benefits at an acceptable level of risk (Pearlman & Speer, 1983).

Although professionals hold positions in which they judge the client's life situation and potentials, in the final analysis clients maintain the responsibility for determining the quality of their own lives. The ability to "get on with life" is one of these inherent qualities. Johnson (1982) recommends methods to achieve acceptance of cancer, a chronic illness, including word desensitization, self-belief, education, and acknowledgment of potential disease outcome. She lists patterns of resistance such as being oneself, guarding against depression, refusing limitations, and resisting isolation. These suggestions apply to other chronic illnesses as well.

Support from Providers

Long-term care responsibility requires varying types of expertise provided by a variety of professionals. Learning to deal with the system is an ongoing accomplishment. Individuals and their families are entitled to information and counseling about the mechanisms for obtaining care. They need access to opportunities to provide feedback on care received and to report problems with the system.

The professional community and society at large have joint responsibility to assist the chronically ill person and family to achieve maximum function and to slow or prevent functional impairment. In the interest of cost containment, health professionals negotiate during each client contact terms of concern and care using parameters of efficiency and effectiveness. Recent studies of techniques now used by these interviewers urge comprehensive history taking and "windows of opportunity" to optimize each interaction (Branch & Malik, 1993), with efforts made to empower patients and their families. The focus is increasingly on changing society's entrenched dependence on health professionals. Self-help classes, often specific to a chronic condition, are offered by hospitals, health maintenance organizations (HMOs), public media, and community agencies. Libraries and newsstands carry books and magazines urging self-education and self-assertiveness. Clients can be helped to know their role and responsibilities in a patient–health-provider relationship through interactive models of care. The Participation Medical Management Model (Doiron, 1993) creates a mind-set for both client and provider of collaborative progress through information gathering, decision making, and treatment options. In other words, the client helps the health care team to help him or her.

A disease-specific focus or cure-oriented model is not practical for long-term care. The dominant issue in chronic illness is management rather than a search for remedial results. Functional improvement and well-being can usually be achieved without curing the underlying disease. Health professionals must examine their reactions to chronically ill persons and recognize feelings of frustration and previous disappointments caused by the impossibility of effecting a total cure. Disease management can be viewed more positively and objectively by emphasizing success in modifying discomfort and disability. The satisfaction of crisis prevention can replace the drama of crisis intervention.

Professional and Community Responsibility

Committed professionals must advocate for commonsense prevention planning. Healthy People 2000, a legislated strategy for improving the health of the nation, provides three broad goals to guide the achievement of 22 priority areas: (1) increase life span, (2) reduce health disparities, and (3) achieve access to preventive services for all (DHHS, 1991). Areas of health promotion and disease prevention that lag in progress are pregnancy and infant health, nutrition, physical fitness and exercise, family planning, sexually transmitted diseases, and occupational safety and health. Areas showing substantial progress are those related to hypertension control, immunization, control of infectious disease, unintentional injury prevention

and control, and substance abuse. To meet the *Healthy People 2000* health goals, persons from the community and professionals need to provide leadership at the local level. Communities can put programs in place and support such activities as walking clubs, telephone contact voluntary services, local health fairs, and health spots in newspapers, supermarkets, and on the radio.

Client Education   Client education has been considered one of the basic components of ensuring self-determined care. Educational programs include preventive health measures to retain function or prevent further disability from other health problems. Since education can pave the way for the individual to assume a greater role in management of chronic illness, the individual and family must be included as participants in the therapeutic decision-making process. A position of mutual trust and respect diminishes the undesirable connotation of long-term illness and care.

Preventive Education for the Client   The primary emphasis of client education is to change opinion about the value of prevention. This effort necessitates putting a positive spin on approaches to living a healthier life-style. For instance, a dinner gathering could feature an array of fresh and whole grain foods, things that are delicious and healthy. In terms of chronic illness, medicine must be seen by the client as primarily for symptom alleviation, since chronic illness, once established, is not cured by medicine or even advanced scientific technology. Prevention is far more desirable (Temple & Burkitt, 1993).

Human behavior is the major factor that determines health. At least 50 percent of deaths can be attributed to behavior and life-styles, abuse of food and drugs, reckless driving of vehicles, and nonadherence to medical treatment (Weiland et al., 1992). Bortz (1992), an outspoken geriatrician, advises that much of the disability associated with aging is caused by disuse. His recommendation to simply move around more could alone change the activity and comfort of thousands of older Americans. Finally, to be fully effective for the client, a preventive campaign must involve all aspects of society: family, community, industry, government, and research agencies. All must recognize opportunities for self-proclaimed contributions to chronic illness prevention while welcoming the benefits of a self-determined healthy life-style.

Preventive Education for the Professional Increasingly, medicine relies on advanced technology to treat health care problems that may be preventable. From the *Nei Ching,* a Chinese medical book compiled around 350 B.C., comes this observation on preventive medicine (Majno, 1975):

> The superior physician helps before the early budding of the disease. . . . The inferior physician begins to help when [the disease] has already developed; he helps when destruction has already set in.

Hence, prevention of disease has long been recognized as a noble endeavor of medicine. In a general practice in Wales, an attempt was made over 25 years to screen for high blood pressure and adverse life-style habits in a working-class population. The aim was to improve health in the individuals in the area by identifying treatable problems at an early, often presymptomatic, stage. The case-finding was relatively easy, but the challenge was follow-up and maintaining high compliance in subsequent management. The report suggests, in summary, that results should be audited and the data shared with the local communities through annual reports that should be acted on by local policymakers rather than filed away. In addition, the report suggests that the physician be allowed, under the health care contract, to spend at least 10 minutes with a patient (Hart et al., 1991).

New models for prevention-oriented education of the professional need to be mandatory, and prevention-oriented education of the professional should be obligatory. A health-oriented education for all care providers would include the totality of preventive measures, including diets as preventive medicine (WHO, 1992), physical fitness (Bortz, 1992), and smoking cessation (CDC, 1991a). New models of education utilize computer software programs featuring preventive care considerations and health promotion measures. Computer capacity frees health professionals from the overwhelming amount of random memory work, client education, and communication inherent in a prevention-oriented practice, as well as assisting communication within offices.

Networking and national conferences are bringing together health professionals for ongoing education. Nurses from many specialties that deal with chronic illness came together at the National Nursing Conference on Chronic Illness (1992). There they shared research, practice modalities, education, and ways to empower patients. Legislatively, the Committee on a National Agenda for the Prevention of Disabilities (Institute of Medicine, 1991) notes that longitudinal care, although having a special appeal to many, has lacked the prestige and recognition of other specialties. Any long-term strategy for prevention of disability must address the educational needs of physicians, nurses, and other allied health professionals.

Educating the Health Professional Student Health educators cite the lack of comprehensive programs for students in medical and nursing schools and propose that classes on chronic illness be a major part of the curriculum. Clinical experiences should relate to the care of long-term illness and disability for all ages. The curriculum must integrate techniques to improve communication between caregivers and clients, families, and allied personnel. Professional caregivers must learn ways to increase individual self-assertiveness and self-care skills. The partnership of client and caregiver can then focus on self-determination.

Attitudinal Change Changing attitudes toward chronicity is a slow process. Television documentaries, newspaper articles, and community hospital and college courses are laying a solid foundation of knowledge about the implications of living with chronic illness. Society's lack of empathy and concern may have been the result of a lack of interaction with those affected. Because of degree of illness and disability, an unfriendly physical environment, and absence from the workplace, in the past the chronically ill were not integrated into the mainstream of society. At present, the chronically ill are still identified frequently by debility rather than ability.

Among the highest rewards of self-determined care are societal recognition and respect for individuals' knowledge of their conditions. These individuals, who also are survivors and equalizers between positive and negative aspects of life, could be valuable resources at all levels of education and legislation to reverse bias and ignorance.

Research: A Key to Change

Research in chronic illness is a key to unlocking evidence that clarifies etiology, treatment, and prevention. Technology allows studies that are both multifactorial in design and interdisciplinary. Resulting data may lead to more complicated questions. Professionals are at the horizon of chronic illness research. A large body of knowledge exists, yet what is still to come may change entirely the perception of chronicity. Research questions about chronicity, its cause and effects, have to be an integral part of medical practice (see Chapter 17, on research).

New Models of Care

Models of care that vary from the prevalent acute illness model give a new perspective to chronicity. Rather than picturing the omnipresent disease or condition centrally, they focus on the function of one's entire life. Two models of interest use family-centered approaches. The first utilizes intensive specialist help; the second, although requiring therapeutic skill, reinforces client self-determination.

The first model, a service management model, describes a life-long, goal-oriented process to comprehensively meet the needs of the family, often through a high degree of social worker involvement. In this model, families received respite care, nursing services, training in child care, educational services, and transportation to school. There were unmet family needs, including recreational activities, life planning, regular day care, legal services, and speech therapy (Marcenko & Smith, 1992).

The second model, the social constructivism interventions model, focuses on creating shared meanings about the client's health problem through conversations with the client and family; therapeutic conversations were used to help families construct and solve their own problems (Cox & Davis, 1993).

Other models of care stress the development and utilization of particular services. As one example, Project School Care provides consultation to school systems for the integration of disabled children who are assisted by medical technology. Because of the complexity of machines and procedures, particular emphasis is placed on upgrading skills at all medical and educational levels (Palfrey et al., 1992).

A collaboration of client and professional caregivers defines health service needs and methods for meeting them. In a nursing HMO model, nurse practitioners working with adults through case management help people promote their own health and learn to live with any disability (Ethridge & Michaels, 1993).

Client-Centered Alternate Models Professionals now provide outreach care, which is making a difference with client access and compliance. For instance, nurse practitioners serve as case managers in nursing centers that not only offer clinical experiences for students but meet a required component of the national Medicaid program for screening, diagnosis, and treatment of persons under 21 years of age. One such program, The Nursing Center in Clemson, South Carolina, is located near the population of greatest need for services (Barger, 1993). Transportation services, expanded hours for appointments, and use of a mobile clinic unit bring services even closer to the client, thereby improving utilization of the Nursing Center's services (Barger, 1993). As health care providers successfully use flexibility in approaches, networking for increased collegial relationships, and implementation of federal policies at state and local levels, the once designated alternate model becomes the mainstream.

At-home care, regardless of complexity of condition, is becoming increasingly important to client and family and attractive to health care cost payers. Nonprofessionals now carry out

CASE STUDY

The Client and the Computer

T. R., 36, became a paraplegic through a traffic accident. Because he is a type I diabetic, his brittle control and probable insulin reaction contributed to the accident. Following stabilization of the paraplegia and a program of rehabilitation, professionals and T. R. felt he was ready for home care. In collaboration with T. R., the physician facilitated a computer analysis using educational level, culture, life-style preferences, medical history, and laboratory and treatment information. The following care program was listed in the computer: basic instructions for the medical regimen, information on expected or adverse reactions to treatment and medications, appropriate diet program, and all resources pertinent to the client's care.

T. R.'s prior employment as a telephone lineman was no longer possible. A telecommuter schedule with a terminal in his home enabled him to contact a vocational economist, have an employment assessment, and receive retraining. He was also able to schedule his infrequent in-office visits through the computer. Utilizing the terminal tied into an outpatient diabetic program, T. R. made daily adjustments of insulin dosage based on serum glucose levels until his condition was stable. He has referred himself to a listed nutritionist and podiatrist. All referrals and their reports are printed out for the monthly meeting with his health team.

---

parenteral nutrition, renal dialysis, ventilator-dependent care, maintenance of aseptic living quarters, and a myriad of other complicated procedures. A well-coordinated system of support services facilitates these at-home procedures, and efforts to increase feasibility of home care are increasing.

Through involvement in health planning at local and regional levels, professional caregivers and chronically ill persons can work to meet the social and personal needs of individuals. The deficiencies and inefficiencies of health services can be brought to the attention of those who make policy and write legislation.

Effects of Computerization Computerization of administration, research, education, and practice is affecting all aspects of medical care. Automated processing is capable of dealing with the complex and detailed recordkeeping and health planning that advanced medical technology necessitates. The presence of computer-based client care data systems improves accuracy, so that the chronically ill person can receive enhanced care and individualization of health planning and promotion. The case study of T. R. and his computer illustrates the application of computer technology.

Social scientists continue to be concerned about whether computers are tools of social reorganization with great promise or dehumanizing machines of social disorganization. At this time, however, more than any other modern implement, computers allow for creativity, networking, and ongoing evaluation of traditional methods of health management not previously possible. *The Post Physician Era*, published in the 1970s (Maxmen, 1976), projects a 21st century with a medi-computer model of client care where various health profession roles would diminish or extend, and computers would supply most of the technical diagnostic and treatment "decisions." Presently, there are computer programs for all phases of physician practice and support services. Under health care reform, it is likely that paraphysicians or mid-level practitioners will increasingly deliver larger portions of health care, with general physicians playing the role of guide or consultant (Goldberg & Bonacini, 1993). Specialist advice, in the form of expert software packages, will be embodied in computer programs.

At present, there is computer-assisted management of offices, such as recordkeeping, scheduling, and accessing literature. Multioffice centralization will possibly effect cost containment and lead to higher efficiency. Physicians can now access clinical diagnostic and treatment "consultants" such as the Antibiotic Assistant Program (Schaal, 1993). Neural network technology, a system of input interconnection for identification, is close to actuality.

Of primary and ultimate concern is the effect of computerization on the care of the chronically ill client. Policies are in effect to ensure humane, ethical client services. The accessibility of information through computer technology will transform client treatment and the basic premises for client intervention. Constant updating of ethical concerns will be necessary. Professional caregivers must work to keep a healthy interdependence with machines to maximize human uniqueness while reaping the benefits of machine capabilities.

Changing Focus of Legislation

The American way of medicine has been free enterprise, private insurance, and employer-paid health coverage. Secondary to this, the health system is groaning under the weight of increasing costs and paperwork. The proposed national health care reform has legislators looking to managed competition or managed cooperation systems, which are networks of physicians and patients, both responsible and accountable for the care given (see Chapter 23, on social/health policy). Professional caregivers must act as advocates to ensure that the focus of legislation is on care rather than on a cure orientation. Preventive measures must be built in.

Competition in the marketplace is having an impact on health providers. Physicians are confronted with requests for outcome and utilization data to evaluate practice efficiency (Stevens, 1993). The status and stature of primary care, once below specialist standing in salary and referrals, is enjoying a sudden rebirth of prestige. Managed care requires that physicians and paraphysicians be capable of providing comprehensive primary and preventive care. Whether legislated financial outcomes will become more important than patient care outcomes is the task and responsibility of all health providers.

Summary and Conclusions

Chronicity is a state of unwellness produced by disease or disability and requiring medico-social intervention over an extended interval; it affects many aspects of an individual's life. In fact, many human beings may be chronically ill to some extent at all times. The chronically ill person exerts efforts to survive with self-determination and quality of life in what is often an unaware society. One of the most pressing obligations professional caregivers have toward chronically ill persons is to make society recognize that this struggle is being waged.

The degree of an individual's health may be determined by interventions caregivers make at the most primary levels. Accident and disease prevention lower the incidence of future chronic conditions. Changes in life-style with reduction of stress and smoking play a major role in lowered heart disease incidence. The recommendation for a diet of healthy food choices may lessen bodily destruction and, ultimately, redesign health roles and concerns of professional caregivers. The world of prevention contains great power and potential for eliminating some diseases and reducing the impact of others.

A challenge to all levels of health service workers is an increase in empathy for chronically ill people through direct involvement with them. The tendency may be to stand back and diagram chronically ill individuals and their needs as students once diagrammed sentences. However, people and their environment are not that elemental. To be effective, we, as professional caregivers, must be part of that diagram. A partnership of care requires information exchange and mutual decision making and offers an opportunity to share a part of courageous, creative lives.

Because of tumultuous effects of technology, constant change in disease and disability states, and efforts to meet resulting needs, a partnership with computers has become necessary and desirable. Computers release caregivers from mundane and highly complex work to concentrate on heightening the unique human qualities in the care of the ill.

A partnership in health care also changes societal focus from the chronically ill as dependent victims to persons inconvenienced but responsible. Chronically ill or disabled persons benefit from expanded rehabilitation, education, employment, and recreation opportunities.

Caregivers promote full partnership in society of individuals with chronic illness through the support of research, legislative advocacy, application of technology, and networking communication.

NURSING DIAGNOSIS[2]

A taxonomy provides (1) the language for classifying phenomena in a discipline, (2) new ways of looking at the discipline, and (3) a direction toward concept derivation. The North American Nursing Diagnosis Association's (NANDA) Taxonomy I evolved over a number of years and is still in the process of change. A modified version has been proposed for inclusion in the World Health Organization International Classification of Diseases.

The first national conference to identify, develop, and classify nursing diagnoses was held in 1973 in St. Louis, Missouri. A number of diagnoses were identified by the nurses who were invited to attend this conference. No scheme for classification was agreed upon, so an alphabetical listing was used. A conceptual framework using nine broad patterns focusing on unitary man was proposed as a structural basis.

A taxonomy interest group evolved and was charged with the task of generating an initial taxonomy. The group divided the existing list of nursing diagnoses, using the patterns of unitary man, into four levels of abstraction, with Level I subsuming the other three. Level IV is the least abstract, is more clinically specific, and is seen as most useful for the practicing nurse.

In 1982, the conferences were opened to the nursing community at large. In 1986, Taxonomy I was endorsed by the membership of NANDA for development and testing. Consequently, these diagnoses are subject to change. The term

"human response patterns" was substituted for the less familiar term "patterns of unitary man." The nine patterns currently in use are Level I concepts, and they provide an organizational framework for the rest of the taxonomy. The draft version of Taxonomy II was presented at the conference in 1990.

None of the nine patterns of Taxonomy I is considered better than any other, and numbering was determined by the order in which they were developed. Each diagnosis is numbered by its level of abstraction (general to specific) to determine placement within the taxonomy. The diagnoses noted in many of the chapters of this text are listed with the numbering, definitions, defining characteristics, and related factors as listed in the *NANDA Nursing Diagnoses: Definitions and Classification 1994*.

The nine human response patterns are[3]

1. *Exchanging:* mutual giving and receiving
2. *Communicating:* sending messages
3. *Relating:* establishing bonds
4. *Valuing:* the assigning of relative worth
5. *Choosing:* the selection of alternatives
6. *Moving:* activity
7. *Perceiving:* the reception of information
8. *Knowing:* the meaning associated with information
9. *Feeling:* the subjective awareness of information

[2] Nursing diagnoses used throughout this book come from *NANDA Nursing Diagnoses: Definitions and Classification 1994*. Used with permission.

[3] From NANDA Taxonomy I, 1987.

STUDY QUESTIONS

1. How do the many factors and conditions (technological, historical, and so on) lead to the increase in chronicity that exists today?
2. In what ways do statistics influence our perspective of chronic illness positively and negatively?
3. What factors should be considered in defining chronicity?
4. How do age and developmental level influence an individual's response to being chronically ill?
5. From a sociocultural and political perspective, how does society in general react to and treat the person who is chronically ill? How does this approach differ from treatment of acutely ill people?
6. How can a person come to terms with his or her chronicity?
7. What roles and actions can professional health care workers take to influence and implement local, state, and national policies regarding preventive health issues?
8. How can computers or new models of care enhance or improve the care of the chronically ill?
9. What is the role of research in answering questions about chronicity?
10. In what way can the professional serve as an advocate to secure changes in the focus of legislation?

References

Abram, H. (1972). The psychology of chronic illness, Editorial. *Journal of Chronic Diseases, 25,* 659-664.

Bachrach, L. (1992). "The chronic patient": In search of a title. *Hospital and Community Psychiatry, 43,* 867-868.

Barger, S. (1993). The delivery of early and periodic screening, diagnosis, and treatment program services by NPs in a nursing center. *Nurse Practitioner, 18,* 65-68.

Binstock, R., & Post, S. (Eds.) (1991). *Too old for health care: Controversies in medicine, law, economics, and ethics.* Baltimore: John Hopkins University Press.

Bortz, W. (1988). Geriatrics: Through the looking glass, Commentary. *Medical Times, 117,* 85-92.

——— (1990). The trajectory of dying: Functional status in the last year of life. *Journal of the American Geriatrics Society, 38,* 146-150.

——— (1992, Nov./Dec.). Use it or lose it. *The Saturday Evening Post,* pp. 62, 64, 84.

Branch, W., & Malik, T. (1993). Using "Windows of Opportunities" in brief interviews to understand patients' concerns, Brief report. *Journal of the American Medical Association, 269,* 1667-1668.

Buergin, P. (1979). Chapter 29 in W. Phipps, B. Long, & N. Woods, *Medical-surgical nursing.* St. Louis: C.V. Mosby.

Cadman, D., Rosenbaum, P., Boyle, M., & Offord, D. (1991). Children with chronic illness: Family and parent demographic characteristics and psychosocial adjustment. *Pediatrics, 87,* 884-889.

Centers for Disease Control and Prevention (1991a). Chronic disease prevention and control activities—U.S. 1989. *MMWR, 40,* 697-700.

——— (1991b). Consensus set of health status indicators for the general assessment of community health status—U.S. *MMWR, 40,* 449-451.

——— (1992). Years of potential life lost before age 65, by race, Hispanic origin and sex—United States, 1986-1988. *MMWR, 41,* 13-23.

——— (1993). Emerging infectious diseases. *MMWR, 42,* 257-263.

Cipolla, C. (1992). *Miasmas and disease: Public health and the environment in the pre-industrial age,* New Haven: Yale University Press.

Cluff, L. (1981). Chronic disease, function and the quality of care, Editorial. *Journal of Chronic Diseases, 34,* 299-304.

Cohen, M. (1993). The unknown and the unknowable: Managing sustained uncertainty. *Western Journal of Nursing Research, 15,* 77-96.

Community Resource Committee of the Infant-Toddler Interagency Collaboration Project of San Diego and Imperial counties. (1992) Pamphlet #15: "Parenting the child with chronic illness, a balancing act."

Connell, C. (1993, September). National center for health statistics. Associated Press.

Cox, R., & Davis, L. (1993). Social constructivist approaches for brief, episodic, problem-focused family encounters. *Nurse Practitioner, 18,* 45-49.

Department of Commerce (1992). *Statistical abstract*

of the United States, 1992 (112 ed.) Washington, D.C.

Department of Health and Human Services (DHHS) (1991). *Healthy people 2000: National health promotion and disease prevention objectives* (Publication No. (PHS) 91-50212). Washington, D.C.: Government Printing Office.

Directory of Medical Rehabilitation Programs (1990). Phoenix: Orynx Press.

Doiron, R. (1993, April). Teach your patients to better use the healthcare system. *Physician's Management,* pp. 66-70, 76-78, 83.

Dowling, C., & Hollister, A. (1993, June). The rebirth of an artist. *Life,* pp. 77-80.

Emanuel, E. (1982). We are all chronic patients. *Journal of Chronic Diseases, 35,* 501-502.

Estes, C., Swan, J., et al. (1993). *The long term care crisis: Elders trapped in the no-care zone.* Newbury Park, CA: Sage.

Ethridge, P., & Michaels, C. (1993). Community nursing network: Bridging the gap in long-term care, Long-term care currents. *Ross, 16,* 5-8.

Fee, E., & Fox, D. (1992). *AIDS: The making of a chronic disease.* Berkeley: University of California Press.

Feinstein, J. (1993). The relationship between socioeconomic status and health: A review of the literature. *The Milbank Quarterly, 71,* 279-322.

Feldman, D. (1974). Chronic disabling illness: A holistic view. *Journal of Chronic Diseases, 27,* 287-291.

Fries, J. (1989). The compression of morbidity: Near or far? *The Milbank Quarterly, 67,* 208-232.

Goldberg, M., & Bonacini, M. (1993, August). The computer age: Impact on medicine and physicians. *Medical Tribune,* p. 17.

Gortmaker, S., Walker, D., Weitzman, M., & Sobol, A. (1990). Chronic conditions, socioeconomic risks, and behavioral problems in children and adolescents. *Pediatrics, 85,* 267-276.

Guralnick, J., LaCroix, A., Branch, L., Kasl, S., & Wallace, R. (1991). Morbidity and disability in older persons in the years prior to death. *American Journal of Public Health, 81,* 443-447.

Hamera, E., & Shontz, F. (1978). Perceived positive and negative effects of life-threatening illness. *Journal of Psychosomatic Research, 22,* 419-424.

Hart, J., Thomas, C., Gibbons, B., et al. (1991). Twenty-five years of case finding and audit in a socially deprived community. *British Medical Journal, 302,* 1509-1513.

Hein, K. (1993, July). HIV in teens exploding: We need rapport badly, Editorial. *Medical Tribune,* pp. 8, 12.

Institute of Medicine (1991). *Disability in America: Toward a national agenda for prevention.* Washington, D.C.: National Academy Press.

Jackson, P., & Vessey, J. (1992). *Primary care of the child with a chronic condition.* St. Louis: Mosby Year Book.

Johnson, J. (1982). Call me healthy. *Oncology Nursing Forum, 9,* 73-76.

Kelley, M., Alexander, C., & Morris, N. (1991). Maternal satisfaction with primary care for children with selected chronic conditions. *Journal of Community Health, 16,* 213-224.

Levy, N. (1979). The chronically ill patient. *Psychiatric Quarterly, 51,* 189-197.

Lobato, D. (1990). *Brothers, sisters, and special needs: Information and activities for helping young siblings of children with chronic illnesses and developmental disabilities.* Baltimore: Paul H. Brookes.

Lowenstein, J. (1992, November). Can we wipe out disease? *Discover,* pp. 120-125.

Lubeck, D., & Yelin, E. (1988). A question of value: Measuring the impact of chronic disease. *The Milbank Quarterly, 66,* 444-464.

Majno, G. (1975). *The healing hand.* Cambridge: Harvard University Press.

Marcenko, M., & Smith, L. (1992). The impact of a family-centered case management approach. *Social Work in Health Care, 17,* 87-100.

Maxmen, J. (1976). *The post-physician era: Medicine in the 21st century.* New York: John Wiley and Sons.

Mazzuca, S. (1982). Does patient education in chronic disease have therapeutic value? *Journal of Chronic Diseases, 35,* 521-529.

Meyer, C. (1993). End-of-life care: Patients' choices, nurses' challenges. *American Journal of Nursing,* February, 40-47.

National Nursing Conference on Chronic Illness (1992). Unpublished Workshop notes. National Institutes of Health, Clinical Center, Nursing Department. Bethesda, Maryland.

National Health Survey (1993). *Vital and health statistics: Health promotion and disease prevention United States, 1990.* (DHHS Publ. No. (PHS) 93-1513). Department of Health and Human Services.

Newacheck, P., & Taylor, W. (1992). Childhood chronic illness: Prevalence, severity and impact. *American Journal of Public Health, 82,* 364-371.

Palfrey, J., Haynie, M., Porter, S., et al. (1992). Project school care: integrating children assisted by medical technology into educational settings. *Journal of School Health, 62,* 50-54.

Pearlman, R., & Speer, J. (1983). Clinical conferences: Quality-of-life considerations in geriatric care. *Journal of the American Geriatrics Society, 31,* 113-120.

Peto, R. (1992). Statistics of chronic disease control. *Nature, 356,* 557-558.

Ries, A. (1993). Preventing COPD: You can make a difference. *The Journal of Respiratory Diseases, 14,* 739-749.

Roberts, D. (1954). The overall picture of long-term illness. Address given at a conference on problems of aging, School of Public Health, Harvard University, Massachusetts, June 1954. Subsequently published in *Journal of Chronic Diseases,* February 1955, 149-159.

Schaal, D. (1993, August). Program pulls patient's profile, picks antibiotic. *Medical Tribune,* p. 17.

Stein, R. (Ed.) (1989). *Caring for children with chronic illness: Issues and strategies.* New York: Springer.

Strauss, A. (1975). *Chronic illness and the quality of life.* St. Louis: C.V. Mosby.

Stevens, S. (1993). Managed-care plans seem more selective in choosing doctors. *Physicians Financial News, 11,* 1, 29.

Temple, N., & Burkitt, D. (1993). Toward a new system of health: The challenge of Western disease. *Journal of Community Health, 18,* 37-46.

Verbrugge, L. (1982). Sex differentials in health. *Public Health Reports, 97,* 417-437.

Weiland, S., Pless, I., & Roghmann, K. (1992). Chronic illness and mental health problems in pediatric practice: Results from a survey of primary care providers. *Pediatrics, 89*(3), 445-449.

WHO (1992). *World health statistics annual 1991.* Geneva: World Health Organization.

Bibliography

Blancquaert, I., Zvagulis, I., Gray-Donald, K., & Pless, I. L. (1992). Referral patterns for children with chronic diseases. *Pediatrics, 90,* 71-74.

Cassetta, R. (1993, July/Aug.), Opportunities on the rise in long-term care. *The American Nurse,* 13-14.

Conant, S. (Ed.) (1990). *Living with chronic fatigue: New strategies for coping with and conquering CFS.* Dallas: Taylor Publishing Company.

Johnson, J. (1993). Medical news and perspectives report: Hispanic/Latino health issues explored. *Journal of the American Medical Association, 269,* 1603.

Weiland, S., Pless, I., & Roghmann, K. (1991). Diet, nutrition, and the prevention of chronic diseases: A report of the WHO study group on diet, nutrition and prevention of noncommunicable diseases. *Nutrition Reviews, 49,* 291-301.

CHAPTER 2

Growth and Development

Diane Peters

Introduction

The interaction of growth and development on the course of chronic illness is complex and should not be underestimated. In fact, it is impossible to address one aspect without the other in a comprehensive approach to health care.

Technological advances of recent years have lead to an increased life expectancy for individuals ranging from premature infants to octogenarians. Caring for this greatly increased cohort of chronically ill individuals presents challenges in all aspects of care, from diagnosis to long-term management.

Individual and Family Developmental Tasks

Erikson's theory of individual psychosocial development (1963) involves progressive steps toward the achievement of independence and a sense of well-being throughout the life span (see Table 2-1). As developmental tasks are accomplished, the individual moves to a higher level of independence and self-esteem. Inherent in this approach is the idea that mastery is cumulative; that is, a higher-level task cannot be satisfactorily accomplished without adequate mastery of the preceding tasks. These tasks are somewhat culturally bound in that they are set by societal norms (Hymovich & Hagopian, 1992).

Family developmental tasks, also called life-cycle stages, are summarized in Table 2-2 beginning with a newly married couple. The family's general tasks to be achieved include (1) meeting basic physical needs, (2) developing individual potential, (3) providing emotional support and effective communication, (4) adapting to changing needs, and (5) functioning within the larger community (Hymovich & Hagopian, 1992). Alternative family styles may fit with this broad sequencing if children are a part of the family. In marriages without children, or in childless alternative family structures, the tasks more easily fit with Erikson's completed life-cycle retrospective view of maturation, as seen in Table 2-3.

Illness Life Cycle

Rolland (1987) proposes a framework for studying chronic illness from both the individual and the family process perspectives. His topology of illness uses four categories: onset, course, outcome, and degree of incapacitation. By looking at all of these areas, it is possible to think about important developmental and family issues so that the effect on individual and family function becomes the focus, instead of specific diseases, as in the more traditional medical model.

TABLE 2-1.   Erikson's stages of development

Stage	Conflict	Developmental Task (sense to be achieved)	Approximate Age (years)	Behavior(s) Indicating Mastery
I	Trust versus mistrust	Trust	1	Separates from mother, explores environment, is not overly anxious or fretful
II	Autonomy versus shame and doubt	Autonomy	2-4	Feeds self, is toilet trained, has good control of gross motor function
III	Initiative versus guilt	Initiative	4-8	Adjusts to school and social spheres outside the home, plays cooperatively with peers
IV	Industry versus inferiority	Industry	8-12	Demonstrates school performance appropriate to age, follows instructions taking task to completion, participates in organized peer activities, is responsible for personal hygiene
V	Identity versus role confusion	Identity	13-20	Develops peer relationships with both sexes, defines goals in life, selects and prepares for vocation, gains independence from family
VI	Intimacy and solidarity versus isolation	Intimacy	20-30	Completes education, achieves economic independence through vocation, selects relationship partner and lifestyle, contributes to society (socially responsible)
VII	Generativity versus self-absorption and stagnation	Generativity	30-60	Stabilizes career, demonstrates concern for family and next generation, participates in community activities
VIII	Integrity versus despair	Integrity	60-death	Serves as counselor and advisor to younger generations, develops interests and abilities according to physical functioning, enjoys accomplishments

SOURCE: Reproduced by permission from Potter, P., & Perry, A. (1993). *Fundamentals of nursing.* St. Louis: The C.V. Mosby Co.

TABLE 2-2.   Stages in family life cycle

Stage	Meet Basic Physical Needs of Family	Assist Members to Develop Potential	Provide Emotional Support and Communicate Effectively	Maintain Organization and Management	Function within the Community
	General Tasks				
Married couple	Find, furnish, maintain first home. Establish mutually satisfying way of supporting selves.	Become established in occupation(s). Plan for possible children.	Establish mutually acceptable personal, emotional, sexual roles. Maintain motivation, morale.	Allocate responsibilities	Interaction with in-laws, relatives, community.
Childbearing	Adapt housing arrangements. Meet present, future costs of childbearing.	Facilitate members' role learning.	Communicate with one another. Maintain motivation, morale.	Assume mutual responsibility. Develop family rituals, routines.	Relate to relatives, others.
Preschool stage	Supply adequate space, facilities, equipment.	Rear, plan for children. Motivate family members.	Maintain mutually satisfying intimate communication.	Assume more responsible roles.	Relate to relatives. Tap outside resources.
School-age stage	Provide for children's activities, parents' privacy.	Further socialization of family members.	Upgrade communication in family. Develop morally, build family morale.	Reassign role responsibilities.	Establish ties with life outside family.
Teenager stage	Provide facilities for widely different needs. Work out ever-changing financial problems.	Widen horizons of teens, parents.	Keep marriage relationship in focus. Bridge communication gap between generations. Maintain ethical, moral stance.	Reassign role responsibilities as appropriate.	Keep in touch with relatives.

TABLE 2–2. *Continued*

	General Tasks				
Stage	*Meet Basic Physical Needs of Family*	*Assist Members to Develop Potential*	*Provide Emotional Support and Communicate Effectively*	*Maintain Organization and Management*	*Function within the Community*
Launching young adults	Rearrange physical facilities, resources to meet expenses.	Come to terms with selves as husband, wife.	Maintain open systems of communication within family, between family, others. Reconcile conflicting loyalties, philosophies of life.	Reallocate responsibilities among grown, growing children.	Widen family circle through release of young adult children, recruitment of new.
Middle-aged parents in an empty nest	Provide for comfortable, healthful well-being. Allocate resources for present, future needs.	Develop patterns of complementarity. Undertake appropriate social roles.	Assure marital satisfaction. Affirm life's central values.	Establish new routines.	Enlarge family circle. Participate in life beyond the home.
Aging family members	Make satisfactory living arrangements as aging progresses. Adjust to retirement income. Safeguard physical, mental health.	Keep active, involved.	Maintain love, sex, marital relationships. Find meaning in life.	Establish comfortable routines.	Remain in touch with other family members.

SOURCE: Reproduced by permission from Hymovich, D., & Hagopian G. (1992). *Chronic illness in children and adults.* Philadelphia: W.B. Saunders Co.

Onset of the disease may be either acute or gradual. Acute onset, such as with head injury, calls for immediate response from the individual and family. Families with clearly defined roles and effective problem-solving experience will have an easier time adjusting to an acute-onset situation. Gradual-onset illnesses, such as liver disease, present themselves insidiously over time, allowing for a longer period of adjustment. Acute onset is felt to be more stressful because of the sudden nature of the crisis situation.

The *course* of the illness can be progressive, constant, or relapsing/episodic. A progressive course, such as with Alzheimer's disease or

TABLE 2-3. The completed life cycle

In Erikson's view, each stage of life is associated with a specific psychological conflict and a specific resolution. In a new application, lessons from each of the earlier stages mature into the many facets of wisdom in old age, shown in column at right.

Conflict and Resolution	Culmination in Old Age
Old age Integrity vs. despair: wisdom	Existential identity; a sense of integrity strong enough to withstand physical disintegration
Adulthood Generativity vs. stagnation: care	*Caritas,* caring for others, and *agape,* empathy and concern
Early adulthood Intimacy vs. isolation: love	Sense of the complexity of relationships; values of tenderness and loving freely
Adolescence Identity vs. confusion: fidelity	Sense of complexity of life; merger of sensory, logical, and aesthetic perception
School age Industry vs. inferiority: competence	Humility; acceptance of the course of one's life and unfulfilled hopes
Play age Initiative vs. guilt: purpose	Humor; empathy; resilience
Early childhood Autonomy vs. shame: will	Acceptance of the cycle of life, from integration to disintegration
Infancy Basic trust vs. mistrust: hope	Appreciation of interdependence and relatedness

SOURCE: Based on ideas from Erikson (1986) and Goleman (1988).

multiple sclerosis, is typified by a worsening of symptoms over time that requires relentless care-taking, even though specific needs may change. A constant course, such as a cerebral vascular accident (stroke), is more predictable, as it is manifested by an acute event followed by a stable period. Usually, life does not return to a precrisis state because of a permanent limitation. Diseases with a relapsing/episodic course, such as asthma, are unpredictable, often causing dramatic emotional swings as the individual and family try to live a normal life under the certainty of eventual crisis.

Outcome refers to the likelihood of an illness causing death or shortening life span. Rolland (1987) states that the most crucial factor in outcome is the initial expectation about the life-threatening nature of the disease. The major characteristic along this continuum is the degree to which the family continually anticipates the most negative outcome.

The level of cognitive, sensory, or motor *incapacitation* resulting from an illness can lead to various adaptive responses from the family. A cumulative effect can be seen if more than one of the client's faculties are impaired. The social stigma related to some impairments only magnifies the effects of the incapacitation. In fact, the degree of uncertainty or predictability of the disease affects all four categories, especially in relation to the nature of the disease and in the rapidity of change (Collier, 1990).

Time Phases and Transition Periods Rolland (1987) also incorporates *time phases* as another dimension to this framework. Time phases include the crisis, chronic, and terminal phases of chronic illness (also see Chapter 4, on illness roles). Individual and family responses to these phases vary according to the coping skills and cohesiveness of the family unit prior to the diagnosis.

Transition periods exist between phases of the illness in the same way they are present between individual developmental levels. A transition period is the time for evaluating the situation and planning for the future as much as possible (Rolland, 1987). If the crisis, or beginning, phase of a chronic illness comes during a developmental transition period for the individual or family, both illness and expected developmental adjustment may be adversely affected.

Illness has a *centripetal,* or drawing in, effect on family members. Development normally has a *centrifugal,* or liberating, effect. An illness diagnosed at a centrifugal period (such as the first week of school for a child) leads to an incongruity of events resulting in ensuing problems being compounded (Rolland, 1987). During a time when independence is being encouraged, physical as well as emotional, the family is forced to respond to a crisis and may react either by getting back on track fairly quickly or by being distracted for prolonged periods of time and, possibly, never completely recovering. The case study about J. S. demonstrates the impact of a centrifugal period for this family.

Problems and Issues Relating to Growth and Development

Every member of a family system is affected when one member is diagnosed with a chronic illness. Family dynamics, physical changes, and psychosocial adaptation particularly need to be examined in relation to developmental stages and cultural expectations. The extent of any impact that occurs will be determined by developmental levels, past coping skills, and overall stamina of the family in adversity.

Family Dynamics

Each family member brings strengths, limitations, and unresolved personal issues into the system. This is true whether the family consists of only two adults or comprises a large extended family with adults and children of varying ages. Health care providers must assume that each family member desires the best possible interpersonal relationships for the family unit. If it were a matter of choice, families would all get along in an ideal, supportive manner. More realistically, people respond to situations and to each other by using behaviors they have learned in previous years, whether those behaviors worked at the time or not. For this reason, relationships are not often optimal for every family member in every situation. The greater the stress associated with an event, the less able each member is to respond in an ideal manner (Rolland, 1987).

Most family systems adjust to a crisis fairly well. They approach a problem in an organized fashion, the members relying upon each other for support as they work together toward resolution and eventual return to normalcy. The degree of difficulty experienced in this process depends on the strengths and limitations the family brings to the situation as well as the severity of the crisis as perceived by the family. In facing the diagnosis of chronic illness, the type of onset, course of illness, and expected outcome very much affect the family's response (Rolland, 1987).

The dynamics of individual and family behavior depend upon the achieved developmental level of each person. Emotional, cognitive, and social development usually does not happen simultaneously. Individuals mature at varying rates according to opportunities within the environment. Therefore, family members struggle with their own issues at the same time the family group is attempting to perform collective tasks. Even the most advantaged families experience dissonance along the way (Eisenberg et al., 1984).

Roles The roles of individual family members evolve over time as they learn to live with each other. In the past, in traditional families, husbands worked outside the home, wives worked in the home, and children or elders were expected to perform whatever helpful chores they could in order to contribute. Now, alternative family styles result in variations of traditional roles. Family structure can include any two or more people (adult or child) living together who are concerned for each other and who share common goals (Giger & Davidhizar, 1991).

CASE STUDY

Injury During Transition

As a result of a self-inflicted gunshot wound, J. S., a 15-year-old female, was left with a C5-level spinal cord injury. Her suicide attempt came after being confronted about illegal behavior that could have resulted in police action. By responding in this way, she demonstrated poor problem-solving skills and a pattern of negative coping skills. Her family responded by blaming her and withdrawing their support during her rehabilitation. Although cheerful and outgoing, especially with friends who visited, she resisted attempts to teach her activities of daily living (ADLs) in order to increase independence.

At the time of the injury, J. S.'s family was in the process of placing a relative in a nursing home. It was a troubled time for J. S., who was attempting to gain independence, experiment with sexuality, and establish self-esteem as a young individual working toward adulthood. Her active, healthy preinjury life-style had allowed her to form friendships, date, and form a positive body image. As a result of the injury, she was forced to become totally dependent with little hope of regaining preinjury health status. Previous strides made toward independence were negated.

During rehabilitation, J. S. became unusually resistant to any treatment attempts focused on learning new skills. Challenging authority and testing limits are expected reactions to this type of injury for an adolescent. Her resistance persisted until the health care team decided to focus on only a few essential skills that she or her family had to learn prior to discharge in order to prevent further deterioration of her health.

Although minimally involved in the beginning, J. S.'s family began to participate in the teaching plan that would result in her discharge. Once they resolved the stressful event going on at home (nursing home placement), they were able to become more involved as a support system for J. S. The combination of her developmental stage, the family's stressful life event, and the prospects of this type of injury (acute, constant, severely incapacitating) made for a rocky adjustment for all.

J. S. was eventually discharged home, but only after staff expectations were reduced to a minimum for both client and family. The focus changed from resistance to rewarding positive accomplishments by both J. S. and her family.

SOURCE: Adapted from Kurtz (1993).

In a single-parent household, the remaining parent is forced to assume the role of both father and mother because there is no other adult to help. A healthy resolution of this dilemma might be to involve a friend willing to participate in some appropriate functions. Another possible solution would be to participate in formal support groups such as the Big Brother/Big Sister organization, whose purpose is to provide adult role models for children from single-parent or dysfunctional families.

Mastery Dysfunctional families are those that, for some reason, are unable to provide the necessary nurturance to family members (Falvo, 1991). Again, the problem is not one of motivation but, rather, of ineffective coping skills necessary for the physical and emotional development of family members. In this event, the limitations

brought into the family group outweigh the strengths.

Lack of mastery of individual developmental tasks results in compounding deficiencies as the person ages. The extent to which individual problems exist will necessarily affect family development. If the family is functioning minimally prior to the diagnosis of a chronic illness, they will demonstrate even weaker coping skills as they attempt to respond to the crisis situation (Falvo, 1991).

Mobility Limitations

Physical limitations are the most common cause of growth and development difficulties in persons with a chronic illness throughout all developmental stages (see Chapter 6, on altered mobility). This is especially true if they have a condition that is a visually noticeable deviation (Anderson & Bury, 1988). The extent to which physical achievement signals success in development will determine the likelihood of problems developing.

Infancy Beginning with the infant's need to explore the environment, mobility is central to both physical and psychosocial development and influences all future development. The infant experiments with distance and separation from the caregiver; such action becomes part of its psychosocial ability to achieve independence. The achievement of rudimentary trust then becomes the impetus for risk taking and even greater physical accomplishments (Miller, 1992). In addition, if the infant and parent are separated for periods of time, the natural building of trust and experimentation with control and distance cannot take place for either of them.

Toddler The toddler works at refining this beginning sense of separateness and autonomy by trying to gain control in every event. Physical mobility is perhaps the most important tool used to experiment with this control. If the toddler's physical limitation is incapacitating, a sense of helplessness results that is difficult to overcome later on. Toddlers and young adolescents experience the most anxiety related to immobility because of their need to seek adventure (Miller, 1992).

School Age School-age children are primarily concerned with learning to take initiative as they work at their job of school. They are industrious, interactive, and in almost constant motion. When physical limitations keep them from moving about freely, the numbers and types of interpersonal contacts that they normally would have become restricted. Likewise, they are inhibited in the testing of their physical ability against the ability of others as they strive to feel good about accomplishments. Instead, they may feel as if they are always behind, trying to catch up (Eisenberg et al., 1984).

The school-age child becomes increasingly responsible for self-care activities such as grooming, toileting, and often choosing what clothes to wear. Organized peer activities become essential. The development of self-esteem for this age group involves mobility, competition, mastery of physical and cognitive skills, and an overall feeling of competence. Severe mobility limitations may mean the child will need to excel in a different area where success is possible, or it may result in the child no longer attempting to interact with peers but withdrawing into the safety of family (Eisenberg et al., 1984).

Adolescence The adolescent focuses on peer acceptance and the development of identity. If mobility is limited to the extent that there is dependence on caregivers for basic needs, disruption in normal peer group membership and identity formation is likely. Limitations in mobility can affect opportunities for romantic experimentation, which can have lasting implications for learning to trust and care intimately about another adult (Rankin & Weekes, 1989).

Adulthood Adults are least affected by limitations in mobility unless their ability to be productive is also restricted. During early adulthood, relationships are tested, goals for life are selected, and independence from the nuclear family is realized. The degree of mobility necessary for these activities and the resultant achievement of independence and productivity may vary considerably. An adult who has an insidious, progressive disease, such as multiple sclerosis, can continue to function in the role of parent, worker, and spouse with some adjustment in responsibilities and roles. Even when mobility is limited to a wheelchair, a complete reorganization of family functions may not be necessary (Foxall et al., 1985).

The older adult normally expects to be less vigorous in physical activity. Adaptation to limitations in mobility is part of the elder's anticipated developmental tasks. As physical ability changes, activities need to be revised to accommodate the change. Mobility becomes an issue only if the person can no longer care for himself or herself or for a dependent significant other. Within the role of counselor or advisor to younger people, mobility is not essential. The onset of a chronic illness during this period is usually met with acceptance and a satisfactory adjustment. If, however, the limitation of mobility is severe enough to necessitate a change of residence to a more dependent setting, such as a skilled nursing facility or the home of a child, the adjustment will be less optimal (Corbin & Strauss, 1984).

Body Image

The concept of body image involves the mental perception of how the body looks and functions in relation to others (see Chapter 13, on body image). This concept develops throughout childhood, but is ever changing even for adults.

Infants and Children   An infant has no concept of body image until there is awareness of the existence of others. Psychosocial development of body image begins around nine months of age as infants recognize they are separate from the consistent caregiver (Hymovich & Hagopian, 1992). Toddlers understand they are separate, but they have no sense of their own bodies as right or wrong in relation to others and do not experience difficulty with their perception of body image if they look different from others.

During this time, however, they begin experimenting with control over bodily functions, refusing to do as they are told and testing the limits of their bodies. As they reach school age, children become more aware of their bodies compared to those of their peers. They compete for best jumper, best runner, strongest, and so forth. The feedback they receive from each other, as well as from adults, builds their sense of "good" or "bad" body image (Hymovich & Hagopian, 1992).

Adolescents and Young Adults   Adolescents and young adults who believe their bodies are undesirable become limited in their ability to experiment with intimate relationships. Physical changes that occur secondary to a chronic illness can be interpreted as repulsive by client or peers and can have permanent damaging effects on interpersonal intimacy. For instance, adolescents may see physical changes (such as hair loss) as worse than having cancer itself (Eisenberg et al., 1984).

Older Adults   Middle-aged and older adults are usually more comfortable with their bodies, so illness does not impact body image as much. The challenges of finding a partner, beginning a family, and establishing themselves in a productive role are resolved. In addition, the physiological changes in body image that accompany normal aging also force variations in life-style, so that decreasing ability becomes less influential on how they see themselves as long as they continue to perceive life as meaningful (Putnam, 1987).

Sexuality

Chapter 14, on sexuality, provides helpful information for identifying normal sexual development throughout the life cycle. Achievement of healthy attitudes, including self-confidence, in this area is difficult even in the most ideal situation. The shaping of perceptions, performance, and quality of sexual relationships can be affected by physiological changes, side effects of prescribed drugs, changes in body image, or alterations in the social environment (Eisenberg et al., 1984). Socially, misconceptions about disabled individuals and their capacity for sexual expression often result in a reduction in the number of available partners for these individuals.

Chronic illnesses that involve reproductive organs, such as severe hypospadias or testicular cancer, place the individual, whether child or adult, at risk for developmental problems. Young children may experience delay in sexual development if they cannot privately experiment with increasing levels of intimacy. Older adults may be reluctant to ask questions or seek help related to sexuality for fear of further alienation by younger members of society who think the elderly should no longer be interested in sexual activity (Eisenberg et al., 1984).

Psychological Adaptation

The psychological adaptation of an individual with a chronic illness is best achieved through maximizing independence and self-control. Increased dependence upon others may be necessary through periods of crisis, but it is essential to restore optimum functioning to the highest level as soon as possible.

Loss of Independence   The loss of independence has devastating potential outcomes for any person, regardless of age, who is experiencing a chronic illness. Young children normally work diligently to experiment with self-sufficiency, the achievement of which provides the foundation for the self-confidence necessary to attempt later developmental tasks. Older children master physical and psychological milestones necessary to accomplish their goal of becoming independent adults who are then ready to contribute to the greater society. Obstacles that come in the form of treatment regimens, physical limitations, or absence from school interfere with such mastery (Jackson & Vessey, 1992).

If the illness begins during adulthood, the extent to which the person's independence is limited directly affects his or her response to the illness. Older adults who are already concerned with maintaining their independence secondary to age and possibly chronic illness face a difficult adjustment if they are also presented with the trauma of relocation. This move is a visible signal of loss of independence and is potentially devastating. Confusion, withdrawal, and disorientation are common results. If the move includes admission to a skilled care facility offering no rehabilitative services, the custodial philosophy of the facility may contribute to the client and family's attitude of giving up (Eisenberg et al., 1984).

Compliance and Control   Compliance with prescribed treatment requiring the cooperation of the client often becomes an issue of control (see Chapter 10, on compliance). Responses to compliance vary by developmental level.

Young Children   Normal development includes the child's progression in gaining power and control over the environment. If the opportunities for experimentation are limited, the child will attempt to gain control over whatever is going on in his or her immediate surroundings (Miller, 1992). This may include activities directly affecting the treatment plan, such as refusing to eat

required diets, to take medication, or to cooperate with therapy sessions.

The same problems of control apply to young siblings in the family who may experience increased stress due to the family crisis, especially if they are currently laboring with control issues of their own. Under these conditions, siblings may demonstrate extreme behaviors in order to test their own control limits. In fact, the feelings of loss of control can result in regressive behavior (such as bed-wetting) by either the ill child or the sibling (Miller, 1992).

Adolescents   Adolescents are normally emotionally labile as they fluctuate between extreme opposite feelings. If they become incapacitated in any way with a loss of physical control of their bodies, they may seek control over people and situations. Their responses may include a combination of (1) directive behavior—that is, controlling every aspect of what will be done with or to them; (2) resistive behavior; and (3) compliant behavior, which is apparent by their yielding, consenting, and conforming in all situations (Miller, 1992). Adolescents are more likely to comply with requests if they are able to retain contact with peers and participate in decision making regarding their care.

Adults   Young and middle-aged adults also experience a loss of control when they become permanently ill or disabled and tend to grieve over missed opportunities. Role changes they must undergo often lead them to feel unproductive and unsuccessful in the business of family development. Changes necessitated in marital intimacy also can become predominant control issues for them (Miller, 1992).

Older adults are particularly vulnerable to feelings of powerlessness, as they have already experienced a number of losses leading to fewer intact resources for themselves (Miller, 1992). When they suffer a situational or permanent loss of control they can become depressed and feel hopeless.

Isolation   Individuals, whether children or adults, who are isolated from their peer groups are denied the normal give and take they should have and may therefore not master age-appropriate social skills. For children, normal sibling and neighborhood experiences enhance social feedback and ultimately their sense of self-worth (Stein & Jessop, 1989). For adults, social interactions in the workplace and community provide opportunities for sharing common experiences of family life. This communication with other adults can provide reassurance and a sense of optimism in the management of everyday problems. Socialization with age-appropriate peers should be incorporated as a priority whenever possible.

During periods of crisis and hospitalization of a child, families find that it may be necessary to attend to other priorities. Social isolation for the child at such times can occur if the parents tend to overprotect or shield the child from further harm (see Chapter 8, on social isolation). This desire on the parents' part is certainly understandable. In those instances where the family lacks knowledge about the social component of normal development and the importance of peer involvement, education encourages them to seek opportunities to provide social contact beyond the immediate household (Stein & Jessop, 1989).

Cultural Variations

Culture is the way we live our lives. It is the mechanism by which shared ideas, beliefs, and traditions are maintained throughout generations. Culture implies not only ethnic background but also gender, work groups, religion, class, social groups, or any grouping of people with shared beliefs, including groups of disabled individuals or families. In recent years, it has been acknowledged that the nature of human activity is a function of both cultural and biological assets that afford the individual the means to respond to the challenges necessary for survival (Brookins, 1993). The focus of culturally diverse nursing care needs to be on the individual in the context of his or her culture rather than as apart from it. Brookins (1993) calls for such a focus to be not on deficits or difference but, rather, on the strengths brought to any situation.

Positive growth and developmental outcomes can best be facilitated by biocultural competence (Patterson & Blum, 1993). This does not mean sacrificing a lifetime of cultural experience but, rather, encouraging individuals and families to retain existing cultural ties while incorporating some level of ability to understand and survive in another culture. Included in this blending of cultures is acceptance of both sets of norms as needed to function in either setting. When this level of comfort is accomplished, social development in the form of individual identity is achieved, allowing for psychic energy to be available for the individual's and family's next developmental milestone (Edwards & Polite, 1992).

Cross-Cultural Issues   There are three issues that are consistent in cross-cultural studies of individuals and families experiencing chronic illnesses (Grace & Zola, 1993). First is the culturally perceived cause of the illness or disability. Second are the expectations for survival resulting in the amount of effort expended by the family toward optimum results. And third are the social roles deemed appropriate for those affected.

Culturally Perceived Causes of Disability Chronic illness is identified by some cultures as a form of punishment for wrongdoing. This perception mediates family and community response to the individual. The affected person may be seen as tangible evidence of moral wrongs committed by self or family. Other cultures link disability with witchcraft, particularly if the onset is sudden (Grace & Zola, 1993).

The common thread among such belief systems involves accountability for the illness by the individual or family. Associating with these individuals may be seen as containing a certain risk for members of the community (Grace & Zola, 1993). These beliefs, understandably, can result in a reluctance to assist the family even if they are from the same cultural subgroup. Families may feel shame and seek to hide the disabled person, particularly if the illness includes physical disfigurement or deformity. Children may be kept home from school, distancing them from any form of early diagnosis or treatment programs and adversely impacting their developmental tasks (Grace & Zola, 1993).

However, not all cultures consider the cause of chronic illness in a negative manner. In a recent study of Mexican-American parents of chronically ill children, Madiros (1989) found a common belief that they had been singled out to care for a child with special needs because of a previously demonstrated capacity for compassion. It was seen as an honor rather than a curse.

Expectations for Survival Cultures that traditionally have limited resources may consider it reasonable to deprive the chronically ill family member of needed means in order to ensure the survival of stronger members. This reasoning eventually contributes to an earlier demise of the ill individual, partly because he or she received less than an equal share of resources, or it can lead to a disastrous effect on physical and psychological development (Grace & Zola, 1993).

The cultural belief of how one is restored to health also has implications, especially for long-term planning and education. Hope for miracles or divine intervention, especially when there are strong religious ties, may distract the family from the necessary motivation to institute treatment or become involved in treatment or planning (Grace & Zola, 1993).

Appropriate Social Roles Whether the person with a chronic illness can be expected to function as a contributing member of society may dictate the amount of time, energy, and resources devoted to his or her education or occupational achievements. In some cultures, this is especially true for girls or women. However, the disabled family member, even though kept at home, will usually be expected to contribute to family functioning in whatever custodial role he or she can assume. The dominant culture in America often cannot understand this reluctance to expend significant family resources if a financial cost will not be realized (Grace & Zola, 1993).

Stigma Chapter 5, on stigma, deals with the causes and impact of stigma. Here we will briefly discuss the association of stigma and culture. Stigma associated with chronic illness exists in all cultures, with the stigmatized feature varying according to the norms of the culture. Therefore, it is important to collect information about cul-

tural beliefs as they relate to chronic illness (Giger & Davidhizar, 1991). As an example, McCubbin et al. (1993) identified differences in family belief systems associated with disability in Anglo-American and Aboriginal (native American and Hawaiian) families.

Anglo-Americans Anglo-Americans describe disability by using stigmatizing labels and attributing the cause of an illness to scientific reasons outside the family. The roles of disabled individuals are seen as limited due to the disease, whether this perception is realistic or not, and the person is viewed as different and stigmatized within society. Among Anglo-Americans, chronically ill persons probably experience the most developmental disruption, resulting from societal reactions that attribute negative connotations to them as different. This effect is most important during developmental stages where interpersonal relationships and acceptance by peers are most crucial.

Aboriginal Cultures In Aboriginal cultures, the cause of illness is considered an imbalance within the family or misconduct by one or more members. There are no disparaging words to describe family members who have a disability. Rather, they continue to be valued family members who contribute as they can. Illness is seen as part of wellness or as part of the normal variation of life. Blame for the disability is not directed at the person experiencing the illness.

Socioeconomic Factors

Family systems may be grouped by socioeconomic class rather than race or ethnic background. Social organization is learned by observation, with the most relevant influence on social behavior being the family group regardless of cultural background (Giger & Davidhizar, 1991). Types of family structures often differ for economic reasons. For example, the number of adults in the household working outside the home can vary. If all the adults in a given family work, the increased income can result in better adjustment to the chronic illness because less energy must be devoted to meeting basic needs (Eisenberg et al., 1984). In fact, extended or alternative family structures allow for considerable diversity in the development of roles and the delegation of household tasks.

Individual and group behavior is an outgrowth of socioeconomic status. Families from lower socioeconomic groups are often less organized, less able to problem-solve, or less future oriented. Survival is often on a day-to-day basis, making long-term planning impractical. Roles can become confused as family members come or go in the system. In families of lower socioeconomic status, there is often a sense of an external locus of control—that is, being controlled by an external force. Chronic illness often magnifies disorganization if it exists. However, being poor does not necessarily mean people are unwilling or unable to cope with change (Giger & Davidhizar, 1991).

Middle- and upper-income families benefit in many ways by being more financially stable. Being independent from others for basic needs results in higher self-esteem. These families tend to be fairly well organized, with designated roles and tasks for each member. When confronted with a crisis, such as the diagnosis of an illness that will be chronic or disabling, there is a tendency to respond, at least initially, in a reasonable, appropriate manner (Eisenberg et al., 1984).

Pain and Fear

The expression of pain or fear is often difficult, especially for people who have had limited contact with the health care environment. In addition, an individual's developmental stage and level of acculturation or familiarity with the health care setting affect readiness to share feelings about such personal and sensitive issues. Health care providers must demonstrate a willingness to facilitate communication and need to take time to listen.

Pain It is felt that infants can localize pain between three and ten months of age, and that they begin to have memory of pain after six months (Garrison & McQuiston, 1989). Infants who experience repeated hospitalizations involving separation from their primary caregivers, and who are, in addition, faced with the unpre-

dictability of numerous other care providers and repeated painful procedures are at more risk for future problems in developing trusting relationships (Jackson & Vessey, 1992).

Young Children Toddlers have a grasp of language and are beginning to understand the means-to-an-end concept. They can understand the necessity of pain during procedures or treatment if what is happening is presented in simple terms. Although intellectually the means-to-an-end explanation makes sense, toddlers are not yet able to control themselves when pain is imminent. In addition, while they understand illness only as it interferes with their lives, toddlers are beginning to suspect they are responsible (Garrison & McQuiston, 1989).

Preschoolers more readily assume personal blame for their illnesses. They are magical thinkers who interpret the world from an egocentric view, assuming all things are caused by, or at least relevant to, them. They tend to interpret the infliction of pain as punishment for bad deeds. Older preschoolers begin to reject this self-blame and view illness as coming from the environment, such as in the form of germs. Preschoolers communicate their pain experience through body movements and often loud verbal protest (Garrison & McQuiston, 1989).

School-age children can use their rapidly increasing language skills to describe their pain experience. By age 8 or 9, they can consider several aspects of a situation simultaneously. They have better physical control over themselves as they attempt to be cooperative by holding still. School-age children are able to understand the purpose for therapeutic procedures and are usually more cooperative if allowed to participate in the procedure in some way. Cognitively, they do not understand concepts related to the prevention of illness (Garrison & McQuiston, 1989).

Adolescents By the time children reach adolescence, they can understand the reasons for painful or invasive procedures. Their attempts at cooperation are usually expressed by stoicism, feeling the need to hide emotions in order to be seen as more mature. Aggression toward parents or health professionals may be used as a mechanism for releasing their unexpressed emotion at a later time (Garrison & McQuiston, 1989).

Adults Adults have learned attitudes and reactions to pain within the context of their sociocultural group membership. As children they learned how to respond to pain, what interventions were helpful in relieving pain, and acceptable ways of expressing pain. These values shape not only their perception and expression of pain but the meaning and attitude assigned to it (Villaruel & deMontellano, 1992). These past experiences help determine the adult's response to painful stimuli.

Elderly clients expect to experience degenerative physiological changes accompanied by pain. Because the changes are seen as inevitable, the older person is expected to tolerate this pain and accompanying disability quietly. Even though physical changes are inevitable, the older person can be helped to remain as comfortable and active as possible (Eisenberg et al., 1984). Chapter 7, on chronic pain, addresses many of the myths associated with pain in the elderly as well as more extensive information about dealing with pain.

Fear   Fear is a common occurrence when hospitalized (see Chapter 11, on coping with fear and grief). Even though it occurs frequently, the source of fear differs for each developmental group.

Children It is important to understand the cognitive level and age of the child in order to provide appropriate explanations, safety measures, and reassurance. Very young children's greatest fear is separation from their primary caregiver. Preschoolers fear mutilation and loss of control because they tend to be very concrete in interpretations they make about what is happening, making them especially vulnerable to inaccurate fantasies about mutilation. School-age children and adolescents fear being different and not being able to measure up to their peers. However, a gradual decline in the number of general as well as medical fears can be expected over the school years (Dolgin et al., 1990). Adoles-

cents also fear permanent disability as they strive to become independent adults (Miller, 1992).

Adults Adults, young and old, most often fear losing the ability to carry out self-care and family activities (Miller, 1992). Young adults spend the majority of their time generating income and engaging in activities related to producing healthy, independent offspring. Aging adults focus on self-care and possibly care of dependent spouses. Many fears of this age group can be eased by collaboration with spouse or significant others.

Understanding Death

The ability to grasp death varies in many ways and includes individual and family development factors that have evolved through generations of attempts to cope with explainable and unexplainable life events.

Children   The child's understanding of death is affected by psychological development, emotional maturity, coping ability, previous experience, environment, culture, and parental attitudes (Huntley, 1991). Cognitive maturation of the child along the growth and development continuum determines the impact of death of a family member upon that child. Table 2–4 summarizes the child's concept of time, body parts, and death throughout childhood developmental stages.

Adults   The adult's perception of death is influenced by many factors. The extent to which terminally ill individuals have successfully completed previous developmental tasks will determine their ability to view the significance of their contribution in life. Adults have either a sense of having contributed to society and having had a fulfilling life, or a sense of despair at having been deprived of such a life. When religious beliefs are a factor in their perception of death, they may perceive a rewarding afterlife, regardless of discerned successes in life. Such beliefs offer consolation to the dying person and the family (Dimond & Jones, 1983).

Families are also affected when a productive adult member dies. Not only do such deaths

TABLE 2-4. Factors in the child's understanding of death

Age	Time Sense	Understanding of Body	Death
Birth–18 months: Prelanguage	Lacking	Exploring boundaries of body. Attempting to differentiate self from others.	Experiences as separation.
18 months–5 years: Preschool	Time linked with concrete events. Develops understanding of morning and night. Begins to differentiate yesterday, today, and tomorrow. Does not understand future. Cannot tell time.	Learns names of major body parts first, then minor body parts. Often knows location of heart and stomach. Inside of body unknown. Illness caused by external events, particularly accidents.	Experiences as separation and absence of mobility. Notices that dead things disappear. Feels death is temporary, caused by some external force (accidents, "bogeyman") from which rescue is possible. Feels dead people eat, breathe, move about.
5–9 years: School-age	Begins telling time around age 7. Understands the future as a long time. Clear on yesterday, today, and tomorrow.	Knows location of major internal organs. Begins to correlate functions with specific organs. Illness caused by germs and other external forces. Begins to understand internal causes.	Believes death is selective; only old people die. Understands the physical limitations of death. May perceive death as a spirit or angel.
10 years and above	Can conceptualize future, but tends to think about near future.	Gains adult understanding of body parts and functions. Describes role of external and internal factors causing illness. Realizes that some factors are unknown.	Death is the end of life. It is final and irreversible. Adolescents continue to act on premise that personal death is unlikely.

SOURCE: Reproduced by permission from Foley, G., & Whittam, E. (1990). Care of the child dying of cancer. *Ca—A Cancer Journal for Clinicians, 40*(6), 327-354.

require a reorganization of tasks and relationships, but other members suffer the loss of emotional support normally given by the deceased person, thereby creating a void that can result in withdrawal from interactions with others (Dimond & Jones, 1983).

Even when the death is of an elderly family member and expected, it may be nonetheless traumatic. In many cases, especially when families are close, older adults participate in many daily family activities such as child care. They also provide support and advice to their offspring who seek feedback in decision making with their own children. Loss of this informal support may result in a sense of isolation in addition to emphasizing mortality to other adults (Dimond & Jones, 1983).

Interventions

Effective interventions that influence development in a positive manner can take place at almost any point during the disease process. In order to attain maximum benefit from interventions, the health care provider needs to assess the developmental level of each individual and of the entire family as a developing system. Readers are redirected to Tables 2-1 and 2-2 and reminded that they should familiarize themselves with these data. Table 2-5 contains a suggested format for family assessment that could be used to collect data about specific family developmental needs.

The timing of an intervention can be critical to outcomes, so the transition period between

Table 2-5. Family assessment guide

I. Family formation
  A. Family formation and composition
    1. At what stage in the family life cycle is the family?
    2. What is the family's composition?
    3. What is the family's social class, and how is this related to the family's health care?
    4. What is the family's religious orientation? How actively involved are they?
    5. What is the family's ethnicity and cultural heritage? To what extent have ethnicity and cultural heritage been maintained? How does this relate to health status?
  B. Developmental history
    1. What is the developmental history of the family, and how is it related to family health and illness values?
    2. To what extent has the family been crisis-prone in the past?
    3. What current stresses is the family reacting to?

II. Socialization
  A. Role models
    1. To what extent are cultural values carried on to each succeeding generation?
    2. Who are the role models for each family member?
  B. Family attitudes toward health and illness
    1. What are the family's definitions of health and illness?
      a. What are the family's own health care practices?
    2. For what kinds of illness does the family consider professional care necessary?
    3. What are the family's drug habits? use of alcohol? dietary habits? hygiene and cleanliness? exercise? recreation? values?
  C. What are the family's child-rearing practices?
    1. Who assumes responsibility for child care?
    2. How are the children regarded in the family?

III. Marital and family role structure
  A. Family role structure
    1. To what extent are the husband-wife roles traditional or modern?
    2. What role does each family member fulfill?
    3. How flexible are family roles?
    4. How are decisions made within the family?
    5. Who holds the power position within the family?
  B. Economic structure
    1. Who is the economic provider in the family? How are decisions made regarding spending?
    2. What is the family's status regarding health care insurance?
  C. Health and illness
    1. Who is the primary person in the making of health care decisions?
    2. Who takes on the therapeutic role in times of illness within the family?
    3. What is the wife-mother's role within the family in relation to health and illness?
    4. Have the family roles changed in the past because of family illness?

Continued

Table 2-5. *Continued*

IV. Institutional interaction

    A. Health care services

        1. To what extent does the family use health care services?

        2. How accessible are health care services to the family?

    B. Home care of sick family members

        1. What types of home remedies are used?

        2. Have sick family members been taken care of in the home in the past?

        3. What types of medications are taken by each family member?

    C. Community resources

        1. How does the family view community resources?

        2. To what extent does the family use community resources?

        3. What social support systems does the family have within the larger community?

V. Interpersonal relationships

    A. Individual versus family emphasis

        1. What is the emphasis in the family on individual versus overall family needs?

        2. Are each family member's needs respected by other family members?

    B. Closeness of family relationships

        1. How close are family ties between family members?

        2. To what extent do family members depend on each other for support in times of crisis?

        3. What are the communication patterns between family members?

SOURCE: Adapted from Dimond and Jones (1983).

the crisis and chronic phases of illness needs to be assessed. Rolland (1987) refers to this transition period as a window of opportunity for correcting problems of individual or family development that have begun to appear. For example, if a young child is diagnosed with a chronic illness at a transitional family developmental phase, the father might withdraw from the wife and child during the initial hospitalization, forcing the mother to become the parent with exclusive knowledge about the disease and the only one who provides comfort in the hospital setting. Such behavior might have an adverse impact on continued family development. Noticing this type of behavior and addressing it during the crisis phase allows the health professional an opportunity to intervene early.

Cultural Assessment

It is the responsibility of health care providers to educate themselves about the cultural beliefs and social expectations of the individuals and families they work with. Unfortunately, health care providers often do not pay adequate attention to the social and cultural context in which families operate (Ridley, 1989). The individual's ethnic background, social class, and even recent immigration status influence his or her health care beliefs. The dominance of such beliefs signals major cultural differences requiring sensitive evaluation (Kleinman, 1988). Evaluation of the client's growth and developmental achievements can only be completed after comparison for norms within the cultural group.

A thorough psychosocial history that includes cultural factors should be taken soon after admission to the hospital. Table 2-6 contains suggestions for useful information relevant to such a cultural assessment. Greater participation by client and family takes place if the health care team recognizes and attempts to accommodate differences in a nonjudgmental manner (Guendelman, 1983). It should be assumed that families care for their chronically ill member and want to contribute in whatever way they can to the well-being of that person.

Table 2-6. Psychosocial assessment

1. Country and region of origin; number of years in the United States.

2. Degree of acculturation in the American culture.

3. Family structure and role distribution.

4. Ease of access to the hospital in terms of child care, lodging, transportation, financial resources.

5. Availability and quality of supports, both within the family and in the community. Linkages with other health and social agencies.

6. Proficiency in English.

7. Understanding of the client's condition. Cultural beliefs associated with it.

8. Capacity to function in a complex hospital environment.

9. Legal status.

10. Concurrent problems that the family encounters.

SOURCE: From Guendelman (1983).

Teaching and Education

In the lifelong quest for independence and a sense of well-being and self-worth, knowledge is essential. This applies to both individuals and families. Without assistance, few families have the internal resources to investigate disease, methods of effective coping, and community support systems needed to deal with chronic illnesses or disability.

Teaching and the Developmental Levels of the Family Members   The approximate functional developmental level of any individual determines the quantity and sophistication of the material he or she is capable of learning, with cultural background serving as the lens through which new information is filtered. Information should be presented at a cognitive level that is understandable to the age group. New information cannot be attended to unless the learner desires the knowledge and participates in the process (see Chapter 16, on teaching).

Young children are often overlooked when families are assessed for learning needs. The as-

sumption is that they are either too young to understand or that others in the family will pass on the information. However, children need developmentally appropriate information about what is going on around them. They are able to sense emotional changes within the family system and need explanations for why people are spending more time with the person who is ill. Preschoolers, for instance, need explanations for illness and behavior changes in order to minimize their tendency to assume responsibility as punishment for deeds they feel guilty about (Garrison & McQuiston, 1989).

Information provided to young children should be simple, concise, and honest, even if the news is not positive. Questions should be answered openly, since children need answers to questions they are capable of asking. If they are ignored or have no confidence in the answer given, the only option left open to them is to relate their experience to something seen on television or fantasized. If young children let it be known they do not want to know more, then their wishes should be respected until they do wish to learn more (Craft & Craft, 1989). Being included as part of the family reassures young children about their worth within the system.

Anticipatory Guidance: A Teaching Strategy
Anticipatory guidance refers to information given in advance of a potentially stressful event in order to make the event more predictable and to facilitate adaptation to a desired outcome (Hymovich & Hagopian, 1992). Care should be taken, however, to describe events in general terms in order to allow for normal variation. Children should not be promised anything in advance when individual differences may necessitate change.

Anticipatory guidance has been identified as the most helpful intervention used in working with families coping with chronic illness (Rankin & Weekes, 1989). People seek practical guidance when facing unknown situations. In unknown situations planning for the future becomes less predictable. It is common to hear expressions indicating that the family feels they can learn to live with unanticipated changes if they know what is normally expected. The answers given to their questions are not always clear; however, it is beneficial to them to have at least some idea of the range of outcomes that are possible.

Counseling

Counseling can be used with all members of a family. It is especially important as an intervention with families where children have chronic illnesses, since there are often concerns about genetic factors, growth and development, and so forth. For instance, children with chronic illnesses and their families have a higher risk of psychosocial problems than those without such conditions (Jackson & Vessey, 1992). The actual impact they sustain depends on the type of illness and pre-illness roles practiced by the family members (Rolland, 1987). The severity of the condition, individual personality traits, and the availability of social supports all influence the risk for negative developmental effects. Counseling services for these individuals can provide information as well as the social support necessary for optimum functioning within limits imposed by the chronic illness.

Individual Counseling Individual counseling for chronically ill persons may be available in some settings through a multidisciplinary team approach. These teams often include professionals trained to identify potential problems associated with disease progression, functional status, and social interactions. Individualized intervention strategies include therapeutic management, education, and advocacy—all of which can be designed and implemented to assist individuals to reach their developmental potential (Jackson & Vessey, 1992). Individual therapy can vary in length of treatment needed based on previously achieved development and the amount of energy needed to meet ongoing physical challenges.

If appropriate counseling within the team is not available, referral to other local sources should be made. There are therapists who specialize in treatment of distinct interest areas, such as those who counsel only women. For instance, individual counseling for women with disabilities may be the intervention of choice when other members of the family do not see the need to participate. Because some women with disabilities have had limited life opportunities, basic issues involving relationships and rights and responsibilities need to be approached over a period of time (Power et al., 1988).

Older adults often are neglected as a population who could benefit from individual counseling. Few therapists have formal training in gerontology, which adds to the tendency to view elderly clients as poor candidates for positive change (Eisenberg et al., 1984). Some clients have incorporated these negative cultural views of themselves, which leads to a decrease in self-esteem and discouragement about the prospects of treatment that could help. However, many of these clients are capable of learning new skills and taking positive action on their own behalf. Therapists who have expertise in working with elderly clients often help them set realistic goals for achieving a maximum level of functioning.

Family Counseling Family counseling is the preferred approach if all family members are willing to make changes in themselves. If the family has coping strategies that were at least adequate in the past, they have a good chance of working together to overcome new obstacles. New problem-solving skills may need to be developed as situations arise. If chronically ill individuals have limitations that preclude resuming all or some of their previous roles, the family can discuss how to reassign portions of the responsibility. On the other hand, the disabled individual may voluntarily assume alternative responsibilities formerly carried out by another member. The extent of the disability, of course, will have a great effect on the amount of exchange that is realistic (Collier, 1990).

Children and extended family members such as grandparents should have the opportunity to participate in planning if they are to be involved in coping with long-term effects of an illness. Otherwise, unspoken blame or other unresolved feelings can result in the slow erosion of relationships that will eventually interfere with adaptation of all family members (Collier, 1990). Regardless of the format used, engaging everyone who will be involved can only increase the likelihood of a positive adjustment.

Support Groups

Increased stress resulting from the inherent demands of a chronic illness can be moderated through sharing and comparing personal experience (Phillips, 1990). Support groups developed from the need to talk with others who have been through the same process and who can comprehend on a level beyond just trying to understand. Within a group's boundaries, emotional expression is encouraged rather than suppressed, as occurs in public (Strauss et al., 1984). Disclosure of emotions and experiences to other group members substitutes for interactions within the family (Anderson, 1990).

There are several types of support groups. *Relations groups,* such as those available for the children of disabled adults, are facilitated by a professional with expertise in disability issues. They are for clients and significant others to meet for the purpose of supporting one another as they learn about the illness. Relations groups usually have a preset number of sessions with a definitive beginning and end (Power et al., 1988).

Family support groups involve two or more entire families who discuss the personal needs and concerns of all group members. These groups may be planned around a social activity without a preset agenda other than to provide an opportunity for sharing needs and frustrations (Power et al., 1988) or they may have agendas and be more structured depending on the purpose of the particular group. For example, parents of children with genetic disorders may be helped in assuaging guilt associated with passing the disease on to their children when they can interact with other similarly impacted families (Gagliardi, 1991).

Informal support groups have grown in numbers during recent years. They often are formed as a result of families with similar problems meeting one another through an informal network. Professionals may or may not be involved. If they are, it is usually for the purpose of providing information about group process.

For example, several benefits of such groups were identified by participating parents who had chronically ill children (Phillips, 1990). The parents noted that having someone to talk to decreased their sense of isolation and stress. Their feelings of being unique were decreased, and they were able to establish some sense of normality through comparisons with each other. Parents felt they received accurate information from other group members resulting in the possibility of improved care for their children. Socialization and support for anticipated changes were also noted as important benefits. In addition, parents who participated in these groups identified one of their greatest needs as the desire to understand the impact of chronic illness on growth and development (Phillips, 1990).

Unfortunately, since so many support groups are informal and have no follow-up, it is difficult to measure any impact on adjustment that results from participation. In spite of this, families should be encouraged to participate as a way of meeting others with similar problems who may be able to offer help when needed. Verbal reports of benefit from the support group experience are evidence of the benefit. If families do not find the group helpful, they have the option of no longer attending.

Encouraging Balance

The family best able to maintain a balance between changes necessary to accommodate illness and individual needs of family members will experience the fewest long-term developmental difficulties (Stein & Jessop, 1989). In general, families manage well on their own by mobilizing resources and reorganizing priorities as they arise. However, they can benefit from specialized help to negotiate with outside resources for services when that becomes necessary.

Sharing Control Control can become an issue in family life when a family member has a chronic illness. To encourage optimum development, all family members, from the beginning, should be involved in decision making and taking responsibility (Eisenberg et al., 1984). Even young children can be involved in family discussions about the changes needed to be made if provided with a rationale. Children also benefit if given chores or responsibilities of some kind within the home.

The person who is ill can contribute by acknowledging the needs of others. As an example, hospitalized school-age children should be encouraged to consider the needs of both siblings and parents (Jackson & Vessey, 1992). These children need to understand that parents are unable to be continually at their side, that they need to take care of themselves, and that they have a responsibility to other siblings (Jackson & Vessey, 1992). When these children accept that others have needs, the parents need not feel guilty, and the family has the best chance of maintaining balance.

Although there are advantages to seeing the family as the primary unit of care, we must acknowledge the differences individuals bring to the unit. Therefore, it is important to inquire about the beliefs of each family member in order to have the most complete plan for assisting the family to achieve optimum balance in their lives (Whyte, 1992). For instance, each parent may have a different perspective on illness and whether or not the child is seen as normal. Knafl and associates (1993) found that when both parents viewed their child as other than normal, the child had lower scores on self-worth measures than either children whose parents viewed them as normal or those whose parents had conflicting views.

Respite for the Family

Respite allows caregivers to take time away from their responsibilities; it is a service for the entire family designed to support people living in their own homes (Stein & Jessop, 1989). In even the most ideal situations, parents and siblings need time away from caregiving to allow for their own growth and development (Gagliardi, 1991). The respite service may be a formal arrangement with an agency, or it may be provided by trained community volunteers.

In addition to offering relief for caregivers, respite services can provide relief for clients who are concerned about the impact of their illness upon other family members (Capelli et al., 1989). Clients who feel as if they are preventing their caregivers from achieving their own potential may welcome an opportunity to see the family enjoy themselves at an activity that would not otherwise be possible.

Disease-specific camps for children are helpful in ameliorating the feeling of difference from peers (Gagliardi, 1991). In a camp for adolescents with cancer, for instance, everyone has experienced similar physical changes resulting from treatment. In the camp setting, everyone can feel normal if even for a brief time. They are able to compare themselves with their true equals in a way they otherwise cannot. This type of camp is not commonly available for adults, but perhaps should be.

Summary and Conclusions

Reactions to the onset of a chronic illness vary according to an individual's and family's stage of development. Normal development is a continuous process, each stage having its own built-in stressors, and is interrupted to the extent that the illness creates barriers to mastery of important tasks. Family members ordinarily adjust to developmental changes as they occur, but in the presence of chronic illness, expectations are sometimes modified, adding to the difficulty of developmental achievement.

If the onset of illness occurs during early infancy, the greatest developmental hazards include separation from a consistent caregiver, physical limitations of environmental exploration, and the parental tendency to overprotect the infant. The school-age child is at risk for decreased interactions with peers, which can result in lack of acceptance by them. Adolescents are especially at risk if the illness results in alterations in physical appearance; a decrease in positive body image can lead to problems in sexual identity and self-concept.

Young adults are most affected by limitations in career goals and the ability to function as contributing members of the family. Middle-aged adults may be faced with economic changes and identity and self-esteem implications. Older adults are confronted with physical or cognitive limitations in addition to those of normal aging; the economic drain can quickly deplete life savings.

The family as a unit normally meets the basic needs of individual members to develop their full potential. The family unit provides emotional support, an organizational structure, and a means of functioning within the community. The extent to which these tasks are interrupted will either temporarily or permanently impact the ability to complete the family life-cycle tasks.

The illness life cycle, as described by Rolland (1987), offers a framework for evaluating severity of the illness in reference to type of onset, course of the illness, outcome potential, and the degree of expected incapacitation. When the onset of illness occurs during a period of family transition toward independence, the unit is least prepared to accommodate the adjustment necessary for effective coping.

Cultural variations present challenges to health care professionals. Psychosocial and cultural assessment can provide information about the strengths and needs brought with the family to the illness setting. It is the responsibility of health care providers to become aware of sociocultural beliefs related to the client, illness, and outcome expectations. Good communication with feedback for understanding allows health professionals to avoid withdrawal or resistance to health-promoting behaviors.

Interventions for promoting uninterrupted growth and development during illness periods include teaching through anticipatory guidance, individual or family counseling, support groups, respite for the family, and encouraging balance within the family.

NURSING DIAGNOSIS

Editor's Note: The following nursing diagnoses were selected by the author of this chapter as appropriate to the content herein. Her preferred source book is one written by McFarland and McFarlane (1993), which lists different definitions and defining characteristics than those found in the NANDA source book. The reader may wish to review this other source.

6.6 Altered Growth and Development

Definition: The state in which an individual demonstrates deviations from norms for his/her age group.

Defining Characteristics:

Major: Delay or difficulty in performing skills (motor, social, or expressive) typical of age group; altered physical growth; inability to perform self-care or self-control activities appropriate for age.

Minor: Flat affect; listlessness, decreased responses.

Related Factors: Inadequate caretaking; indifference, inconsistent responsiveness; multiple caretakers; separation from significant others; environmental and stimulation deficiencies; effect of physical disability; prescribed dependence.

3.2.1.1.1. Altered Parenting

Definition: The state in which a nurturing figure(s) experiences an inability to create an environment which promotes the optimum growth and development of another human being.[1]

Defining Characteristics:[2] Abandonment; verbalization; runaway; cannot control child; incidence of physical and psychological trauma; lack of parental attachment behaviors; inappropriate visual, tactile, auditory stimulation; negative identification of infant/child's characteristics; negative attachment of meanings to

---

[1]It is important to state as a preface to this diagnosis that adjustment to parenting in general is a normal maturational process that elicits nursing behaviors of prevention of potential problems and health promotion.

[2]The asterisk indicates a critical defining characteristic.

infant/child; verbalization of resentment toward the infant/child; verbalization of role inadequacy; *inattentive to infant/child needs; verbal disgust at body functions of infant/child; noncompliance with health appointments for self and/or infant/child; *history of child abuse or abandonment by primary caretaker; verbalizes desire to have child call him/herself by first name versus traditional cultural tendencies; child receives care from multiple caretakers without consideration for the needs of the infant/child; compulsively seeking role approval from others.

Related Factors: Lack of available role model; ineffective role model; physical and psychosocial abuse of nurturing figure; lack of support between/from significant other(s); unmet social/ emotional maturation needs of parenting figures; interruption in bonding process, i.e., maternal, paternal, other; unrealistic expectation for self, infant, partner; perceive threat to own survival, physical and emotional; mental and/or physical illness; presence of stress (financial, legal, recent crisis, cultural move); lack of knowledge; limited cognitive functioning; lack of role identity; lack of or inappropriate response of child to relationship; multiple pregnancies.

5.1.2.1.2 Ineffective Family Coping: Compromised

See Chapter 12, on family caregivers, for definition, defining characteristics, and related factors.

STUDY QUESTIONS

1. Describe Rolland's illness life-cycle framework. How can it be used to view chronic illness from a growth and development perspective rather than a disease perspective?
2. Discuss the cumulative effect of mastery in developmental stages.
3. How do family dynamics influence adaptation to chronic illness of any member?
4. What negative impact can a chronic illness have on the psychological well-being and compliance of individuals through the life cycle?
5. Discuss cultural variations that should be assessed to better understand how a client from another culture perceives illness. What are the implications when planning care?

6. Compare factors involved in a child's understanding of death from infancy to school age. How can you talk with each age group about death?
7. What influence does altered mobility have on the growth and development of individuals who have a chronic or disabling disorder? Discuss this across the life cycle.
8. How does chronic illness influence body image through the life cycle? Sexuality?
9. How does teaching help individuals at different developmental levels adapt to chronic illness? Help families?
10. How can counseling be used to help family members deal with chronic illness? Support groups?

References

Anderson, G. R. (Ed.) (1990). *Courage to care: Responding to the crisis of children with AIDS.* Washington, D.C.: Child Welfare League of America.

Anderson, R., & Bury, M. (Eds.) (1988). *Living with chronic illness: The experience of patients and their families.* London: University in Hyman Ltd.

Brookins, G. K. (1993). Culture, ethnicity, and bicultural competence: Implications for children with chronic illness and disability. *Pediatrics, 91*(4), 1056-1062.

Capelli, M., McGrath, P. J., & Heick, C. E. (1989). Chronic disease and its impact: The adolescent's perspective. *Journal of Adolescent Health Care, 10,* 283-288.

Collier, J. H. (1990). Developmental and systems perspectives on chronic illness. *Holistic Nursing Practice, 5*(1), 1-9.

Corbin, J. M., & Strauss, A. L. (1984). Collaboration: Couples working together to manage chronic illness. *Image: The Journal of Nursing Scholarship, 16*(4), 109-115.

Craft, M. J., & Craft, J. L. (1989). Perceived changes in siblings of hospitalized children: A comparison of sibling and parent reports. *Child Health Care, 18*(1), 42-48.

Dimond, M., & Jones, S. L. (1983). *Chronic illness across the life span.* Norwalk, CT: Appleton-Century-Crofts.

Dolgin, H. J., Phipps, S., Harow, E., & Zelter, L. K. (1990). Parental management of fear in chronically ill and healthy children. *Journal of Pediatric Psychology, 12*(6), 733-744.

Edwards, A., & Polite, C. K. (1992). *Children of the dream: The psychology of black success.* New York: Doubleday.

Eisenberg, M. G., Sutkin, L. C., & Jansen, M. A. (Eds.) (1984). *Chronic illness and disability through the life span: Effects on self and family.* New York: Springer.

Erikson, E. H. (1963). *Childhood and society.* New York: Norton.

——— (1986). *Vital involvement in old age.* New York: Macmillan.

Falvo, D. R. (1991). *Medical and Psychological Aspects of Chronic Illness and Disability.* Gaithersburg, MD: Aspen Publishing.

Foley, G. V., & Whittam, E. H. (1990). Care of the child dying of cancer. *Ca—A Cancer Journal for Clinicians, 40*(6), 327-354.

Foxall, M. J., Ekberg, J. Y., & Griffith, N. (1985). Adjustment patterns of chronically ill middle-aged persons and spouses. *Western Journal of Nursing Research, 7*(4), 425-444.

Gagliardi, B. A. (1991). The family's experience of living with a child with Duchenne Muscular Dystrophy. *Applied Nursing Research, 4*(4), 159-164.

Garrison, W. T., & McQuiston, S. (1989). *Chronic illness during childhood and adolescence: Psychological aspects.* Newbury Park, CA: Sage.

Giger, J. N., & Davidhizar, R. E. (1991). *Transcultural nursing: assessment and intervention.* St. Louis: Mosby Year Book.

Goleman, D. (1988, June 14). Erikson, In his own old age, expands his view of life. *New York Times,* pp. 13, 16.

Grace, N. E., & Zola, I. K. (1993). Multiculturalism, chronic illness and disability. *Pediatrics, 91*(5), 1048-1055.

Guendelman, S. (1983). Developing responsiveness to the health needs of Hispanic children and families. *Social Work in Health Care, 8*(4), 1-15.

Huntley, T. (1991). *Helping children grieve.* Minneapolis: Augsburg Fortress.

Hymovich, D. P., & Hagopian, G. A. (1992). *Chronic illness in children and adults: A psychosocial approach.* Philadelphia: W. B. Saunders.

Jackson, P. L., Vessey, J. A. (1992). *Primary care of the child with a chronic condition.* St. Louis: Mosby Year Book.

Kleinman, A. (1988). *The illness narratives: Suffering, healing and the human condition.* New York: Basic Books.

Knafl K., Gallo, A., Breitmayer, B., Zoeller, L., & Ayres, L. (1993). Family response to a child's chronic illness: A description of major defining themes. In S. Funk, M. Tornquist, M. Champayne, & R. Wiese (Eds.), *Key aspects of caring for the chronically ill.* New York: Springer.

Kurtz, M. J. (1993). Case study of an adolescent spinal cord injured patient. *Rehabilitation Nursing, 18*(4), 237-239.

Madiros, M. (1989). Conception of childhood disability among Mexican-American parents. *Medical Anthropology, 12,* 55-68.

McCubbin, M. A. (1989). Family stress and family strengths: A comparison of single and two-parent families with handicapped children. *Research in Nursing and Health, 12,* 101-110.

McCubbin, H. I., Thompson, E. A., Thompson, A. I., McCubbin, M. A., & Kaston, A. J. (1993). Culture, ethnicity and the family: Critical factors in childhood chronic illnesses and disabilities. *Pediatrics, 91*(5), 1063-1070.

McFarland, C. R., & McFarlane, Z. H. (1993). *Nursing diagnosis and intervention: Planning for patient care.* St. Louis: Mosby Year Book.

Miller, J. F. (1992). *Coping with chronic illness: Overcoming powerlessness.* Philadelphia: F. A. Davis.

Patterson, J. M., & Blum, R. W. (1993). A conference on culture and chronic illness in childhood: Conference summary. *Pediatrics, 91*(5), 1025-1030.

Phillips, M. (1990). Support groups for parents of chronically ill children. *Pediatric Nursing, 16*(4), 404-406.

Power, P. W., Dell Orto, A. E., & Gibbons, M. B. (Eds.) (1988). *Family interventions throughout chronic illness and disability.* New York: Springer.

Putnam, P. A. (1987). Coping in later years: The reconciliation of opposites. *Image: The Journal of Nursing Scholarship, 19*(2), 67-69.

Rankin, S. H., & Weekes, D. P. (1989). Life-span and development: A review of theory and practice for families with chronically ill members. *Scholarly Inquiry for Nursing Practice: An International Journal, 3*(1), 3-22.

Ridley, B. (1989). Family response in head injury: Denial . . . or hope for the future? *Social Science Medicine, 29*(4), 555-561.

Rolland, J. S. (1987, June). Chronic illness and the life cycle: A conceptual framework. *Family Process, 26,* 203-221.

Stein, R. E. K., & Jessop, D. J. (1989). *Meeting the needs of individuals and families in caring for children with chronic illness.* In R. E. K. Stein (Ed.), *Caring for children with chronic illness: Issues and strategies* (pp. 63-74). New York: Springer.

Strauss, A. L., Corbin, J., Fagerhaugh, S., Glaser, B., Maines, D., Suczek, B., & Wiener, C. L. (1984). *Chronic illness and the quality of life.* St. Louis: C. V. Mosby.

Villaruel, A. M., & deMontellano, B. O. (1992). Culture and pain: A Mesoamerican perspective. *Advances in Nursing Science, 15*(1), 21-32.

Whyte, D. A. (1992). A family nursing approach to the care of a child with a chronic illness. *Journal of Advanced Nursing, 17*, 317-327.

Bibliography

Anderson, S. V. & Bauwens, E. E. (1981). *Chronic health problems: Concepts and application.* St. Louis: C.V. Mosby.

Baker, L. S. (1991). *You and HIV: A day at a time.* Philadelphia: W.B. Saunders.

Bregman, A. M. (1980). Living with progressive childhood illness: Parental management of neuromuscular disease. *Social Work in Health Care, 5*(4), 390-407.

Christ, M. A., & Hohlock, F. (1988). *Gerontological nursing.* Springhouse, PA: Springhouse.

Fowler, M. G., Simpson, G. A., & Schoendorg, K. C. (1993). Families on the move and children's health care. *Pediatrics, 91*(5), 934-940.

Gallo, A., Breitmayer, B., Knafl, K., & Zoeller, L. (1992). Well siblings of children with chronic illness: Parents' reports of their psychologic adjustment. *Pediatric Nursing, 18*(1), 23-27.

Geber, G., & Latts, E. (1993). Race and ethnicity: Issues for adolescents with chronic illness and disabilities. An annotated bibliography. *Pediatrics, 91*(5), 1071-1081.

Kübler-Ross, E. (1987). *AIDS: The ultimate challenge.* New York: Macmillan.

Lambert, V. A., & Lambert, C. E. (Eds.) (1987). Adaptation to chronic illness. *Nursing Clinics of North America, 22,* 3.

Lambert, V. A., Lambert, C. E., Klipple, G. L., & Mewshaw, E. A. (1989). Social support, hardiness and psychological well-being in women with arthritis. *Image: The Journal of Nursing Scholarship, 21*(3), 128-131.

Miles, M., Carter, M., Elberly, T., Henessey, J., & Riddle, I. (1989). Toward an understanding of parent stress in the pediatric intensive care unit: Overview of the program of research. *Maternal-Child Nursing Journal, 18*(3), 181-243.

Newacheck, P. W., Stoddard, J. J., & McManus, M. (1993). Ethnocultural variations in the prevalence and impact of childhood chronic conditions. *Pediatrics, 91*(5), 1031-1039.

Newacheck, P., & Taylor, W. (1992). Childhood chronic illness: Prevalence, severity and impact. *American Journal of Public Health, 82,* 364-371.

Perrin, J. M. (1985). Introduction. In N. Hobbs, & J. M. Perrin (Eds.), *Issues in the care of children with chronic disease* (pp. 1-10). San Francisco: Jossey-Bass.

Pfefferbaum, B., Adams, J., & Aceves, J. (1990). The influence of culture on pain in Anglo and Hispanic children with cancer. *Journal of the American Academy of Child and Adolescent Psychiatry, 29*(4), 642-647.

Reinert, B. R. (1986). The health care beliefs and values of Mexican-Americans. *Home Healthcare Nurse, 4*(5), 23-31.

Richardson, S. A. (1989). Transition to adulthood. In R.E.K. Stein (Ed.), *Caring for children with chronic illness: Issues and strategies.* New York: Springer.

Rodriguez, T. (1983, February). Mexican Americans: Factors influencing health practices. *Journal of School Health,* 136-139.

Romand, J. L. (1989). *Children facing grief: Letters from bereaved brothers and sisters.* St. Meinrad, IN: Abbey Press.

Simon, N., & Smith, D. (1992). Living with chronic pediatric liver disease: The parents' experience. *Pediatric Nursing, 18*(5), 453-458.

Thomas, R. B. & Wicks, K. (1987). Nursing assessment of chronic conditions in children. In M. H. Rose, & R. B. Thomas (Eds.), *Children with chronic conditions: Nursing in a family and community context.* Orlando, FL: Grune & Stratton.

Walker, C. L. (1988). Stress and coping in siblings of childhood cancer patients. *Nursing Research, 37*(4), 208-212.

Wilson, H. S. (1989). Family caregiving for a relative with Alzheimer's dementia: Coping with negative choices. *Nursing Research, 38*(2), 94-98.

CHAPTER 3

Illness Trajectory

Nancy White • Ilene Lubkin

Trajectory 1. The curve that a body (as a planet or comet in its orbit or a rocket) describes in space. 2. A path, progression, or line of development resembling a physical trajectory.
Webster's Ninth New Collegiate Dictionary, 1987

Introduction

Implicit in the preceding definition of *trajectory* are the ideas of direction, movement, shape, and predictability. These four characteristics are apparent when one thinks of some object, such as a missile, hurtling toward a landing site determined by calculating physical properties involved in movement over time and through space. The concept, however, is less obvious in relation to illness.

Yet an illness can be seen as a trajectory if one thinks of it as a process that begins with some physiological change and alteration in health status, which continues through life with a positive or negative resolution. By taking into account a disease's characteristic symptoms, phases, and treatment over time, one can predict potential or probable outcomes. Physicians use knowledge of these outcomes to plan appropriate therapy to correct, reverse, or slow disease progression. Nurses use this same knowledge to plan and perform work necessary to care for and provide support for clients and families experiencing chronic illness.

Glaser and Strauss (1968) introduced trajectory as a concept applicable to illness in a study of the dying client in a hospital setting. They discovered that the process of dying often takes considerable time and affects not only the dying individual but also the family and staff. Their efforts to increase understanding of the distancing that sometimes occurs between staff and the terminally ill client (without placing blame for that unfortunate situation) created an awareness that dying is an event that different people perceive differently. In addition, all involved individuals use many different strategies to manage the dying course.

Strauss spent several years teaching courses in chronic illness and accumulating a significant amount of information about living with chronic illness through case studies of his own and his students (Corbin & Strauss, 1993). The trajectory concept underlying these studies served to provide a sociological perspective on the experience of managing the course of a chronic illness. Trajectories were understood to be something comprising the lives, histories, and attitudes of *all* who are involved in a particular course of illness (Wiener, 1989). Not only does illness trajectory consider the physiological components of the disease, but it also encompasses the total identification of those involved and the organization and performance of work done over the entire course of the illness (Strauss et al., 1985).

For the health professional, trajectory is a relatively unfamiliar psychosocial concept that focuses on the difference in perception, over time, of those involved in the situation (for example, health professionals, clients, and families). It considers the impact on these people and their responses (Strauss et al., 1985). Different diseases have different trajectories, much as they differ in symptomatology; like symptoms, these trajectories are influenced by many factors: the medical plan; each person's background, problems, or complications; interaction among those involved, and so on.

Because of the dynamic nature of illness, trajectories can never be predicted with any certainty. Rather, they constantly change and reorganize based on physiological alterations and the changing responses of the individuals involved. However, illness trajectories do have some characteristic shapes and patterns associated with their projected course. Some may typically be stable with only periodic downward directions characteristic of exacerbations. Others may begin with a sudden downward pattern followed by stabilization and perhaps improvement, such as when associated with rehabilitation following a stroke. In most diseases there is a difference between the actual course of the disease and the perceived course, or between the professional's view of the projected course and the client's view.

Perceptions depend on people's knowledge, experiences, and capabilities (Strauss et al., 1984). Just as several witnesses report varying versions of an accident, so professionals see the progression of a disease somewhat differently from each other and from the client. Once a diagnosis is made, the physician, nurse, or other health professional knows the physiological basis of what is happening, what might happen with treatment, what probably might happen without treatment, the range of possible complications, and procedures necessary to achieve a positive resolution. Each health professional then develops an image of the disease and predicts what can or will happen. If each health team member's perception of a trajectory were graphed onto a transparency, the differences and similarities would become apparent even though they might be minimal. Subtle differences seen in trajectory do not adversely impact necessary work.

The client may have a markedly different perception, focusing not on physiology but on the effects of symptoms, on anxiety and concern over long-term effects, or on a sense of uncertainty secondary to limited understanding of what is happening. With acute illnesses, clients tend to move into the sick role, in which the responsibility of managing the illness rests on the professional staff (see Chapter 4, on illness roles). Chronically ill individuals, on the other hand, have a fuller sense of their disease and its progression and management, and they are aware of what works and does not work for them. Although the actual course of the disease can only be known retrospectively, persons who deal with chronic illness make projections for the future based on their perceptions of what is going to happen. Thus, perceptions are an integral part of illness trajectory. Unlike hospital personnel, who tend to base their perceptions on the episodic nature of disease, chronically ill clients may be focusing not only on the primary condition but on managing secondary, but currently quiescent, illnesses (Fagerhaugh & Strauss, 1977).

Reif's study (1975) implied that individual perceptions lead to responses that are appropriate to those perceptions. The man who is recovering from a myocardial infarction can respond with too much or too little activity based on his perception of his cardiac status. If he considers his heart highly damaged rather than healing, he may see himself as a cardiac cripple and markedly limit his activity. His wife may believe that he is now well and his heart healed, and urge him to return to work. The physician, if conservative in approach, may be concerned about recurrence and encourage the client to take things easy, reinforcing the cardiac cripple status. If, however, the physician feels that activity maximizes recovery, conflict about how much is enough activity can arise between this client and his doctor.

And what about a situation in which the physician, client, and family agree that returning to work is a reasonable choice in the near future, but other individuals involved in the situation disagree? For instance, an employer may consider the person permanently disabled or be concerned about the possibility of another heart attack, which would affect productivity, safety, and disability insurance rates. In either case, a forced early retirement may be in store for this individual, despite his and others' wishes.

Once understood, trajectory can allow analytical ordering of a variety of events that are present and can lead to distancing and perspective on why some problems occur between health professionals, between professional and client and family, or between client and family (Strauss et al., 1985), all of which may provide insight into compliance/noncompliance issues. In addition, professionals may become more sensitive to the health care needs of the chronically ill and more adept at guiding clients through a fragmented health care system, assisting them to make informed decisions regarding treatment options, helping client and family meet the demands of the illness, and assisting them in learning to live with it.

Trajectory Terminology

An adequate understanding of trajectory requires that health professionals understand clearly the terms, concepts, and distinct characteristics involved (see Table 3–1). All trajectories occur over time and move in some direction. Trajectory characteristics can be perceived differently because they are influenced by actions taken by participants or by the contingencies of a given situation. A trajectory requires the combined effort of the affected individual, family, and health care practitioners to determine its eventual outcome, manage any symptoms, and handle associated disability (Corbin & Strauss, 1993).

Phases Trajectory phasing represents the changes in status that a chronic condition can undergo over its course. Phases, called acute,

comeback, stable, unstable, and downward, can have predictable or unpredictable sequences or timing (Corbin & Strauss, 1988). An *acute* phase is one in which the afflicted individual is physically or mentally affected by an illness to a degree that necessitates immediate medical attention and hospitalization to prevent deterioration or death. *Comeback* refers to the overall upward course in which the individual achieves a satisfying life within the boundaries imposed by the limitations of the disease; the goal of management is to regain as much functional ability as possible. A *stable* phase is one in which the illness is in remission, quiet, or changing so slowly that there are few signs. In an *unstable* phase, the illness is persistently out of control. *Downward* phases include progressive deterioration as well as dying when one's life work needs to be finished and closure completed (Corbin & Strauss, 1988).

Rolland's (1987) phases (crisis, chronic, and terminal) can also be viewed from a trajectory perspective and provide a developmental understanding of the natural history of chronic disease. The *crisis* phase consists of the period after the occurrence of symptoms and before a diagnosis has been made, the diagnosis stage, and the initial adjustment period. During this time the client and family are learning to create meaning for the illness event and gain a sense of competency to manage the situation. They grieve for the losses brought on by the condition, but are also moving toward acceptance of a new identity (biography) that incorporates the illness.

The *chronic* phase is the time between the crisis phase and the third phase, when issues of death predominate. Rolland (1987) calls this the "long haul" or the phase of "day to day living with chronic illness" (p. 207). The ability of the family to maintain some semblance of normalcy in the presence of uncertainty is the key task of this period. In cases where individuals require significant caretaking by family members, the situation may be seen as both hopeless and unending.

The *terminal* phase consists of the preterminal stage, death, mourning, and resolution of loss. During the preterminal stage, the inevitability of death is realized and dominates the lives of the individual and family. Individuals may

Table 3-1. Trajectory terminology

Trajectory	A concept that deals with the way disease progression is perceived over time by those involved in the situation, the responses resulting from this perception, and the relationship of these factors to the organization and performance of necessary work.
Participant	Anyone involved in the illness situation. Participants include client, family members, nurses, and physicians, and even friends, neighbors, and employers if they influence the trajectory.
Duration	The time span involved in the trajectory, which may range from swift (as following a fatal accident) to slow and progressively downhill. Duration is not an objective physiological property, since it varies in each situation and is perceived differently by each person.
Direction and movement	The progression of a disease from point A to point B to point C, and so on. Direction and movement occur over time and are influenced by actions taken to manage the trajectory.
Perception/Projection	What participants define as occurring or expect to occur, given their knowledge and experience. Participants' perceptions of events vary, even when their knowledge and experience are similar. "Perception" of what is occurring differs from the "actual" unfolding of a disease.
Predictability	The ability to anticipate the way the trajectory will progress, including the rate at which changes will occur. Some diseases are highly predictable; others are not.
Shape	The mental image that the course of an illness is expected to take. Since shape has direction and movement that occur over time, it can be graphed. Like duration, shape is a perceived property, with each participant having a somewhat different image.
Shaping	Actions that influence the outcome of a disease (different from shape but similar in meaning to management). Management implies successful outcomes, whereas shaping implies that unexpected problems are handled in the best way possible, even when the trajectory is not in full control. Shaping covers the complexity of trajectory work, medical outcome, and consequences to the workers.
Work	Effort directed to accomplishing an objective. Work occurs over time, is diverse, and has complexities related to the tasks involved. Trajectory work includes performing technical chores and providing comfort and clinical safety, managing or supervising machines, coordinating efforts, and so on. Hospital work is done by patients and family as well as staff. At home, the client and family do the work.
Phases	Major divisions of trajectory consisting of stages that contain clusters of necessary interrelated tasks; phases include diagnosis, various therapeutic steps, and recovery. Each phase has points of decision concerning the cluster, sequence, and organization of tasks necessary for that phase. Like trajectories, phases can be certain or uncertain. When phase tasks go awry or conflict with tasks for another trajectory arises, problems that result may affect the shape of the trajectory.
Biographies	The background or life history that makes each individual unique from others (social identity, family and social relationships, work history, lifestyle, and so on); also called social trajectories. Like all trajectories, biographies are perceived; have duration, shape, and predictability; and involve work. All participants (staff, client, and others) bring with them aspects of their biographies (such as attitudes, impressions, and moods) that influence interpretation and reaction to events.

Table 3-1. *Continued*

Contingency	Problems of a medical, interactional, organizational, or biographical nature. Contingencies can be expected (such as side effects of drugs) or unexpected (such as effects of technology whose outcomes are unknown). The former allows for advanced preparation to manage the problem; the latter cannot. Contingencies influence the shape of the trajectory; the interplay between contingencies and efforts at illness control creates the specific details of trajectories.
Balancing	The process of making choices. Often a matter of determining priorities, balancing generally entails giving up some considerations in exchange for others. Families do much balancing at home to avoid adverse physiological aftermaths or to retain some acceptable degree of life-style. Hospital staff also perform balancing tasks.

SOURCE: Lubkin (1990).

experience "anticipatory grief" as they begin to imagine life without their loved one. Following the death of the ill person, the family issues and tasks deal with loss, grief, mourning, and eventually the resumption of family life beyond the loss (Rolland, 1987).

Projection   Trajectory projection refers to the vision, or perception, of the illness course by each individual who comes into contact with the illness and its management. This projection involves trying to ascertain for oneself what will happen in the future, how long it will take, and what action will be taken as a result of the projected trajectory. Involved individuals have their own trajectory projection and ideas about how the illness should be shaped based on their own knowledge and experience (Corbin & Strauss, 1993). *Predictability,* which is an outgrowth of projection, refers to the way the trajectory will progress and includes how closely the projection matches the actual unfolding of the disease.

Shape   The shape of a trajectory results from changes that occur. It may go straight down, vacillate slowly, plateau for periods of time, and then move quickly or slowly in one direction or another (Glaser & Strauss, 1968). The shape can be accurately graphed, but only retrospectively. However, once a diagnosis is made, professionals tend to mentally graph what they feel will probably occur.

The word *shaping* is used rather than *management* because the latter does not adequately cover the complexity of trajectory work, medical outcome, or consequences for the workers. Although health professionals are more comfortable using the word *management, shaping* more accurately reflects the conscientious, but not always effective, efforts to deal with complex trajectories or the iatrogenic effects of new technologies. One can say that shaping the trajectory helps give shape to the course of an illness. Only when illness courses are routine and trajectories are nonproblematic is the term *managing* appropriate.

Work   The work involved in shaping trajectories has temporal relationships (timing, pacing, sequencing), occurs spatially, is diverse, and has complexities in relation to the tasks involved. Work includes not only necessary procedures to control the illness, symptoms, or complications but the management of household and family (Corbin & Strauss, 1988).

Contingencies   Contingencies are problems, expected or unexpected, depending on the nature of the illness or technology. With many diseases, the problems that can arise are known and planned for. With others, especially when modern technology exists, the contingencies have an unknown quality, making predictability impossible.

Biographies Biographies are trajectories in that they are perceived; they have duration, shape, and predictability; and they involve work. Client biographies include previous hospital experiences, usual ways of dealing with symptomatology, feeling tones, and other factors. Staff also have biographies that affect the situation; each staff member's biography includes "a host of individual attitudes, impressions, conceptions, [and] mood changes" that influence much of what happens (Wiener et al., 1979). Biographies should be considered perceptions rather than actualities of personal history, since each individual includes certain components of events and excludes others. As an example, family members and clients recall different information when providing social history on admission.

Balancing Balancing refers to a necessary process to keep symptoms and disease under control, especially when there are multiple chronic illnesses with regimens that have conflicting task requirements (Strauss et al., 1985). Balancing at home helps clients and families deal with the illness in relation to other needs by determining adjustments that must be made in regimens so that they fit into life-style or the timing of other activities. Often balancing occurs without the knowledge or consent of the primary health care provider—for example, the client who omits occasional doses of a diuretic prior to planned outings.

During hospitalization, clients and family continue to do what they see as necessary balancing. The client and family and the health professional may have different perspectives of what should be balanced; that is, clients may weigh options differently from professionals (Strauss et al., 1985), leading to contests over control (Fagerhaugh & Strauss, 1977).

Staff also do balancing in the hospital setting. Balancing in these situations can be adversely influenced by such factors as (1) lack of knowledge—for instance, the side effects of new drugs or other innovative treatment modalities; (2) staff's tendency to focus on the primary trajectory to the exclusion of other currently stabilized disorders; and (3) personnel's actual lack of information about other diagnoses or illnesses

(Strauss et al., 1985). For example, the precarious condition of premature infants in an intensive care nursery (ICN) requires balancing the provision of sufficient oxygen to keep fragile lungs functioning with ensuring that quantity is insufficient to cause blindness (Wiener et al., 1979).

Problems and Issues from a Trajectory Perspective

The ranks of the chronically ill grow not only because there are more chronically ill elderly people but also because of an ever increasing number of middle-aged and young adults, as well as children, who are surviving formerly fatal diseases and trauma. Wiener et al. (1979) point out that the ranks of the chronically ill are even being increased by premature infants, now graduates of ICNs, many of whom need long-term care and treatment. Many illnesses progress in an expected manner, with treatment handled routinely and work patterns anticipated and planned—all without untoward difficulty or problems. Other illnesses, in growing numbers, have multiple problems, which adversely influence perception, increase the number of possible outcomes, and in turn influence the trajectory.

Disease versus Illness Perception

An important distinction should be made between disease and illness, as well as between disease course and illness trajectory. Disease refers to the state of nonhealth in which biological dysfunction is present and is the major focus of the medical model. Illness is the client's personal perspective that relates to the psychosocial impact of disease on the ill individual (Hymovich & Hagopian, 1992). The physician can legitimate that disease is present, but experiencing illness is a personal perspective and may not always be consistent with the disease state. For example, a person with leukemia may be said to have a disease; however, when the person is in remission and experiencing no functional disability or symptomatology, he or she may deny feeling ill.

Similarly, a chronic disease course begins with the development of pathophysiology, is followed by the worsening of the disease, and may end with physiological stabilization or death. *Disease course* is a term used by health care providers to acknowledge the actual progression of the disease and to classify each kind of illness and its characteristics, phases, and symptoms (Strauss et al., 1985). *Illness trajectory,* on the other hand, includes such personal issues as managing the medical regimen, adapting to necessary restrictions on one's life-style, and perhaps living with the accompanying social isolation brought on by the illness.

Rolland (1987) recommends bridging the gap that exists between the biological/medical world and the personal/psychosocial perspectives of chronic illness, so that health care practitioners can begin to comprehend the magnitude of the illness experience on the individual and family, both of whom are necessary for a successful management plan (White & Richter, 1993). Rolland's (1987) psychosocial typology of illness allows a comparison of similar psychosocial issues and demands between people with different chronic diseases, as well as the examination of different issues for people experiencing the same disease. This typology considers information about the onset, course, outcome, and incapacitation experienced as a result of the disease (see Chapter 2, on growth and development). Onset may be acute (as with a stroke) or gradual (as with Parkinson's disease). The disease course may be progressive, constant/stable, or relapsing/episodic. Outcome refers to the degree to which a chronic disease can shorten one's life span, and incapacitation refers to the extent and kind of disability experienced. Using this information to understand and categorize chronic illnesses makes it possible to recognize similarities and differences in issues and illness demands across a wide spectrum of chronic diseases.

Technology as a Contingency

Advances in medical technology have created new contingencies that are often unexpected, are difficult to evaluate, and decrease the ability to predict outcomes. Technological advances have also created alternative lines of action, meaning that choices often must be made to shape the trajectory most effectively (Strauss et al., 1985). In medical centers, where new and often innovative diagnostic and treatment modalities (equipment, medication, and techniques) are devised and tested, uncertainty is anticipated and built into medical and nursing management. Participants accept that details of a disease or treatment may not be within the realm of knowledge. Furthermore, as knowledge has grown, the impact of technology no longer resides exclusively in major medical centers, but has been extended into community-based hospitals and even into the home as the result of the availability of more and more sophisticated equipment and advanced skills (Morris, 1984). In these settings, however, fewer contingencies are anticipated and there is more predictability.

Technology has also prolonged existing trajectories or created new ones, where lives are maintained by machines, procedures, or drugs. Clients who would have died in the past now face uncertain futures, often stemming from iatrogenic effects of treatment that have impacts not only on the originally diseased body system but also on other body systems. For some of these people, long-term complications or contingencies remain unknown; the impact on lifestyles and on the organization of in-hospital or at-home work is often enormous (Strauss et al., 1985).

End stage renal disease (ESRD) is an example of an iatrogenic condition created by technologic developments; ESRD has radically altered the social and illness trajectories of kidney failure (Plough, 1981). Before federal funding, renal dialysis and transplantation were marginal experimental treatments. Once funding became available, these expensive treatments were accessible to all individuals in renal failure (Plough, 1981). Because dialysis and transplants keep people alive but do not cure them, the ESRD client faces the difficult choice of dialysis versus transplant versus dying. Treatment focuses on the pathophysiology of the kidney and physiological complications. Figure 3-1 is a graph reflecting the health professional's view of the ESRD trajectory.

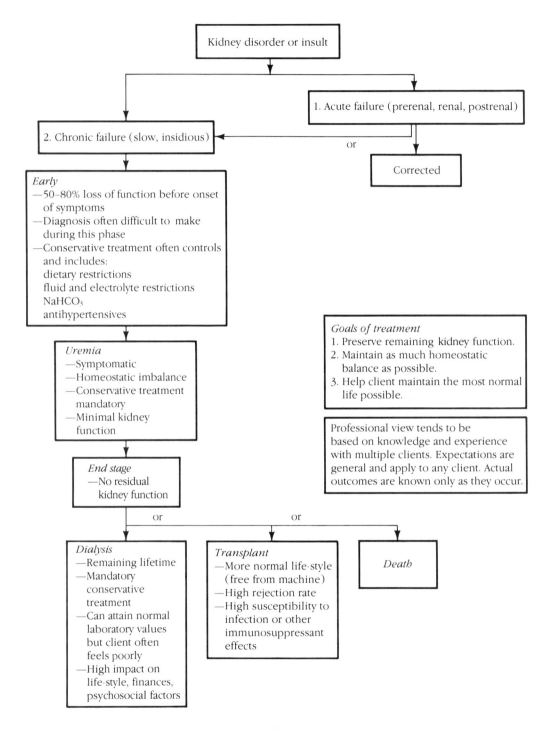

FIGURE 3-1.   Trajectory: Professional Perception of ESRD

SOURCE: Lubkin (1990).

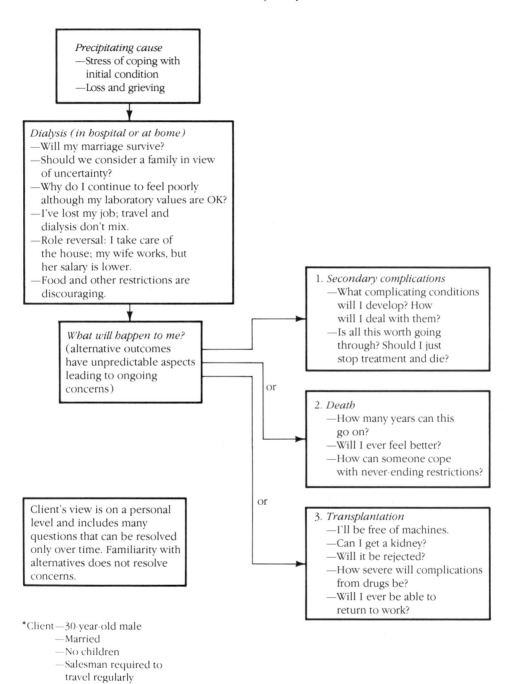

FIGURE 3-2. Trajectory: A Client's Perception of ESRD

SOURCE: Lubkin (1990).

Psychological Impact

Quality of life and the psychosocial impact of chronic diseases are receiving more attention in the literature. Calland (1972), who was both physician and ESRD client, raised a number of questions that evolve from reality-based client problems. How does one deal with fluid and electrolyte restrictions that make meals unpalatable? Should marriage be considered, or is it even possible? Can or should the individual start a family? Is it worth struggling for the rest of one's life with the problems that dialysis creates? Plough (1981) points out that some clients are unable to work because they cannot deal with additional stresses beyond dialysis, and because the time spent on the machines and in commuting blocks many job opportunities. Role changes and role reversal can occur. Expression of problems is not always encouraged by health care providers; clients therefore conceal these problems, and the staff remain unaware of the difficulties they experience (Calland, 1972). Figure 3-2 is a graph reflecting the way that an individual who has ESRD might view the trajectory of this condition.

Families also undergo tremendous stress, as evidenced by the increase in the rate of divorce shortly after treatment begins (Plough, 1981). Social support has been found to diminish with poorer health, perhaps because of limited opportunity to develop and maintain supportive networks (White, Richter & Fry, 1992). The staff may become so involved in the technological management of the disease that they assume that current problems are the result of prior problems and that dialysis is just another event in the client's life (Plough, 1981).

Physiological Impact

Clients and staff perceive physiological responses to ESRD differently. The medical model of health care uses laboratory values to evaluate homeostasis. Clients do not always find laboratory reports in line with the way they feel or are able to function (Calland, 1972), since accumulated fluids, metabolites, and waste products create unpleasant symptoms (Plough, 1981). In addition, dialysis causes secondary illness trajec-

tories, such as cardiac disorders, neuropathies, or atherosclerosis, that nephrologists consider "nonrenal complications."

Many clients see transplantation as a valid alternative to dialysis. Yet when it is possible, the client is not necessarily freed from anxiety or contingencies. The possibility of rejection or of complications from immunosuppressant therapy remains, and the trajectory continues to show uncertainty. Problems may become so severe that the client loses the desire or will to live and refuses continued treatment.

Symptom Awareness and Management

During the early stages of an illness, symptoms may become more evident to the individual, but the meaning of these symptoms may not be understood and frequently tend to be dismissed as common minor ailments. After a while, as symptoms continue and perhaps increase in severity, they become a source of worry and the individual will seek help (see Chapter 4, on illness roles).

Symptom control becomes an important task in shaping an illness trajectory. The recurrence of former symptoms, or the appearance of new symptoms, often signals the beginning of an exacerbation or a worsening of the condition. Some chronic diseases, such as cancer, progress without noticeable symptoms until the disease has spread to an advanced stage. Others, such as chronic skin diseases, have difficult or bothersome symptoms, such as pain, soreness, itching, tiredness, and sleep disturbance often endured for long periods of time with little relief possible (Kirkevold, 1993). For example, the itchiness associated with an outbreak of atopic dermatitis is particularly bothersome because of its unrelenting presence; the scaling of psoriasis, while not as physically disturbing, produces a significant stigma that patients try to conceal (see Chapter 5, on stigma).

Certain versus Uncertain Trajectories

Despite the inability to know an illness trajectory in advance and with any assurance, individuals involved in the management of the illness do project future trajectory shapes and phases based on their previous experience. Some disease processes may be easier to predict than others, but with all chronic illnesses there is a tremendous amount of uncertainty about what lies ahead. Uncertainty is the inability to determine the meaning of illness-related events; it occurs when the decision maker is unable to accurately predict outcomes because cues are lacking (Mishel, 1990). Seeing or speaking to individuals who are ahead of oneself on the illness trajectory provides an opportunity for "rehearsal" in one's mind of the future trajectory (Strauss et al., 1985).

The unpredictability of the psoriasis trajectory was found to be particularly troublesome to patients and staff (Kirkevold, 1993). The only factor known to influence the course of the disease is stress, and total control of stress was considered almost impossible. Even limited amounts of stress could precipitate an exacerbation and set off a vicious cycle: stress leading to worsening disease state leading to increased stress. Uncertainty is also related to a sense that one may be losing control over the disease and the inability to predict a stable course.

Wiener and Dodd's (1993) work among cancer patients led them to recognize several aspects of uncertainty. *Temporal uncertainty* applies to the disruption of one's expectations of the future. The individual also considers the *duration* (How long will the illness last, and when will I begin to feel better?); *pace* (How long do I have to live? How soon before a recurrence develops somewhere else?); and *frequency* (How often must I go for treatment?). The answers to these questions are often tentative at best.

Uncertainty of body functioning has to do with the ability of the body to perform an activity, the appearance of the body to self and others, and the physiological functioning of the body along with response to treatment (Wiener & Dodd, 1993). There is much uncertainty with the appearance of new symptoms: Which ones can be safely ignored, and which ones should be reported? Which symptoms are normal side effects of the therapy, and which ones mean the illness has entered a new phase?

The uncertain temporality and failed body that accompany many chronic conditions ultimately affect the patient's view of self and lead to *uncertainty in identity.* Patients may take on new identities that reflect their changing life course in response to a changing illness course. They may, for example, have to overcome old patterns of self-reliance and noncomplaining, and incorporate into their identity new acceptance of support and help from outsiders. The trajectory framework emphasizes that, for the chronically ill, the interplay between mind, body, work, and behavior is always fluctuating, emphasizing the uncertainty of the disease course and the illness experience (Wiener & Dodd, 1993).

Mishel (1990) addresses the experience of living with continual, constant uncertainty in chronic illness. Although the uncertainty that cannot be eliminated from one's life is likely to enhance the sense of disorganization and instability, uncertainty can move a person toward a new state of adaptation. When someone with a chronic illness achieves this new state, he or she has learned to accept uncertainty as a "natural rhythm to life" and can begin to view it as opportunity rather than danger (Mishel, 1990).

Uncertainty is also problematic for physicians who manage patients' trajectories. Physicians face uncertainty in diagnosing the illness, selecting the treatment alternatives that will keep the course of the disease under control, and anticipating the patient's response to both disease and therapy. Hardesty and Geist (1990) found that in order to manage the uncertainty they face, physicians engage in "self-referencing communication" with specialists, patients, and family members. Self-referencing communication is a style that seeks positive evaluations by others, which help instill in the physician the confidence to make difficult patient care decisions in uncertain illness trajectories.

Work Problems

Trajectory work consists of organizing and performing necessary tasks and actions that shape trajectories. With chronic illness, this work moves from home to hospital and back to home, depending on the phases or contingencies that are currently present in the situation. Such movement makes it obvious that work is shared by clients and families as well as staff in shaping trajectories (Strauss et al., 1982).

Client and Family Work Although health care providers may have the knowledge and compassion important in managing chronic illness, the patient and family are central to illness care. In addition to the daily struggle to manage the disease and its symptoms, they must try to achieve a sense of control and normalcy in their lives. Initially, the patient and family are unskilled, but they receive considerable "on-the-job" training to manage the work necessary to shape the illness trajectory.

Chronic illness disrupts one's biography or self-concept. New conceptions of what and who one is must be created and continually adapted to changes that occur. Biographical work, illness-related work, and everyday life work are essentially self-taught by the chronically ill and achieved with varying degrees of success (Wiener, 1989).

The work that patients do (following prescribed regimens, balancing treatment options, pacing activities, and overcoming disabilities) is devalued, invisible, and unacknowledged by society (Wiener, 1989). Invisibility of work may sometimes be deliberate if the client feels the staff would disapprove of the client's actions. The invisibility of the work that clients do and the extent to which it is not acknowledged or appreciated add to the burden of living with a chronic illness (Wiener, 1989).

Explicit Work Explicit work, which supplements staff work, includes such tasks as monitoring machines, carrying out painful rehabilitation procedures, and providing feedback to teaching done for home management. Staff generally realize that the client is involved, often regarding that participation as cooperation rather than work. Sometimes clients do not identify their own activities as work because they differ from the official work that the staff does (Strauss et al., 1982).

Implicit Work Implicit work tends to be unrecognized; that is, it includes activities not seen as work. Implicit work includes the many activities of daily living performed by the client: providing

information in relation to admission, responding to treatment, and so on. It also includes giving cooperation and maximum performance required by tests, procedures, or interventions. Being uncooperative with such tasks is considered a noncompliant or recalcitrant behavior when the staff deem such cooperation important (Strauss et al., 1982) (see Chapter 10, on compliance).

Family Work in the Hospital Families also do various kinds of work in the hospital: helping clients deal with reactions and maintain the necessary composure required for technical, sometimes painful tasks; providing comfort (positioning, requesting medications); helping with safety (raising bed rails, checking on procedures); and doing much of the necessary legal/administrative work, including filling out forms, signing documents, and so on (Strauss et al., 1984).

Families are often responsible for crucial decision-making work that may require choices among less-than-perfect options. Intelligent decisions are often difficult, since obtaining information may be difficult. Doctors may be hard to reach, or specialists and primary physicians may each feel that the other is responsible for providing information. Moreover, specialists may not agree among themselves about the medical consequences of actions. When all this uncertainty is coupled with new or little-tried interventions, as in large medical centers, it is not surprising that the family is impeded in its decision making (Strauss et al., 1984).

Client and Family Work at Home In the home, someone must take responsibility for all trajectory management as well as the home management that is necessary despite the presence of an illness. The trajectory work includes many of the tasks performed in hospitals, but also involves other tasks such as crisis work (preventing and handling), symptom and regimen management, time management, and providing psychological support (Strauss et al., 1984).

In chronic illness, work of considerable range and complexity goes on 24 hours a day, 7 days a week, often in a setting not designed for such work (Corbin & Strauss, 1988). Families usually have minimal equipment, no shift relief, and little training, which is eventually supplemented by what they learn over time. The way family members share medically related tasks depends on the degree and kind of physical impairment, financial resources, and interpersonal relationships and communication patterns within the family. With each change in the trajectory, the family must reassess social arrangements, daily life, and future development. Trajectory changes can lead to increased physical labor and altered identities (Strauss et al., 1984; Corbin & Strauss, 1988).

When children are ill, physical and psychological problems generally impact on the parents, with most of the work load falling unequally on one parent, usually the mother. For adult clients, the burden of work usually falls on the spouse, especially when children are too young to help or have left home. Home management consists of all the responsibilities and activities that the ill person cannot manage but that are necessitated by both the illness and the requirements of the household.

Collaboration and Coordination Collaboration is the work pattern that explains how couples succeed in working together to effectively manage chronic illness (Corbin & Strauss, 1988). The work necessary to manage an illness trajectory varies by amount, type, degree of difficulty, amount of time it takes to complete, and intensity. What tasks need to be done and by whom has to be negotiated by the couple and is influenced by one partner's willingness to relinquish tasks and the other's willingness to take them over.

Couples also need to collaborate in order to accomplish necessary work. The division of labor is standardized (based on knowledge and ability), flexible (shifts with trajectory changes), and mutually agreed to even if not equally divided. For collaboration to be successful, the couple must be sensitive to the needs of each partner, provide for self-renewal activities, be willing to compromise, perceive a payoff for the work, have a pool of resources to draw from, and trust that each partner is doing everything possible. Collaboration provides choices, a sense of control over the situation, and an increased

feeling of sufficient resources to meet the illness demands (Corbin & Strauss, 1988).

The coordination of necessary work activities is also important—the work has to be done correctly, on time, and without gaps or duplications (Corbin & Strauss, 1988). Coordination also involves the sequencing of tasks according to priorities and the assigning of tasks to specific individuals. Problems in coordinating work activities may arise when there are different perceptions between the couple concerning the illness trajectory and trajectory projections. Failure to take responsibility for planning the work and insufficient resources to meet the work demands may also hinder effective coordination.

Work Overload The amount of work that must be done is often unbalanced, depending on factors such as illness status, availability of outside resources, and presence of contingencies that may increase the work load. The key to balancing is not the actual amount of work being done but the perception of this load and the conditions under which one is working. With adequate support or help, positive change in status, and so on, the amount of work can seem to contract (Corbin & Strauss, 1988).

Managing both illness and home can overwhelm caregivers, causing a sense of being stretched to the limits of energy and tolerance (Strauss et al., 1984) and leading to resentment, anger, or other negative responses. Should the caregiver find no relief, the impact on the family may be devastating; decisions to end the marriage or to place the client in a nursing home may seem to be the only viable alternatives (Corbin & Strauss, 1988; Strauss et al., 1984).

Respite from continuous responsibilities can make the difference in a caregiver's ability to continue. Respite takes various forms and lasts for variable periods of time. The caregiver can try to get a friend or family member to take over responsibility for a short while, to get assistance from outside resources, or to go away temporarily or for several days. This last alternative can sometimes be accomplished by placing the client in a care facility for a few days (Corbin & Strauss, 1988; Strauss et al., 1984) (see Chapter 12, on family caregivers).

Client and Family Work in the Hospital In the home environment, all work involved in trajectory shaping is done by balancing the interplay of technology and bodily reactions (Strauss et al., 1982). In fact, the client has become the expert manager of his or her own care and for the most part has been quite successful. When hospitalization is required, this knowledge goes with the client even though the staff do not always try to gain such information. When hospitalized, clients are expected to delegate the responsibility of their care to the staff and to conform to the medical model in the traditional sick role (see Chapter 4, on illness roles). Such an expectation may be met with variable responses from both the client and family.

Some clients resent relinquishing the control they have attempted to achieve in managing their illness trajectory. They often find it difficult to conform to hospital routines that may not match the established home regimen. Family members may find it difficult to transfer their caregiving roles to staff members and may view the need for hospitalization as some sort of failure on their part to adequately meet the needs of the ill person.

On the other hand, hospitalization may be viewed by some chronically ill persons as a chance to refuel, restabilize, or try out a new treatment (Forsyth et al., 1984), especially when the hospitalization results from a change in the stability of the trajectory. Work done in the hospital consists of buying time, waiting to see if a drug will work or what further testing will show while attempting to reach a functional plateau (Forsyth et al., 1984). In this situation, the client and family work may gladly be relinquished to the staff and hospitalization may be viewed as an opportunity for respite.

Staff Work The diagnostic phase marks the beginning of trajectory work for the health professional. Tests and procedures require time, organization, preparation, and follow-through of the staff. Once the disease is identified, the image of the potential course of the illness helps the physician map out interventions and allows the nurse to plan appropriate care. The occurrence of new symptoms signifies change in the disease trajectory that may require that diagnosis and mapping recur at intervals (Strauss et al., 1985).

In the hospital, the staff often see clients in relation to the amount of work they create for the expected trajectory. "Good" clients are those without problems or complaints, or those who have multiple problems but are cooperative. "Problem" clients are individuals who are uncooperative, complaining, or overly emotional, as well as those who respond poorly to treatment and therefore need a great deal of staff time (Lorber, 1981).

Noncompliance The idea of noncompliance by clients is an aspect of client work (or absence of work) with which staff must reckon. Nurses and physicians often assume that the reason for exacerbation of a disease is related to clients' noncompliance and that additional teaching and reinforcement will correct the problem. If clients remain noncompliant, they are seen as "difficult" and may be harassed or neglected by health care staff (see Chapter 10, on compliance).

In interviews with chronically ill patients and family members, it was discovered that noncompliant behavior reflected an individual's lack of trust in health care professional expertise and increased confidence in his or her own competence to make health care decisions (Thorne, 1990). Noncompliant behavior included modifying treatment regimens without consulting the health care professional (usually in response to some untoward side effect of the regimen), selective compliance with certain aspects of the regimen (recognizing that not all aspects of the regimen were equally valid), and juggling recommendations from a variety of professionals (clients often choosing what they considered to be best for themselves).

Thorne (1990) calls this behavior "constructive noncompliance" because it serves the purpose of self-protection for the individual and maintenance of health care relationships. Self-protection acknowledges the developing expertise of the client and an increasing awareness of the uniqueness of his or her own psychologic and physiologic responses to the disease processes. Recognizing that there were no infallible authorities in chronic illness management, clients began to challenge the decisions of the providers yet recognized the need to maintain a working relationship with them. Noncompliance protected the patient from the perceived problems associated with the treatment without jeopardizing the health care relationship on which the patient depended (Thorne, 1990). Patients view the primary role of the physician as providing symptom control, as being competent, and of giving the best possible care. Patients often stay with physicians who have expertise in symptom control and who provided straightforward information about the disease (Forsyth et al., 1984).

Chronically ill clients often view their problems as not important enough to demand much nursing attention, especially if they believe other hospitalized patients are sicker and require more care. In their study of hospitalized chronically ill patients, Forsyth and associates (1984) found that patients believed that nurses are very busy with multiple tasks and should be called only when the patient is really sick or in pain. Nurses were seen by patients in the role of a subtle support group and not on caregivers or information sources, as nurses see themselves.

Kirkevold (1993) identified two basic values that seemed to undergird the nurses' care of patients with chronic skin diseases. These were *alleviating* the patient of the stress and burdens associated with the disease and *enabling* the patient to manage the disease and its impact via teaching and support. The nurses understood that the patients' experiences of caregiving could be overwhelming at times, leading them to temporarily take over the responsibility for alleviating the bothersome symptoms and managing the disease.

Dying Trajectories

Many chronic illnesses are on some kind of downward spiral; death is a known outcome. Repeated hospitalizations are not uncommon during the course of these illnesses. Often death comes while an individual is hospitalized, but with the advent of home hospice care, more and more chronic illnesses reach termination in the home. Planning care for the dying patient was found to be dependent on the perception of the dying rather than its actual course (Glaser & Strauss, 1968). Participants had varying degrees of awareness and acceptance of the client's dying and expectations of the way the process would progress. Shaping, by professionals, of the dying trajectory tended to focus on the medical aspects of dying (managing the physical dying), since caregivers demonstrated less ability to fulfill psychological than physical needs (Strauss & Glaser, 1970). Today, however, health care providers are better prepared to manage all aspects of terminal care with the entire family.

Types of Dying Trajectories Dying trajectories can be divided into quick and lingering categories (Glaser & Strauss, 1968). Quick dying trajectories occur over relatively short periods of time and may be expected or unexpected. Sometimes it is apparent that death will occur quickly and expectedly within hours or at most a few days (the head trauma client kept alive by life-support systems). Or quick death can come when someone who was expected to die eventually, dies unexpectedly as a result of a sudden deterioration (the terminal cancer client who has a massive myocardial infarction). The quick dying trajectory that is most traumatic for the staff occurs unexpectedly to someone who was not expected to die at all (recovery is expected after surgery, and death results from massive pulmonary emboli).

Lingering trajectories have two major features: long duration and slow but steady downward movement. They have a greater potential for biological, human, or psychological unpredictability than do quick trajectories. If lingering is relatively short (days to weeks), with little pain and a reasonably high level of family acceptance, it is not greatly upsetting (Glaser & Strauss, 1968). When the lingering exceeds perceived reasonable limits, much stress for family and staff results.

Dying in the Hospital Quick deaths in the hospital may sadden the staff, but the sadness passes rather quickly and work resumes. Lingering deaths are different, since dying is a process constantly undergoing change, requiring staff to redefine the trajectory continually to ensure appropriate medical and nursing care for each phase (Strauss & Glaser, 1970; Glaser & Strauss,

1968). Although some degree of certainty is often present, the total length of time involved in the dying may not always be clear to the personnel or the family. Time miscalculations can lead to crises on the unit that necessitate changes in work load (Strauss & Glaser, 1970). For example, the individual who suffers a major cerebral vascular accident may linger for weeks rather than days.

Differences in projection of the dying process can also lead to inconsistencies in care. The nurse who senses that the client is now terminally ill may be more generous with pain medications than the nurse who feels that death is a long way off and worries about addicting the client (see Chapter 7, on chronic pain). Staff often become more involved in the dying of young clients than of the elderly, especially if they themselves are young (Strauss & Glaser, 1970).

Accurate expectations make possible arrangements that provide adequate personnel to perform necessary tasks. As dying moves into the terminal phase, tasks and relationships change (Glaser & Strauss, 1968). Therapy may stop and comfort care increase. The dying client may also have a concurrent pain trajectory that must be considered (Fagerhaugh & Strauss, 1977). Balancing questions arise: Should pain medications be temporarily withheld because they might obscure diagnostic symptoms? Should opiates be given, knowing their administration may hasten death? Is it more important to keep the client pain-free or alert but in some pain? And what are the client's wishes or preferences?

Dying at Home   Clients may prefer to die at home, where time and the work involved in providing care and support allow the family and client to shape the trajectory and gain a sense of control over events (Glaser & Strauss, 1968). The client's dying at home provides the family the satisfaction of knowing that they were able to maintain solidarity and to fulfill obligations they felt toward the dying individual. Problems of management in these situations include the ability of the caregiver to meet the physical needs of the client without becoming exhausted and ill. Assistance from health care providers may

focus on providing care of the caregiver. The case study of D. M. shows the way one individual handled his dying in the environment that met his needs.

The development of the hospice movement has dramatically changed the management of the dying trajectory for client and family. The emphasis has shifted from "curing" to "caring" (Caruso-Herman, 1989). Concern for the family as well as the client has become the focus as issues of anticipatory grief and grief therapy for the surviving family are being addressed. Family members of hospitalized terminal cancer patients, whose treatment was palliative and supportive, said that their own needs were met when their dying family member was getting good care and they were included in giving that care. Further, family members asked to be provided with explanations of procedures and with honest information (Dyck & Wright, 1985). Today most terminal patients are informed of their prognosis and actively participate in decisions about treatments and when to end treatment. Concerns of terminally ill individuals may include loss of control, pain management, sexuality, and dealing with grief (Caruso-Herman, 1989).

Interventions That Consider the Trajectory Concept

The trajectory concept furnishes the professional with an alternative perspective on problems or conflicts: a way of highlighting the entire environment and the participants within. The concept can lead to a greater depth of understanding of disease processes in relation to both client and work done to manage the disease regardless of setting. This perspective can promote greater accountability and development of interventions that are more humane and improve the client's quality of life. In addition, professionals might well find themselves in a better and more effective work environment. Strauss et al. (1984) also feel that a greater awareness of the influence of illness perception on actions could lead to a broader-based national social policy: a policy that relieves individual providers of sole responsibility for components of health care, such as

---

CASE STUDY

Dying at Home

D. M. knew that he was dying long before anyone else did. In spite of having non-insulin-dependent diabetes, mild hypertension, and chronic constipation, he saw himself as well until he passed his 75th birthday. Each year after that, he developed another medical problem. One year he had problems with his ear, the next year, a prostatectomy, and the following year, cataract surgery. Then came the painless hematuria, but no definitive diagnosis was made. At age 79 he began to feel "poorly" and was diagnosed as having pancytopenia, cause unknown.

When his condition deteriorated to the point that death would have ensued within a matter of weeks, he finally agreed to have a splenectomy. D. M. realized that he might well die on the operating room table but decided that it was worth the risk for the probable 18 months of relatively comfortable living the doctor told him was the alternative. He survived the surgery without any complications but never fully recovered. Over the next six months he lost weight slowly but continuously.

Shortly after his 81st birthday he developed severe low back pain, which the doctor diagnosed over the phone as a lumbar strain.

But he knew he was dying. He finally persuaded his physician and wife that a trip to visit his daughter would be beneficial. His real goal was to die in his daughter's home rather than in a hospital. He threw a pulmonary embolus shortly after arriving and had to enter the hospital again. There a diagnostic workup revealed pathological fractures of the lumbar spine and other bony involvement secondary to metastatic prostatic cancer. His request to die at his daughter's home was honored, and he was subsequently discharged. The visiting nurse and hospice program in that area made it possible for his wish to be fulfilled. Pain control was the greatest problem his family faced. Surrounded by his wife, his daughter, and her family, D. M. died 3 weeks later. Even though his dying lingered over several months, awareness of the process for family and health providers involved only a few weeks.

SOURCE: Lubkin (1990).

---

maintaining the terminally ill with machines, by establishing national guidelines for consistency of care and sharing of responsibility.

Accountability

In addition to health professionals' sense of responsibility, hospital policy requires professional accountability of physician and nurse, especially in relation to proper diagnosis, following medical orders, and performing medically supported tasks (Strauss & Glaser, 1970). There is little required accountability for ensuring that knowledge about the client's biography or experiential history with disease and pain is gathered or reported (Strauss et al., 1984), and only limited amounts of social and psychological information are collected systematically.

The acute illness orientation of most hospital settings serves to block accountability in issues other than those of a medical nature (Fagerhaugh & Strauss, 1977), in spite of the fact that the chronically ill individual often enters the hospital with multiple trajectories related to illness state(s) that should be considered. The complexity involved in a client's long-term management and hospital experiences can lead to a great variation in the client's responses to the staff's handling of the current acute problem. When clients are "difficult," the staff tend to organize efforts to collect data that will help them solve the immediate problem(s). However, since the same problems arise repeatedly, staff would find permanent solutions or interventions more beneficial than repeatedly gaining and analyzing information and selecting appropriate solutions. The repeated need to resolve the same kind of problem indicates little accountability for nonmedical aspects of care (Strauss et al., 1984).

Personnel tend to focus on the reason for the admission and not on other existing illnesses that may impinge on trajectory management (Strauss et al., 1985; Fagerhaugh & Strauss, 1977). With the advent of Diagnostic Related Groups (DRGs), accountability in relation to the primary illness has increased. Ironically, if quiescent illnesses flare up or complicate the situation, their importance to the staff grows and the primary illness can even become secondary. For example, the older person admitted with a fractured hip whose chronic pulmonary problems become acute presents two trajectories the staff must consider.

Biography: Seeing the Whole Client

Chronically ill individuals who manage their own care at home frequently find delegating full responsibility to hospital personnel difficult, especially since personnel tend to lack knowledge about the intricacies of disease regimens carried out at home. A rational approach to easing this transitional phase is to allow the client greater participation in decisions while in health care facilities or to extend the health care system so that personnel can play more of a role in helping the chronically ill and their families inside and outside the hospital setting (Strauss et al., 1984). Such an approach requires inclusion of a more extensive client biographical history than is usually obtained.

Importance of Biography Ordinarily, biographical material collected by hospital personnel pertains to current work, not to the total identity of the client. For instance, the client who has long managed chronic pain can have difficulty trusting the staff when they change the frequency, amount, or even the medication itself without gaining information about prior experiences with medication effectiveness, sensitivity, or alternative methods for minimizing pain. Prior hospital experiences have conditioned chronic pain sufferers to expect that the staff will not attend to their long-term needs and that requests for medication will be periodically delayed or unanswered. This mismanagement contributes to the creation of somewhat difficult clients (Strauss et al., 1984).

Interviewing is an effective way to obtain biographical information that can be collected while care is given or during multiple short sessions, which is less tiring for the client. Family members should also be interviewed, since they often have additional information or a different perspective that may provide insight into family dynamics (Strauss et al., 1984).

Biographical information can be used in several ways. First, it can help shape work and responses in terms of specific information about the client. Second, information gathered over time from multiple clients can be used in planning care for the types of individuals who generally enter that specific unit. Finally, this information can help determine the proportion of responsibility the client should retain and the proportion the staff must assume. These actions lead to more individualized care and provide support for the client in dealing with disease and contingencies.

Dealing with Uncertainty

Uncertainty is a significant and sometimes very difficult factor for those involved with shaping the chronic illness trajectory. It is important to find ways to successfully manage uncertainty so it does not become overwhelming to the individual, family, or health care provider.

Several strategies have been identified that cancer patients use to reduce uncertainty and maintain some control over their lives (Wiener & Dodd, 1993). These strategies include *pacing* (modifying or cutting back on activities), *becoming professional patients* (learning the appropriate medical language), *seeking reinforcing comparisons* (finding "worse-case" comparisons), and *engaging in reviews* (looking back on the onset of symptoms and giving meaning to them in light of present knowledge). Nursing activities should facilitate the chronically ill person's acceptance of uncertainty by helping the client and family consider new ways to accomplish the things they value and consider different ways to adjust to the changing nature of the illness (Mishel, 1990).

Improving Care for the Dying

Currently, accountability required in relation to the dying client includes maintaining a reasonably pain-free environment, notifying the family of the impending death, pronouncing the individual dead, and informing the family of the death—tasks that are often performed in a perfunctory manner. Personnel are less accountable for providing the client with information about his or her status or the way work is done around the dying person. Accountability is also affected by the distancing between staff and the terminal client that can be triggered by awareness of one's own mortality (Strauss & Glaser, 1970).

When hospital staff face unexpected client or family responses, their discussions recalling similar situations can lead to problem solving and betterment of care for the client, family, and staff. Unfortunately, after the death and postmortem care, this learning does not lead to a set of permanent approaches, but seems to disappear until another crisis or negative situation occurs (Strauss & Glaser, 1970).

Terminal care should be directed toward easing inconsistency of interactions and improving accountability to the dying client on a personal level. This goal can be accomplished by increased sensitivity to the process of dying and by an increased awareness of one's own perceptions and feelings about dying. Within the hospital setting all staff members need training in terminal care to enhance their understanding of the social relationships associated with lingering deaths. This training should not be limited to hospitals, but should be integrated into medical and nursing schools' educational programs (Glaser & Strauss, 1968; Strauss & Glaser, 1970).

Accountability requires familiarity with the social and psychological needs of the client and family. Hospitals can increase accountability to the dying by explicitly reviewing social, psychological, and organizational aspects of terminal care, as well as by focusing on nursing and medical matters (Strauss & Glaser, 1970). Increased accountability requires that the hospital take responsibility for such actions, which are currently left to personal discretion and are therefore unreported.

For most people having a lingering trajectory, the dying process often requires multiple admissions to the hospital between stays at home. Home hospice care is not uniformly available throughout the country, and government policy toward financial support limits the availability of hospice care for prolonged periods. Advocacy by the health care provider could help ensure a national policy that would provide money to train personnel and to make hospice care available throughout the country. The entire cost in money, time, and energy would be lower in the home environment, and the presence of support would decrease the anguish for those involved (Strauss & Glaser, 1970).

Also needed in the public domain is a policy governing issues that transcend professional responsibilities for terminal care—for example, on withholding addicting drugs or prolonging life when it results in increased agony or financial ruin (Strauss & Glaser, 1970). Medical and nursing personnel should encourage public discussion of these issues (see Chapter 23, on social/health policy).

Applying Trajectory to Nursing Practice

Illness trajectory is an important aspect in understanding and managing chronic illness for which limited resources are available. Gathering and utilizing more complete information and respecting the client's and family's knowledge about management of the disease provide a basis for determining work that must be done. The use of biographical data enhances quality care by increasing awareness of the whole person. Understanding the interaction between illness, biography, and everyday activities sensitizes health care providers to the complexity of illness trajectory management (Corbin & Strauss, 1993).

Trajectory management is the process by which the illness course is shaped, through all its phases, by controlling symptoms and treating side effects, handling crises, preventing complications, and dealing with limitations and disabilities (Corbin & Strauss, 1993). The overall goal is to maintain quality of life throughout the shaping process. Of all the health care providers, only nurses have the skills, knowledge, and vision to organize and provide for the comprehensive and technologically complex care that chronically ill clients require (Corbin & Strauss, 1993).

Unless an individual is hospitalized, the everyday trajectory management takes place in the home. Consequently, the home should be conceived as the center of care (Corbin & Strauss, 1988); the hospital should be a backup resource to supplement home care during illness instability or when the patient or family need time to refuel or restabilize (Forsyth et al., 1984).

Those who manage the chronic illness trajectory (client, family, and health care provider) must consider the specific tasks to be done and arrange for who will perform what tasks, in what setting, and with what needed resources. With time, these arrangements usually become routinized, and participants become rather adept at incorporating trajectory management into their everyday activities (Corbin & Strauss, 1993).

Nurses provide "supportive assistance," which includes direct care, teaching, counseling, making referrals and arrangements, and monitoring the trajectory and response to medical treatment. Nursing care should adjust to changes in clients' illnesses and families' living conditions, keeping in mind the clients' past experiences and future trajectories (Corbin & Strauss, 1993).

Summary and Conclusions

Trajectory is a sociological concept that broadens understanding of client problems and needs beyond the acute medical model. It deals with individuals' perceptions of situations, their responses to those perceptions, and the organization of work that is involved. The various kinds of trajectories—illness, biographical, dying, and so on—all have the qualities of duration, movement, predictability, and shape. Work that is necessary to shape or manage the trajectory is performed by staff and by clients and their families.

The management problems of chronic illness have increased as trajectories have become more complex, which leads to decreased predictability and changes in work and organization. Technological advances impact on trajectory because they add to the numbers and kinds of chronically ill individuals.

The episodic nature of some illnesses may necessitate admission to acute care settings and lead to conflict between hospital personnel and chronically ill individuals who are experienced managers of their own illnesses. When the staff manage illness without adequate awareness of client biographies and experiences, care that is less than satisfactory may result. Staff, clients, and families participate in work, both in the hospital and at home, although staff may have different goals from those of clients and families. The willingness of health care providers to relinquish some of the control and responsibility for managing the illness is critical.

Clients and families must cope with the physiologic aspects of illness as well as a host of health-related social problems that affect roles, relationships, and adjustments. The business of the chronically ill is to live as normally as possible despite the symptoms and the disease. Therefore, chronic illness must be integrated into the lives and needs of the client and family, not the reverse (Strauss, 1981).

The professional must focus beyond the medicophysiological perspective of illness to take into account the lives and expectations of the client and family; compassion and medical or nursing competence are not sufficient. Through an awareness of such concepts as trajectory, professionals can expand their knowledge and sensitivity to the social aspects of symptom control, regimen management, and crisis prevention, as well as to the management of dying (Strauss, 1981). Integrating social concepts into their work will allow professionals not only to develop strategies or tactics beneficial to the client but to influence public policy to gain a more humane approach to all who are affected by chronic illnesses.

NURSING DIAGNOSIS

Editor's Note: There are no specific nursing diagnoses based on the trajectory concept. A possible diagnostic category that could be implied from this chapter follows:

5.3.1.1 Decisional Conflict (specify):

(See Chapter 9 on quality of life for a definition, defining characteristics, and related factors.)

Since trajectory deals with differences in perspective, none of the listed related factors apply as causative or contributing to difficulties arising from this concept. This author suggests that "differences in perspective" be considered as a valid related factor. Solutions for decisional conflicts secondary to trajectory difficulties require resolution of these different perspectives.

Since the client and professional see the situation differently, the professional might *assume* either of the following nursing diagnosis categories:

5.1.1.1 Ineffective Individual Coping

Definition: Impairment of adaptive behaviors and problem-solving abilities of a person in meeting life's demands and roles.

Defining Characteristics:[1] *Verbalization of inability to cope or inability to ask for help; in-

[1]The asterisk indicates a critical defining characteristic.

ability to meet role expectations; inability to meet basic needs; *inability to problem-solve; alterations in societal participation; destructive behavior toward self or others; inappropriate use of defense mechanisms; change in usual communication patterns; verbal manipulation; high illness rate; high rate of accidents.

Related Factors: Situational crises; maturational crises; personal vulnerability.

5.2.1.1 Noncompliance (specify):

(See Chapter 10, on noncompliance for definition, defining characteristics, related factors and comments about use of this category.)

Client behavior should not be interpreted as ineffective coping without validation from the client and/or family, since critical characteristics of this category require the client's verbalization of not being able to cope or problem-solve. Without validation, the use of this category is not client-centered because of possible differences in perspective. Essential to such a validation would be a trusting relationship, which is hard to obtain when individuals perceive things differently.

Premature diagnostic decisions should be avoided. Adequate assessment is necessary to ensure that the difference in the client/family perspective from that of the professional is clearly understood.

STUDY QUESTIONS

1. How would you define trajectory as it relates to illness?
2. What is the difference between the actual course of chronic illness and its perceived course? How does the latter relate to trajectory?
3. Define the following terms in relation to trajectory: *participants, duration, perception, predictability, shape, shaping, work, phases, biographies, contingency, balancing.*
4. How does technology influence trajectory? How does this influence affect staff and client?
5. In the hospital, how does the work of staff and client differ? What work does a family do in the hospital? What influences staff's awareness of client work?
6. What kinds of work do the client and family do at home when they have a regimen that must be followed?
7. What are the contingencies that impact on the effectiveness with which client and family manage at home? How do they lead to work overload?
8. What difficulties may arise because of the "vagueness" of symptoms associated with

chronic illness and difficulty arriving at a specific diagnosis?

9. Discuss what is meant by *uncertainty* as related to illness trajectories and how it impacts on the individual and family with a chronic illness as well as the health care provider.

10. What two categories of dying trajectories have Glaser and Strauss identified? What are their characteristics?

11. Why are lingering dying trajectories more prone to contingencies? What are these contingencies?

12. How can health professionals increase their accountability to clients in the hospital setting? How do biographical data influence this accountability?

13. How can care for the dying client improve in the hospital setting?

14. What reasons that would encourage health professionals to serve more readily as client advocates can you identify? What issues deserve emphasis?

15. If you could set up a unit to increase clients' involvement in their own care, how would you go about doing this?

References

Calland, C. H. (1972, August 17). Iatrogenic problems in end-stage renal failure. *New England Journal of Medicine, 287,* 334-336.

Caruso-Herman, D. (1989). Concerns for the dying patient and family. *Seminars in Oncology Nursing, 5*(2), 120-123.

Corbin, J., & Strauss, A. (1988). *Unending work and care: Managing chronic illness at home.* San Francisco: Jossey-Bass.

——— (1993). A nursing model for chronic illness management based upon the trajectory framework. In P. Woog (Ed.), *The chronic illness trajectory framework.* New York: Springer.

Dyck, S., & Wright, K. (1985). Family perceptions: The role of the nurse throughout an adult's cancer experience. *Oncology Nursing Forum, 12*(5), 53-56.

Fagerhaugh, S. Y., & Strauss, A. L. (1977). *Politics of pain management: Staff-patient interaction.* Menlo Park, CA: Addison-Wesley.

Forsyth, G., Delaney, K., & Gresham, M. (1984). Vying for a winning position: Management style of the chronically ill. *Research in Nursing and Health, 7,* 181-188.

Glaser, B., & Strauss, A. (1968). *Time for dying.* Chicago: Aldine.

Hardesty, M., & Geist, P. L. (1990). Physicians' self-referent communication as management of uncertainty along the illness trajectory. *Advances in Medical Sociology, 1,* 27-55.

Hymovich, D. P., & Hagopian, G. A. (1992). *Chronic illness in children and adults.* Philadelphia: W. B. Saunders.

Kirkevold, M. (1993). Toward a practice theory of caring for patients with chronic skin disease. *Scholarly Inquiry for Nursing Practice, 6*(1), 37-52.

Lorber, J. (1981). Good patients and problem patients: Conformity and deviance in a general hospital. In P. Conrad & R. Kern (Eds.), *The sociology of health and illness: Critical perspectives.* New York: St. Martin's.

Lubkin, I. (Ed.) (1990). *Chronic illness* (2nd ed.). Boston: Jones and Bartlett.

Mishel, M. (1990). Reconceptualization of the uncertainty in illness theory. *Image: The Journal of Nursing Scholarship, 22*(45), 256-262.

Morris, E. M. (1984). Home care today. *American Journal of Nursing, 84*(3), 340-347.

Plough, A. (1981). Medical technology and the crisis of experience: The costs of clinical legitimation. *Social Science and Medicine, 15F,* 89-101.

Reif, L. (1975) *Cardiacs and normals: The social construction of a disability* (unpublished). Abstracts, UCSF.

Rolland, J. S. (1987). Family illness and the life cycle: A conceptual framework. *Family Process, 26,* 203-221.

Strauss, A. L. (1981). Chronic illness. In P. Conrad, & R. Kern (Eds.), *The sociology of health and illness: Critical perspectives.* New York: St. Martin's.

Strauss, A., Corbin, J., Fagerhaugh, S., Glaser, B., Maines, D., Suczek, B., & Wiener, C. (1984). *Chronic illness and the quality of life.* St. Louis: C. V. Mosby.

Strauss, A., Fagerhaugh, S., Suczek, B., & Wiener, C. (1982). The work of hospitalized patients. *Social Science and Medicine, 16,* 977-986.

——— (1985). Illness trajectories (Chapter 2). In *Social organization of medical work.* Chicago: University of Chicago Press.

Strauss, A., & Glaser, B. (1970). *Anguish: A case history of a dying trajectory.* Mill Valley, CA: The Sociology Press.

Thorne, S. (1990). Constructive noncompliance in chronic illness. *Holistic Nursing Practice, 5*(1), 62-69.

White, N., & Richter, J. (1993). Response. *Scholarly Inquiry for Nursing Practice, 7*(1), 53-57.

White, N., Richter, J., & Fry, C. (1992). Coping, social support, and adaptation to chronic illness. *Western Journal of Nursing Research, 14*(2), 211-224.

Wiener, C. (1989). Untrained, unpaid, and unacknowledged: The patient as worker. *Arthritis Care and Research, 2*(1), 16-21.

Wiener, C., & Dodd, M. (1993). Coping amid uncertainty: An illness trajectory perspective. *Inquiry for Nursing Practice, 7*(1), 17-31.

Wiener, C., Strauss, A., Fagerhaugh, S., & Suczek, B. (1979). Trajectories, biographies and the evolving medical scene: Labor and delivery and the intensive care nursery. *Sociology of Health and Illness, 1*(3), 263-283.

Bibliography

Davis, M. A. (1980). The organizational interactional and care oriented conditions for patient participation in continuity of care: A framework for staff intervention. *Social Science and Medicine, 14A,* 39-47.

Stewart, D. R., & Sullivan, T. J. (1982). Illness behavior and the sick role in chronic disease: The case of multiple sclerosis. *Social Science Medicine, 16,* 1397-1404.

Strauss, A. (1980). Editorial comment. *Social Science and Medicine, 14D,* 351-353.

CHAPTER 4

Illness Roles

Patricia Lewis • *Ilene Lubkin*

Introduction

Living together in social groups, as most of us do, requires guidance so that interactions do not lead to chaos. Society establishes guidelines, which in turn influence the responses and behaviors of group members. *Role theory,* based on the premise that most of the time, most people define most important situations approximately the same way (Berger, 1963), provides a vehicle for understanding these guidelines. According to role theory, society defines every recognized position and assigns roles that contain a set of *norms,* or behavioral rules, that are socially accepted (Wu, 1973; Berger, 1963).

Roles not only include norms for behaviors, actions, emotions, and attitudes, but lead to the emergence of identities that others recognize and that help maintain one's self-image (Berger, 1963). The mechanism by which socially assigned identities are learned is called *socialization,* which Mead (1934) explains as a process in which the individual discovers self and society at the same time. Interactions with and direction from significant others (parents, teachers, friends, and others) reflect the expectations and recognition of society at large. Each role exists in relationship to another. For example, the role of parent requires that there be a child; the role of nurse requires that there be a patient. Associated with learning each role is a set of expectations about how a person in the complementary role will behave (Andrews, 1991).

Children play at different roles, practicing behaviors inherent in these roles. Over time, a person becomes a repertoire of multiple roles, much as an actor in the theater does, with the ability to focus on behaviors that are part of the individual role appropriate to a given situation. For example, the young mother who is also a nursing student utilizes appropriate but different role behaviors in each of her life situations.

Socialization to roles is a continuous and cumulative process throughout the life cycle. Both normal development and life events stimulate *role transitions,* or changes in roles (Hurley-Wilson, 1988). As roles emerge, they are seen in terms of the roles of significant others and are validated by the acceptance of those significant others.

During periods of illness, role expectations must change so that the affected individuals can move from daily responsibilities to behaviors deemed appropriate to their changing health status. The individual who fully recovers returns to prior behavior and roles. However, when there is only partial recovery or residual pathology, the individual has to modify or adapt prior roles to accommodate both social expectations and the illness. The nurse who is aware of the roles that occur during illness, the behavior appropriate to these roles, and interventions that can support the client during and after these role transitions is in a position to help the client and significant others.

Illness Behavior

The onset of symptoms leads to a response, called *illness behavior,* that helps individuals determine their own state of health and need for treatment (Wu, 1973). Illness behavior has been defined as "the way in which given symptoms may be differentially perceived, evaluated and acted (or not acted) upon by different kinds of persons" (Mechanic, 1961).

Viewed from this perspective, illness behavior is limited to help-seeking behavior that either identifies and assesses changes that are occurring or searches for solutions. Because it is health seeking, illness behavior can be triggered whenever an individual feels that a symptom demands explanation, desires a means of managing the underlying disorder, or disagrees with current treatment. For example, the client with recurring, nonspecific neurological symptoms may consult many physicians and receive several diagnostic opinions and treatment plans before multiple sclerosis is finally confirmed. Or a family who finds that current medical treatment is not helping their dying child may move to Mexico to try laetrile treatments.

In 1966 Rosenstock formulated a *health belief model* (HBM) to explain the way one's beliefs about health and illness can predict health service consumption. The HBM showed that attitudes, personal values, beliefs, previous life experiences, and present life stresses may alter actions, choices, and responses to illness (Rankin & Duffy, 1983). Although the HBM is more useful in evaluating preventive health teaching and in assessing compliance with treatment regimens, it also clarifies illness behavior. According to Rosenstock's model, individuals are not likely to choose a health-promoting course of action unless (1) they believe that they are susceptible to the disease in question, (2) they believe that the disease is harmful and will have a serious

effect on their lives, (3) they believe that certain actions can reduce their likelihood of contracting the disease or reduce the severity of the disease, and (4) they believe that taking action is not as threatening as is contracting the disease (Rankin & Duffy, 1983; Redman, 1993).

Sociocultural factors also influence beliefs and illness behavior. People tend to be internally consistent with their own cultural system; that consistency can result in a gap between the values and beliefs of segments of the population and those of health practitioners (Redman, 1993). As an example, Mexican-Americans who believe that illness is a result of life-style and an imbalance in the body between "hot" and "cold" will carry out treatment at home, seeking outside advice only when such treatment proves ineffective (Gonzalez-Swafford, 1983).

Another factor influencing health behavior is economic status, which affects educational level, economic level, family structure, and so forth. The poor, who often have less knowledge of preventive measures and know of fewer resources to obtain services, tend to delay seeking medical help until symptoms interfere with daily independence or ability to function in usual daily roles (Helman, 1990). Table 4–1 lists many determinants or influences that can affect illness behavior.

The Sick Role

The *sick role* was introduced in juxtaposition to the physician's role by Talcott Parsons (1951). These two roles were not seen as equal, since the physician retained leverage to influence client movement toward a positive health change (Cockerham, 1989). In fact, the physician–client dyad presented by Parsons contains a quality of the parent–child relationship, despite the more limited involvement the physician has with the client than the parent has with the child (Parsons & Fox, 1952).

Parsons saw illness as a response to social pressures (for example, evading responsibilities) and therefore as both biologic and sociologic in nature. Anyone could take on the role he identified; therefore, the role was *contingent*—that is, negatively achieved through failure to keep well. In addition, the role also carried with it the

TABLE 4-1. Determinants of illness behavior

Recurrence of the aberrance	The more frequent a symptom, the more an individual feels that help is needed. If relief is obtained from home remedies, less outside help is sought.
Visibility and consequences	Symptoms that are more apparent lead to more illness behavior. However, if the individual feels that the disorder will lead to stigma, there may be less tendency to seek help. Community tolerance toward certain symptomatology will allow for less help being sought, whereas a prejudice against a symptom or disease forces help-seeking behavior. When a symptom is seen as life-threatening, help will usually be sought regardless of other factors. Also influencing a person's willingness to seek help are the consequences on other roles or significant others.
Perceived seriousness or severity	How overt or life-threatening are the symptoms? What influences do they have on social or work relationships? Are they associated with stigma or guilt? What organs are involved? What is the prognosis or rate of recovery? Disorders seen as serious lead to earlier illness behavior. However, how serious or severe a person considers an illness may differ by social class and by health belief system. In addition, when seriousness is viewed on a hierarchy of other needs and desires, symptoms may be considered to have lesser consequences.
Influences of availability of treatment and the medical care system	Distance, costs, convenience, time, effort, and fear of outcomes all influence a person's willingness to seek help. In addition, the health care system tends to subordinate the individual's needs, requires conformity, removes personal identity and privacy, and places the client in a situation similar to that of parent/child. Such subordination can influence willingness to begin illness behavior.
Knowledge and significance of symptoms	Lack of knowledge of the significance of symptoms can influence help seeking. For example, older, symptomatic individuals can interpret their symptoms as illness or as part of the aging process.
Cultural and social expectations	Cultural and ethnic variations in symptom interpretation and notions of what is acceptable health care all serve to guide individuals toward or away from seeking help from a physician. Socioeconomic class, age, and sex influence how symptoms are interpreted. Lower classes give more credence to symptoms that interfere with important roles; the aged utilize more health services; women seek more medical care than men.

SOURCE: Compiled from Wu (1973) and Alonzo (1980).

connotation that individuals were not competent to help themselves (Parsons, 1951). Table 4–2 lists the four major components or characteristics of this role.

Like all roles, the sick role is learned and is influenced by evaluation and legitimization from others (Alonzo, 1980). One assumes the sick role when one has accepted being ill, initiated some form of action, and demonstrates a desire to be well again. Should the individual continue to seek another more acceptable diagnosis or treatment, then illness behavior continues.

The Impaired Role

The sick role assumes major importance in medical sociology on the basis of its reasonableness in relationship to acute illness and its focus on

TABLE 4-2.   Characteristics of the sick role

Component of the Role	*Associated Expectations and Behaviors*
RIGHTS Exemption from normal responsibilities	Dependent on the nature and severity of illness. Requires legitimization (validation) by others and by physician, thus discouraging malingerer. Once legitimization is obtained, individual is obligated to avoid responsibilities.
Right to be cared for	The individual is not expected to get well by an act of will or decision. Not responsible for becoming sick, the individual therefore has a right to be cared for. Physical dependency and the right to emotional support are therefore acceptable.
OBLIGATIONS Obligation to want to become well	Being ill is seen as undesirable. Since privileges and exemptions of the sick role can become secondary gains, the motivation to recover assumes primary importance.
Obligation to seek and cooperate with technically competent help	The patient needs technical expertise that the physician and other health professionals have. Cooperation with these professionals for the common goal of getting well is mandatory.

SOURCE: Adapted with permission from Talcott Parsons's *The social system,* 1951. New York: The Free Press, a Division of Macmillan, Inc.

movement toward recovery. However, it has little applicability to chronic illness.

Gordon (1966) carried out the first study that identified behaviors applicable to chronically ill clients when he examined responses and expectations of several socioeconomic groups toward illnesses that differed in severity and duration. He found, among all groups, that prognosis was the major factor in defining someone as "sick," and that once someone was so defined, acceptable behaviors were consistent with Parsons's model. When prognosis worsened, all groups encouraged increased exemption from social responsibility. Socioeconomic groups varied in terms of *who* was defined as sick, with members from lower socioeconomic groups equating sickness with functional incapacity. In addition, Gordon found that individuals and their families made illness-related decisions primarily during either the early, nonhelpless stages or the recuperative stage; they made few of these kinds of decisions during the highly dependent phase.

Gordon identified two illness role statuses. The first was the *sick role,* as presented by Parsons, which was seen as valid when the prognosis was grave and uncertain. When this role was deemed appropriate, all social groups felt pressure should be applied to insulate the client from usual role responsibilities. The second role, which Gordon called the *impaired role,* was considered appropriate for disorders in which the prognosis was known and was not grave. When individuals were seen in the impaired role, social expectations supported normal behavior and usual role involvement (Gordon, 1966). In other words, the study showed that social pressure would discourage normal behavior if the individual were considered sick, but would encourage an individual who was disabled and was not experiencing illness to maintain normal behavior, within the limitations of the condition.

The impaired role assumes the following characteristics:

1. The individual has an impairment that is permanent.
2. The individual does not give up normal role responsibilities but is expected to maintain normal behavior within the limits of the health condition. Modification of life situations may be necessitated by the disability.

3. The individual does not have to "want to get well," but rather is encouraged to make the most of remaining capabilities. The individual must realize potentialities while accepting the existence of the impairment and recognizing limitations and performance commensurate with the disability (Wu, 1973).

Inherent in the impaired role is the attitude that retaining sick role behaviors prevents the disabled from taking over their own management of care. However, once the impaired role is accepted, any activity that helps maintain control of the condition, prevents complications, leads to resumption of role responsibilities, and results in full realization of potentialities is acceptable (Wu, 1973). The impaired role incorporates both rehabilitation and maximization of wellness. If the individual retains sick role behaviors at this time, such action is considered deviant and inconsistent with the medical condition (Wu, 1973).

The use of the term "at risk" has also been suggested to describe the role assumed by the individual with a chronic illness (Loveys, 1990; Meleis, 1988). This label puts emphasis on the ongoing health or optimal functioning of the person who has an increased risk of disability. The individual with a chronic illness engages in some illness behaviors and some health behaviors. Perception of risk (a perceived susceptibility) has been shown to be predictive of preventive health behaviors (Janz & Becker, 1984). The at-risk role is pervaded by uncertainty. The possibility of progression or recurrence of illness is present, as is the relative effectiveness of recommended treatment regimens. This relates to the HBM concepts of perceived susceptibility and perceived benefits.

The individual attaches probabilities to the risk of illness versus the chance of continuing health. The at-risk role is seen as a transitional state, one in which individuals make changes in a variety of role behaviors that they enacted prior to the illness. This role has some obligations (a certain regimen, a diet, and so forth) and requires much less reduction in other social roles than does the sick role, but it is more uncertain than the sick role. It lacks the clarity of signs, symp-

toms, and time boundaries that are found in the sick role (Meleis, 1988).

Problems and Issues Related to Illness Roles

Parsons's sick role model, which was presented as an ideal type (Segall, 1976), was accepted on its reasonableness and logic (Cockerham, 1989). Most research that has explored its various components in relation to the acutely ill tends to support Parsons's basic assumptions (Steward & Sullivan, 1982). However, the nature of some illnesses is such that there is no clear societal agreement over when the person should be admitted to the sick role (Segall, 1976). The behaviors Parsons identified provide limited insight into the process of assuming the sick role or the variations that can be observed in that process. The concepts of sick role and illness behaviors have also been criticized as too disease oriented and too focused on short-term role changes (Kasl & Cobb, 1966; Meleis, 1988).

Criticisms of Parsons's Model

The major deficiency of the sick role model is that it is based on acute episodic illness. Consequently, it overlooks chronic illness characteristics: the long-term rather than temporary nature of the illness, the reality that full recovery is not a reasonable expectation, acknowledgment that management is often the responsibility of the client or family, and the individual must adjust to a permanent change. The chronically ill often are unable to resume prior roles fully and need to focus on retaining (not regaining) optimal role performance, restricted only in relationship to limitations imposed by the disease (Kassenbaum & Baumann, 1965). Yet society does not provide a clear and acceptable role for this group (Segall, 1976).

Sociocultural Limitations   Application of the sick role model also has limitations among different sociocultural groups in relation to attitudes toward sickness. Many populations have distinct concepts of the way illness is defined and the sociocultural behaviors that are valid for themselves or others (Helman, 1990). The only universal agreement seems to be that the sick role is undesirable (Segall, 1976). Behaviors described in Parsons's model have a middle-class orientation; the impact of poverty on people's responses is ignored. The poor, who have to work to survive, often deny sickness unless it entails functional incapacity (Helman, 1990). In spite of symptoms, people who are poor may not move into the sick role.

Although sociocultural differences have been identified in responses to illness (Helman, 1990), studies have more often focused on illness behavior than on the sick role itself or on the relationship of role expectations regarding appropriate behavior for sick persons and those with whom they interact. A recently proposed model for achieving cultural sensitivity while studying health and illness behavior includes components such as consequential beliefs, social influences, and environmental resources (Facione, 1993). This sort of model holds promise for the development of explanations of differences related to ethnicity as well as gender and social class.

Seeking and Cooperating with Competent Help The four components of the sick role have been studied quite extensively, especially the component that deals with seeking out and cooperating with technically competent helpers. Often missing from discussion of this component is the idea that defining oneself as "ill" is a social process, one that involves both subjective experiences of physical or emotional changes and the confirmation of those changes by other people (Helman, 1990). Cultural factors determine which symptoms or signs are perceived as abnormal and the appropriate response that is expected. Other criticisms concern the oversimplification of behaviors and the model's failure to take into account the personality and orientation of the individual, aspects that influence dependence, knowledge, psychological needs, and so forth (Helman, 1990).

Also missing from this component of the model is a "healthy stage" when individuals may seek contact with the health care system for purposes other than treatment of illness (Hover & Juelsgaard, 1978). Many people are less

dependent than Parsons's model would indicate (Hover & Juelsgaard, 1978). Mechanic (1961, 1972) takes issue with the assumption that seeking professional care and legitimization is always a condition of assuming the sick role. He demonstrated that individuals can assume a sick role that may or may not include medical treatment.

Exemption from Role Responsibilities Studies dealing with role responsibilities and performance assume that the person who is willing to consult the doctor is ready to adopt the sick role (Segall, 1976), although the individual's willingness to give up normal work responsibilities or to become dependent on others has not been studied.

Exemption from role responsibilities also requires legitimization, or validation, from others to prevent malingering by those who are not truly ill (Cockerham, 1989). Parsons's model appears to view individuals as helpless victims of illness who have only to seek care and then to cooperate with that care. However, changing health care values have led to the assumption by many Americans that much of the responsibility for health lies with the individual. Studies have not analyzed legitimization when a social question of personal responsibility for causing the health condition is involved.

Alcoholism and mental illness are both disorders in which obtaining release from role responsibilities can be difficult (Segall, 1976). Although alcoholism is now considered a disease needing treatment, most people, including most health professionals, still feel that legitimizing this disorder removes the responsibility that society believes alcoholics should take for their behavior. Consequently, alcoholics are frequently denied the legitimacy that allows them to take on the sick role.

Mental illness presents a somewhat different perspective of social role exemption. The literature shows that the mentally ill are not exempt from performance of normal roles and responsibilities while they are trying to get well (Segall, 1976). Hospital treatment programs include work incentives and activities that are similar to those found in the community. The mentally ill are expected to be active, independent, and self-directed in their interaction with the physician and other health care providers. They are not expected to be helpless, passive, submissive, or dependent. When mental illnesses, such as depression, are treated in community settings, these individuals are encouraged to maintain their normal roles while undergoing outpatient treatment. Once recovered, the mentally ill, especially those who have been hospitalized, must prepare for the stigma and rejection associated with being labeled as "formerly mentally ill" (see Chapter 5, on stigma).

Who Legitimizes Chronic Illness?   Parsons's model emphasized the physician's role in legitimizing illness; it did not deal with the roles of nurses, social workers, and other health care providers in the process. Legitimizing actions by family and others were also considered less significant. Although the physician may give the final validation with acute illnesses, one must question whether this prerogative applies to situations involving the chronically ill or permanently handicapped.

Health care management of chronic illnesses occurs primarily in the home, a situation that results in increased dependency on nonprofessional sources for evaluating client status. Helman (1990) points out that in order for an individual to adopt the rights and benefits of the sick role, the cooperation of his or her social group is required. Once members of the social group deem an individual "sick," they feel obligated to provide care. Honig-Parnass (1981) found that a "more crucial role in their treatment was assigned [by patients] to the lay significant others than to professionals." In other words, care and support by lay caregivers were felt to be more important legitimizing criteria for the chronically ill than was medical care in relation to managing their daily activities.

With some illnesses, especially when early symptoms are not well defined, receiving legitimization from the physician, other health professionals, or nonprofessionals can be difficult and frustrating. Denial of opportunity to move into the sick role leads to "doctor hopping," placing clients in problematic relationships in which they must "work out" solutions alone (Steward & Sullivan, 1982). As a result, symptomatic persons may be left to question the truth of their own perceptions. The case of J. A. is an illustration.

Multiple sclerosis (MS) demonstrates this difficulty in obtaining legitimization. MS takes about five years from onset of symptoms to diagnosis. Initially, the lack of definitive tests makes obtaining a diagnosis difficult; visits to doctors result in a multitude of incorrect diagnoses. If significant others accept these initial diagnoses, the still-complaining client is viewed as a hypochondriac or malingerer. Because the individual is not socially defined as sick, in spite of increasing symptoms and increasing need for the sick role, the lack of a diagnosis and legitimization prevents the individual from adopting the role.

When diagnosis is finally made, the client frequently shows an initial somewhat joyous response to having a name for the recurrent and troublesome symptoms. This initial reaction results from the decrease in stress over the unknown. In addition, professional legitimization and greater social support from significant others now follow.

Delay in Seeking Help

Symptomatic people are sometimes reluctant to seek medical care. Such delay can prove detrimental when illnesses that require early consultation and diagnosis are not identified so that effective, and sometimes lifesaving, treatment can be instituted. Delay can also have an adverse economic effect if it results in treatment that is prolonged or less efficient, or if correcting or minimizing the condition consequently requires more time. At times, delay can even affect the total community's health. For example, should active tuberculosis remain untreated, others might contract the disease (Blackwell, 1963)

Psychological stress can serve as the trigger to action. Crisis, as the capacity to adapt is lessened, can cause enough disequilibrium to make the individual seek help (Stoeckle et al., 1963). Care seeking is also associated with family or friends' evaluation of a situation, when they decide that symptoms represent an illness requiring expedient medical intervention (Alonzo, 1980).

In spite of factors that move clients to seek health care, delays having potential adverse ef-

CASE STUDY
Trying to Obtain Legitimization

Because of their vague nature, 24-year-old J.A. paid little attention to her symptoms. When the weakness and numbness in her left leg continued for several weeks, abated, and then recurred, she decided to consult her physician. Her history and clinical manifestations were so vague that the physician felt that nothing was physiologically wrong with her, and she accepted the evaluation. Over the next year she developed two episodes of diplopia and some spasticity in the left leg, followed by scotomas and vertigo. Each time, although symptoms did not persist, they were more severe. Repeated visits to J.A.'s family physician did not result in a diagnosis. In fact, the physician believed that J.A. had a "pseudoillness" and recommended that she talk to a psychiatrist because she had recently undergone a traumatic breakup with her boyfriend of several years. Because her initial symptoms predated this breakup and because each recurrence of symptoms was slightly more pronounced, she interpreted her findings as more significant than the physician did. She went to another physician, who treated her for a low-grade infection. Treatment seemed

to help at first, but when symptoms again recurred, J.A. rejected the diagnosis and actions as ineffective.

J.A.'s parents, who had no reason to question the ability of their long-time family physician, supported his suggestion that she seek psychiatric help, although her symptoms were growing worse with each exacerbation. This attitude was very upsetting to J.A. because she felt she was losing vital support in her efforts to find out what was wrong with her. She began keeping records of tests and findings and asking more and more questions. Her goal was to assist, not to impede, the physician.

In addition to being time-consuming, the uncertainty caused her to doubt her own mental state. Her distress continued as her search proved fruitless. She eventually was referred to a medical center, where a diagnosis of multiple sclerosis was made. Her initial response was a sense of relief, although she soon found out that treatment would not lead to cure but only to some symptomatic relief. J.A. was 28 when diagnosis was finally made.

SOURCE: From Lubkin (1990).

---

fects on the outcome of the disease process occur. Choosing to become a patient or to remain a nonpatient does not necessarily depend on the nature or quality of the distress, the seriousness of the complaint, or the ability to treat the disorder. Some sociocultural groups allow delay until symptoms interfere with relationships, others until physical or functional activity is prevented, and still others until after approval or decisions of the family or group (Stoeckle et al., 1963).

Blackwell (1963), analyzing studies dealing with delays involving cancer patients, points out that these studies primarily indicate that delay does exist and that many people are not saved because they postpone seeking diagnosis and treatment. Individuals with mental problems often remain at home and do not seek treatment. Once their families feel they have reached the

limits of tolerance, they demand that the individual seek medical care, which often moves the client into therapy.

Three features seem to influence help seeking (Stoeckle et al., 1963). These are the client's (1) perception, knowledge, beliefs, and attitudes about the objective clinical disorder or symptom; (2) attitudes toward and expectations of the physician and medical services; and (3) personal definitions of health and sickness and beliefs about when medical care is necessary (see Table 4-3).

It seems clear that help-seeking behavior is a culturally and socially learned response. An individual responds to his or her personal definition of the situation (Cockerham, 1989). To understand the behavior, a health care professional must develop an understanding of the individual's view of the situation.

TABLE 4-3.   Influences: Delay in seeking help

Symptoms are a normal part of life	The presence of symptoms of one kind or another is so widespread, that it is considered a norm in most populations. In fact, total absence of any complaints even among the "healthy" over a long period of time may be the exception. Respiratory, abdominal, and muscular-skeletal symptoms occur on a regular basis, and are generally treated by the individual or family with home remedies or over-the-counter medications. What the individual identifies as "sickness" requiring medical intervention may differ from what the health professional defines as illness in relation to signs and symptoms alone. It is a fact of life that a large percentage of those people with illnesses do not seek medical assistance.
Type of onset	Concern about symptoms often depends on whether onset is acute or slow and insidious, or on the individual's perspective of the significance of the symptom(s). Rapidly developing, acute symptoms such as bleeding, crushing chest pain, or severe trauma lead people to seek medical care. Care may not be sought with slow insidious symptoms.
Significance of "chief complaint"	Medical significance of a symptom is not the criterion used by individuals in seeking help. Health care is sought if the client's *chief complaint* or concern about a symptom is distressing to that individual. For instance, the individual who focuses on edema that causes leg discomfort rather than on other nephrotic signs and symptoms may be more concerned about impairment of his or her social roles than about the meaning of physical symptoms. When symptoms are seen as indicative of possible incurable disorders, the individual might choose to avoid the "truth" about the illness, especially if there is a feeling that the health care provider cannot help.
Differences in symptom perception	Different cultural, ethnic, or social groups perceive and respond to symptoms differently. What may be operating is a difference in the definition of what constitutes a symptom. The same symptom can lead to different courses of action. Some cultural groups may see the onset of pain as requiring immediate attention and be concerned about physical and social effects of the illness; others may be more concerned with the functional impact of the disease. Socioeconomic status also influences whether the individual will seek medical care. For example, a well-off individual will seek treatment for "nervousness," but this problem might be ignored by someone with little money or free time as of little significance.
Attitudes and expectations of the health care provider	The acceptance and use of a particular caregiver are frequently determined by the client's reason for seeking health care or the client's perspective and attitude toward health providers. People who only want to be reassured about the disease and symptoms, or who rate "personal interest in the patient" as more important than technical competence, delay seeking help from health providers who emphasize technical competence. Primary providers may be seen as less influential than caregivers who seem more helpful. The advice of the physical therapist who helps in the rehabilitation of the stroke patient may carry more weight than that of the physician.

TABLE 4-3. *Continued*

| Definitions and beliefs regarding health care | The stages that people go through in the process of health care, from deciding something is wrong to doing something about it, may depend on their definitions of and beliefs about health and illness. Individuals who see avoidance of disease as an achievement undergo more health checkups to assure such attainment; others who show more apathy regarding health may make fewer visits. People who are concerned about anything that interferes with their usual activities will seek care when they develop ailments that impede such activities. |

SOURCE: Summarized with permission from *Journal of Chronic Diseases, 16,* Stoeckle, J. D., Zola, I. K., & Davidson, G. E. On going to see the doctor, the contributions of the patient to the decision to seek medical aid: A selective review. Copyright 1963, Pergamon Press.

Who Seeks the Sick Role?

Individuals gauge sickness more by the disruption of their ability to function than by organic parameters. Psychological factors such as anxiety and fear play a role. Individuals may have to experience a crisis or realize that symptoms interfere with important activities before they will seek help (Redman, 1993).

Another factor may be previous associations with the sick role. One study found that individuals who, as children, received rewards (toys, food, and so on) when they were sick tended to move into the sick role more readily, voiced more somatic complaints, made more doctor visits, had more acute and chronic illnesses, and missed a greater number of work days (Whitehead et al., 1982).

Other factors that influence moving into the sick role include economic ability to pay for medical care; a sense of responsibility to one's own health; and personal views of medicine, professionals, surgery, and the body itself (Redman, 1993). As an example, the elderly often see bodily changes as a "natural" part of aging rather than as symptoms, and this attitude adds to their reluctance to seek care, especially when it is coupled with economic concerns.

Mechanic (1972) points out seven important variables that influence an individual's willingness to move into the sick role; some of them tie into an individual's health beliefs:

1. Number and persistence of symptoms
2. Individual's ability to recognize symptoms
3. Perceived seriousness of symptoms
4. Available information and medical knowledge
5. Cultural background of the defining person, group, or agency in terms of emphasis placed on qualities such as tolerance or stoicism
6. Extent of social and physical disability resulting from the symptoms
7. Available sources of help and their social and physical accessibility

Role Changes

Transition into the sick role, sudden or gradual, is not easy. Such movement, which includes loss of some current roles during the acquisition of new roles, requires the person to incorporate new knowledge, to alter behavior, and to define self in a new social context (Meleis, 1975).

Although a chronically ill client takes on either the sick or the impaired role, such roles may be enacted in ways that are not effective in achieving the individual's goals for well-being, either voluntarily or involuntarily. For example, a rehabilitating cardiovascular client may not be following the exercise, diet, and work schedule regimen that has been prescribed. This behavior is voluntary if the client has weighed the rewards to be derived against the costs to be incurred and does not feel the gains are worth the costs. Involuntary role behavior, on the other hand, may be related to lack of knowledge and understanding of expected role behaviors or related to role conflicts.

Role Insufficiency Problems that arise in making role transitions can result in role insufficiency. Role insufficiency describes any difficulty in understanding or performing role behaviors and indicates that one's role performance is seen as inadequate by oneself or by others (Meleis, 1975). Role insufficiency may arise from a variety of sources, including role conflict.

Role Conflict Role conflict is a broad term used to describe an individual's experience of conflicting role demands. In *intrarole conflict* the individual fails to demonstrate role mastery because of conflicting expectations of others for the enactment of a particular role (Nuwayhid, 1991). An example of this type of conflict is a new mother who is trying to adjust to the role of motherhood and is receiving strongly conflicting messages from her own mother and her mother-in-law about how she should care for her child. In *interrole conflict* the individual fails to demonstrate appropriate role behaviors as a result of occupying two roles that require behaviors that are incompatible with each other (Hardy & Hardy, 1988). An example of this type of conflict is a woman with a chronic illness who fails to take on the self-care behaviors required for the impaired role because she sees the demands of caring for her children as incompatible with taking the time to care for herself.

Role Ambiguity Role insufficiency may also be linked to role ambiguity, which describes a situation in which there is a lack of clarity about the expectations of a role (Hardy & Hardy, 1988). This situation arises when the individual has little information about the behaviors expected in a particular role or when members of an individual's social system do not communicate clear expectations for a particular role.

Role Strain When faced with role uncertainty of any kind, the individual may exhibit psychological and physiological signs of role strain. Role strain is the response to feelings that role obligations are difficult or impossible to carry out. Symptoms of role strain may include anxiety, irritation, resentment, hostility, depression, grief, and apathy, as well as typical physiological stress responses (Hardy & Hardy, 1988; Meleis, 1975).

Secondary Gains

The desire to get well is an essential aspect of Parsons's model, but at times clients choose to remain in the sick role; many of their reactions and responses to illness are influenced by premorbid personality, life-type, and level of psychosocial competence (Feldman, 1974). Almost everyone, at some point, welcomes illness as a temporary release from stressful situations. Young children quickly discover the manipulative possibilities of sore throats and stomachaches vis-à-vis school, and adults frequently welcome a day in bed with "a touch of the flu" as a sanctioned break from normal pressures.

Byrne, Whyte, and Butler (1981) found that only 85 percent of their patients who had been working prior to a myocardial infarction (MI) returned to work. The objective severity of the infarct showed no relation to their resumption of employment. Those who had not returned to work eight months after their MI were more likely to have remained in the sick role. Anxiety influenced movement back to prior activities. Individuals whose anxiety predated the MI and persisted over time showed reluctance to engage in social activities (Byrne, 1982). This group tended to show a level of concern for aspects of bodily functioning and well-being that reflected affective responses rather than recognition of physical symptoms. Reigel (1989) also found that psychological factors were predictors of return to work versus prolonged dependency in patients who had MIs.

The uncritical assumption that "everybody wants to be healthy" can blind us to important aspects of health and illness behavior. Few, if any, people want good health at all costs, particularly if the enjoyment of good health seriously curtails all pleasures. Each year millions of Americans smoke, drink, and eat fatty foods in spite of the overwhelming evidence that these behaviors increase the likelihood of illness. Good health competes as a priority with all nonhealth activities, and individual behavior can be understood only in the larger context of life goals.

Life-Cycle Differences

Responses to illness differ, depending on people's developmental stages, tasks, and roles (see Chapter 2, on growth and development). Each age group deals with illness roles, especially the impaired role, differently. Such variations are best reflected in the responses of children and the elderly to illnesses.

Children and Chronic Illness   Research demonstrates that the chronically ill child is at significant risk for emotional maladjustment (Pless & Nolan, 1991). Problems include behavioral difficulties, low self-esteem, and poor resolution of developmental tasks. Evidence suggests that a child's risk for development of psychosocial problems is not linked to specific diagnoses or severity of illness (Breslau & Marshall, 1985; Heller et al., 1985), although children with central nervous system involvement (especially mental retardation) do seem to be at higher risk (Breslau, 1982; Breslau & Marshall, 1985). In addition, the age and developmental stage of a child influence the resources that can be brought to the process of adjustment to chronic illness.

Work with diabetic children and adolescents demonstrates the way children cope with illness (Grey et al., 1991). Preadolescents were less depressed and anxious, coped in more positive ways, and were in better metabolic control than were adolescents. Adolescents, already under stress due to development and role changes, demonstrated more avoidance and depression and poorer metabolic control.

The social environment of children with chronic illness, especially the family environment, is very important in their adjustment (Harris et al., 1991). Chronic illness management is a way of life, and the ability of the family to respond to these demands dictates the quality of the child's and the family's life (McCarthy & Gallo, 1992). A change in the role of one person within the family (the chronically ill child) necessitates changes in the roles of all members of this social system (Meleis, 1975). Christian's (1989) work with families of children with cystic fibrosis suggests that an understanding of the family system is an important framework for explaining the family's adaptation to chronic illness.

It is often difficult, however, to draw conclusions about the direction of the relationship between family problems and maladjustment in chronically ill children. Family dysfunction is often shown to be associated with emotional problems among children with chronic illness (Pless & Nolan, 1991). However, the research has generally focused on families already impacted by the stress of chronic illness and does not measure family functioning prior to the onset of the problem.

The Elderly   The aged, who are involved in many role changes—often in a negative way—also illustrate the interaction of illness and life-cycle roles. Although our society purports to value each individual, many societal actions do not support this contention. Our society values youth, productivity, and independence, and many of these values no longer exist for the elderly as they face more and more role and responsibility losses. The loss of esteemed roles forces the elderly into dependent positions in which they receive little of the positive feedback that allows individuals to consider themselves valued (Kiesel & Beninger, 1979). Being old is sometimes similar to being ill, even for a person who is physically and mentally able (Gilles, 1972). In fact, some social attitudes toward aging and retirement are more appropriate with respect to the soon to be terminally ill than to those who have many long years ahead (Clark & Anderson, 1967).

These role losses impact on physical and emotional well-being (Robinson, 1971). Given the greater number of illnesses found among the aged, and given that the sick role is a socially acceptable one, albeit of lower status than others, the aged sometimes find focusing on symptoms easy.

In the elderly, illness can be precipitated by many factors aside from physical and mental deterioration. Limited finances, poor housing and nutrition, social devaluation, and multiple losses all contribute to social isolation and illness (Robinson, 1971). Despite acute onset, most of these illnesses are chronic in nature. Being ill,

CASE STUDY
The Elderly and the Sick Role

A.B. had passed most of her adult life without serious health problems. At 68 she was widowed, 3 years after retirement from her job as a candy maker. Her children had long since married and left home, and only one daughter lived in the same community. Her former activities as wife and mother and her involvement with her work had ended. In spite of adequate income to meet her needs and occasional phone contact from her children, A.B. felt lonely and deprived of a meaningful role.

A.B. had some long-standing but mild symptomatology that her physician had evaluated and treated: dysphagia (never diagnosed), mild coronary artery disease, and occasional low back pain. She had also been overweight most of her adult life. Within months of her widowhood, A.B. began making more frequent visits to her physician for evaluation of any symptom, regardless of how minimal. This illness behavior brought forth concerned responses from her family and pro-

vided her with a topic of conversation and a socially acceptable behavior: waiting in the doctor's office. She also enjoyed striking up conversations with others who were waiting as a change from her daily routine of cleaning house and watching television. No suggestions by her family that she would feel better if she would lose weight and increase her activity were effective. She insisted that the doctor would help her "get well." Visits to the doctor every month or two went on for several years.

By the time A.B. developed a terminal illness, her physician had become insensitive to her ongoing complaints of weakness, pain, fatigue, and so on. At age 74, A.B. consulted another physician, who became concerned by her insistence that she had been growing more fatigued over the last several months. A diagnostic workup revealed acute leukemia, and she entered a true sick role. She died two weeks later while undergoing chemotherapy.

SOURCE: From Lubkin (1990).

which allows dependency without obligation, contains many features already present in their lives. For older persons who are alone even when they have families, the onset of symptoms can bring more attention from family members, attention that is unwarranted by the illness but that is considered culturally appropriate behavior (Hyman, 1971). This preferential treatment may become symbolic to the elderly client in two ways: (1) it indicates that some changes in status have occurred, and (2) it reinforces the sense of the sick role. The coupling of a socially acceptable role with the lack of other positive roles for the aged leads to a cycle in which the person adopts the sick role as normal and ongoing, as the case study of A. B. illustrates.

Professional Responses to Illness Roles

Health providers generally expect those entering the acute hospital setting to conform to sick role

behaviors. Most people entering the hospital for the first time are quickly socialized and expect to cooperate with treatment, to recover, and to return to their normal roles. Provider expectations and client responses are in line with social expectations and fit with the traditional medical model of illness as acute and curable, and discharge is frequently equated with cure. When clients are compliant and cooperative, health providers communicate to them that they are "good patients" (Lorber, 1981). When clients are less cooperative, the staff may consider them problematic.

But the percentage of chronically ill individuals entering hospitals is increasing. Such admissions occur when symptoms flare or acute illnesses are superimposed. Many of these people have had their chronic illnesses for indefinite periods of time and have had prior hospital experiences. Multiple contacts with the health care system result in loss of the "blind faith" that the individual once had in that system. Chronically ill individuals are seeking a new kind of relationship with health care providers (Thorne & Robinson, 1988).

Being in the impaired role is integral to the daily lives of the chronically ill. Although willing to delegate some responsibility for care to health care personnel, they prefer to retain some control of their regimens when possible. These clients have developed their own competence over time spent dealing with their illnesses, and they have come to expect acknowledgment of that competence in their health care relationships (Thorne & Robinson, 1988).

Thorne's (1990) study of chronically ill individuals and their families found that their relationships with health care professionals evolved from what was termed "naive trust" through "disenchantment" to a final stage of "guarded alliance." She proposed that the "rules" that govern these relationships should be entirely different for acute and chronic illness. While assuming sick role dependency may be adaptive in acute illness, where medical expertise offers hope of a cure, it is not so in chronic illness. Chronically ill individuals are the "experts" on their illnesses and should have the ultimate authority in managing them over time.

When chronically ill individuals are hospitalized, they view the situation quite differently from the health care providers with whom they interact. Clients with multiple chronic disorders may focus on maintaining stability of quiescent conditions to prevent unnecessary symptomatology, whereas staff most likely focus on managing the current acute disorder (Strauss, 1981). In addition, clients who have had multiple prior admissions are more likely to use their hospital savvy to gain what they want or need from the system (Glaser & Strauss, 1968). During hospitalization, these individuals may demand certain treatment, specific times for treatment, or specific routines. They may keep track of times that various routines occur or complain about or report actions of the staff as a means to an end they consider important. All of these demands increase staff work and stress, and frequently the client is labeled a "problem patient" (Lorber, 1981). Table 4-4 compares acute and chronic illness behaviors seen in hospitals.

Health care providers also receive secondary gains from their work, manifested in a sense of

TABLE 4-4. Comparing acute and chronic illness behavior in hospitals

Acute	Chronic
1. Passive, dependent, regressive	1. Positive dependency[1]
2. Predictable symptoms and outcome	2. Symptoms variable, progressive, difficult to assess
3. Illness temporary	3. Illness permanent or long-term
4. Return to normal responsibilities	4. Modified responsibilities
5. Desire to get well	5. Accepts inability to get well
6. Role less desirable but acceptable since temporary	6. Role inferior, some nonperson status
7. Limited experience with this role in this setting	7. Knowledgeable about patient role because illness is full-time
8. Decision making by staff	8. Retains much of decision-making power; wants familiar patterns followed
9. Sick role behavior reinforced by staff	9. Often seen as "problem" patient

[1]Recognizes and accepts help to achieve maximum function.
SOURCE: From Lubkin (1990).

accomplishment and the personal satisfaction that comes from witnessing a client's recovery. The goals of acute care (cure and full restoration of all faculties) provide a subconscious motivation or reward for many nurses, making them feel that they are healers (Wesson, 1965) and generating a sense of omnipotence and self-fulfillment (see Table 4-5). The grateful client who recovers makes hospital work worthwhile for those who provide this care.

But cure is not possible for the chronically ill; only stabilization is. Frequent readmissions, often for recurrence of the same problems, can create a sense of frustration for the staff

TABLE 4-5. Professional Role: relationship to the acute and chronically ill

Acute	Chronic
RESPONSIBILITY	
Responsibility for patient health management	Directs care plan but not responsible for it
ACCOUNTABILITY	
Held accountable for care by patient (i.e., lawsuits)	Holds patient accountable for managing own care. Sees patient as problem; easily irritated by patient's use of manipulation or by patient demands
SECONDARY GAINS	
Many for the staff:	Limited for the staff:
1. Patients' gratitude satisfying to staff	1. No available cures; only ability to stabilize condition
2. Feelings of omnipotence when helping to "save" others	2. Repetitive recurrences become tiresome to caregivers
3. Seeing results of efforts through relatively rapid recovery	3. Long-term interactions can lead to valuable relationships

SOURCE: From Lubkin (1990).

and require repetitive, tiresome care that may become boring. Long-term goals focus on maximizing remaining functional potential and minimizing further deterioration (see Chapter 24, on rehabilitation). These tasks do not provide the dramatic secondary gains that acute care does.

Feelings of frustration and dissatisfaction on the part of the caregiver often lead to avoidance of chronically ill patients. Caregiver attitudes may demonstrate a lack of sensitivity to the meaning of illness to the long-term client and to the client's perspective of his or her own best interest. Results of treatment are less predictable, undermining the health care providers' sense of power and efficacy. Power struggles can ensue between clients and providers (Thorne, 1990).

Lack of Role Norms for the Chronically Ill

Chronic illnesses require that a variety of tasks be performed to fulfill the requirements of both medical regimen and personal life-style. In spite of residual disability that limits activity, society does not identify the chronically ill as individuals who are experiencing illness. Assuming sick role behaviors is discouraged. These individuals enter and remain in the impaired role, but implicit behaviors for this role are not well defined by society, leading to a situation of role ambiguity. Given this lack of norms, influences on the client include the degree of disability (with different attributes of disability producing different consequences), visibility of the disability (the lower the visibility, the more normal the response), self-acceptance of the disability (resulting in others' reciprocating with acceptance), and societal views of the disabled as either economically dependent or productive (Wu, 1973). Without role definition, whether disability is present or not, the individual is unable to achieve maximum levels of functioning. Table 4-6 outlines tasks chronically ill individuals must perform.

Interventions Based on Illness Role Theory

The sick role and the impaired role are sociological explanations of behavior responses of individuals; they are states of being, not problems requiring interventions per se. Through knowledge of these roles, health providers can help their clients cope more effectively with appropriate dependency and can gain a better understanding of the relationship between client and health professional, as well as between those roles and social expectations. Because the application of illness role theory to clinical practice has not been fully explored, it provides fertile ground for research. As with the sick role model, which was accepted on its "reasonableness and logic" rather than on empirical validation, this section considers actions in terms of personal experience and is not all-inclusive. Where it exists, research supporting the validity of a pro-

TABLE 4-6. Tasks required of the chronically ill

1. *Carrying out the medical regimen* Learning the amount of time, energy, and often discomfort required to carry it out. Following the regimen is influenced by its visibility and its effectiveness in preventing symptoms.

2. *Controlling symptoms* Learning to plan ahead, to modify the environment, and to plan activities when symptom-free.

3. *Preventing and managing crisis* Learning what a crisis is, recognizing signs and symptoms, preventing its occurrence, and evolving a plan for handling it.

4. *Reordering time* Adjusting schedules to cope with too much or too little time that occurs with trying to manage health regimens along with other life experiences.

5. *Adjusting to changes in course of the disease* Learning to deal with predictable and unpredictable situations or symptoms and adapting to deterioration.

6. *Preventing social isolation* Preventing self-withdrawal or withdrawal by others.

7. *Normalizing* Learning to hide disabilities, manage symptoms, find ways to be treated as normal.

SOURCE: Adapted from Strauss, A.L., et al. (1984). *Chronic illness and the quality of life* (2nd ed.). St. Louis: The C.V. Mosby Company. Used with permission.

posed course of action is noted. It is hoped that readers will find many applications of illness role theory to their own clinical practice.

Dealing with Dependency

As noted, dependency is an inherent part of the sick role. But health professionals are not always comfortable about the client's being in this dependent role without making some effort to help him or her move back to independence. Take, for instance, the practice of beginning discharge planning soon after admission, even for the critically ill. Such action is based on several factors: first, the societal expectations that the sick should want to get well; second, wariness of the malingerer or the patient who might want to stay ill for various secondary gains; and third,

the pressure created by the economics of our health care system to move clients out of the hospital as quickly as possible. For the client whose disease improves as expected, malingering is generally not a problem, but at times individuals, whether suffering from acute or chronic illnesses, remain in dependent states longer than expected.

Severely ill patients are more concerned with physical than psychosocial aspects of care (Hover & Juelsgaard, 1978) and are incapable of making many decisions (Gordon, 1966). Emphasis on the physical aspects of care with these individuals is compatible with Maslow's *Hierarchy of Needs* model, which emphasizes that meeting physiological and then safety needs precedes the emergence and fulfillment of higher, psychosocial needs. One client noted that during her hospitalization she did not have enough energy to want to survive and was incapable of extending any efforts to improve her condition. Given these factors, the health professional must be able to recognize and accept even total dependency.

Miller (1992) discusses dependency in the chronically ill and links it with the sense of powerlessness that these individuals often confront. Chronic illness is fraught with unpredictable dilemmas. Even when an acute stage is past, the client's energy for recovery may be sapped by the uncertainty about the illness's future course, the effectiveness of medical regimens, and the disruption of usual patterns of living. Awareness of behavioral responses and when they occur can help the professional avoid premature emphasis on independence until the client can collaborate in working toward a return to normal roles.

Miller (1992) recommends several strategies for decreasing client's feelings of powerlessness once they can work toward independence. They are

1. Modifying the environment to afford clients more means of control
2. Helping clients set realistic goals and expectations
3. Increasing clients' knowledge about their illness and its management

4. Increasing the sensitivity of health professionals and significant others to the powerlessness imposed by chronic illness
5. Encouraging verbalization of feelings

Utilizing knowledge of illness roles in planning interventions allows the health professional to maximize time spent with the client. One such intervention that could benefit from integrating knowledge of illness roles is teaching (see Chapter 16, on teaching). The client who is still in the highly dependent phase cannot benefit from teaching. As improvement in physical status occurs, emphasis on the desire to return to normal roles creates motivation to learn about the condition and necessary procedures for maximizing health. As the client moves into the impaired role and becomes aware of the necessity to maximize remaining potential, teaching provides a highly successful tool both in the hospital and at home.

Role Supplementation

Role supplementation is the process through which the sick role or the impaired role is clarified by the use of planned interventions (Meleis, 1988). Role supplementation strategies help individuals who are dealing with intrarole conflicts because they are aimed at clarifying roles. Since the individual is dealing with a problem with incompatible role expectations, strategies that clarify alternatives and help the individual to "try them on" may be useful. There are several role supplementation strategies that health professionals can use to help individuals take on new roles successfully.

Role Clarification Role clarification involves identifying and defining the knowledge, skills, and boundaries of a role (Meleis, 1988). It includes making explicit the expectations of self and others in a new situation through education and the explanation of behaviors expected in the new role. Role clarification is further enhanced when the chronically ill individual successfully rehearses some of the behaviors expected in the new role. For instance, the newly diagnosed diabetic can practice self-injection of insulin.

Role rehearsal enables the individual to anticipate behaviors and feelings associated with a new role (Meleis, 1988). This process can be enhanced if the individual's significant others are identified and included in the rehearsal. Mutually agreed upon roles can then evolve smoothly.

Role Modeling While information about a role and associated new behaviors may help an individual to clarify ideas about the role, exposure to role models is also an important strategy in helping an individual take on a role. *Role modeling* occurs when an individual is able to observe a role being enacted and thus learn to understand and emulate the role (Hardy & Hardy, 1988). Health professionals can act as role models themselves or promote contacts with relevant role models (Meleis, 1975). Examples of such contacts might be the Reach to Recovery program for breast cancer patients or Alcoholics Anonymous for the alcoholic.

Role Taking Role taking focuses on developing an individual's ability to imagine the responses to his or her behavior (Meleis, 1988), to view his or her behavior through the eyes of another, and to adjust his or her performance accordingly (Hurley-Wilson, 1988). Through role taking, behaviors may be rehearsed through fantasies in which patients imagine themselves acting out new roles and also imagine the responses of significant others. Anticipating the responses of others is an important component of taking on a new role, since roles are never enacted in isolation. Patients can then adjust their own role behaviors accordingly (Hurley-Wilson, 1988).

Dealing with Interrole Conflict An individual experiencing interrole conflict needs help with conflict resolution strategies. Appropriate interventions include teaching relative to the problem-solving process and to time management, teaching significant others, and support provided by the health care professional during the problem-solving process (Nuwayhid, 1991).

Norms for the Impaired Role

As mentioned earlier, chronically ill individuals do not have clear role norms to help them define themselves socially, especially since the impaired role, which continues as long as residual pathology or disability does, may limit activity in a variety of ways. For the chronically ill, adaptation requires learning new behaviors, accepting some congruence between old and new behaviors, and being motivated to take on new roles.

The need to adapt has led the chronically ill to evolve some unique roles (Wu, 1973). The *handicapped performer* develops a different and more limited repertoire than that of a well person. Goal achievement may require innovative approaches, and other role needs may require modified activities. The individual who has an *instrumental dependency* required to complete tasks needs to learn to be an object of aid, despite negative feelings about accepting such aid. The *co-manager* becomes actively involved in care by making decisions and assuming responsibility for controlling, maintaining, or improving current status. Finally, the role of *public relations* person includes the necessity of explaining one's health condition at times. Maintaining good public relations enables the person to receive aid and to satisfy the curiosity of others. It also helps to resolve inconsistencies between self and others who are not impaired, to focus on abilities relevant to employment or admission to college, to lessen social prejudice through education, and to maximize individual potential (Wu, 1973).

But self-definition of roles is not adequate for meeting the challenges of our society. We all need to know the behaviors that society expects and accepts. The political activism of disabled, handicapped, and elderly advocacy groups is creating new norms. These groups are demanding a greater voice in society and more meaningful lives. Their activism has resulted in legislation such as the Americans with Disabilities Act that took effect in 1992 and assures disabled citizens of access and equal opportunity under the law. Each professional can also help promote the development of norms that lead to greater productivity of a growing segment of the population.

Assisting Those in the Impaired Role

Some studies of the relationship of illness response, personality, and stress have found unique responses to specific diseases, as well as variations in affective behavior and cognitive meaning of specific illness (Byrne & Whyte, 1978; Pilowsky & Spence, 1975). These studies, using the same tool, found that individuals who had myocardial infarctions (MIs) had different patterns of concerns regarding their bodily functioning, recognition of the gravity of their illness, and responses to stress from those individuals experiencing intractable pain. In fact, patients with MIs initially had difficulty accepting the sick role (Byrne & Whyte, 1978). Such information can be useful in planning care and in devising programs of rehabilitation and prevention. The practicing professional also can consider utilizing such tools to identify characteristics of other chronically ill people in order to plan their short- and long-term care.

Other studies have found commonalities across illnesses in adjustment to the impaired role. Viney and Westbrook (1982) examined psychological reactions of clients who had newly diagnosed chronic illnesses and found that type of illness did not seem to determine client reaction. The best index of patients' emotional reaction to a chronic illness was their perception of how the illness would handicap them. This corresponds closely to work done by Benner and Wrubel (1989) that points out that symptoms are laden with meaning and that getting in touch with this meaning and context of the experience of the illness is essential to caring for clients.

Pollack, Christian, and Sands (1990) established that psychologic adaption did not correspond directly to measures of physiologic well-being in chronically ill individuals, regardless of type of illness. Rather, psychologic adaption corresponded to a specific style of handling stress known as the "hardiness characteristic." The personality dispositions of hardiness are specific attitudes of commitment, control, and challenge that mediate the stress response, again indicating individual differences in adjustment to chronic illness (Pollack, 1989).

Not only is ongoing treatment necessary, but individuals in the impaired role are "continually threatened by a decrease in function related to the chronic illness" (Monohan, 1982). This characteristic has led to a modification of the impaired role described as the *at-risk role*, mentioned earlier. Clients who perceive themselves as being at risk of having complications are more highly motivated to greater compliance with regimens (see Chapter 10, on compliance). To encourage movement into this modified role, the health provider needs to persuade the client that compliance is valuable in maximizing health and wellness when developing symptoms or complications without such adherence is a possibility. The goal should be retaining, not regaining, optimal physical functioning. Helping the client decrease the risks of complications requires that the professional assess the following factors: health beliefs, environmental factors (family setting, role, and composition; medical and social supports; sociocultural factors), and present functioning level and symptoms.

Learning to Deal with Personal Biases

Professionals who have limited awareness of illness roles are often insensitive to these roles, their meaning, and the ways their own responses are affected by and affect the client. The health professional in the hospital setting deals with clients on an episodic basis and often has limited knowledge of the entire situation that these individuals must live with on a daily basis. This limited perspective may hamper efforts to promote recovery or rehabilitation, especially for the chronically ill.

The problem is compounded because chronically ill clients, who are experienced with hospital settings, are not always compliant (Thorne, 1990). Since these individuals are responsible for self-management at home, they may be unwilling to delegate control over all their care and have acquired ways of continuing aspects of their regimens that they consider important, even though they are in the hospital for other reasons. The chronically ill individual may never fully move into the dependency of the sick role, except during the most acute phases of illness. Health care professionals dealing with such clients often are frustrated because the client is not taking on the expected "sick role." Power struggles may develop between provider and client.

Caring for individuals who have frequent recurrences of the same health problems can lead the provider to feel the same sense of powerlessness over the illness that the chronically ill person feels. Both groups realize that the client will never fully recover. At times, health care providers express their frustration by blaming the client. Such negative feelings about clients inevitably influence interactions with them.

To be truly helpful, health professionals must focus on feelings and responses triggered by the client's need to retain autonomy. Only awareness of how these feelings impact on patient care can allow the provider to achieve an objective view of the situation and the realization that chronically ill persons are trying to manage their symptoms and lives and to maximize their remaining potential. Staff members must realize that demands for autonomy indicate that the client is adapting to the illness and its accompanying role while striving to achieve holistic wellness.

Once health care professionals are able to restructure their view, joint goal setting and planning are possible; power becomes shared and a satisfying relationship of reciprocal trust develops between health care provider and client (Thorne & Robinson, 1988). Feeling trusted and respected both fosters satisfaction with the relationship and helps promote and maintain the competence of the chronically ill clients.

The Need for Research

Although research related to chronic illness is increasing (see Chapter 17, on research), the preponderance of studies focus on the relation of illness to clinical practice. Most research on the sick role has emphasized the theoretical perspective. More research on clinical application of the sick role needs to be carried out by clinical practitioners. Two instances of the application of role theory research to clinical practice are noteworthy.

Personality and Illness Behavior   Theoretical research can have clinical application even if it was not specifically designed for that purpose. As an example, extensive worldwide research has analyzed the relationship of the Type A personality and illness behavior to the person who has a myocardial infarction (Byrne & Whyte,

1978; Byrne et al., 1981; Heller, 1979; Hackett, 1982; Byrne, 1982; Appels et al., 1982). These studies were intended to verify the role of personality factors in this condition and to determine whether the tool that was developed had international application. Outgrowths of this research led to the development of preventive programs for Type A personalities, application of this information in post-MI teaching, and the integration of knowledge about personality with patient care and rehabilitation programs.

Identified Subroles One qualitative study that considered the dialysis patient's ability to assume or reject the sick role identified several subroles (Artinian, 1983). The *undecided role* is usually assumed by the newly diagnosed individual who is still questioning the necessity of dialysis; eventually the individual moves to one of the other roles. The *worker role* fits the individual who rejects the sick role, continues to define himself or herself as normal, and finds ways to fit dialysis into other life activities. The patient does this by cooperating with dialysis and selecting the type of dialysis most suitable to life-style. The *waiter role* is adopted by the person who does not accept the sick role but finds dialysis unacceptable as a way of life. This individual waits for a transplant or death, is least informed about the process, is least compliant, and feels trapped and deprived of a future. The *true dialysis patient* accepts the sick role and centers life around dialysis, which becomes his or her "job." This person is knowledgeable about the disease and its management, arrives early for treatment, and stays late to socialize. The *emancipated role* is not a dialysis role, since an individual assumes it only after being freed from dialysis through transplantation.

Artinian notes that individualization of care is essential to fulfilling the physical and self-esteem needs of each role group. The *undecided* needs time without pressure to accept dialysis. Expeditious service allows the *worker* to feel in control. The *waiter* needs to have a nonhostile environment even when being noncompliant. The *true dialysis patient* needs praise for successfully managing the dialysis regimen, as well as opportunities for companionship.

Summary and Conclusions

When symptoms strike, the affected individual generally takes action to identify and correct the cause. This *illness behavior* is influenced by many variables, including the client's health beliefs. At some point along the illness behavior continuum, the acutely ill individual enters the *sick role,* in which it is acceptable to be dependent on others while being relieved of social responsibilities. In exchange, one is obligated to want to become well and to seek and cooperate with technically competent professionals. This role is more applicable to acute, rather than chronic, disorders. According to the *impaired role* model, chronically ill or disabled persons must be responsible for their own health management and can meet normal role expectations within the limits of their health condition. In other words, the impaired role entails adapted wellness.

The sick role was postulated on the basis of reasonableness and logic rather than on research. Studies have investigated its four major components, and results indicate that although it has some weaknesses, the model is validated in relation to acute illness. Its lack of usefulness to chronic illness is a major drawback, especially in light of increasing numbers of chronically ill people. The impaired role is problematic in that society has yet to define role norms clearly that maximize social integration of impaired individuals. The nurse can promote such integration by supporting individualized strategies for each affected person.

Health professionals must also come to terms with the differences in behavior of acutely ill and chronically ill clients in the hospital setting by recognizing the internal aspects of their relationship to the client. Using illness roles as a basis for clinical practice currently has a strong experiential component, since research data are limited. In the meantime, knowledge of illness roles can provide some direction for the health professional.

All theorists agree that illness is not only an individual matter but a biological and sociological event. Since social systems depend on individuals, the health status of all members is a matter of group concern. Society's responses to illness depend on many sociocultural factors, which are not always logical or scientifically based (Helman, 1990). The health professional needs to be aware of the many factors that influence the chronically ill, including the roles assumed during acute illness and when residual disorders remain.

NURSING DIAGNOSIS

3.2.1 Altered Role Performance

Definition: Disruption in the way one perceives one's own role.

Defining Characteristics: Change in self-perception of role; denial of role; change in others' perception of role; conflict in roles; change in physical capacity to resume role; lack of knowledge of role; change in usual patterns of responsibility.

Related Factors: To be developed.

Editor's Note: Several of the defining characteristics above are unclear based on the definition of this diagnostic category. For example, how can one perceive one's role as different when in denial? Or how does one perceive a difference in one's role if the characteristic is that others perceive the role as different? The difficulty lies in the category not being clinically specific enough.

Some of the defining characteristics could be modified to become definitions of categories that are at a more clinically specific level. The following are suggestions for further development.

1. Role Insufficiency

Definition: Lack of understanding or performing of role behaviors so that one's role performance is inadequate (such as a client hospitalized for the first time).

OR

Role Ambiguity

Definition: Lack of clarity about the expectations of a role, preventing its integration into one's role repertoire.

Editor's Note: Although role insufficiency and role ambiguity seem interchangeable, role insufficiency is a broader term. The literature seems to support the more specific term of role ambiguity.

2. Interrole Conflict (or Role Conflict: Own Perspective)

Definition: Perception of incongruity, incompatibility, or contradictory expectations of one's own roles.

3. Intrarole Conflict (or Role Conflict: Perspective of Others)

Definition: Others' perception that a client's role has changed, which the client does not acknowledge.

Other clinical categories to consider under this level, but not based on existing defining characteristics, are

4. Role Strain

Definition: The experience of stress when one feels that role obligations are difficult or impossible to carry out.

5. Secondary Gains:[1]

Definition: Unconscious need to retain inappropriate role behaviors for other advantages or benefits appropriate to the role situation

---

[1]Secondary gains need to be differentiated from *malingering,* which involves *knowingly* wishing to enter or remain in an inappropriate role.

STUDY QUESTIONS

1. What is illness behavior, and what factors influence the symptomatic individual to adopt illness behavior?
2. What are the characteristics of the sick role? When do symptomatic individuals take on this role?
3. How does the impaired role differ from the sick role? What are the characteristics of the impaired role?
4. What problems have been identified in relation to the sick role and its characteristics? Discuss them.
5. What other problems may cause individuals to delay seeking help or moving into the sick role?
6. What role difficulties might an individual encounter when moving into the sick or impaired role? Differentiate them.
7. How do children differ in role response to illness? How do the elderly respond?
8. In what ways do professionals' expectations influence their response to clients?
9. In what way does the lack of clarity regarding role norms for the impaired role influence clients' behavior?
10. Consider a client you have cared for in the hospital setting. What criteria could you see in determining whether the individual is in a dependent role? ready to move toward greater independence?
11. How can you use knowledge about illness roles in planning your time and work? in helping the client adapt to the sick role? the impaired role?
12. Why is it important that nurses understand themselves and their personal biases?
13. What problems arise from an inadequate societal role for chronically ill or impaired people?
14. What value does research have for relating the sick role to clinical practice? Identify areas in which such research would be beneficial.

References

Alonzo, A. A. (1980). Acute illness behavior: A conceptual exploration and specification. *Social Science and Medicine, 14A,* 515-526.

Andrews, H. A. (1991). Overview of the role function mode. In C. A. Roy & H. A. Andrews, *The Roy Adaption Model: The definitive statement* (pp. 347-361). Norwalk, CT: Appleton & Lange.

Appels, A., Jenkins, C. D., & Rosenmann, R. H. (1982). Coronary-prone behavior in the Netherlands: A cross-cultural validation study. *Journal of Behavioral Medicine, 5*(1), 83-88.

Artinian, B. M. (1983, May/June). Role identities of the dialysis patient. *Nephrology Nurse, 5*(30), 10-14.

Benner, P., & Wrubel, J. (1989). *The primacy of caring: Stress and coping in health and illness.* Menlo Park, CA: Addison-Wesley.

Berger, P. L. (1963). *Invitation to Sociology: A Humanistic Perspective.* Garden City, NY: Anchor Books.

Blackwell, B. (1963). The literature of delay in seeking medical care for chronic illness. *Health Education Monographs, 16,* 3-31.

Breslau, N. (1982). Psychiatric disorder in children with physical disabilities. *Journal of the American Academy of Child Psychiatry, 24,* 87-94.

Breslau, N., & Marshall, I. A. (1985). Psychological disturbance in children with physical disabilities: Continuity and change in a 5-year follow-up. *Journal of Abnormal Child Psychology, 13,* 199-216.

Byrne, D. G. (1982). Illness behavior and psychosocial outcomes after a heart attack. *British Journal of Clinical Psychology, 21,* 145-146.

Byrne, D. G., & Whyte, H. M. (1978). Dimensions of illness behavior in survivors of myocardial infarction. *Journal of Psychosomatic Research, 22,* 485-491.

Byrne, D. G., Whyte, H. M., & Butler, K. L. (1981). Illness behavior and outcome following survived M.I.: A prospective study. *Journal of Psychosomatic Research, 25*(2), 97-107.

Christian, B. J. (1989). *Family adaption to chronic illness: Family coping style, family relationships, and family coping status—implications for nursing.* Unpublished doctoral dissertation, University of Texas, Austin.

Clark, M., & Anderson, B. G. (1967). *Culture and aging.* Springfield, IL: Charles C. Thomas.

Cockerham, W. C. (1989). The sick role. In *Medical sociology* (4th ed.). Englewood Cliffs, NJ: Prentice-Hall.

Facione, N. C. (1993). The Triandis model for the study of health and illness behavior: A social behavior theory with sensitivity to diversity. *Advances in Nursing Science, 15*(3), 49–58.

Feldman, D. J. (1974). Chronic disabling illness: A holistic view. *Journal of Chronic Diseases, 27,* 287–291.

Gilles, L. (1972). *Human behavior in illness.* London: Faber & Faber.

Glaser, B., & Strauss, A. L. (1968). *Time for dying.* Chicago: Aldine.

Gonzalez-Swafford, M. J. (1983). Ethno-medical beliefs and practices of Mexican-Americans. *Nurse Practitioner, 8*(10), 29–30, 32, 34.

Gordon, G. (1966). *Role Theory and Illness: A sociological perspective.* New Haven, CT: College and University Press.

Grey, M., Camerson, M. E., & Thurber, F. W. (1991). Coping and adaption in children with diabetes. *Nursing Research, 40*(3), 144–149.

Hackett, T. P. (1982). Sociocultural influences, the response to illness, Editorial comments. *Cardiology, 69,* 301–302.

Hardy, M. E., & Hardy, W. L. (1988). Role stress and role strain. In M. E. Hardy & M. E. Conway (Eds.), *Role theory: Perspectives for health professionals* (2nd ed.). Norwalk, CT: Appleton & Lange.

Harris, J. A., Newcomb, A. F., & Gewanter, H. L. (1991) Psychosocial effects of juvenile rheumatic disease: The family and peer systems as a context for coping. *Arthritis Care and Research, 4*(3), 123–130.

Heller, R. F. (1979). Type A behavior and coronary heart disease. *British Medical Journal, 280,* 365.

Heller, A., Rafman, S., Zvagulis, I., & Pless, I. B. (1985). Birth defects and psychosocial adjustment. *American Journal of Diseases of Children, 139,* 257–263.

Helman, C. G. (1990). *Culture, health and illness: An introduction for health professionals* (2nd ed.). London: Wright.

Honig-Parnass, T. (1981). Lay concepts of the sick role: An examination of the professional bias in Parsons's model. *Social Science and Medicine, 15A,* 615–623.

Hover, J., & Juelsgaard, N. (1978). The sick role reconceptualized. *Nursing Forum, XVII*(4), 406–415.

Hurley-Wilson B. A. (1988). Socialization for roles. In M. E. Hardy & M. E. Conway (Eds.), *Role theory: Perspectives for health professionals* (2nd ed.). Norwalk, CT: Appleton & Lange.

Hyman, M. D. (1971). Disability and patient's perceptions of preferential treatment: Some preliminary findings. *Journal of Chronic Diseases, 24,* 329–342.

Janz, N. K., & Becker, M. H. (1984). The health belief model: A decade later. *Health Education Quarterly, 11*(1), 1–47.

Kasl, S. V., & Cobb, S. (1966). Health behavior, illness behavior, and sick role behavior. I. Health and illness behavior. *Archives of Environmental Health, 12,* 246–266.

Kassenbaum, G. G., & Baumann, B. O. (1965). Dimensions of the sick role in chronic illness. *Journal of Health and Human Behavior, 6*(1), 16–27.

Kiesel, M., Sr., & Beninger, C. (1979). An application of psycho-social role theory to the aging. *Nursing Forum, XVIII*(1), 80–91.

Lewis, S. M., & Collier, I. C. (1991). *Medical-surgical nursing: Assessment and management of clinical problems.* New York: McGraw-Hill.

Lorber, J. (1981). Good patients and problem patients: Conformity and deviance in a general hospital. In P. Conrad & R. Kern (Eds.), *The sociology of health and illness: Critical perspectives.* New York: St. Martin's.

Loveys, B. (1990). Transitions in chronic illness: The at-risk role. *Holistic Nursing Practice, 4*(3), 56–64.

Lubkin, I. (Ed.) (1990). *Chronic illness: Impact and interventions* (2nd ed.). Boston: Jones and Bartlett.

McCarthy, S. M., & Gallo, A. M. (1992). A case illustration of family management style. *Journal of Pediatric Nursing: Nursing Care of Children and Families, 7*(6), 395–402.

Mead, G. H. (1934). *Mind, self & society.* Chicago: University Press.

Mechanic, D. (1961). The concept of illness behavior. *Journal of Chronic Diseases, 15,* 189–194.

——— (1972). *Public expectations and health care.* New York: John Wiley.

——— (1978). *Medical sociology* (2nd ed.). New York: Free Press.

Meleis, A. I. (1975). Role insufficiency and role supplementation: A conceptual framework. *Nursing Research, 24*(4), 264–271.

——— (1988). The sick role. In M. E. Hardy & M. E. Conway (Eds.), *Role theory: Perspectives for health professionals* (2nd ed.). Norwalk, CT: Appleton & Lange.

Miller, J. F. (1992). *Coping with chronic illness: Overcoming powerlessness* (2nd ed.). Philadelphia: F. A. Davis.

Monohan, R. S. (1982, May). The "at-risk" role. *Nurse Practitioner,* pp. 42–44, 52.

Nuwayhid, K. A. (1991). Role transition, distance and conflict. In C. A. Roy & H. A. Andrews, *The Roy Adaption Model: The definitive statement* (pp. 363–376). Norwalk, CT: Appleton & Lange.

Parsons, T. (1951). *The social system.* New York: The Free Press.

Parsons, T., & Fox, R. (1952). Illness, therapy and the modern urban American family. *Journal of Social Issues, VIII,* 31–44.

Pilowsky, I., & Spence, N. D. (1975). Patterns of illness behaviour in patients with intractable pain. *Journal of Psychosomatic Research, 19,* 279–287.

Pless, B., & Nolan, T. (1991). Revision, replication, and neglect—research on maladjustment in chronic illness. *Journal of Child Psychology and Psychiatry, 32*(2), 347–365.

Pollack, S. E. (1989). The hardiness characteristic: A motivating factor in adaption. *Advances in Nursing Science, 11*(2), 53–62.

Pollack, S. E., Christian, B. J., & Sands, D. (1990). Responses to chronic illness: Analysis of psychological and physiological adaption. *Nursing Research, 39*(5), 300–304.

Rankin, S. J., & Duffy, K. L. (1983). A model for patient decision making and mutual goal setting. In *Patient education: Issues, principles, and guidelines.* New York: J. B. Lippincott.

Redman, B. K. (1993). *The process of patient education.* St. Louis: Mosby.

Reigel, B. (1989). Social support and psychological adjustment to chronic coronary heart disease: Operationalization of Johnson's behavioral system model. *Advances in Nursing Science, 11*(2), 74–84.

Robinson, D. (1971). *The process of becoming ill.* London: Routledge and Kegan Paul.

Segall, A. (1976). The sick role concept: Understanding illness behavior. *Journal of Health and Social Behavior, 17,* 163–170.

Steward, D. C., & Sullivan, T. J. (1982). Illness behavior and the sick role in chronic disease: The case of multiple sclerosis. *Social Science and Medicine, 16,* 1397–1404.

Stoeckle, J. D., Zola, I. K., & Davidson, G. E. (1963). On going to see the doctor, the contributions of the patient to the decision to seek medical aid: A selective review. *Journal of Chronic Diseases, 16,* 975–989.

Strauss, A. L. (1981). Chronic illness. In P. Conrad, & R. Kern (Eds.), *The sociology of health and illness: Critical perspectives.* New York: St. Martin's.

Strauss, A. L., Corbin, J., Fagerhaugh, S., Glaser, B., Maines, D., Suczek, B., & Wiener, C. (1984). *Chronic illness and the quality of Life.* St. Louis: C. V. Mosby.

Thorne, S. E. (1990). Constructive noncompliance in chronic illness. *Holistic Nursing Practice, 5*(1), 62–69.

Thorne, S. E., & Robinson, C. A. (1988). Reciprocal trust in health care relationships. *Journal of Advanced Nursing, 13,* 782–789.

Viney, L. L., & Westbrook, M. T. (1982). Psychological reactions to the onset of chronic illness. *Social Science and Medicine, 16,* 899–905.

Wesson, A. F. (1965). Long-term care: The forces that have shaped it and the evidence for needed change. In *Meeting the social needs of long-term patients.* Chicago: American Hospital Association.

Whitehead, W. E., Winget, C., Federactivius, A. S., Wooley, S., & Blackwell, B. (1982). Learned illness behavior in patients with irritable bowel syndrome and peptic ulcer. *Digestive Diseases and Sciences, 27*(3), 202–208.

Wu, R. (1973). *Behavior and illness.* Englewood Cliffs, NJ: Prentice-Hall.

Bibliography

Bawwens, E. E., Anderson, D. V., & Buergin, P. (1983). Chronic illness. In W. J. Phipps, B. C. Long, & N. E. Woods (Eds.), *Medical surgical nursing: Concepts and clinical practice* (2nd ed.). St. Louis: C. V. Mosby.

Blackwell, B. (1967). Upper middle class adult expectations about entering the sick role for physical and psychiatric dysfunctions. *Journal of Health and Social Behavior, 8,* 83–95.

Carasso, R., Yehuda, S., & Ben-uriah, Y. (1981). Personality type, life events, and sudden CVA. *International Journal of Neuroscience, 14,* 223–225.

Erikson, K. T. (1957). Patient role and social uncertainty: A dilemma of the mentally ill. *Psychiatry, 20,* 262–272.

Fross, K. H., Dirks, J., Kinsman, R. A., & Jones, N. F. (1980). Functionally determined invalidism in chronic asthma. *Journal of Chronic Diseases, 33,* 485–490.

Jelnick, L. J. (1977, Jan./Feb.). The special needs of the adolescent with chronic illness. *Maternal Child Nursing,* 57–61.

Johnson, D. (1967, April). Powerlessness: A significant determinant in patient behavior? *Journal of Nursing Education,* 39–44.

Jourard, S. (1968). *The transparent self* (2nd ed.) (pp. 3–18). New York: Van Nostrand.

Kawash, G., Woolcott, D. M., & Sabry, J. H. (1980). Personality correlates of selected elements of the Health Belief Model. *Journal of Social Psychology, 112,* 219–227.

Lawson, B. A. (1977, Jan./Feb.). Chronic illness in the school-aged child: Effects on the total family. *Maternal Child Nursing,* pp. 49–56.

Lewis, B. L., & Khaw, K.-T. (1982). Family functioning as a mediating variable affecting psychosocial adjustment of children with cystic fibrosis. *The Journal of Pediatrics, 101*(4), 636-639.

Linn, M. W., Linn, B. S., Skylar, J. S., & Harris, R. (1980). The importance of self-assessed health in patients with diabetes. *Diabetic Care, 3,* 599-606.

Longenecker, G. K. D., & Woods, N. F. (1991). Health and illness: The human experience. In W. J. Phipps, B. K. Long, N. F. Woods, & V. L. Cassmeyer (Eds.), *Medical-surgical nursing: Concepts and clinical practice* (4th ed.). St. Louis: C. V. Mosby.

Neff, E. J. A., & Dale, J. C. (1990). Assessment of quality of life in school-aged children: A method—phase I. *Maternal Child Nursing Journal, 19*(4), 313-320.

Papper, S. (1970). The undesirable patient. *Journal of Chronic Diseases, 22,* 777-779.

Petroni, F. A. (1971). Preferred right to the sick role and illness behavior. *Social Science and Medicine, 5,* 645-653.

Pilowsky, I., & Spence, N. D. (1976). Illness behaviour syndromes associated with intractable pain. *Pain, 2,* 61-71.

Pond, H. (1979). Parental attitudes toward children with a chronic medical disorder: Special reference to diabetes mellitus. *Diabetic Care, 2*(5), 425-430.

Pritchard, M. (1977). Further studies of illness behaviour in long term haemodialysis. *Journal of Psychosomatic Research, 21,* 41-48.

CHAPTER 5

Stigma

Coleen Saylor

My car came to a stop at the intersection. I looked around me at all the people in the other cars, but no one there was like me. They were apart from me, distant, different. If they looked at me, they couldn't see my defect. But if they knew, they would turn away. I am separate and different from everybody that I can see in every direction as far as I can see. And it will never be the same again.

Cancer patient

Introduction: The Significance of Stigma

This chapter demonstrates how the concept of stigma has evolved and acts as a significant factor in many chronic diseases and disabilities. It also explores the relationship of stigma to the more common concepts of prejudice, stereotyping, and labeling. Since stigma is socially constructed, it varies from setting to setting. In addition, individuals and groups react differently to the stigmatizing process. Those reactions must be taken into consideration when planning strategies to improve the quality of life of individuals with chronic illnesses.

The word *normals* is used in this chapter to designate people without the stigmatizing characteristic under discussion. If one person has been diagnosed as arthritic and another has

not, the designation of "normal" simply refers to the one without arthritis. However, the normal person may have other characteristics that could be stigmatized, such as being hypertensive, grossly obese, or abnormally tall. Further, one should not infer that normal is "better" or "physically perfect," although the tendency to attach these value judgments is evident in the historical beginnings of the concept of stigma.

Not all persons attach a stigma to disease or deformity, even though the stigmatizing process is very common. This chapter does not assume that all who come into contact with those who deviate from normal devalue them; rather, it insists that each of us examine our thoughts and actions carefully.

Webster's Third New International Dictionary (1986) defines stigma as a "mark of shame or discredit." *Roget's International Thesaurus* (1977) lists synonyms such as *blemish* and *disre-*

pute. Goffman (1963) traces the historic use of the word to the Greeks, who referred to "bodily signs designed to expose something unusual and bad about the moral status of the signifier" (p. 1). These signs were cut or burned into a person's body as an indication of being a slave, a criminal, or a traitor. Notice the moral and judgmental nature of these stigmata. The disgrace and shame of the stigma became more important than the bodily evidence of it.

To illustrate the way a concept used by the Greeks relates to chronic disease, the next section explores social identity and the discrepancies that exist between expectations and actuality. This section discusses Goffman's (1963) view of stigma as a spoiled social identity.

Social Identity

Society teaches its members to categorize persons and defines the attributes and characteristics that are ordinary for persons in those categories (Goffman, 1963). Daily routines establish the usual and the expected. When we meet strangers, certain appearances help us to anticipate what Goffman calls "social identity." This identity includes personal attributes, such as competence, as well as structural ones, such as occupation. For example, university students usually tolerate some eccentricities in their professors, but stuttering, physical handicaps, or diseases may bestow a social identity of incompetency. Although this identity is not based on professional criteria, it may be stigmatizing.

One's social identity may include (1) physical activities, (2) professional roles, and (3) the concept of self. Anything that changes one of these, such as a disability, changes the person's identity and therefore creates a stigma (Hooper, 1981).

Goffman's study (1963) used the idea of social identity to expand previous work done on stigma. His theory defines stigma as something that disqualifies an individual from full social acceptance. Goffman argues that social identity is a primary force in the development of stigma because the identity that an individual conveys categorizes that person. Social settings and routines tell us which categories to antici-

pate. Therefore, when individuals fail to meet expectations because of attributes that are different and/or undesirable, they are reduced from accepted people to discounted ones—that is, stigmatized.

Stigma as a Discrepancy

Society defines the attributes expected of ordinary people, such as personal attributes, accomplishments, and health. When these structural expectations are met, one evaluates those individuals as "good," "valuable," or "worthwhile." If these expectations are not met, judgments are negative. Therefore, these judgments, as well as the attributes, are an essential part of one's social identity.

Individuals are often unaware of their expectations until a situation arises in which those expectations are not fulfilled (Goffman, 1963). If a professor stutters or arrives in a wheelchair, students realize that they held unmet expectations. Likewise, people expect others to be healthy and free from a debilitating condition. When deviations from this expected norm occur in any situation, the discrepancy between actual and expected is highlighted. These expected character attributes are called *virtual social identity* (Goffman, 1963) and are different from the attributes that the individual actually possesses. The latter are an individual's *actual social identity.*

Stigma is defined as the discrepancy, or difference, between virtual and actual social identity. That is, evidence exists of an attribute that makes an individual both different from and less desirable than others in his or her category (Goffman, 1963). More specifically, stigma can "be considered the negative perceptions and behaviors of so-called normal people to individuals who are different from themselves" (English, 1977). Goffman (1963) states it in a slightly different way: Stigma is "undesirable attributes incongruous with our stereotype of what a given individual should be" (p. 3). Both authors see stigma as a discrepancy between what is desired and what is actual by noting a special relationship between an attribute and a stereotype. This discrepancy "spoils" the social identity, isolating the person from self-acceptance and societal acceptance (Goffman, 1963).

A Spoiled Identity   In the past, the words *shame* and *guilt* were used to describe a concept similar to stigma: a perceived difference between behavior or attribute and an ideal standard. From this perspective, guilt is defined as self-criticism, and shame results from the disapproval of others. Guilt is similar to seeing oneself as discredited. Shame is a painful feeling caused by the scorn or contempt of others (Lynd, 1958). For example, an alcoholic may feel guilty about drinking and also feel ashamed that others perceive his or her behavior as less than desirable.

Most stigmata are considered threatening to others. We stigmatize criminals and social deviants because they create a sense of anxiety by threatening our values and safety. Similarly, encounters with sick and disabled individuals also cause us anxiety and apprehension, but in a different way. The encounter destroys the dream that life is fair. Sick people remind us of our mortality and vulnerability; consequently, normal people often avoid contact with individuals with chronic diseases (Katz, 1981). Further, normals may make negative value judgments about persons who are ill or disabled. For example, some may regard blind people as being very dependent or unwilling to take care of themselves, an assumption that is not based on what the blind person is willing or able to do. Individuals with AIDS often are subject to a moral judgment in addition to being sick. Those with psychiatric illness have been stigmatized since medieval times (Fabrega, 1991). As a result, these individuals have to contend with more than the loss of sight or the symptoms of AIDS; some people perceive them as less worthy or valuable: They possess a stigma.

The attribute that provides the stigma need not be undesirable in itself. If everyone in town had diabetes, it would be expected and no discrepancy would exist. There would be no stigma; the condition would be normal. Only when expectations differ from actual experiences is a stigma possible. The difference between expected attributes and actual attributes provides the deficit and spoils the identity.

Furthermore, the concept of *deviance* versus *normality* is a social construct. That is, individuals are devalued because they display attributes that some communities have chosen to call deviant (Katz, 1981). Indeed, old age, which will one day characterize all of us, is often stigmatized (Luken, 1987). Further, since stigma is socially defined, it can differ from setting to setting. Although many cultural values are constant, others may vary from group to group. Use of recreational drugs, for instance, may be normal in one group and taboo in another.

Whenever a stigma is present, the devaluing characteristic is so powerful that it overshadows other traits and becomes the focus of personal evaluations (Volinn, 1983). This trait, or differentness, is powerful enough to break the claim of all of the other attributes (Goffman, 1963). The fact that a nurse is a brittle diabetic may cancel the remaining identity as a competent health provider. A professor's stutter may negate academic competence.

Although a stigma can be powerful, the extent of stigma resulting from any particular condition cannot be predicted. Individuals with a specific disease do not universally feel the same degree of stigma. On the other hand, very different handicaps may possess the same stigma. In writing about individuals who are mentally handicapped, Dudley (1983) describes great variations in intellectual ability among them; however, normals did not take the variation into account. All those who were handicapped shared the same stigma—mental retardation—regardless of their capabilities. That is, people responded to the Down's syndrome stereotype rather than to actual physical ability. The actual physical ability, or lack of it, was not solely responsible for the social reaction.

Similarly, Piner and Kahle (1984) report a study of the stigmatizing effects of the label of mental illness or mental disorders. Half of the subjects were told that they were interacting with mental patients; the other half were told they were interacting with physically injured patients. The results indicate that the label of mental illness was stigmatizing even in the absence of any unusual behavior. In a study by Cash, Briddell, Gillen, and MacKinnon (1984), the label of alcoholic negatively affected responses to both normal and excessive drinking behavior. The subjects' perceptions were negatively affected by the label of alcoholic, rather than the behavior, which was normal in half of the participants.

This point is an important one in understanding the concept of stigma. The label produces the negative response from normals rather than some aberrant or inadequate behavior. Therefore, the diagnosis or label and associated stigma of a disability or disease exclude individuals from social interaction; their intellectual or physical handicaps may or may not (Hainsworth, et al., 1993). This example of a spoiled identity that leads to stigma excludes the individual from the societal interaction that would have otherwise been expected.

Discredited versus Discreditable Goffman (1963) distinguishes between two classifications of stigma: discredited and discreditable. Some discrepancies between actual and virtual social identities are obvious; others are not. A discredited condition is one with visible cues. Limping, shortness of breath, physical deformity, and wheelchairs are immediately apparent. These and other kinds of clues identify an individual who is different from the expected norm. As soon as these clues are seen, the individual may be discredited in the eyes of others.

In other circumstances, the discrepancy may be hidden. An individual without obvious clues to a defect is known as discreditable. Diabetes, positive AIDS antibody test results, or a hearing impairment are not readily apparent; the differentness is not visible. However, if others knew about the hidden condition, stigmatization could occur. Nevertheless, as long as the condition is hidden, the individual is not discredited.

A discreditable condition creates the problem of whether or not to reveal the defect. The issue becomes one of managing information about the failing. One must decide whether the defect should be displayed or not; should others be told or not? Is it worth lying about? (Goffman, 1963). The dilemma of managing this information will be discussed later in the chapter.

Types of Stigma

Stigma is a universal phenomenon; every society stigmatizes certain conditions. Goffman (1963) distinguishes among three types of stigma. The first is the stigma of physical deformity; the actual stigma is the deficit between the expected norm of perfect physical condition and the actual physical condition. For example, many chronic conditions create changes in physical appearance or function. These changes frequently create a difference in self-perception (see Chapter 13, on body image). Changes of this kind also occur with aging. The normal aging process creates a body far from the television commercial "norm" of youth, physical beauty, and leanness, although this norm is changing to include mature and elderly individuals.

The second type of stigma is that of character blemishes, such as rigid beliefs or dishonesty. This type may occur in individuals with AIDS, alcoholism, or mental illness. Many obese individuals carry this type of stigma because others assume they could lose weight "if they only had will power."

The third type of stigma is tribal in origin and is known more commonly as *prejudice*. This type originates when one group perceives features of race, religion, or nationality of another group as deficient compared to their socially constructed norm. Although society is increasingly aware of job discrimination against women and African-Americans, we may be less sensitive to discrimination against handicapped persons or former psychiatric patients (Katz, 1981).

Most health professionals agree that prejudice, the third type of stigma, has no place in the health care delivery system. Although some professionals display both subtle and overt intolerance, others strive to treat persons of every age, race, and nationality with individual sensitivity. However, we may be surprised to find that prejudice against chronically ill persons exists as surely as racial or religious prejudice.

The three types of stigma may overlap and reinforce each other (Volinn, 1983). Individuals who are already socially isolated because of race, age, or poverty will be doubly hurt by the isolation resulting from another stigma. Those who are financially disadvantaged or culturally distinct (that is, stigmatized by the majority society) will suffer even more should they become disabled or handicapped.

Furthermore, not only is stigma ever present, once it occurs it is irreversible (Link, Mirotznik, & Cullen, 1991). If the cause of stigma is removed, the effects are not easily overcome. Social identity is influenced by a history of a stigmatizing attribute. The alcoholic or former mental patient continues to carry a stigma in the same way that a former prison inmate does. One's identity is not only spoiled, it is spoiled permanently.

Chronic Disease as Stigma

Persons with chronic diseases present daily examples of deviations from what we normally expect in our daily social interchanges. Most people do not expect to meet a person in a wheelchair or one with an insulin pump in ordinary personal or business encounters. Persons with speech or visual handicaps are not expected at most social functions.

American values contribute to the perception of chronic disease as a stigmatizing condition. That is, the dominant culture emphasizes qualities of youth, attractiveness, and personal accomplishment. The work ethic and heritage of the western frontier provide heroes who are strong, productive, and healthy. Television and magazines demonstrate, on a daily basis, that physical perfection is the standard against which all are measured. Yet these societal values collide with the reality of chronic conditions. A great discrepancy exists between the realities of chronic conditions, like arthritis and AIDS, and the social expectation of physical perfection.

Characteristics such as an unclear etiology can contribute to the stigma of many chronic diseases. In fact, any disease having an unclear cause or ineffectual treatment is suspect (Sontag, 1977). Diseases that are somewhat mysterious and at the same time feared are often felt to be morally contagious.

Stigma can be associated with inequitable treatment. The seriously mentally ill are covered by medical insurance at a rate often below that for physical illness. This situation not only stems from stigma, but adds to it (Domenici, 1993).

So far this chapter has defined stigma as a perceived deficiency between expected and actual characteristics. What is the impact of stigma on chronically ill people who possess less than desired characteristics such as physical deformity, shortened life span, reduced energy level, and medical and dietary requirements? All types of stigma share a common tie: In every case an individual who might have interacted easily in a particular social situation now may be prevented from doing so by the discredited trait. The trait may become the focus of attention and can actually turn others away. The following section describes the way many individuals respond to stigma.

Impact of Stigma

A stigmatizing condition has a profound impact on both the affected individual and on normals; the effects must be confronted when these people encounter each other. The stigmatized individual is often unsure about the attitudes of others and therefore may feel a constant need to make a good impression. At the same time, normal individuals may worry about whether to acknowledge the deficiency; they may be concerned about making unrealistic demands (Goffman, 1963). Individuals with a chronic condition may not be included in groups because others do not know how to act toward them. Responses to stigma vary. These responses will be discussed from the perspective of the stigmatized individual, the normal individual, and the professional.

Responses of Stigmatized Individuals to Others

The way an individual deals with the reactions caused by a stigma varies depending on the length and nature of the condition as well as on the individual's personal characteristics. Dudley (1983, p. 64) eloquently identifies how the stigmatized often feel when he states:

A depreciating remark, cold stare, willful disregard of a person's viewpoint hurts in unimaginable ways. The pain derives not only from each stigma-producing incident, but also from the cumulative effect of numerous previous incidents, with the latest one serving as a further reminder of their inferior status.

In addition to the stigmatized individual, family members, who often acquire what Goffman calls a courtesy stigma as a result of association, have to deal with their responses to normals. Well siblings, for example, must learn how to reveal the details of their chronically ill sibling to others (Gallo, Breitmayer, Knafl, & Zoeller 1991). Likewise, family members who care for persons with AIDS share the stigma of AIDS and are likewise discredited, resulting in rejection, loss of friends, and harassment (Powell-Cope & Brown 1992). Stigmatized individuals respond to the reactions of others in a variety of ways.

Disregard   A person's first response to a stigmatizing reaction may be disregard. Individuals may choose not to reflect on or discuss the painful incidents. Well-adjusted individuals who feel comfortable with their identity, have dealt with stigma for a long time, and choose not to invest much effort in responding to the reaction, may disregard it (Dudley, 1983). For example, many proud and confident people of color disregard demeaning comments directed toward their group.

A different example of disregard is provided by wheelchair athletes. They disregard perceptions that their disabilities prohibit them from participating in strenuous, athletic endeavors. Any normal who has observed these wellconditioned athletes racing their wheelchairs up hills in competitive meets may find it difficult to consider them discounted.

Going public with the diagnosis of AIDS is another example of acting in the face of negative consequences. In one study of family caregivers, going public entailed selecting appropriate persons to tell and formulating the approach, while considering the risks and benefits of this action (Powell-Cope & Brown, 1991). One positive aspect of going public is the potential for assertive political action and social change.

Isolation   Human beings have a proclivity for separating themselves into small subgroups. This tendency may not necessarily signify prejudice, since staying with one's own group is easier and requires less effort, and, for some individuals, is more congenial. However, this separation into groups tends to emphasize differences rather than similarities (Allport, 1954).

Once a group has been set apart, a strategy of closed interaction may occur. In this process an ingroup seldom invites outsiders to participate and interaction is contained within the group itself. Closed interaction from within enhances one's feelings of normality because the individual is surrounded by others who are similar. This process can occur any time outsiders are seen as threatening or are reminders that the world is different from the ingroup.

Staying with others who are similar is a source of support, but *similar* does not always mean disabled or ill. Individuals who have a sense of normality, even though disabled or ill, may feel more comfortable when they are surrounded by normals. One young woman, handicapped from a birth defect, feels better around normal people because she has always considered herself as normal. Other handicapped people sometimes made her feel uncomfortable (S. Saylor, personal communication, December 1988). Her attitude reminds us to use caution when making assumptions about the perceptions of others.

Secondary Gains   Another possible response is to seek secondary benefits (Dudley, 1983). If the deviance and its stigma are great enough, the individual may try to derive maximum benefit from the situation (Lemert, 1972). For instance, Dudley describes a docile, dependent mentally retarded individual who behaved in such a way as to gain favors. Health professionals are familiar with individuals who capitalize on their conditions in order to achieve special favors. They rarely value such behavior, but it is one real alternative for a stigmatized individual.

Some secondary gains from a chronic condition may be desirable (Dudley, 1983). For example, sheltered workshops are places to foster social relationships, an important secondary benefit. Most individuals benefit greatly from these sheltered environments; however, the rewards can deter a person from progressing beyond the sheltered environment itself. Caution must be applied if the benefits discourage growth.

Resistance Another response to a stigmatizing situation is resistance (Dudley, 1983). Individuals may speak out and challenge rules and protocol if their needs are not met. For how many years were wheelchair-bound individuals unable to reach pay telephones? But the wheelchair-bound and others united in voicing their protests of the situation, and now lower pay telephones are a much more common sight, as are ramps on stairs and curbs. Anger often serves as a catalyst for those seeking change. Dudley sees this resistance, at least in the case of mentally retarded individuals, as an important step toward autonomy.

Passing An important potential response is *passing:* pretending to have a less stigmatic identity or even a normal one (Dudley, 1983; Goffman, 1963). If the attribute is discreditable (not readily visible), such as being a type II diabetic or having a positive AIDS antibody test, passing is a viable option. It may begin accidentally and be strongly reinforced. As time goes on, individuals become proficient at performing activities as though they were normal. Consider, for example, the illiterate individual who bought and carried a newspaper on the bus in order to appear normal (Dudley, 1983) or the person with a hearing impairment who pretends to be daydreaming in order to pass (Goffman, 1963). This process may also include the concealment of any signs of the stigma. Some individuals refuse to use physical equipment, such as hearing aids, because this will notify others of their disability.

In addition to visibility, obtrusiveness determines the ability to pass. In other words, how much does the condition interfere with normal functioning? For the individual in a wheelchair, being behind a desk or conference table makes this differentness easier to ignore (Goffman, 1963). A person with a speech impediment has no visible symbol of stigma, but whenever he or she speaks, others are reminded of the disability.

Discreditable persons often divide the world into a large group to whom they tell nothing and a small group who are aware of the stigmatizing condition. Further, medical practitioners often recommend this type of information management (Goffman, 1963). For example, the diagnosis for leprosy may be listed as Hansen's disease or mycobacterial neurodermatitis. The client then has the option of revealing the alternate name of *leprosy,* with its accompanying historical stigma. Intimates who know of the stigmatizing condition often protect and help the stigmatized individual. Another common example is the alcoholic's spouse who provides necessary explanations for periods of absence from work or social occasions.

The final step in passing is for the stigmatized individual to move completely into the normal world (Goffman, 1963). An epileptic or mildly retarded individual may live, work, and function completely in a normal social context. Only selected people may be aware of the stigmatized condition and offer assistance in helping the person pass.

Learning to pass is one phase of a stigmatized person's career. However, acceptance and self-respect will mitigate the need to hide the defect. Voluntary disclosure is a sign of a well-adjusted phase, "a state of grace" (Goffman, 1963).

Covering Because of the potential threat and anxiety-provoking nature of disclosure of a stigmatizing defect, most people deemphasize their differentness. This response, called *covering,* is an attempt to make the defect seem smaller or less significant than it really is (Goffman, 1963). Like passing, this process involves understanding the difference between visibility and obtrusiveness; that is, the condition is openly acknowledged, but its consequences are minimized. The object is to reduce tension. We have all observed persons with special dietary requirements who, in a social situation, deny the importance of maintaining the restriction even though they follow it. Minimizing the importance diverts attention from the stigma or defect and creates a more comfortable situation for all.

Another way in which visible stigma becomes less anxiety-producing is the skillful and often light-hearted manner in which the stigmatized individual handles it. The defect is deemphasized by joking about it, thereby reducing the anxiety of normals during the encounter. "I make a joke about my wheelchair and that lets others know it's OK to talk about it" (S. Saylor, personal communication, 1988). The anxiety-producing subject is therefore no longer taboo and can more easily be managed.

Responses Toward Self: Changes in Attitudes

Societal norms and values are a major determinant of an individual's self-esteem and self-worth. Children are socialized to adopt the attributes of their particular sociocultural group. Most of our standards of what is normal or expected from our particular society are derived from this socialization. To use Goffman's terms, we expect of ourselves what is expected of those in our particular social category. Specifically, in the United States achievement and attractiveness are commonly held values.

The person who does not possess the expected attribute is quite aware of this discredit as an equal and desired individual in the society. In addition, individuals with chronic diseases or conditions may find that their own deformities or failings decrease their self-respect. That is, not only do stigmatized individuals have to deal with the responses of others, but some find their own attributes undesirable. This self-imposed cloak of discredit may be heavier than the illness or handicap itself.

In contrast, some individuals can accept deviations from expected norms and feel relatively untouched. A strong sense of identity protects them, and they are able to feel acceptable in the face of the stigma (Goffman, 1963). This is true in groups of culturally distinct individuals such as Jews and Mennonites who have pride in the group identity of their members. Similarly, strong extended families and cultural pride provide a strong identity for members of the African-American and Hispanic communities.

This identity belief system, also called *cognitive belief patterns,* refers to a person's perspective. It includes one's perceptions, mental attitudes, beliefs, and interpretations of experiences (Burns, 1980). Individuals who are stigmatized by the major society may believe and perceive that their groups are actually superior

or at least preferable. These belief patterns offer protection from the stigmatized reactions of others.

In chronic disease, cognitive belief patterns help individuals achieve identity acceptance and protection in the face of stigmatizing defects. For example, after mutilating cancer surgery, patients may consciously tell themselves that they are full human beings because the missing part was diseased and useless. The body, although disfigured, is now healthy, whole, and totally acceptable. Similarly, wheelchair athletes take pride in their superb physical condition and competitiveness (see Chapter 6, on mobility and Chapter 13, on body image). That is, one's perception of self-worth influences one's reactions to disease or disability. An individual's question, "Am I worthwhile?" is answered by determining his or her own values and perspective. Therefore, clients' definitions of themselves are crucial factors in self-satisfaction.

In describing studies of cerebral palsy, cancer, facial deformity, arthritis, and multiple sclerosis clients, Shontz (1977) noted that the personal meaning of the disability to each client was uniformly regarded as crucial. For example, individuals who feel valuable because they are healthy and physically fit suffer feelings of worthlessness if they contract a chronic condition. But the diabetic will never be without a regimen and the necessary paraphernalia; visually impaired individuals will never see normally again. Therefore, the individuals' reactions and ability to accommodate these discrepancies from normal determine their attitudes of worth and value.

Responses of Normals to Stigmatized Individuals

Responses of normals to a stigmatized individual vary with the particular stigma and the "normal" person's past conditioning. Because society specifies the characteristics that are stigmatized, it also teaches its members how to react to that stigma. One study found men more likely than women to state they would avoid persons with AIDS (Herek & Capitanio, 1993). Differences between groups based on nationality have been found in attitudes toward those with disabilities (Westbrook et al., 1993). Children learn to interact with others who are culturally different by watching and listening to those around them. In the same way, we learn how to treat chronically ill or disabled individuals by incorporating societal judgments. Unfortunately, these reactions are usually negative, since the stigma usually identifies an individual as discredited.

Devaluing   Normals often believe that the person with the stigma is less valuable, less human, and/or less desired. Many of us practice more than one kind of discrimination and by so doing effectively reduce the life chances of the stigmatized individual (Goffman, 1963). Many tend to stigmatize persons as inferior or even dangerous and use such words as *cripple* or *moron*. Those who accept the devaluing effect of the physical changes see the stigmatized person as having a spoiled social identity.

Stereotyping   Categories simplify our lives. Instead of having to decide what to do in every situation, we can respond to categories of situations. Most of our life's events fall into general categories, and the responses are therefore simplified (Allport, 1954). University classes are punctual. Church occasions require appropriate dress. Sometimes, however, the inclination to categorize leads to restricted and inaccurate thinking, such as assuming that the handicapped are incompetent.

Stereotypes are a negative type of category. They are a social reaction to ambiguous situations and allow us to react to group expectations rather than to individuals. When normal people meet impaired people, expectations are not clear (Katz, 1981). Normal people often are at a loss as to how to react. Placing the chronically ill individual in a stereotyped category reduces the ambiguousness toward him or her and makes the situation more comfortable for those doing the stereotyping. However, categories not only lead to dangerous thinking, but they are difficult to change. Much less effort is required to sustain a bias than is required to reconsider or alter it.

Using categories and stereotypes to understand people decreases our attention to other characteristics (Lynd, 1958). If we are unaware of a person's positive attributes or capabilities, the negative characteristics become the major

social identity. When people are put into categories, normal others often are blinded and look no further.

Categorizing tends to make one see the world as a dichotomy. This is true of both normals and impaired people. For example, people are categorized as either mentally retarded or normal, even though mental handicaps exist on a continuum, with all of us falling somewhere along the line. Often stigmatized people may see themselves as more similar to normals than different from them.

Responses such as scapegoating and ostracism to those with AIDS have increased the impact of this disease (McGrath, 1992). Indeed, these responses impede appropriate health education aimed at prevention. Regardless of categories, individuals from different groups are similar in some ways and dissimilar in others.

Labeling   The label attached to an individual's condition is crucial and influences the way we think about that individual. For example, the diagnosis of AIDS is a powerful label resulting in the loss of relationships and jobs not warranted by symptoms or the possibility of infection.

Mentally handicapped individuals sometimes do not mind being called *slow learners,* but are startled by being called *mentally retarded* (Dudley, 1983). Their response indicates that they see this term as a taboo. Mentally handicapped individuals go to great lengths to explain why they are not retarded when they note that they work, fix their own meals, clean up after themselves, and so on. Their definition of this state is that it is less than human: "Mentally retarded, that's for very low people" (Dudley, 1983, p. 38). That is, the inability to perform certain functions is not as traumatizing to these individuals as the connotations inherent in the negative label.

Professional Responses: Attitudes Toward Stigma

Health care professionals share the values and expectations of their society (Allen & Birse, 1991). Most nurses, physical therapists, and allied health workers share the American dream of achievement, attractiveness, and a cohesive, healthy family. These values influence perceptions of individuals who are disabled, impaired, or otherwise "less than normal."

Society's values and definitions of stigma affect professionals' attitudes. These attitudes are also influenced by professional education; students in health professional schools are enormously affected by their faculty and staff (Cohen et al., 1982). Cohen et al. (1982) describe how faculty influenced medical students in developing attitudes toward cancer clients: Students assimilated the attitudes they saw around them, so if faculty treated clients with intolerance or a demeaning attitude, the students often adopted that behavior. On the other hand, if humane acceptance of all kinds of clients was observed, that behavior was more likely to be copied.

In addition to the influences of faculty and staff, attitudes were also changed by interactions with clients and chronically ill acquaintances (Cohen et al., 1982). Students' confidence in clients' ability to cope with the disease increased with professional experience. In a similar manner, knowing someone with a chronic condition increased positive attitudes.

Health professionals display all the reactions that any unstigmatized person has toward those with discrepancies of some sort. Therefore, caregivers need a thorough understanding of potential responses toward individuals with stigma if they are to overcome the effects of this stigmatizing behavior. Understanding the concept of stigma will increase our ability to plan interventions for chronic diseases (Siminoff et al., 1991).

Interventions: Dealing with Stigmatized Individuals

A handicap imposes various kinds and degrees of constraints on a person's life. The stigma of that disorder adds additional burdens, often far greater than those caused by the disorder itself (Domenici, 1993). Individuals with chronic conditions usually receive medical treatment, but few interventions may be directed at reducing the effects of the associated stigma.

Helping others to manage the effects of stigma is not simple and should be approached with care. At best, change will be slow and uneven. However, consistent and knowledgeable interventions aimed specifically at reducing the impact of stigma are as crucial as those that reduce blood pressure or chronic pain. The following section discusses appropriate strategies for managing stigma.

Developing a Support Group of One's Own

Those who share the same stigma can offer the "tricks of the trade," acceptance, and moral support to a stigmatized person. Goffman (1963) used the term *the own* for those who share a stigma. Groups of like-afflicted individuals enable the stigmatized person to feel like any normal person. Self-help groups are examples of persons who are *the own*. Alcoholics Anonymous, for instance, provides a community of *own* as well as a way of life for its members. Members speak publicly, demonstrating that alcoholics are treatable, not terrible, people. They act as *heroes of adjustment*, to use Goffman's term.

Groups composed of people with similar conditions can be formal or informal and are enormously helpful. First, peer groups can be used to explore all the potential response options previously discussed, such as resisting and passing. Second, problem-solving sessions in the groups explore possible solutions to common situations (Dudley, 1983). Finally, others who share the stigma provide a source of acceptance and support for both the individuals with the disease or disability and their families.

One word of caution is appropriate. Sometimes stigmatized individuals feel more comfortable with normals than with like others as a result of a closer identity with the normals. For example, not all women respond positively to Reach to Recovery groups; some may feel more discomfort than support. The "best" solution varies from individual to individual.

Developing Supportive Others

Supportive others are persons who do not carry the stigmatizing trait but are knowledgeable and offer sensitive understanding to individuals who do carry the trait. These people are called *the wise* by Goffman (1963) and are accorded acceptance within the group of stigmatized individuals. The wise, who see the stigmatized as normal others and do not make affected individuals feel shame, treat such individuals in a normal fashion. One handicapped college student, asked what behaviors she liked from others, indicated a preference for knowledgeable acceptance:

> I like to look people in the eye, but that means they need to sit down and come close. I like to be touched. Other students slap each other on the back, why not me? I really feel accepted when they ask to ride with me in my chair up and down the halls. Some people see *me,* not my wheelchair. (S. Saylor, personal communication, 1988)

Short of riding in wheelchairs with clients, these desired behaviors are simply the ones two friends or acquaintances would use. The stigmatized person must be seen and treated as normal, viewed as more than body changes or orthopedic equipment, seen as a person who is more than a stigmatized condition.

The AIDS epidemic has added to the impetus for the development of groups of supportive others. In many cities, the model of care for those with AIDS depends on volunteer, community-based groups that supply food, transportation, in-home care, acceptance, and support. This community network is an adjunct to hospital care and provides a vivid example of wise others who are essential to the care of these individuals.

The process of becoming wise is not simple; it may mean offering oneself and waiting for validation of acceptance. Health care professionals who encounter chronically ill individuals cannot prove themselves as wise immediately. Validation requires consistent behavior by the professional that is sensitive, knowledgeable, and accepting.

One way an individual can become wise is by asking straightforward, sensitive questions, such as inquiring about the disabled person's condition. Many disabled individuals would be delighted to have the opportunity to disclose as much or as little as they wish, since that would mean that the disability was no longer taboo. For example, the disabled person may prefer that others ask about a cane or a walker rather than

ignore it. This opportunity allows the disabled individual to reply with whatever explanation he or she wishes. Thus, the disability is acknowledged, not ignored.

Wiseness can come from working around individuals with a particular stigma. Health professionals can acquire real-life knowledge about problems, effective strategies, and concerns of a particular illness. This knowledge can enable them to offer the sensitive understanding and practical suggestions of the wise to chronically ill individuals. Nurses who work with AIDS clients, for instance, have the opportunity to find out which behavior is really effective and can learn about outcomes and clients' reactions. This information is extremely valuable to similar clients and their families.

Caring, close friends or relatives are another type of wise. Siblings, spouses, and parents have the opportunity to be powerfully wise because they can see beneath the disorder to the human being and show that they see ill persons as persons first. However, not all relatives and friends become wise. Many cannot deal with the stigmatizing condition and tend to separate themselves from the ill individual.

Neither are all health care providers wise. Many people who work with the chronically ill or handicapped compound the stigmatization of clients by their lack of acceptance and insensitivity.

Being wise is not a new role for nurses or other caring health professionals. Nurses have traditionally worked in medically underserved areas with discredited persons and are accustomed to treating clients as people, not as conditions. Nurses often assume the predominant role of gatekeepers to the health care delivery system for many devalued individuals. Often, clients with chronic diseases receive effective and efficient care from these and other health professionals, who have great opportunities to perform the role of the wise.

Advocacy

Others who demonstrate the concept of the wise are client advocates: persons who support the right of clients to make informed decisions and to determine the treatment they will accept. The client advocate supports that right by speaking on behalf of someone in need, combining professional expertise with a sensitive understanding of an individual or group of individuals. Advocacy is a demonstration of wiseness because both processes require treating the individual as valuable and worthwhile.

Such an act of advocacy is obvious when lay persons and professionals speak out against proposed legislation or health policies that unnecessarily deprive those with AIDS or positive HIV antibody tests of their rights. As another example, groups of British psychiatrists launched a campaign to decrease the stigma of depression by improving public awareness of the condition and improving practitioners' knowledge of it (Sims, 1993).

Changing Definitions of Disability

One way to change stigmatized persons' perceptions of self-worth is to reassess the criteria by which they determine what is normal. This is also applicable to normals. For example, people with healthy minds and bodies can be crippled by an inability to enjoy happiness (Goffman, 1963). Other people, such as those who have had life-threatening accidents or diseases, often reorder life's priorities. Absence of disease or disability is no longer their sole criterion for self-worth. Rather, an alternate ideology develops to counter the ideologies that discredit them.

Family, friends, and health care providers who interact with the stigmatized person are powerful influences in the self-perception of value and worth (Becker, 1981). Being treated as valuable and acceptable by significant persons enhances one's self-esteem. Stigmatized persons may find that this healthy perception of self counteracts the negative reactions from others. Some individuals who are disabled but who have always been treated as if they were normal do not feel devalued.

Individuals whose self-esteem or identity is dependent on an occupation or hobby may lose these attributes as a result of a chronic condition. Just as a parent whose children are grown may find previously undeveloped personal attributes to fill the lost sense of identity, so many individuals with chronic conditions may find new sources of identity to replace lost functions.

A person should be able to feel intrinsically worthwhile without fulfilling any particular conditions. For instance, a nurse who can no longer work because of a chronic condition may enjoy leisure time with professional friends and former colleagues without suffering a complete loss of self-identity. In the same way, changes in body image may not be catastrophic for those who answer the question, "Who am I?" with intrinsic values rather than physical attributes.

Nonacceptance versus Nonparticipation

The distinction between nonacceptance and nonparticipation is important in caring for stigmatized individuals. *Nonparticipation* is a reasonable abstinence from social activities based on limitations caused by the handicap or illness. *Nonacceptance,* on the other hand, is a negative attitude—a resistance or reluctance to admit the handicapped person to various kinds and degrees of social relationships (Ladieu-Leviton et al., 1977). A disabled person who chooses not to join a camping trip is a nonparticipant; the physical disability serves as the basis for that person's decision not to participate. Deciding not to invite that person to join the group, whether or not participation seems possible, is nonacceptance, preempting the person's choice.

Commonly, normal people cannot correctly estimate the limits of potential participation by those having a disease or disability. Usually, the physical limitations imposed by a disability are overestimated. If normals incorrectly assume that an individual is not able to participate, that is a form of nonacceptance. Such nonacceptance is created by the difference between the degree of participation that is actually possible and the degree assumed possible by normals. If the difference can be resolved, nonacceptance ceases to be a problem.

The remedy can be simple. Normals can simply indicate that they want the individual to participate, leaving to him or her the decision of whether or not to become involved. Perhaps the disabled individual would like to participate in a different way. The young adult who has juvenile arthritis may not regret being unable to go fishing if he or she can elect to go along and spend time socializing with friends (Ladieu-Leviton et al., 1977).

Professional Attitudes: Care versus Cure

Traditionally, the goal of health care has been to cure the client. Even today, health care providers tend to measure success in this way. Since chronic disease is now more prevalent than infectious disease or acute illness, this criterion of success may be inappropriate. Cure is neither essential nor necessary in order that the client benefit (Kübler-Ross, 1969). Rather, caring should be the criterion. With the increasing number of people who have chronic diseases, providers must learn to accept the characteristics of chronic disease: an indeterminate course of disease, relapses, and multiple treatment modalities. Today cost containment is a central focus in health care delivery. But providers must not lose sight of health policy considerations that include ideas of personhood and equitable health care sensitive to the reality of stigmatizing chronic illness (Mechanic, 1991).

Selecting an Appropriate Model for Health Care Delivery The manner in which health care is delivered may increase or decrease the effects of stigma. Encouraging a client's participation in health care decision making is an outward demonstration of respect and regard for that person. Treating a client as a partner in establishing goals demonstrates one's acceptance of the individual as valuable. On the other hand, when health providers make decisions regarding treatment or goals without consulting a client, they reinforce the clients' feeling of being discredited. Therefore, any mode of delivery that increases client participation enhances that person's perception of self-worth and therefore reduces the effects of stigma.

All provider–client encounters fall into one of three basic health care delivery models (Szasz & Hollander, 1956). For reasons of stigma management as well as chronic disease manage-

ment, it is wise to determine which model of health care delivery is most appropriate for chronic conditions.

Active–Passive The active-passive encounter is not really an interaction, since the client is acted upon and makes no contribution to decision making; the provider is the only active participant. This model is analogous to the relationship between a helpless infant and its parent. In emergency situations, this model may be the most appropriate one, but this form of encounter essentially says that the client is unable to participate in decision making.

Guidance–Cooperation A client seeks help from a provider and is willing to cooperate in the guidance-cooperation model. This model implies that the client is expected to respect and obey the health provider; the power is unequal because the client is not expected to question the provider's recommendations. This model of health care delivery makes up the majority of traditional client–provider encounters and is valuable with many acute illnesses. However, it allows little, if any, room for clients' expectations or goals, which may be different from those of the provider.

Mutual Participation Mutual participation divides power between provider and client evenly and leads to a relationship that can be mutually satisfying. In other words, the client should be as satisfied with the recommendations and decisions as the provider is. In addition, each party depends on the other for information culminating in that satisfactory solution. The client needs the provider's experience and expertise; the provider needs not only the client's history and symptoms but his or her priorities, expectations, and goals. Sometimes a choice between treatments with relatively equal mortality rates is necessary—for example, surgery or radiation for cancer treatment. The physician can offer expert knowledge regarding long-term effects of radiation and changes in body image due to surgery. The client must decide the relative value of side effects of the alternative proposed treatments. Because the "right" decision depends on the individual, input from both client and health care provider is necessary to produce a course of action that is mutually acceptable.

An important factor in combating stigma is to allow individuals who have limitations the opportunity to become "central participants in the battle" (Dudley, 1983). If the provider dominates the interaction, fuller client involvement does not result. The traditional models of client–provider interaction that give power and the right to decision making to the provider must give way to one that allows increased client participation.

When providers become more comfortable with allowing clients a greater range of participation and decision making, the relationship decreases some of the stigmatizing effects of the disability. Wise health professionals create an atmosphere in which individuals with chronic conditions not only are expected to cooperate, but are encouraged to express their concerns, observations, expectations, and limitations.

The mutual participation model is the model of choice in stigmatizing chronic diseases, since it enhances the client's feelings of self-worth. The client is responsible for long-term disease management, and the health care provider is responsible for helping the client help himself or herself (Szasz & Hollander, 1956). Together, they explore alternative strategies and decide on one that is agreeable to both.

Attempts to shelter or protect clients may well decrease participation and therefore perceptions of worth and value. When a client's priorities and goals are valued and incorporated into the regimen, an increased sense of acceptance emerges. Therefore, the respect and regard for clients demonstrated by this model provide an effective tool to counteract some stigmatizing effects of illness.

Another benefit of a mutual participation model is increased compliance with medical regimen. In chronic disease, the client carries out the regimen; therefore, compliance becomes a particularly important issue (see Chapter 10, on compliance). Relationships between clients and practitioners that are collegial rather than authoritarian are associated with more compliance. The need for compliance provides further rein-forcement for the use of a mutual participation model that increases the client's responsibility for health care. Thus, instead of wondering why the client does not comply with recommendations, providers might consider recommending an acceptable plan.

Inservice Training   Health care providers' attitudes are representative of general societal views and so can be expected to include prejudices. Since health professionals have prolonged relationships with chronically ill individuals, the impact of these prejudices can be great. Training programs to teach professional and nonprofessional staff to identify and correct preconceived and often unconscious notions of categories and stereotypes deserve high priority (Dudley, 1983).

One study of stigma-promoting behaviors provides ideas for health care providers who wish to change their attitudes (Dudley, 1983). The most frequent stigma-promoting behaviors included the following: inappropriate language in referring to clients, inappropriate restrictions of activities, violation of confidentiality, physical abuse, denial of opportunities for clients to present views, ignoring clients, and staring.

An effective way to increase awareness is through planned contact with stigmatized individuals. This approach should be preceded by group work with a knowledgeable leader who can help identify and work through attitudes and reactions. For example, many nursing students do not like skilled nursing facilities (SNFs) because elderly clients are seen as unappealing. A gerontological nurse specialist spent time with such a group of students before they began working in the facility. Her slides of faces etched with character and stories of interesting experiences helped the students see the elderly as human beings. A group discussion confronted myths and stereotypical thinking regarding the stigma of aging. As a result, these students had a more positive experience at the facility. Knowledgeable preparation for contact with stigmatized individuals does not solve all problems; it is, however, one way to expose stigmatized reactions such as stereotypes, to examine them, and to provide information to caregivers.

CASE STUDY
Dealing with Stigma

As the result of an auto accident, Jo, a 44-year-old homemaker with two children, was left with residual neurological damage to her legs. Ten days after the accident, she was in a rehabilitation hospital being trained to stand, walk, and perform activities of daily living. Her prognosis for a full recovery was guarded. Jo had been a jogger and had enjoyed backpacking with her family. She was now faced with a wheelchair, a walker, decreased sensation and movement, and an inability to care for herself, much less her family. Her familiar sources of identity, self-worth, and satisfaction were severely challenged.

Fortunately for Jo, many of the caregivers were direct and shared realistic information with her. These caregivers treated her as a normal person, rather than a discredited one. The rehabilitation center's counselor immediately began a series of therapy sessions and acted as one of the "the wise." No subject was taboo as the two confronted sexuality, body image, and self-esteem. She did not feel rejected by the nursing staff, nor was she allowed any secondary gains at this institution. She was treated as a person who would take care of herself to the maximum of her capabilities—a worthwhile individual, not a stigmatized one.

Her family was intimately involved in Jo's care. They participated in physical therapy so that they would know what to expect and would not be afraid or overprotective; they and Jo were also involved with long-term planning. Exercise regimens and medications for muscle spasm, for instance, were planned *with* Jo, not *for* her.

As time passed, Jo regained enough function to walk with a cane and supportive shoes, although she was slow and awkward. There were fewer stigmatizing orthopedic appliances at this stage, but everyone realized Jo would never run again. She was supported by others who have gone through catastrophic events of many sorts—

"the own." Friends and family have become "wise" by continuing to acknowledge that the important parts of Jo have not changed; that is, the physical limitations are not relevant to the quality of interpersonal relationships. She was supported by friends and family who did everyday tasks—errands, cleaning, food preparation. She did not need and would not have appreciated being smothered with their kindness, however. Further, as she grappled with all of these adjustments, she was relieved of an enormous emotional burden by a husband who continued to accept her.

Everyone, however, did not react to Jo in a supportive manner. Some people, upon seeing her cane or walker, began to speak to her as though she were mentally handicapped. Others ignored this equipment completely, probably out of an intention to treat her kindly. Jo prefers that people ask about her cane. An inquiry provides an opportunity for her to reply as she chooses. She suggests, "Acknowledge, don't ignore."

Now, four years later, Jo continues to have muscle weakness, muscle spasm, and pain. She walks with low-heeled shoes, sometimes using a cane. She has resumed cooking and light housekeeping and recently began graduate school to become a counselor. The family spends more time attending musical performances and eating out at restaurants, all of which Jo can manage quite well. She has rejoined her church activities, as well as neighborhood social groups.

The residual pain and limitations are not trivial. However, these problems would be compounded if they were coupled with the burden of stigma. Fortunately, the reactions of health care professionals, family, and friends have greatly reduced the effects of stigma. This direct, accepting response may well have contributed to Jo's determination to focus on the positive and the possible.

The attitudes of nonprofessional staff also must be included, since they provide much of the care, in community and agency settings. The attitudes and behaviors of these caregivers can promote or decrease the process of stigmatiza-

tion (Volinn, 1983). Providing intensive staff education for the purpose of reducing stigma perception by all employees in any particular agency is beneficial. The group sessions described earlier may be appropriate for both nonprofessional and professional caregivers. In addition, professional staff are in a position to practice role model behavior and to give informal information to help nonprofessional staff treat clients in an accepting manner.

Community Education Programs

Educational programs that reduce the effects of stigma can be carried to the community at large. Many organizations, such as the American Cancer Society and the American Diabetes Association, provide speakers or literature in the community. Educational programs for young children, who are still being socialized, would be effective in preventing the formation of stigma-producing attitudes (Dudley, 1983). Schools, scout troops, and church groups are ideal settings for sensitive introductions of individuals who have many positive values and characteristics but do not meet normal health expectations. For instance, individuals with AIDS have been the focus of group discussions in which children learn to see them simply as other human beings. Educational programs, such as ones that dispel the belief in a moral nature of alcoholism, reduce the stigmatizing effects of that disease (Moore, 1992).

In addition to formal community education programs, society's attitudes might be changed by increasing contact with disabled individuals. The amount of rewarding, mutual interaction between normal and chronically ill individuals can be increased. For instance, one might encourage service projects, pen pals, and outings between groups of normals and the disabled such as the blind or deaf.

The media can be influenced to present a more positive portrayal of chronically ill people. Providers and others can write to commend television networks that show disabled individuals functioning well. Finally, the client's family must be involved in the treatment program, both for short-term and long-term planning.

Summary and Conclusions

This chapter has followed the evolution of the concept of stigma to its present meaning: a mark of discredit. Stigma is caused by a discrepancy between an expected, socially defined norm and an actual attribute. This discrepancy, or defect, attaches a value judgment to its owner: It becomes the stigma. The person is discredited and less valuable. The discrediting and socially isolating effects of stigma transcend any limitations imposed by the actual disease or disability.

Chronic diseases are an everyday example of stigmatized conditions. Shortened life span, physical deformities, medical and dietary requirements, and other limitations are not considered normal and cause anxiety among others who do not have these characteristics. This anxiety is met with the same kinds of prejudicial responses that have occurred throughout the ages: stereotyping, devaluing, and labeling. The affected individuals, in an effort to limit the impact of such responses, use techniques such as resisting and passing.

Several helpful interventions have been discussed. All individuals must redefine the criteria by which they value others and themselves, reexamining their definition of a person's worth. The stigmatized individual benefits from the support of like others and from learning to cope with negative responses. Health care providers are encouraged to become "the wise" and to act as knowledgeable and sensitive advocates for individuals bearing the stigma of chronic disease. In addition, a model of health care delivery characterized by a more equitable sharing of power and goals must be developed. Teaching becomes a valuable tool to create change. Inservice education for professionals and nonprofessionals can increase sensitivity to behaviors that encourage stigma-producing attitudes. Societal education is also necessary to make inroads into underlying causes of stigma.

The preceding are general ways of dealing with stigma. As mentioned earlier, helping others to manage the effects of stigma is not simple. The health care provider who tries to deal with this problem in toto may be wrestling with overpowering problems. However, choosing a single technique that reduces stigma's effects and devoting one's energy to improving or correcting that particular component can produce positive results.

NURSING DIAGNOSIS

Editor's Note: There are no specific diagnostic categories for stigma. However, the following diagnostic categories could be implied from the content of this chapter.

3.1.2 Social Isolation

(See Chapter 8, on isolation, for definition, defining characteristics, related factors, and discussion about this category.)

OR

3.2.1 Altered Role Performance

(See Chapter 4, on illness roles, for definition, defining characteristics, related factors, and discussion about this category.)

OR POSSIBLY

7.1.2.2 Situational Low Self-Esteem

Definition: Negative self evaluation/feelings about self that develop in response to a loss or change in an individual who previously had a positive self-evaluation.

Defining Characteristics:

Major: Episodic occurrence of negative self-appraisal in response to life events in a person with a previous positive self-evaluation; verbalization of negative feelings about the self (helplessness, uselessness).

Minor: Self-negating verbalization; expressions of shame/guilt; evaluates self as unable to handle situations/events; difficulty making decisions.

Related Factors: None noted.

A differential diagnosis would need to be made among the three nursing diagnoses noted above, depending on assessment of the client or situation. With each of these the causative or contributing (related) factor would be the stigma itself or the basis for the individual being stigmatized, such as being stereotyped.

STUDY QUESTIONS

1. How would you use Goffman's theory to identify potential sources of stigma in a population of nonwhite, low-income individuals with high rates of hypertension, diabetes, and arthritis?
2. What strategies would you use to reduce the effects of stigma in a specific client family? Use the example of a child who has cerebral palsy and whose mother is responsible for his exercises and special care. Identify strategies to reduce the effects of stigma for the mother and for the child.
3. What stigmatizing situations could arise for disabled individuals at a summer outing that involves food, games, and outdoor activities? What procedures could prevent or reduce the effects?
4. How do various client participation models of health care delivery differ in terms of their effect on potential or actual stigma?
5. What are the benefits and costs of increasing client participation in health care delivery? If a client chooses not to accept a recommended diet or exercise regimen, how can this choice be managed so that stigma is not increased?
6. What reactions to personal and clinical experiences of stigma has a chronically ill person of your acquaintance had? What strategies does this person use to lessen the effects of the stigma?

References

Allen, M., & Birse, E. (1991). Stigma and blindness. *Journal of Opthalmic Nursing and Technology, 10*(4), 147-152.

Allport, G. (1954). *The nature of prejudice.* Reading, MA: Addison-Wesley.

Becker, G. (1981). Coping with stigma: Lifelong adaptation of deaf people. *Social Science and Medicine, 15B*(1), 21-24.

Burns, D. (1980). *Feeling good: The new mood therapy.* New York: William Morrow.

Cash, T., Briddell, D., Gillen, B., & MacKinnon, C. (1984). When alcoholics are not anonymous: Socioperceptual effects of labeling and drinking patterns. *Journal of Studies on Alcohol, 45*(3), 272-275.

Cohen, R., Ruckdeschel, J., Blanchard, C., Rohrbaugh, M., & Horton, J. (1982). Attitudes toward cancer. *Cancer, 50,* 1218-1223.

Domenici, P. (1993). Mental health care policy in the 1990s: Discrimination in health care coverage of the seriously mentally ill. *Journal of Clinical Psychiatry, 54,* 5-6.

Dudley, J. (1983). *Living with stigma: The plight of the people who we label mentally retarded.* Springfield, IL: Charles C. Thomas.

English, R. W. (1977). Correlates of stigma toward physically disabled persons. In R. Marinelli & A. Dell Orto (Eds.), *The psychological and social impact of physical disability.* New York: Springer.

Fabrega, H. (1991). The culture and history of psychiatric stigma in early modern and modern Western societies: A review of recent literature. *Comprehensive Psychiatry, 32*(2), 97-119.

Gallo, A., Breitmayer, B., Knafl, K., & Zoeller, L. (1991). Stigma in childhood chronic illness: A well sibling perspective. *Pediatric Nursing, 17*(1), 21-25.

Goffman, E. (1963). *Stigma: Notes on management of spoiled identity.* Englewood Cliffs, NJ: Prentice-Hall.

Hainsworth, M, Burke, M., Lindgren, C., & Eakes, G. (1993). Chronic sorrow in multiple sclerosis: A case study. *Home Healthcare Nurse, 11*(2), 9-13.

Herek, G., & Capitanio, J. (1993). Public reactions to AIDS in the United States: A second decade of stigma. *American Journal of Public Health, 83*(4), 574-577.

Hooper, S. (1981). Diabetes as a stigmatized condition: The case of low income clinic patient in the United States. *Social Science and Medicine 15B*(1) 11-19.

Katz, I. (1981). *Stigma: A social psychological analysis.* Hillsdale, NJ: Lawrence Erlbaum Associates.

Kübler-Ross, E. (1969). *On death and dying.* New York: Macmillan.

Ladieu-Leviton, G., Adler, D., & Dembo, T. (1977). Studies in adjustment to visible injuries: Social acceptance of the injured. In R. Marinelli & A. Dell Orto (Eds.), *The psychological and social impact of the physical disability.* New York: Springer.

Lemert, E. (1972). *Human deviance, social problems, and social control* (2nd ed.). Englewood Cliffs, NJ: Prentice-Hall.

Link, B., Mirotznik, J., & Cullen, F. (1991). The effectiveness of stigma coping orientations: Can negative consequences of mental illness labeling be avoided? *Journal of Health and Social Behavior, 32*(3), 302-320.

Luken, P. (1987). Social identity in later life: A situational approach to understanding old age stigma. *International Journal of Aging and Human Development, 25*(3), 177-193.

Lynd, H. M. (1958). *On shame and the search for identity.* New York: Harcourt Brace Jovanovich.

McGrath, J. (1992). The biological impact of social responses to the AIDS epidemic. *Medical Anthropology, 15*(1), 63-79.

Mechanic, D. (1991). Changing perspectives in the study of the social role of medicine. *Milbank Quarterly, 69*(2), 215-232.

Moore, J. (1992). Conceptions of alcoholism. *International Journal of the Addictions, 27*(8), 935-945.

Piner, K., & Kahle, L. (1984). Adapting to the stigmatizing label of mental illness: Foregone but not forgotten. *Journal of Personality and Social Psychology, 47*(4), 805-811.

Powell-Cope, G., & Brown, M. (1992). Going public as an AIDS family caregiver. *Social Sciences in Medicine, 34*(5), 571-580.

Roget's International Thesaurus (4th ed.) (1977). New York: Thomas Y. Crowell.

Shontz, E. (1977). Physical disability and personality: Theory and recent research. In R. Marinelli & A. Dell Orto (Eds.), *The psychological and social impact of physical disability.* New York: Springer.

Siminoff, L., Erien, J., & Lidz, C. (1991). Stigma, AIDS and quality of nursing care: State of the science. *Journal of Advanced Nursing, 16*(3), 262-269.

Sims, A. (1993). The scar that is more than skin deep: The stigma of depression. *British Journal of General Practice, 43*(366), 30-31.

Sontag, S. (1977). *Illness as metaphor.* New York: Farrar, Straus & Giroux.

Szasz, T., & Hollander, M. (1956). A contribution to the philosophy of medicine. *American Medical Association Archives of Internal Medicine, 97,* 585-592.

Volinn, I. (1983). Health professionals as stigmatizers and destigmatizers of diseases: Alcoholism and leprosy as examples. *Social Science and Medicine, 17*(7), 385-393.

Webster's Third New International Dictionary (1986). Springfield, MA: G. & C. Merriam.

Westbrook, M., Legge, V., & Pennay, M. (1993). Attitudes toward disabilities in a multicultural society. *Social Sciences in Medicine, 36*(5), 615-623.

CHAPTER 6

Altered Mobility

Katheliene Kohler •
Mary Therese Schweikert-Stary • *Ilene Lubkin*

Introduction

To observe people is often to observe them in motion: children running and jumping, adults walking and jogging. Being in motion is a natural state of the human body. Imagine not being able to move freely or pick up objects with your hands. Picture yourself bedridden or dependent on an assistive device. Think of yourself as restricted because you are unable to see where you are going or hear the sound of danger. In all these situations some kind of mobility has been lost.

Without the ability to move, we lose independence and our world shrinks. Mobility allows us to function independently and to enjoy leisure and recreational activities at will. Participation in formal education is enhanced and enriched by independent mobility; employment often requires the ability to get around, especially to and from the work setting. Access to medical services and health resources may be limited for an individual who is unable to get to them freely.

Mobility can be defined as "the act of going from one place to another safely and effectively . . . making full use of whatever mechanical, technological, or human resources that are needed" (Goodman, 1989). These needs tend to change throughout life. Children are usually active, whereas adults lead a more sedentary, but still mobile, existence. Most aged individuals are still active and involved, despite the common association of aging with lessened activity and often chronic illness.

Diseases, especially chronic ones, may affect mobility. How does the person who has undergone a change in mobility make necessary adjustments? How does society treat such a person? What are the potentially ego-shattering and psychological effects on human beings who have lost some degree of mobility? How do these changes effect family relationships, self-esteem, and self-motivation? And how can people deal with societal and environmental barriers that inhibit maximum independence? Within the person's environment, impaired physical mobility creates potential or actual limitations on independent physical movement (Carpenito, 1989).

Problems of Altered Mobility

Health professionals usually think of altered or impaired mobility in terms of bedrest, "confinement" to a wheelchair, or loss of the use of upper or lower body extremities. In other words, mobility changes are seen as apparent musculoskeletal impairment.

But mobility alterations can involve other aspects of an individual's life. Mobility can be influenced by sensory loss, pain, or energy depletion, none of which directly involve the musculoskeletal system. A person's freedom of movement is restricted by almost any kind of disability or chronic illness, and this restriction becomes a common underlying theme of almost any illness (Goodman, 1989). In addition, mobility loss tends to occur in patterns: intermittent, progressive, or permanent, or combinations thereof. Regardless of pattern, alterations in mobility are associated with psychosocial problems that affect the client and significant others. This chapter touches on these factors.

Bedrest

First we should look at the effects of bedrest. Although illness is often measured by the length of time spent in bed (Asher, 1983), extended periods of bedrest may not always be efficacious because, beneath the comfort of the blanket, there lurks a host of formidable dangers. Even a few days of bedrest result in adverse effects on body systems and on psychosocial equilibrium (Groer & Skekleton, 1989; Kemp & Pilloterri, 1984; Olsen et al., 1967; Sorenson & Luckman, 1986). This observation has prompted physicians to insist that their bedridden patients sit up as soon as possible. Interestingly, altered physiological responses associated with bedrest are not abnormal; they are the body's attempts to optimize its functions and to enhance its survival potential (Greenleaf & Kozlowski, 1982). (See Table 6-1.)

Bedrest is a restricted level of activity often necessitated by illness, either acute or chronic. In acute illness, for example, when surgery is necessary, periods of bedrest tend to be temporary, improvement is expected, and complications are uncommon. Recovery and rehabilitation are relatively short in duration, with body functions quickly regained: The individual rapidly regains mobility, independence, and, by society's standards, productivity.

Unlike acute illness, many chronic disease states demand longer or more frequent periods of bedrest. For long-term bedrest, the effects may be irreversible. Through selected interventions, nursing goals may consist of maintaining homeostasis and some functional capacity. Such interventions may include the prevention of complications of decreased mobility, increased endurance, and the promotion of an optimal level of mobility (Carpenito, 1989).

Cardiovascular Effects Even three days of bedrest cause changes in the cardiovascular system. These changes include decreased venous flow with increased probability of thrombus formation and decreased orthostatic tolerance, resulting in dizziness or fainting upon resuming an upright position. Following prolonged periods of bedrest, fatigue or weakness results from limited periods of exertion (Olson et al., 1967). Goldman (1977) found that healthy young adult males, after three to six weeks of bedrest, required at least six weeks to regain full cardiac function.

Respiratory Effects The respiratory system shows a decrease in oxygen transport capacity after short-term bedrest. In his study of healthy young adult males, Goldman (1977) found that respiratory deconditioning included an 18 percent decrease in maximum oxygen uptake. The increased oxygen debt led to lactic acidemia and symptomatic fatigue with exertion. Recovery of respiratory function required two to five weeks (Goldman, 1977). Lack of oxygenation and fatigue, coupled with decreased coughing ability and increased hypostatic pooling, can lead to increased risk of atelectasis (Olson et al., 1967).

Musculoskeletal Effects Regardless of age, musculoskeletal changes can significantly reduce the ability of the client to resume normal activity. Demineralization of bone is thought to be secondary to the decreased stress on long bones in the upper and lower legs (Olson et al., 1967). Muscle mass and strength diminish without frequent stress and work demands on the muscle. An aged individual with decreased bone density and muscle mass has increased risk of fractures. A decreased ability to resume activities of daily living leads to slower recovery. Limited joint mobility results in decreased range of motion and lack of joint stability, and leads eventually to contractures (Olson et al., 1967). Prolonged

TABLE 6-1. Effects of bedrest

CARDIOVASCULAR
1. Hypotension: neurovascular reflex control decreases, producing decreased muscle tone and decreased muscle action on veins.
2. Increased workload on heart: Changes in resistance and pressures lead to redistribution of blood and increased circulation. The Valsalva maneuver increases intrathoracic pressure.
3. Thrombus formation: Thrombi form secondary to venous stasis, hyper-coagulability, external pressure on legs.

PULMONARY
1. Decreased basal metabolism reflects a lessened cellular oxygen need; carbon dioxide production decreases.
2. Chest expansion is limited (compression), muscle power and coordination diminish, and compliance and elastic recoil decrease.
3. Increased secretions resulting from less effective coughing, pooling, and thickening lead to hypostatic pneumonia.
4. Poor ventilation and gas exchange results in carbon dioxide retention and hypoxemia with eventual respiratory acidosis.

MUSCULOSKELETAL
1. Contractures: Disuse leads to atrophy and loss of muscle tone and mass. The integrity of muscle function (lengthening and shortening of muscle fibers) lessens, leading to an imbalance between opposing muscles (spasm) and decreased function of ligaments, tendons, and joint capsule (decreased range of motion).
2. Osteoporosis: The absence of weight-bearing stress on the skeleton causes a decrease in osteoblastic function; osteoclastic action continues.
3. Decubitus: Increased pressure and decreased circulation lead to decreased nutrition and ischemia; necrosis and ulceration can develop with eventual osteomyelitis or systemic infection.

GENITOURINARY
1. Calculi: Stasis occurs when urine must move against gravity; infection can result. Urine becomes more alkaline. Stasis and alkalinity plus protein breakdown and bone demineralization increase minerals and salts that need to be excreted; any particle can become the nucleus for formation of a renal calculus.

2. Voiding: Difficulty relaxing the pelvic muscles for micturition causes distention and overflow incontinence, leading to skin breakdown and lowered self-esteem; voiding difficulties can lead to reflux and kidney damage. In-dwelling catheters help drain the bladder, but invariably lead to infection.

GASTROINTESTINAL
1. Negative nitrogen balance results from increased catabolic activity (protein breakdown) and anorexia (common with many illnesses). Stress (parasympathetic stimulation) can lead to dyspepsia, distention, anorexia, diarrhea, or constipation.
2. Constipation is secondary to several factors: Malnutrition and decreased exercise cause muscle atrophy and loss of tone; decreased response to defecation reflex occurs secondary to unnatural position and disruption of familiar patterns, and withdrawal of water from fecal material in the bowel causes hard, dry stools.

METABOLISM
1. Decreased metabolic rate, tissue atrophy, and protein catabolism occur. There is bone demineralization; anabolic processes are retarded while catabolic activity accelerates.
2. Body temperature: Heat conduction and radiation are lessened by bed clothing. Sweating increases wherever skin surfaces touch, contributing to fluid and electrolyte loss.
3. The supine position reduces the production of adrenocortical hormones, which affects the metabolism of carbohydrate, protein, and fat, and affects electrolyte balance.

PSYCHOLOGICAL
1. Motivation and ability to learn and retain information decrease; ability to problem-solve lessens.
2. Emotional behavior becomes exaggerated and manifests as apathy, withdrawal, anger, aggression, or regression; drives are diminished.
3. Body image is altered. There is a loss of feelings of self-esteem, self-worth, and pride.
4. Efficiency of sensory processes is reduced, leading to sensory deprivation that in turn causes a decrease in perception. Time distortion occurs.
5. Role activities and drives change; roles are altered, reversed, or eliminated.

SOURCE: Summarized from Olsen et al. (1967).

pressure, inadequate nutrition, and other factors lead to decubitus ulcers; often slow to heal, such open wounds make the body susceptible to systemic infection (Olson et al., 1967).

Genitourinary Effects Bladder emptying is incomplete in the supine position. An indwelling catheter aids in draining the bladder, but may result in infection and perhaps bladder dysfunction such as incontinence. Urinary stasis in the renal pelvis due to dorsal recumbency fosters both infection and calculi formation (Goldman, 1977). The kidneys filter larger amounts of minerals and salts, which are released into the blood plasma as a consequence of hemo-dynamic and metabolic changes. The passing of renal calculi, usually composed of calcium salts, may injure the mucosal lining and increase the urinary tract's susceptibility to infection (Olson et al., 1967).

Gastrointestinal Effects Bedrest leads to psychological and mechanical effects on gastro-intestinal function, especially ingestion and elimination (Olson et al., 1967). The loss of appetite, perhaps initially from stress or pain, leads to anorexia, which in turn results in a negative nitrogen balance (Greenleaf & Kozlowski, 1982). Bowel dysfunction, constipation, and fecal impactions, along with accompanying discomfort, may well undo many of the goals that necessitated bedrest.

Metabolic Effects Immobility markedly reduces both the energy requirements of cells and their metabolic processes. Bedrest interferes with metabolic homeostasis, influencing the efficiency of homeostatic mechanisms. Functional changes include reduced metabolic rate, tissue atrophy, protein catabolism, bone demineralization, alterations in the exchange of nutrients and other substances between extracellular and intracellular fluids, fluid and electrolyte imbalance, and gastrointestinal hyper- or hypomotility (Olson et al., 1967).

Psychosocial Effects Dependency, depression, and dissociation are common. Changes in body image also occur. The dependent person often overreacts to perceived threats to self-image. The anxious or depressed person interprets required bedrest as serious illness. Problem-solving ability decreases, motivation lessens, and discriminatory ability decreases (Olson et al., 1967). When bedrest is prescribed for aged individuals, hazards become much graver because of reduced reserve; death is frequently an outcome (Goldman, 1977). Immobility often sets the stage for the expression of either exaggerated or inappropriate emotional reactions; for example, individuals may voice expressions of loss of personal worth, fear, wounded pride, guilt, disgust, or anger.

Patterns of Mobility Alteration

In most chronic illnesses, bedrest is only a temporary phase. Most of the time people with chronic illnesses follow patterns of activity and altered mobility; some of these patterns are quite characteristic of certain diseases. Although each of these patterns is described here as if it were a separate entity, one must remember that affected individuals may fluctuate between patterns, depending on the activity of the disease or on the current situation. As an example, the client with Type II diabetes shows *intermittent* changes in mobility patterns when blood sugar levels vary radically, resulting in hyper- or hypoglycemia. Later, when chronic complications set in, the same individual either shows a *progressive* pattern or stabilizes at a *permanent* level. Such movement between patterns of mobility is demonstrated in most chronic illnesses.

Intermittent Changes in Mobility Intermittent changes come and go, often at unpredictable times (see Figure 6–1). This unpredictability creates difficulty for client or family in planning activities of any kind because of the ambiguity of tomorrow. Holding a job, participating in social events, or planning other activities becomes uncertain.

Frequently, intermittent mobility patterns have a variety of recurrent physiological responses or effects. As an example, the client with arthritis may experience episodes of weakness, pain, and swelling of joints. Classically, clients with intermittent mobility have sporadic rises in energy and activity occurring during phases of

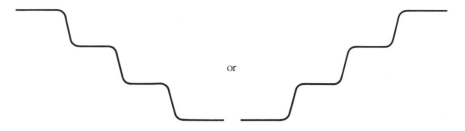

FIGURE 6-1.   Intermittent Pattern of Altered Mobility

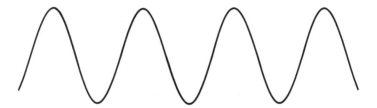

FIGURE 6-2.   Progressive Pattern of Altered Mobility

remission or when the client feels better. In other words, overactivity becomes an overcompensation for the function loss that occurs at other times. This behavior pattern tends to exhaust the individual and in turn leads to more episodes of bedrest than might otherwise be necessary.

Progressive Changes in Mobility Progressive changes continue over time in a given steplike direction (see Figure 6-2). A negative progression has continuous downward steps; a positive direction demonstrates some kind of improvement. An individual with multiple sclerosis (MS), for example, may show steplike deterioration over time, whereas a person with a myocardial infarction may progress to increased activity. Stabilization at a plateau sometimes occurs, providing opportunities for client and family to adjust before another change occurs. In some disease states, progressive immobility is associated with physical or functional decline, pain, or fatigue.

Psychological responses are associated with the steplike quality of progressive changes. Downward progression often has physical and emotional components that make client or family coping difficult. Should the strain become excessive, major disruption of family cohesiveness may result. Some families have greater adaptive ability than others and are less disrupted by these changes. Even positive progression can have adverse effects. Expectations for continued improvement can exceed the client's potential or ability; client and family may be greatly disappointed when their hopes are not realized.

For example, multiple sclerosis is a chronic, complex neurological disease, characterized by exacerbations and remissions, that primarily affects young adults with a mean age of 33 (Clark, 1991). The nerves affected, the seriousness of the symptoms, and the pattern of recovery or deterioration vary from one person to another. Coping with the unpredictability of this disease presents its own source of stress, making it difficult to plan ahead with any certainty and requiring most affected people to take one day at a time (Trieschmann, 1987).

Permanent Change in Mobility Permanence refers to mobility loss that does not vary, assuming that good maintenance care is provided (see Figure 6-3). Permanent change can occur after a period of intermittent or progressive change, but frequently results from sudden

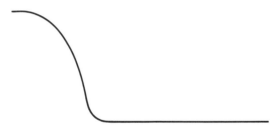

FIGURE 6-3. Permanent Pattern of Altered Mobility

trauma or injury, as with spinal cord injuries (SCIs) or cerebral vascular accidents (CVAs). Damage to the central nervous system, with its instantaneous effect of paralysis, results in major life-style disruption and thus places a heavy burden of financial, emotional, and psychosocial demands on the client and significant others, especially in the beginning. Adjustment may be slow and painful; however, if it is achieved, the family functions in a reasonably stable way.

The client with rheumatoid arthritis (RA) is representative of changes from one mobility level to another. Some forms of RA are chronic systemic disorders associated with restricted activity, deformity or disfigurement, expense, and physical and emotional pain.

Pam's case study, which illustrates the effects of changes in mobility, demonstrates movement from one level to another. (We will return to Pam's case throughout this chapter.)

Sensory Loss

Generally, one does not associate mobility alteration with sensory problems, since loss of sensory function does not directly affect the musculoskeletal system. However, inability to see or to hear has a great impact on ability to move freely in one's environment. The more severe the loss, the more it affects mobility (Goodman, 1989).

Visual Loss Visual loss alters mobility indirectly. Ease of travel decreases, since most of our cues for moving about are visual. Diminished cues prevent individuals with partial visual loss from having full awareness of stairs, pathways,

curbs, or obstacles. Loss of access to visual information is restricting because if one is unable to read signs, directions, and printed material, the ability to act on that information is lost.

Visual impairment adversely impacts independent living; loss of the ability to perceive the environment makes ambulating precarious. Eye changes can also cause light and glare sensitivity and reduced color perception (Genesky, 1981). Visual impairment reduces grooming skills and can cause hesitancy in going out in public.

The impact of visual loss depends on visually impaired people's development of spatial ability (Pick, 1980). *Spatial ability* encompasses organizing information so that the individual senses how to get from one area to another by interpreting incoming nonvisual stimulation. Additionally, the selection of travel aids (a cane, a guide dog, or a sighted guide) affects potential travel routes. For example, an individual who has a guide dog moves about comfortably in familiar territory but may experience difficulty when traveling in unfamiliar territory.

Hearing Impairment Persons with hearing loss usually have few mobility problems in the physical environment. However, they experience indirect obstacles to mobility because they frequently do not possess high oral or written language skills, so communicating their mobility needs is difficult. Even those who are proficient in lip or speech reading are limited in their ability to communicate, since a person with good skills usually understands only about 30 percent of a conversation. As an example, sign language incorporates visual concepts rather than the verbal language structure familiar to those who can hear. Persons with a hearing impairment may be reluctant to solicit needed help or information because of this difference in language skill. They may choose to remain silent if they think their speech is difficult to understand (Goodman, 1989).

Individuals who have hearing losses may be vulnerable to danger because they are unable to hear warning signals. In an emergency they may be immobilized, not knowing what is happening or the best way to move out of danger. Some hearing-impaired persons have less experience in traveling independently if their family and

CASE STUDY
Pam: Changes in Mobility

Pam, now 28, was 13 years old at the onset of juvenile arthritis (JA), rheumatoid type. At age 25, she developed Sjogren's syndrome, manifesting as diminished glandular secretion, resulting in dryness of mucous membranes. During the early years of her illness, Pam had difficulty keeping up with her friends' activities because her levels of energy were lower than theirs. She often found herself bedridden after an active day. Recently, while vacationing in Japan, Pam enthusiastically decided to participate in mountain climbing during a "good" day. She spent the following two days in bed recuperating rather than sightseeing.

As her arthritis progressed, Pam developed ulnar deviation of her hands and finger joints,

necessitating extensive changes in the way she used her hands. She needed a large ring on her keys to allow her to pick up and turn them, kitchen utensils adapted for her use, and so on. Initially, Pam's husband had difficulty understanding her need for these adaptations, but with time they both adjusted.

The permanent quality of changes she faced created problems for Pam, her husband, and her parents. With specialized counseling over several years, Pam eventually accepted her disease and has come to terms with these irreversible changes. Pam realizes that JA is a part of her identity, not a foreign element. Her adaptations are now integrated into everyday living.

---

friends are overprotective (Welsh & Blasch, 1980) and therefore may lack confidence in their ability to travel on their own.

In addition to its obvious adverse effects on mobility, hearing impairment can lead to psychosocial isolation and depression (Herbst, 1983). In the Framingham cohort, 41 percent of those 65 years of age and older admitted to hearing difficulty, but only 10 percent had ever used a hearing aid (Gates et al., 1990).

Pain and Loss of Energy

Pain can be an invisible handicap that becomes a disabling condition in itself. Fatigue or energy loss (for example, caused by multiple sclerosis or rheumatoid arthritis) can be so overwhelming that even being with other people becomes unbearable. Opening doors, driving, and carrying items are tasks that may intensify pain or, because they require energy and agility, become impossible.

Pain   Chronic pain can make life's tasks even more difficult. Everyone feels and responds to pain differently, and because pain is invisible, it may not be understood by others (see Chapter 7, on chronic pain). Some people withdraw from activities because of the unpredictability of the

pain experience. Others try to "tough it out" or may feel guilty for resting on a bad day. Still others may use chronic pain to get special attention or as an excuse for not doing certain things (Arthritis Foundation, 1992; Slonaker, 1992).

PAM: Pain is physically and emotionally draining. Even if you try to keep up with others to the point of total exhaustion and great physical pain, there is no one to confide in about your great emotional pain.

Children suffer from almost the same variety of chronic pain that occurs in adults. Even though effective techniques for pain management in children are available, studies indicate that their pain is not managed as well as pain in adults (U.S. Department of Health and Human Services, 1992). Inadequate pain relief in the young may be due more to a lack of knowledge than to a lack of concern (McCaffery & Beebe, 1989).

Loss of Energy   Many chronic conditions, such as myocardial infarction or chronic obstructive pulmonary disease, cause fatigue that makes mobility more difficult. Although many of these energy-depleting conditions have no visible manifestations, they are nevertheless incapacitating. Even a simple thing such as stepping up onto a curb can seem impossible to a person whose body is receiving inadequate oxygenation.

Energy loss can also develop directly from musculoskeletal problems. Small, simple movements may demand great effort when arthritis has reduced flexibility and range of motion. Painful joints and weak muscles cause an extra work load for normal joints and muscles, so that unaffected areas must "take up the slack" and therefore tire more rapidly. The cyclic nature or intermittent pattern of some diseases increases fatigue because of the tendency to compensate by overexerting when one is feeling well (Gould, 1982).

Depression and frustration, which often accompany chronic diseases, can cause energy loss. The accompanying fatigue may heighten feelings of depression—for example, when the ill individual is unable to complete a favorite activity or to participate in events with friends as in the past. Thus, a vicious circle is created (Arthritis Foundation, 1992; Tack, 1991).

> PAM: It's hard to justify my fatigue to friends and relatives; my husband often asks, "Why are you so tired?" It took an article in the *National Arthritis News* to finally help me convince myself and him that my fatigue was real, physiologically as well as emotionally.

Psychosocial Aspects

Altered mobility affects the total person. Human beings experience life not solely in physical terms but also in psychological and social terms. Decreased mobility impedes one's sense of independence and productivity and ultimately one's sense of worth and social value.

Psychological Effects When physical ability to move changes, a psychological adjustment must occur. Adjustment is a process of redefining self that requires reconstruction of self-image. The mobile, ambulatory person who has difficulty accepting changes in locomotion or agility finds that adaptation rarely entails an agreeable, acceptable, or easy change.

Clients have compared times of adjustment to riding on a roller coaster: constantly challenged or angered by the uphill struggles, never

knowing when another curve will come, and unable to stop the motion. They have a sense of instability during this period of mixed and conflicting emotions, of bewilderment, of helplessness. The process does not move easily or steadily from one stage to the next, but is usually one of inconsistency, questioning, and occasional hopelessness.

Chronically ill children face the same developmental tasks and challenges that healthy children face. The ongoing presence of a disease can significantly alter the child's physical and mental functions as well as their interactions with the environment. Chronically ill children may experience frequent hospitalizations, disruptions in daily living, and alterations in family life (Garrison & McQuiston, 1989).

Loss The emotional response to loss of mobility expresses itself as grieving. This is a process unique to each person, developing at an individual pace, that must be understood as such. Behavioral responses may seem irrational and inappropriate to both client and health provider; the health professional should be aware that this behavior accompanies psychological adaptation. In addition, somatic manifestations (pain, loss of appetite, sleep disturbances, slowed thinking and action) may be symptoms of the grieving and adjustment process (see Chapter 11, on coping with fear and grieving). Guilt, or a sense of needing to be punished, is usually characteristic of this loss (Walker & Lattanzi, 1982): "If only I had done (or had not done) this, then I would not be sick/paralyzed/bedridden." Of course, sorrow accompanies loss—loss of physical function, body image, social status, employment, familiar life-style, or previously stable emotions.

Chronic progressive diseases cause emotional readjustment each time the person must adapt to a new loss of mobility state, just as readjustment may become necessary at each new growth and development level. Recovery from loss (sometimes referred to as *acceptance*) is indicated when the person becomes more open to change, is able to use the experience for personal goals, and again welcomes life (Lattanzi, 1983).

Self-Image One's perspective of self has many components. Body image changes are common when mobility is altered (see chapter 13, on body image). When changes are visible, the client may deny the reality of the visible outer body, viewing it as perfect and totally functioning or as ugly and deformed. Other people may perceive the client's outer body differently and interact on the basis of that perception. When these viewpoints of the body contradict, the client's concept of self may become confused.

Contradictions may also exist in cases of nonvisible chronic illnesses, such as some cardiovascular or respiratory diseases. Although outwardly others may perceive the individual as actively mobile, the inward physique may be intensely altered by illness. The expectations of the client and others may exceed the client's ability to perform many functions.

Self-esteem is also affected. Earle and associates (1979) compared people having RA to those not having the disease and found that subjects with more severe joint disease showed more feelings of lower self-esteem and meaninglessness than those who had less active disease or who were disease free. Such feelings can lead to difficulties in dealing with the disease and can result in depression.

Isolation Impaired mobility may result in a decreased opportunity to socialize. Although client responses and behaviors vary, one can see a host of behaviors that are less acceptable to others: depression, hostility, belligerence, withdrawal, confusion, anxiety, apathy, regression, a decreased ability to concentrate and problem-solve, altered time perception, and increased dependency on others (Potter & Perry, 1991; Olson et al., 1967; Miller, 1975; Stewart, 1986). Clients who exhibit these behaviors may be excluded from social interaction leading to isolation (Mobily & Kelley, 1991). (See Chapter 8, on social isolation.)

Because of the emotional and physical stress associated with relating to others who have a negative or misinformed attitude, individuals may isolate themselves to avoid stigma (see Chapter 5, on stigma). It may appear easier and healthier for a client to remain at home where the social atmosphere is recognizable and the physical environment is constant and manageable. Clients may become passive, less outgoing,

and unable to reach out to others (Goodman, 1989).

> PAM: I had a poor self-image because I was so depressed about the chronic, painful JA and its disfigurement. It's hard when you're a teenager and can't keep up with your physically energetic friends. I spent much of my life in total isolation with no one to talk to about my disease. I consequently denied my JA to myself and to my friends, who couldn't or wouldn't understand.

Fear Fear is a common psychological barrier and interferes with mobility (Goodman, 1989). It emerges when the body suddenly or gradually transforms from functioning in its usual expected manner to responding in an unexpected way to an unknown disease. Anger may erupt because of limited choice. Many individuals have the feeling "Why me?" Fear of rejection and abandonment is common. According to Marsh, Ellison, and Strite (1983), many individuals fear that other people consider them abnormal, deformed, or contagious. Themes include frustration at being handicapped and dependent on others for meeting some needs, frustration and anger concerning disabilities and insensitive treatment by others, reluctance to assert oneself, faulty communications with family members, and an unrealistic expectation that other people should "understand."

An underlying fear may be that of asking for help. For example, an assumed barrier to mobility for the visually impaired is stairs or an inability to read a sign, but the real reluctance in asking for help may be the desire to "pass" as sighted. The hearing impaired may be afraid that others will misunderstand their voice or gestures. Practical fears emerge when one is uncomfortable asking for help—for example, being fearful of getting lost or of not finding a needed restroom—which could lead to embarrassment and hinder further mobility attempts (Goodman, 1989).

Travel The client's ability to move from one location to another is a complex interaction between independent travel and psychological factors (Welsh & Blasch, 1980). Lack of independent travel may lead to increased dependency, isolation, hopelessness, and poor self-concept. The process becomes cyclic, with these factors serving as obstacles to independent movement. On the other hand, successful independent travel improves self-concept, gives a greater sense of independence, and improves motivation for other tasks. Overcoming fear of independent travel requires the development of self-confidence and the acquisition of new mobility skills.

Stress Altered mobility seems to directly increase psychological stress (Goodman, 1989). Stress can exacerbate disease activity or associated pain, as in systemic lupus erythematosus (SLE), and in turn affect mobility. The client is consequently in a double bind: trying to avoid stress because it intensifies the disease, yet experiencing stress by the very nature of the disease. Loss of control produces an attitude of helplessness and depression and may generate a setback in psychological and physical well-being. In the case of SLE, for example, depression may be magnified by emotional stress, normal life tensions, and steroid therapy. For this reason, emotional adjustment to the disease and its effects is very important (Lewis, 1984).

Sociological Effects Disability frequently includes necessary dependence on relatives and professionals. In addition, architectural barriers impact on sociological well-being by preventing access. It is not only pathology that affects the individual, as the medical model suggests; it is also the physical, social, political, and economic environment that limits choices (DeJong & Lifchez, 1983).

Family Family members may face life-style changes necessitated by the immobilized member. Altered home life strains all family members by causing adjustments to accustomed routines. Financial concerns are common, and family members may feel frustrated by an inability to meet the special needs of the ill individual.

Family and client may be at odds in their assessment of the role of independent travel as a contributing factor to a healthy adjustment. Members of the family can be fearful, overprotective, or embarrassed to "expose" the client to the world (Welsh & Blasch, 1980). Because

such fears are real and understandable, health professionals must help the family to overcome their anxieties so they can understand the client's need for independence (see Chapter 12, on family caregivers).

Role Changes Throughout all life stages, mobility allows individuals the opportunity to take on roles set out for them by society; in this way it allows needs satisfaction. Our American culture reflects its value orientation, social attitudes, and norms through role behaviors centering on wellness, work, individual independence, social justice, and social responsibility.

When mobility is altered, accustomed roles may change or appear to change from a familiar status to a perceived dependent role, creating anxiety and a sense of hopelessness. This change occurs through modified physical and occupational activity and through altered sensory and motor interaction (Olson et al., 1967). Concomitantly, leisure time for the recreational role increases, but with diminished physical ability and energy to expend on recreation. The roles of spouse, parent, sibling, sexual partner, and provider may be altered, reversed, or eliminated.

Altered mobility also influences social mobility, since it has consequences of psychological and sociological deprivation that lead to downward movement. In a society that places prime value on the worker role, the nonworker role is generally interpreted as a lesser position, with a consequent lowering of status in the societal hierarchy (Olson et al., 1967); the disabled person experiences diminished personal worth.

Sexual Functioning Mobility changes influence sexual behavior. Depending on the physiological impact of the chronic disease and its physical effects, the individual may be limited in sexual functioning (see Chapter 14, on sexuality). For example, a decreased range of motion, an inability to assume sexual positions or to shift to another position, or the presence of paralysis may cause the person to perceive his or her body as asexual or undesirable. The loss of visual or auditory acuity may impede the ability to see or hear sexual cues. Physical pain may accompany any movement, or chronic fatigue may hinder sexual interest or arousal. If movement changes greatly, the individual may feel unable to "perform" sexually. Guilt or fear can result from an inability to satisfy self or partner.

The altered mobility of one person has an impact on the sexual partner as well. The partner may need a time to adjust to physical differences and may also be affected by psychological reactions the client experiences. The partner may be afraid of causing pain, hesitating to initiate sex or changes in position. A visible mobility aid (braces or a wheelchair) may hinder the "sexual overtones" of sexual cues and arousal.

> PAM: It is difficult to express sensual pleasures—intercourse, touching, holding, hand-holding, hugging—when the body hurts. I often feel pain when trying new positions, which is also affected by my limited range of motion. Sjogren's Syndrome causes dysfunction of saliva and mucous glands, leaving the vagina excessively dry and painful.
>
> Sexual expression was limited. My husband was afraid to try new things and positions sometimes because of fear he might physically hurt me. I was afraid of trying new things because I might hurt myself or cry out in pain and spoil the mood or feel embarrassed. I am now able to tell my husband, either verbally or through gestures, if I feel like assuming other positions—for I do worry about our sex life being boring.

Aging The aging process also effects a decrease in mobility. This change is gradual and is often coupled with psychological adjustment to the aging process itself. The aging client may have decreased vision or hearing or be "slowing down," unable to walk long distances, negotiate stairs or uphill grades, or drive an automobile. The possibility of injury from falling restricts mobility. The previously accessible environment may now contain barriers erected by the elderly person's lessened agility or increased vulnerability to attacks. The elderly may be embarrassed in public situations, feeling that they look older, are less agile, and are not the people they used to be (Welsh & Blasch, 1980; Vandervoort et al., 1990).

Add a chronic disease to these elements, and the problem is multiplied. Since aging and illness often accompany each other, the elderly person may lose the ability, desire, or encouragement to maintain a previous state of mobility. The fear of falling, for example, is a common deterrent to ambulation. Even though most falls do not cause injuries, one fall can be devastating to an individual's pride and confidence (Ham, 1984). The case study of Grandpa illustrates the impact of aging and illness on mobility.

Barriers: Societal and Architectural Barriers diminish an individual's quality of life. In the broadest sense, they include physiological, psychological, and social difficulties that limit chronically ill persons whose mobility is altered. Depending on perspective, they may be environmental or architectural obstacles only, or they may encompass social attitudes as well. Even though societal and architectural barriers seem to be mutually exclusive, there is a tremendous overlap that affects employment, education, transportation, and social activities.

Attitudes Of all the barriers that disabled or chronically ill people experience, the strongest and most difficult to eliminate are societal attitudes. One's feelings about oneself are often affected by the attitudes of others; one's behavior is ruled by attitudes. Even more so, laws, rules, and even etiquette are governed by individual or group attitudes.

Family attitudes can prevent the client from achieving his or her maximum potential. Sometimes people close to the person with limited mobility may foster dependency, believing that doing so reduces injury (Goodman, 1989). A study of attitudes of spouses of stroke patients found that the spouses responded primarily with overprotective and unrealistic attitudes rather than expected feelings of rejection or guilt (Kinsella & Duffy, 1980). This response was usually based on anxiety about the client's condition: Sometimes overprotecting was the only way the worried spouse could cope with the situation without being overwhelmed. Although an expression of loving concern, overprotection can impede adjustment because it tends to hinder one's attempts to function independently.

Stigma Stigma is a reflection of societal attitudes. Often changes in mobility are visible to

CASE STUDY
Aging, Illness, and Mobility Changes

Grandpa's progressively decreasing mobility was first noticed at age 75 with a significant difference in his gait. He was diagnosed as having a partially occluded left femoral artery, diminishing his endurance and distance while walking, causing a discouraging change in his life-style.

Grandpa experienced a major stroke at age 84 that interfered with his sense of balance. Transient ischemic attacks (TIAs) occurred occasionally throughout the next nine years. At age 86, Grandpa fell, suffering a fractured hip. During his hospital stay, he progressed to the use of a walker, which he chose to place in the basement after he returned home. Grandpa learned to ambulate with a cane; his movements were cautious and hesitant, overcompensating so he wouldn't fall forward. He progressively became slower and slower.

A few months later Grandpa fractured his pelvis, forcing him to use the walker he so disliked. His pride and confidence interfered with his acceptance of the wheelchair, except when necessary for mobility beyond a short distance—for example, to go to the doctor's office.

At age 92 Grandpa had a minor cerebral vascular accident (CVA), followed by bronchitis. He chose to remain bedridden except to use a commode or to make rare trips outdoors in the wheelchair. He lost strength and agility in his hands and upper body, further limiting him. Although he refused further physical therapy, he continued to maintain control of his personal life. During his remaining years, he felt secure in his environment at his daughter's home.

---

others—a different gait, use of walking aids, or a wheelchair. Since society expects perfection, youth, and beauty (note advertising messages), gaining social acceptance and approval is extremely difficult for an individual who is visibly different. A person who was previously perceived as "normal," "mobile," or "agile" may be avoided, even by acquaintances or friends. People are not always able to ignore the external differences (see Chapter 5, on stigma).

The individual tends to internalize society's stigma (Welsh & Blasch, 1980). Even assistive devices may appear to the individual to reflect stigma, as do the ongoing problems associated with fear of falling or losing one's balance in public or crossing the street before the light changes. This attitude can be further complicated by the need for assistance in certain situations, such as entering inaccessible buildings, boarding a bus, or walking up stairs. When clients lack appropriate or effective communication skills to solicit needed assistance, the feelings of stigma intensify, causing difficulty in accepting offers of help or expressions of curiosity or sympathy.

PAM: How I felt had a lot to do with social nonacceptance. It is difficult to be a young woman in this society and have a disfiguring but sometimes hidden disability—no one could believe the difficulties I have, and would say things like "you're too young to have arthritis," "you look like you're healthy," "why can't you keep up—all you have are minor aches and pains," and "why are your hands crooked?"

Language Use The way that people use language reflects their attitudes and perceptions of other people. Terms with negative connotations directed toward chronically ill persons stigmatize them and influence others' attitudes toward them. When persons who have chronic illnesses are described as "victims" "suffering" with the "tragedy" of a disease or as having "agonizing" pain that "cripples" or "deforms" the body, "confining" them to a wheelchair, they become the object of a negative social stereotype of sorrow and pity (Brady, 1984). Society, through its members, then judges and alienates. Self-image and self-esteem drop, and altered mobility becomes a greater handicap. One can even say that the health professional is a "victim" of this insensitivity, "suffering" from terminology that "confines" "cripples" to an "unfortunate affliction," dehumanizing them.

The use of inappropriate language or behavior reflects a lack of sensitivity or ignorance. People often have difficulty speaking to someone with altered mobility. This difficulty becomes apparent when conversation is directed through a third person or through comments such as "How well you look" when the person looks and feels awful. Ignorance is apparent when one assumes that being in a wheelchair means paralysis without other physical problems (Gould, 1982). People who use wheelchairs are not "wheelchair bound" or "confined" to them— they don't sleep in them—rather, they use them for mobility (Johnson et al., 1992).

Environmental and Architectural Barriers Although physical barriers continue to exist, we are currently witnessing an increase in access to public areas, offering freedom of mobility for those who may be limited in movement. As these changes are being made, clinicians need to remain alert for stairs, narrow doorways, inclines, and lack of visual or auditory cues that still exist as architectural barriers in the environment. These barriers not only are safety hazards for people with altered mobility but are obstacles that limit their quality of life, restricting their opportunities, limiting their choices, and increasing their dependency.

Architectural barriers also compound the problems of gaining adequate housing. Choices are limited when apartments or houses have lengthy entrance stairways, when heavy security doors may be locked or impossible to pull open, or when tall cabinets are difficult to reach.

Van de Ven's study of lower-limb amputees (1982) observed that individuals who used wheelchairs encountered many architectural barriers. Most subjects lived in homes with steps leading outdoors that restricted access to their external environment; several subjects lived in homes that had steps indoors. Indoor mobility was further impeded by narrow corridors and doorways. Of those who used protheses, few were able to successfully negotiate the environment that included steps and other architectural barriers.

Social mobility is limited by architectural barriers. Travel can be difficult, requiring an accessible mode that is not overly fatiguing. When lodging is necessary or desired, it must be accommodating. Facilities that have stairs, limited bathroom space, or unmaneuverable water faucets prevent use. Attendance at many functions is difficult and therefore avoided by persons who do not own a car, do not live near a bus route or bus stop, or live where bus service stops too early. Seating arrangements might not allow for wheelchairs or provide room for storing a walker or crutches. Social life with friends is also impacted when a friend's home has many stairs to climb or a bathroom lacking devices for allowing the person to sit down on or rise from the toilet or use the water faucet.

> PAM: Architecture is a real physical barrier; the wheelchair disabled aren't the only "cripples" who face architectural barriers. Doors, curbs, car doors, opening jars, turning keys, eating (holding utensils), cooking, dressing, driving—*everything* is difficult when you have pain everywhere and arthritis makes it harder to do everything.

Transportation For people accustomed to driving a car, being unable to drive can be very difficult to accept and limits their participation in activities, thus affecting their social esteem and self-concept (Welsh & Blasch, 1980). The advent of hand controls, special mirrors, automatic shifts, and other devices, as well as the necessary training on these devices, has made automobile driving accessible to many (but not all) people with altered mobility.

Public transportation is a necessity for many, yet it is not always accommodating. Limitations include lines that are not reachable, infrequent schedules, limited routes, early termination, and lengthy travel. Without wheelchair lifts, many buses have limited accessibility. Worse yet is the attitudinal barrier presented by a bus driver who refuses to use the lift, claiming it is broken. Other people are restricted because they use devices that impede use of public transportation or must depend on others for assistance.

PAM: It is very difficult to handle money for public transportation like buses or the rapid transit system. The usual public routes are not that helpful for me. Standing is very tiring, and bus stops usually have no benches to sit on or shelter from the weather. When no seats are available on the bus or train, it is difficult for me to hold on to handles; I am embarrassed to ask for a handicapped seat because my disability is almost invisible. I'm able to get around only because I drive an automatic car.

Impact of Barriers Employment and education are prime examples of the impact of barriers on individuals and their families. Employment is limited when a person cannot enter an employment site because of stairs or toilet stalls that are difficult to use. Because of altered mobility, an individual may not be able to accomplish a task as rapidly as co-workers or may need someone else to read work material. Since transportation to the workplace is necessary for most people, those who can no longer drive or use a bus because there is no public transportation available are prevented from gaining self-esteem through being employed.

Also limiting are the attitudes of employers, many of whom still believe the myths that discredit the ability of disabled persons to function in the workplace. Employers have been known to discriminate against a person who uses a wheelchair or guide dog. They often feel that accommodating altered mobility is expensive or that having a disabled person on the payroll will increase their insurance premiums. However, most often the needed accommodations do not require money but a change in attitude (Johnson et al., 1992).

On the positive side, the growing role of computerization has had a positive impact on creating home-based employment. Positive change will continue with ongoing input and involvement from physically disabled persons who help create avenues that reach into the business community.

Formal education is carried out at various schools, public and private. Getting an education has been a cherished expectation in America, one that is considered available to all citizens. Because of architectural barriers and social attitudes, many individuals with altered mobility have found the educational process barred to them. Current federal and state laws now mandate equal access to education, requiring accommodations for mobility differences and demanding high-quality teaching to enable disabled persons to learn and to progress. Nevertheless, many schools and campuses still have numerous architectural barriers that impede access to classes and facilities. Moreover, stigma that adversely affects the disabled person who wants to learn still prevails.

PAM: Note taking was hard, as was getting around campus and into classes. I was afraid to ask for help because I thought my disability was not bad enough. I was initially advised to major in business administration because I was told that this was something that could get me a job behind a desk, since I "would probably be in a wheelchair." These courses were easier for me but not mentally challenging.

Much work has been done to improve these obstacles through the national efforts of the disabled population and their fight for a barriers-free life (DeJong & Lifchez, 1983; Johnson et al., 1992). The passage of the Americans with Disabilities Act (ADA) in 1990 provided legal means to "assure equality of opportunity, full participation, independent living, and economic self-efficiency for persons with disabilities" (Johnson et al., 1992). The ADA is taken very seriously by local, state, and federal governments; schools; businesses; and the public sector. As its impact is experienced in the 1990s, the lives of persons with chronic illness will become more integrated with the rest of society in all dimensions (see Chapter 24, on rehabilitation).

Interventions for the Client with Altered Mobility

A major goal of the health care practitioner is to help the client gain maximum mobility. This requires initial and ongoing detailed assessment of physiological, psychosocial, and environmental factors that limit mobility. Such an assessment should also consider positive steps that can be integrated into any plans that are developed.

Coping with altered mobility depends on many elements that are not always considered in the early stages of disability management: health, accommodations, family, outside support, finances, and individual motivation. For example, Van de Ven (1982) notes that it seems foolish to fit a person with prostheses if he or she cannot put them on and live alone or is confronted with unmanageable stairs inside the home. The client who becomes exhausted by the effort to get to a physical therapy clinic finds the time spent there far from productive (Burnfield & Burnfield, 1982). Assessment would indicate the need for a physical therapist who makes home visits so that therapy can be provided to a more energetic client.

Realistic treatment goals should be developed. Goal setting should take into account the client's objectives and set a series of successive goals on which success can be built. For example, the homebound client may wish to walk around the block. First, the professional needs to note the environment as well as the client's stamina, agility, and self-confidence in walking. Properly fitted walking aids may need to be incorporated in the plan. The client may first need to increase stamina within living quarters, and furniture arrangements may have to be altered. Then compensation is made for stairs or other impeding barriers. Finally, the client will be able to walk around the block.

Interventions should focus on correcting or compensating for daily problems: physical limitations, barriers in the environment, and psychosocial components of living. An awareness of the ADA regulations, as well as technological and computer resources, is suggested. Health professionals already have a large repertoire of interventions at their disposal or easily available in texts (medical-surgical, rehabilitation, psychology or psychiatry, and so forth) to assist the client and family. Although some specific interventions are discussed here, the major thrust of this section is to suggest ways in which the health professional can increase self-awareness in order to find creative ways of improving client mobility or quality of life.

Dealing with Physiological Aspects of Altered Mobility

As we have seen, the most complete form of altered mobility is long-term bedrest, which impacts on most body systems as well as on psychological well-being. Interventions for the problems of bedrest (Olsen et al., 1967) are summarized in Table 6-2. Regardless of which body system is affected, adequate fluids and some kind of movement (range of motion, turning, sitting up, or ambulating) are essential to reverse adverse effects. Other interventions mentioned are more specific to the system involved.

Most chronically ill individuals, however, are relatively mobile except when their diseases require restrictions. Even those having permanent disabilities tend to use crutches or wheelchairs or are ambulatory in a modified way. It is beyond the scope of one chapter to deal effectively with the many ways to compensate for musculoskeletal limitations. Here again, the health professional should consult the rehabilitation literature to address specific needs or should plan interventions with specialists who have the expertise to maximize mobility.

Regardless of whether physical limitations manifest themselves during intermittent, progressive, or permanent levels of change, interventions should be geared to maintaining function and maximizing the home environment. The health professional should remember that most people are creative in meeting their own mobility needs; given time and opportunity, they develop satisfactory ways of managing obstacles. Teaching, resources, and equipment should be provided to meet physical and emotional needs, but their ultimate utilization depends on client and family interpretation, layout of the home, preferred life-styles, and coping and adaptation skills.

People who have difficulty in walking frequently develop creative ways of ambulating. Unless another method is simpler or safer, the method used should not be discouraged. Ascending and descending stairs in the traditional fashion may not be possible in light of pain or hip and knee contractures. Some individuals can descend stairs only by grabbing

TABLE 6-2. Interventions to avoid complications from bedrest

CARDIOVASCULAR
1. Position changes, including from horizontal to vertical, alter intravascular pressure and stimulate neural reflexes and help prevent hypotension.
2. Progressive activity and exercise, including active or passive range of motion, isometrics, and so on, prevent loss of muscle tone and improve flow of blood to heart.
3. The Valsalva maneuver should be avoided when moving.
4. Adequate fluids prevent hypercoagulability.

PULMONARY
1. Accurate periodic observation of respiratory function (rate, depth, accessory muscles, neurological signs, hypoxia signs) is preventive.
2. Increased activity helps move secretions. Activity includes activities of daily living and position changes (including the upright position if possible).
3. Routine turning, coughing, and deep breathing benefit chest and lung expansion, move secretions, and facilitate gas exchange.
4. Increased fluids thin secretions.

MUSCULOSKELETAL
1. Weight bearing and muscle movement help increase osteoblastic activity and lessen decalcification. Increased calcium is not recommended, since it ends up excreted in urine or deposited in muscles and joints.

2. A functional position should be maintained. Hip and knee flexion should be avoided (no pillows or gatch). A firm mattress, bed or foot board, shoes, and/or padded splints help maintain body alignment.
3. Range of motion, position changes, and exercise prevent contractures.
4. Regular turning and skin care help prevent decubitus ulcers; alcohol (drying) or doughnuts (decrease circulation) should not be used. Toilet schedules help decrease incontinence that contributes to skin breakdown. Maintaining healthy tissue or regeneration requires adequate protein, carbohydrates, and fats in the diet.
5. If ulcers form, infections should be prevented and healing measures instituted promptly.
6. Teaching the client to shift body weight, perform range of motion, and so forth assists in prevention.

GENITOURINARY
1. Around-the-clock activity (exercises, turning, ambulation, positioning) help prevent urinary stasis.
2. If incontinence occurs, a check for bladder distension should be done; normal urination is facilitated if women sit and men stand to void.
3. Adequate fluid intake must be maintained to keep urine dilute, limit precipitates, and decrease stasis. Recording intake and output may be necessary.

the railing with two hands and going down backwards.

Getting into and out of bed can also be difficult. A variety of home adaptations usually are devised by clients or their family, such as the use of an adjacent door or a strap attached to a radiator or headboard. If their own techniques for bed mobility are safe and satisfactory, a more traditional method (such as an overhead trapeze) need not be utilized. For example, an 85-year-old woman who has bilaterally fused hips from previous inflammatory arthritis uses a belt attached to the headboard to pull herself onto her four-poster bed. She gets out of bed by wiggling on her back to the edge of the bed so that her knees extend over the side, and then digging

a cane into the mattress to thrust herself upright (Liang et al., 1983).

Since grooming can enhance one's self-esteem, professionals should intervene to encourage such self-care. This in turn creates a willingness to interact with others or be seen in public. A shower seat and a spray hose may facilitate bathing, and support in getting into and out of the tub or shower can be attained by use of a handrail and a nonskid mat. The psychological benefits of dressing oneself each day should not be overlooked because self-dressing provides exercise and promotes a sense of independence and purpose.

Children are sometimes dependent on assistive devices to maintain ambulation. Concern

TABLE 6-2. *Continued*

4. An acid-ash diet will lower the urine pH. Cranberry juice also decreases the pH. Low calcium intake helps decrease stone formation.
5. If catheterization is necessary, in and out catheterization every six to eight hours leads to fewer infections than does a foley catheter. Scrupulous aseptic technique should be maintained for any catheterization.

GASTROINTESTINAL

1. Sufficient nutrient intake maintains the basal metabolic rate and compensates for catabolism. Diet should have increased protein (to overcome protein breakdown) with adequate amounts of carbohydrates and fats.
2. Small frequent feedings that include liked foods compensate for anorexia.
3. Stress and tension reduction techniques help alleviate parasympathetic nerve stimulation.
4. Foods with bulk and cellulose material (bran, prune juice) help elimination. Stool softeners or gentle digital stimulation may be necessary to maintain bowel habits or decrease straining at stool. Regular use of enemas and laxatives are not recommended.
5. Adequate fluids stimulate reflex activity and provide enough water in the feces.
6. Prior bowel habits should be incorporated into the nursing care plan (most people defecate after meals). Adequate time should be allowed for defecation, and, if possible, a position that promotes evacuation should be assumed; the environment should be modified to provide privacy.
7. Exercises can strengthen abdominal muscles.

METABOLISM

1. Sitting up or having the head of the bed elevated helps alleviate many of the basal metabolic and hormonal level changes.
2. Minimal but adequate bed covering enhances body heat loss.
3. Increased fluid intake and high protein nutrition hasten healing and help maintain electrolyte balance.
4. Range of motion, exercise, and weight bearing prevent atrophy and help limit elevated serum calcium levels.
5. Stress reduction helps maintain metabolic homeostasis.

PSYCHOSOCIAL

1. Reminders about reality, clocks, calendars, and so forth, help maintain orientation.
2. Planning and participating in care promote independence and a sense of control.
3. Increased sensory stimulation and physical activity provide spatial mobility, help reconstruct body image and ego identity, and enhance roles.
4. Promoting independence stimulates physiologic and psychologic mobility.

SOURCE: Summarized from Olsen et al. (1967).

over the cost of providing such devices is understandable, but consideration should also be given to the cost of not providing them. It is more expensive to keep a child dependent on an adult caregiver than to provide him or her with proper devices and training time needed to allow maximum independence (Korpela, Sisstola, & Korrikko, 1992).

Aids for Sensory Impairment

Professionals should become sensitized to the stigma of visual and auditory impairment. They should be informed about causative diseases and preventive measures and about services available to those who need them. Health professionals should increase their awareness of resources for technological assistive devices as they become more available and affordable (Johnson et al., 1992). The ability to interact effectively with those experiencing sensory loss is another essential quality for professionals in human service settings (Welsh & Blasch, 1980). Teaching and modifying the environment are two ways in which the health care provider can best assist with sensory problems.

Visual Impairment For people with visual impairment, many services to help in the performance of daily living skills are available, especially in major metropolitan areas. In fact, formal instruction in independent travel is more extensively developed for visually impaired people than for any other disability group (Welsh & Blasch, 1980). Information about such services should be provided, and client and family should be encouraged to use them.

When an individual has partial vision, improved lighting, especially floor lighting, helps reduce falls or other home accidents. Steps with edging colors, vibrant contrasting colors to mark changes in height or location, or enlarged lettering can alert the person to surroundings and enhance mobility.

For general safety with any degree of visual impairment, it is necessary to reduce the hazards of loose rugs, telephone cords, and waxed or wet floors. Things should be left in the same place rather than moved around, since rearranging creates new obstacle courses for the client.

Tactile or auditory interventions generally are useful. Tactile aids include raised lettering or braille to designate doorways, business locations, elevator floors, and so on. Technology will continue developing aids for visual impairment: Taped books are everywhere, photocopy machines to enlarge print are increasingly common, computer fonts print larger sizes, computer disks have voice output, and braille printers compensate for visual impairments. All are becoming more affordable (Johnson et al., 1992). Auditory information can be provided by a sound system, such as bells to sound alarms or tweeters to indicate that traffic lights have changed.

Hearing Impairment Interventions to compensate for hearing loss increase willingness to initiate independent travel in public places, thereby increasing mobility. Effective interventions require attracting the attention of those with auditory impairments through visual cues (blinking lights and hand and facial gestures) or tactile cues (touching the individual to gain attention or creating vibratory contact such as pounding on a table or floor). General measures include facing the auditorily impaired person to allow him or her to focus on the speaker's face and gestures. Speech should be natural but slow, although not too slow. Care providers should enunciate clearly but without exaggeration, using simple terms and short sentences. When writing any kind of note, professionals

must use simple language because hearing-impaired individuals may have only limited understanding of written language.

Telecommunication devices for the deaf (TDD) allow easy telephone communication for persons with hearing or speech impairments. The nationwide deaf relay service, in effect since the early 1990s, provides communication when a hearing person does not have a TDD, translating the message by TDD to the TDD user. FAX machines transmit written messages quickly. Televisions, films, and videotapes can be subtitled. Assistive listening devices amplify sound, sending the audio message to a hearing aid or small receiver. Many emergency alarm systems already give both auditory and visual warnings; public areas are now required to do so (Johnson et al., 1992; Goodman, 1989).

Hearing aids are helpful, but can create problems. Although sounds are amplified, the ability to make sense of these sounds requires a new mode of concentration (Liang et al., 1983). The health professional and family need to encourage the patience necessary to master the use of hearing aids.

Interventions for Pain and Loss of Energy

The client must learn that chronic pain may not be correctable and that depleted energy may never be regained. However, some interventions or actions can help decrease pain or increase energy enough to enhance mobility.

Pain Pain control exhibits both physical and psychological perimeters. The challenge for clinicians is to balance pain control with concern for client safety and the side effects of pain treatment. The health professional must learn to listen actively to the client's description of the type and quality of experienced pain in order to take effective action, especially when analgesics (both narcotic and nonnarcotic) are to be used (McCaffery & Beebe, 1989). People are more receptive to suggested interventions when they feel that the health provider is genuinely interested in seeking joint solutions (McCaffery & Beebe, 1989). For example, arthritic pain varies, as do individuals having arthritis. Pain management requires individualized interventions (see Chapter 7, on chronic pain).

Despite the availability of effective techniques for pain management in children, studies indicate that their pain is not managed as well as pain in adults (U.S. Department of Health and Human Services, 1992). There are many misconceptions regarding pain felt by children, including the assumption that infants do not feel pain or that being "busy" implies a lack of pain. The health professional needs to better assess children, using adapted tools that are age appropriate, and to advocate for more intervention for this age group (McCaffery & Beebe, 1989).

In research on endorphins and their action in relieving pain, West (1981) points out that many of the traditional nursing techniques of comfort may indeed have physiological as well as psychological effects. Specific comfort techniques, such as relaxation, positioning, massage, acupressure, and distraction, stimulate endorphin release, providing pain relief (West, 1981; Lewis, 1984; McCaffery & Beebe, 1989). Thus, these time-honored comfort techniques are now proved as physiologically sound as well.

When pain is severe, the client tends to become less active in an effort to gain control. Inactivity increases fatigue, weakens muscles, stiffens joints, and decreases circulation (Lewis, 1984). Unless bedrest is medically necessary, the client must be as mobile as possible. When pain is responsive to analgesics, they should be used appropriately to decrease the fear or anxiety that accompanies the pain (McCaffery & Beebe, 1989). This should be done in conjunction with the comfort measures discussed previously. When specific medications such as anti-inflammatory drugs for arthritis can ease pain, they should be used.

Some disorders, such as arthritis, are characterized by pain associated with even simple tasks such as using the toilet, turning in bed, or moving a hand. Except during exacerbations, a properly designed and implemented exercise program should be followed to help keep joints flexible, maintain muscle strength, and build overall stamina (Becker, 1984; Gall & Minor, 1991; Slonaker, 1992). Such general conditioning and maintenance can be accomplished by frequent repetitions of normal activities within the energy and comfort limits of the person. The process can include walking or simple exercises such as raising the arms and straightening the legs (Liang et al., 1983). Exercise helps to develop a more positive mental attitude by improving self-image and reinforcing a sense of worth (Becker, 1984).

When hospitalization becomes necessary, successful home medication routines that control pain should continue. Such regimens can differ from the hospital's scheduled medication times, but the staff should nevertheless integrate these proven methods into their plan of care for the client, with the physician's approval as necessary. Such actions do not release the nurses from their responsibilities to ensure that medications are taken properly and regularly.

Loss of Energy   Clients must understand that energy loss frequently accompanies many diseases and that different disease processes have different bases for energy loss. Fatigue usually demands an altered life-style, requires a conscious effort to assess one's own energy flow, and demands learning how to balance fatigue and needed rest with activities.

When energy is affected by long-term decreased cardiac output or oxygen intake, strategies should limit any decrease in functional capacity. When medically possible, energy should be rebuilt by progressive increments of activity. An initial program may involve walking slowly each day, gradually increasing the distance for improved exercise tolerance. Riding a tricycle is a form of exercise that also serves as a mode of transportation in accomplishing errands. Meals should be eaten at the table with the family rather than in bed, and the client should dress each day. These techniques enhance self-esteem as well as increase activity. In the home, walking should take precedence over using a wheelchair.

For energy that is decreased by inflammatory processes, rest and prescribed medications can reduce the inflammation. Complete bedrest is needed only during disease activity. After a flare-up, average daily activities should resume slowly, guided by attention to the body's responses. Allow time to adjust: A few months may be necessary for resuming all previous activity levels. The client should be attentive to fatigue as a signal to rest and not overexert, maintaining a regular schedule to provide a structure for monitoring activity and rest. Even when an individual is bedridden, some types of exercise should be maintained (Lewis, 1984).

Various energy conservation techniques provide methods for coping with energy loss (Arthritis Foundation, 1992; Gall & Minor, 1991; Tack, 1991). Such techniques should also be provided for senior citizens who deserve opportunities for prevention-oriented exercises aimed at keeping them as mobile and active as possible to delay or minimize the effects of a complex interaction of aging and chronic disease (Vandervoort et al., 1990). Physical therapists can serve as resources for teaching implementing techniques:

1. Exercise program: Exercise to strengthen muscles and increase range of motion.
2. Pacing: Avoid overactivity when feeling good, since it can increase pain and fatigue.
3. Modifications: Adapt the environment by various means, such as constructing ramps, rearranging frequently used rooms, and utilizing assistive devices.
4. Body awareness: Be attentive to body and energy levels. Plan around times of high energy for tasks and low energy for rest periods.
5. Be realistic: Since frustration results from not acknowledging limitations, develop activity alternatives.
6. Teaching others: Educate support persons about fatigue and its effects.

Overcoming Barriers

The presence of barriers, both physical and social, impacts adversely on many individuals with mobility problems. These people want to interact with society, and barriers make such interactions difficult. The professional who is not a rehabilitation counselor or therapist can help these clients by developing a sensitivity to barriers. In this way, the professional can become an advocate by encouraging agencies to move toward greater accessibility and finding creative and workable alternatives for the client and other involved individuals.

The professional has a responsibility for advocacy. This requires a genuine empathy with the client's status, physically and psychosocially. Many disabled people have become politically active to obtain changes regarding all barriers and to achieve recognition as valued citizens who can contribute to society constructively and meaningfully (DeJong & Lifchez, 1983). The professional needs to initiate advocacy projects by becoming knowledgeable of their impact on clients and supporting client self-help and advocacy groups.

Environmental Barriers Many interventions specific to environmental or architectural barriers have already been addressed. There are many other interventions, but addressing them all is beyond the scope of this chapter.

Awareness of the multiple aspects of barriers is enhanced if the health professional develops insight into the difficulties that barriers produce. Sensitivity to such barriers is best achieved by personal experience of mobility problems. One can simulate situations limiting one's mobility in several ways. Although a simulated experience provides a limited perspective on living with disabilities, it does give some insight into the emotional as well as the physical barriers that many individuals experience. Health professionals can try the activities suggested here during their normal daily routines.

Increasing awareness of sensory deprivation can be accomplished by wearing a blindfold or glasses that do not fit one's prescription; ear plugs will block out most auditory input, and finger movement and tactile input can be restricted by mittens or gloves that are oversize and bulky. Limiting upper-body mobility can be accomplished by handcuffs or a sling; the lower body can be restricted by crutch travel. Using a wheelchair in the work environment or at a favorite restaurant enhances one's awareness of obstacles and the attitudes the user encounters.

Once health professionals have experienced these obstacles and the responses they engender in ill persons and those they encounter, sincere empathy and understanding in their interactions with affected individuals will come more readily and meaningful alterations for the client follows. In the home, this may mean access to other rooms or the outside: ramps, wider doors, reachable shelves, handrails on stairways, and so forth.

For example, a woman with decreasing mobility from osteoarthritis and hypertension found herself forced to consider a move to a more functional apartment on the second floor of her building. This move would mean she no longer could go outside, further reducing her incentive to remain active. Aware of difficulties that the woman would encounter in a second-floor unit, a health professional initiated efforts to adapt her current apartment to her needs by a raised toilet seat, bathroom hand bars, raised chair blocks, and so on.

Outside the home, barriers restrict access to the rest of the world. Effecting change in these areas often requires adopting the role of advocate for the client: lobbying for ramps where even one step prevents entrance, having doors widened, altering bathroom space to accommodate a wheelchair, or placing some water fountains at an accessible height. Continued advocacy and knowledge of the ADA regulations by health professionals can further support and enforce such adaptations.

Social Barriers The greatest degree of sensitization must be achieved in the area of social barriers. Sensitivity includes an awareness of the attitudes that the professional projects to clients. Language reinforces our perceptions of people (California Governor's Committee for Employment of People with Disabilities, 1984), and words with negative connotations carry negative expectations and attitudes. Professionals should listen to what they are saying, hearing their words and tone of voice, being alert to subtle implications that stigmatize. Others, including nonmedical professionals, family, friends, and acquaintances, imitate the language used by health professionals, who are seen as role models. Words that contain negative inferences present a model of negative attitudes, subtly reinforcing stigma. Care in choosing words and developing techniques to alert and educate peers about their language use helps deter unhealthy attitudes.

Psychosocial Interventions

Any program of care should clearly address the psychosocial needs of clients and their significant others (Baum & Rothschild, 1983) to make these needs more manageable and less overwhelming. The health professional already has, or can attain, a number of skills to assist the client with many of the adaptations necessary in chronic illness.

Dealing with Psychosocial Difficulties
People have different coping styles (Walker & Lattanzi, 1982) and adjust at individual rates appropriate to them. The health professional should encourage clients to be responsible for their own courses of adjustment (Arthritis Foundation, 1992). Positive support includes acknowledging that adjustment is hard work. A willingness to listen to the client conveys that the professional recognizes feelings of depression and helplessness, but is not trying to change these feelings. For example, it is not helpful to say "You just have to accept it" or "It will be all right" when the client is not feeling that way.

Since feelings of insecurity and worthlessness often surface when a person is coping with mobility alterations, the health professional should nurture the individual's self-confidence. A positive, realistic perception of abilities as well as limitations can support self-confidence. Focusing on physical limitations can become frustrating and overwhelming, yet it is part of the adjustment process.

Coping with Social Problems Prior roles may no longer be possible or may be drastically altered. A change in employment, responsibilities, or home life may be necessary. Rehabilitation assists the client and family in establishing a new life-style (Lewis, 1984) by providing information relative to mobility accommodations and offering emotional support. A positive perspective of fulfilling certain role responsibilities can also increase a feeling of self-worth and meaning.

Coping with social problems caused by mobility differences demands that clients clearly communicate their own needs and abilities (Apple, Apple, & Blasch, 1980; Welsh, 1980; Arthritis Foundation, 1992). Since social attitudes toward people with altered mobility tend to be negative and misinformed, assertive communication by the client provides accurate and useful information. The professional can encourage "assertiveness training"; such self-advocacy is needed and influences the attitudes surrounding the individual.

Clients may need encouragement to be socially active. Perhaps their old social roles have been altered by their mobility changes, or they may be isolated and need to develop new relationships. It is important to be sensitive to their feelings of readiness; social interaction can be encouraged but not pushed. Being able to communicate mobility difficulties effectively facilitates social interaction. Such communication can sometimes be enhanced by dialogue with others in similar situations.

Family The client's entire network of caring others requires support. A realistic understanding of the client's limits, abilities, and goals assists these individuals in working together cohesively. A proper assessment of the family situation and the emotional status of significant others can facilitate meeting their needs as a unit.

Roles within the family may change as a result of the client's situation or modified responsibilities. Such change may be necessary to ensure family harmony. Each individual within the family may have a unique style of adjusting; these various styles may not progress in a similar manner or time frame. Respite time may be advisable, providing family members time away from responsibilities that may seem overwhelming (see Chapter 12, on family caregivers). The financial situation may be burdensome and may create tremendous anxiety; referral to assistance such as an appropriate agency might be helpful. Spiritual affiliations should not be overlooked; support from a minister, priest, rabbi, or religious community may accelerate psychological and social adjustment.

Aging Client Caring for older clients requires sensitivity to meet their needs as well as the needs produced by a chronic condition. Professionals must become aware of their own aging process, identifying and anticipating needs. This awareness is transferred to the aging client with increased empathy.

Research by Rosenbloom (1982) indicates that many individuals who are elderly tend to view the gradual loss of mobility functions as an expected part of aging. Accepting this loss as inevitable, they are less likely to seek assistance or communicate their needs effectively. Yet older clients merit the same sensitivity and advocacy interventions that are given to younger ones. Health professionals should respect the aging client's accomplishments, nurturing the client's self-respect and sense of control over his or her life (Trieschmann, 1987).

Other Interventions

Support Groups Health care providers need to encourage clients to create and nurture their own support group (Arthritis Foundation, 1992). By talking about their problems, individuals who are physically disabled overcome fear of the unknown and find compatible life-styles, satisfaction, and an extension of their productive years (Marsh et al., 1983). Relationship mending occurs, and employment opportunities are extended. They learn to educate others as well as themselves about their chronic illnesses and ensuing mobility difficulties.

> PAM: Support groups showed me I was not alone in my pains—emotional and physical—by grouping me with others who had the same disease. Different people react differently to the same disease. I met a young woman my age who had JA as long as I, and I realized that we had different concerns as young women with arthritis: childbirth/rearing, dating, sexual relations, and so on.
>
> You learn a lot about yourself in a support group. I learned to take responsibility for my own health care, along with the health professional, and to live with daily activities more easily. Sharing showed that we are all individuals and have control over our lives and how we choose to cope with pain and disability.

Outside Resources One final suggestion to help those with mobility problems is to utilize the many helpful agencies that exist outside the health profession. These agencies offer advocacy and additional means of support that are beneficial. Informed professionals can be the hub of a wheel of resources by eliciting the skills and expertise within their own community. (See

Chapter 21, on the agency maze.) The Appendix includes a partial list of agencies that work with mobility difficulties.

Summary and Conclusions

Activity is part of everyday life. Disease states alter mobility adversely. The professional thinks of these alterations as affecting primarily the musculoskeletal system and leading to bedrest. Bedrest is often effective for acute illness, but in chronic illness it usually is a temporary state. Mobility tends to follow several patterns: intermittent, progressive, permanent, or combinations of these patterns. It can also be lost by indirect alterations of the external structure of the body. Visual loss, hearing loss, pain, and depleted energy hinder mobility as well.

Of greater concern is that the individual with a mobility alteration has problems that transcend the disease state. A goodly number of psychological and sociological adjustments become necessary. Psychologically, the individual must handle loss (sometimes again and again), face changes in self-image (body image and self-esteem), and overcome fear and stress. Sociologically, client and family face a myriad of problems. Families and clients may experience role and life-style changes and need to face and resolve differences in perspective. The aging members of our society encounter the double problems of mobility changes: those of aging overlaid with chronic illness.

Barriers, both social and environmental, prevent the individual from gaining maximum mobility. Physical barriers include steps, inadequate facilities within buildings, and so forth. In overcoming these barriers, the disabled have led the way in gaining change through legislative action. But the greatest impediment continues to be the attitudes of others, including health care providers. Negative attitudes, often verbally expressed in our choice of language, create stigma that handicaps the chronically ill.

Many available interventions are known to the health care provider or are readily accessible through sources such as rehabilitation texts. Some of the specifics discussed relate to visual and hearing loss, pain, energy depletion, and ways of overcoming barriers. Health professionals need to develop insight into problems created by loss of mobility, best accomplished by their sensitizing themselves through experiencing, even for a short while, some of the difficulties caused by limited mobility. Health professionals also need to become sensitive to their own attitudes, which often manifest as stigmatizing behavior and language. Given that health care providers often are seen as role models by others, they must observe the stricture "Know thyself." In this way, they treat the *person,* not the disease.

NURSING DIAGNOSIS

6.1.1.1 Impaired Physical Mobility

Definition: A state in which the individual experiences a limitation of ability for independent physical movement.

Defining Characteristics: Inability to purposefully move within the physical environment, including bed mobility, transfer, and ambulation; reluctance to attempt movement; limited range of motion; decreased muscle strength, control, and/or mass; imposed restrictions of movement, including mechanical, medical protocol; impaired coordination.

Related Factors: Intolerance to activity/decreased strength and endurance; pain/discomfort; perceptual/cognitive impairment; neuromuscular impairment; musculoskeletal impairment; depression/severe anxiety.

Suggested Functional Level Classification[1]

0 = Completely independent.

1 = Requires use of equipment or device.

2 = Requires help from another person for assistance, supervision, or teaching.

3 = Requires help from another person and equipment or device.

4 = Dependent; does not participate in activity.

Editor's Note: Decreased strength is listed as both a defining characteristic and a related factor. Assessment should determine if it is a manifestation of the diagnostic category or a contributing factor. A number of the related factors do not fall in the realm of independent nursing intervention, since they can not be altered or eliminated by independent nursing decisions.

Since nursing care of the client on bedrest often focuses on the prevention of many other problems, each of these problems could be noted as separate diagnostic categories. These include the following but are not all inclusive. (The parentheses are my addition.)

1.1.2.2 (High Risk for) Altered Nutrition: Less Than Body Requirement

1.4.2.1 (High Risk for) Decreased Cardiac Output

1.5.1.1 (High Risk for) Impaired Gas Exchange

[1]Functional level classification adapted from Jones E. et al., (1974, November). *Patient classification for long-term care: Users' manual* (Publication No. HRA-74-310). Washington, D.C.: HEW.

1.6.1 High Risk for Injury (2nd to Decreased Bone Density and Muscle Mass)

1.3.2 (High Risk for) Altered Urinary Elimination

9.3.1 Anxiety

Current working conditions, which put limitations on the time and energy nurses can expend on any one patient, make it impossible for them to address each category separately. The following is a better choice, since it focuses on one diagnostic category for all possible and potential complications of immobility secondary to bedrest. Since it is a high-risk problem, the defining characteristics list the risk factors that can be causative of mobility problems. The editor suggests that others should be added that are more amenable to independent nursing actions.

1.6.1.5 High Risk for Disuse Syndrome

Definition: A state in which an individual is at risk for deterioration of body systems as the result of prescribed or unavoidable musculoskeletal inactivity.[2]

Defining Characteristics: Presence of *risk factors such as:* Paralysis; mechanical immobilization; prescribed immobilization; severe pain; altered level of consciousness.

Related Factors: See Risk Factors.

[2]Complications from immobility can include pressure ulcer, constipation, stasis of pulmonary secretions, thrombosis, urinary tract infection/retension, decreased strength/endurance, orthostatic hypotension, decreased range of joint motion, disorientation, body image disturbance, and powerlessness.

STUDY QUESTIONS

1. What are the primary concerns of clients and significant others among the problems that result from altered mobility?
2. Which physiological systems are effected by bedrest? Describe these effects.
3. How would you describe the patterns that characterize mobility alterations? Select a

chronic medical condition. How would this condition "fit" into these patterns?
4. What are the major psychological areas that impact on a person with altered mobility? Describe the way this individual is affected.
5. What are the major sociological barriers resulting from altered mobility? How many can

you identify? What are the effects of these barriers?

6. How can the health care practitioner help the client with altered mobility meet some of the physiological, psychological, social, and environmental limitations that are present? How can the health provider help clients meet their own mobility needs creatively?

7. What interventions are common to all the problems of bedrest? Which are specific to individual systems?

8. What interventions can help satisfy the needs of the sensorially impaired? Discuss some.

9. How do pain and loss of energy affect mobility? What interventions help manage pain or energy loss?

10. In what ways can the health professional develop sensitivity to barriers the immobile person faces? In what way can such sensitivity help the individual? family? society?

11. What skills in the health professional's repertoire assist the client in adapting and adjusting to changes in life-style? in meeting psychosocial needs?

References

Apple, M. M., Apple, L. E., & Blasch, D. (1980). Low vision. In R. L. Welsh, & B. B. Blasch (Eds.), *Foundations of orientation and mobility.* New York: American Foundation for the Blind.

Arthritis Foundation (1992). *Taking charge: Learning to live with arthritis* (booklet). Atlanta, GA: Arthritis Foundation.

Asher, R. (1983). The dangers of going to bed. *Critical Care Update, 10*(5), 40-41.

Baum, H. M., & Rothschild, B. B. (1983). Multiple sclerosis and mobility restriction. *Archives of Physical Medicine and Rehabilitation, 64*(12), 591-596.

Becker, M. (1984, September 12). Therapist tells arthritics to exercise regularly. *Physical Therapy Forum.*

Brady, T. J. (1984). Arthritis has an image problem. *National Arthritis News, 5*(2), 4.

Burnfield, A., & Burnfield, P. (1982). Psychological aspects of multiple sclerosis. *Physiotherapy, 68*(5), 149-150.

California Governor's Committee for Employment of the Disabled (1984). *Language guide on disability.* CA CCEH 3, Sacramento Employment Development Department.

Carpenito, L. (1989). Mobility, impaired physical. *Nursing diagnosis: Application to clinical practice* (3rd ed.). Philadelphia: J. B. Lippincott.

Clark, C. (1991, Jan./Feb.). Nursing care for multiple sclerosis. *Orthopedic Nursing, 10*(1), 21-24.

DeJong, G., & Lifchez, R. (1983). Physical disability and public policy. *Scientific American, 248*(6), 40-49.

Earle, J. R., Perricone, P. J., Maultsby, D. M., Perricone, N., Turner, R. A., & Davis, J. (1979). Psycho-social adjustment of rheumatoid arthritis patients from two alternative treatment settings. *Journal of Rheumatology, 6*(1), 80-87.

Gall, V. & Minor, M. (1991). *Exercise and your arthritis* (booklet). Atlanta, GA: Arthritis Foundation.

Garrison, W. M. T. & McQuiston, S. (1989). *Chronic illness during childhood and adolescence: Psychological aspects.* Newbury Park, CA: Sage.

Gates, G. A., Cooper, J. C. Kannel, W. B. et al. (1990). Hearing and the elderly: The Framingham cohort 1983-85. Basic auditromic test results. *Ear and Hearing, 11*(4), 247-256.

Genesky, S. (1981). Data concerning the partially sighted and the functionally blind. *Visual Impairment and Blindness, 72,* 177.

Goldman, R. (1977). Rest: Its use and abuse in the aged. *Journal of American Geriatrics Society, 25*(10), 433-438.

Goodman, W. (1989). *Mobility training for people with disabilities.* Springfield, IL: Charles C. Thomas.

Gould, J. (1982, November 27). Disabilities and how to live with them. Multiple sclerosis. *Lancet* 1208-1210.

Greenleaf, J., & Kozlowski, S. (1982). Physiological consequences of reduced physical activity during bed rest. *Exercise and Sport Sciences Review, 10,* 84-119.

Groer, N. M. & Skekleton, M. E. (1989). *Basic pathophysiology: A holistic approach* (3rd ed.). St. Louis: Mosby.

Ham, R. J. (1984). Problems of rehabilitation: Many can be prevented. *Generations: Quarterly Journal of the Western Gerontological Society, 8*(4), 14-17.

Herbst, K. G. (1983). Psychological consequences of disorders of hearing in the elderly. In R. Hinchcliffe (Ed.), *Hearing and balance in the elderly.* New York: Churchill Livingstone.

Johnson, M., & the Editors of the *Disability Rag* (1992). *People with disabilities explain it all for you.* Louisville, KY: The Avocado Press.

Kemp, B. & Pilloterri, A. (1984). *Fundamentals of nursing.* Boston: Little, Brown.

Kinsella, G. J., & Duffy, E. D. (1980). Attitudes towards disability expressed by spouses of stroke patients. *Scandinavian Journal of Rehabilitative Medicine, 12*(2), 73-76.

Korpela, R. A., Sisstola, T. O., Korrikko, M. I. (1992, October). the cost of assistive devices for children with mobility limitations. *Pediatrics, 90*(4).

Lattanzi, M. (1983). Coping skills: Working with grief, a workshop, Oakland, Calif., December 6.

Lewis, K. S. (1984). Systemic lupus erythematosus: The great masquerader. *Nurse Practitioner, 9*(8), 13-22.

Liang, M. H., Partridge, A. J., Gall, V., & Eaton, H. (1983). Management of functional disability in homebound patients. *Journal of Family Practice, 17*(3), 429-435.

Marsh, G. G., Ellison, G. W., & Strite, C. (1983). Psychosocial and vocational rehabilitation approaches to multiple sclerosis. *Annual Review of Rehabilitation, 3,* 242-267.

McCaffery, M., & Beebe, A. (1987). Pain: Clinical manual for nursing practice. St. Louis: C. V. Mosby.

Miller, M. B. (1975). Iatrogenic and noniatrogenic effects of prolonged immobilization of the ill aged. *Journal of the American Geriatric Society, 23,* 360-369.

Mobily P. R., & Kelley, L. S. (1991). Iatrogenesis in the elderly: Factors of immobility. *Journal of Gerontological Nursing, 17*(9).

Olson, E. et al. (1967). The hazards of immobility. *American Journal of Nursing, 67*(4), 779-796.

Pavlou, M., & Counte, M. (1982). Cognitive aspects of coping in multiple sclerosis. *Rehabilitation Counseling Bulletin, 25*(3), 138-145.

Pick, H. L., Jr. (1980). Perception, locomotion, and orientation. In R. L. Welsh & B. Blasch (Eds.), *Foundations of orientation and mobility.* New York: American Foundation for the Blind.

Potter, P. & Perry, A. (1991). *Fundamentals of nursing: Concepts, process, and practice.* St. Louis: Mosby.

Rosenbloom, A. A. (1982). Care of elderly people with low vision. *Journal of Visual Impairment and Blindness, 76*(6), 209-212.

Slonaker, D. (1992). *Using your joints wisely* (booklet). Atlanta, GA: Arthritis Foundation.

Sorenson, K. C. & Luckman, J. (1986). *Basic nursing: A psychophysiologic approach* (2nd ed.). Philadelphia: W.B. Saunders.

Stewart, N. (1986). Perceptual and behavioral effects of immobility and social isolation in hospitalized orthopedic patients. *Nursing Paper, 18*(3), 59-74.

Tack, B. (1991). *Coping with fatigue* (booklet). Atlanta, GA: Arthritis Foundation.

Trieschmann, R. B. (1987). *Aging with a disability.* New York: Demos Publications.

Vandervoort, A., Hill, K., Sandrin, M., & Vyes, M. (1990). Mobility impairment and falling in the elderly. *Physiotherapy Canada, 42*(2).

Van de Ven, C. M. C. (1982). Management of bi-lateral lower limb amputees: An investigation. *Physiotherapy, 68*(2), 45-46.

U.S. Department of Health and Human Services (1992). Infants, children & adolescents: Clinical practice guidelines, a quick reference guideline for clinicians (Pamphlet #AHCPR 92-0020). Rockville, MD: Public Health Services, Agency for Health Care Policy and Research.

Walker, J. R., & Lattanzi, M. (1982). *Understanding loss and grief.* Boulder, CO: Boulder County Hospice.

Welsh, R. L. (1980). Psychosocial dimensions. In R. L. Welsh & B. B. Blasch (Eds.), *Foundations of orientation and mobility.* New York: American Foundation for the Blind.

Welsh, R. L. & Blasch, B. B. (1980). Training for persons with mobility limitations. In R. L. Welsh & B. B. Blasch (Eds.), *Foundations of orientation and mobility.* New York: American Foundation for the Blind.

West, B. A. (1981). Understanding endorphins: Our natural pain relief system. *Nursing 81, 11*(2), 50-53.

Bibliography

Brackett, T. O., Condon, N., Kindelan, K. M., & Bassett, L. (1984). The emotional care of a person with a spinal cord injury. *Journal of the American Medical Association, 252*(6), 793-795.

Brown, E. L. (1978). Psychosocial needs of the aged: What nurses can do. In E. Seymour (Ed.), *Psychosocial need, of the aged: A health care perspective.* Los Angeles: The University of Southern California Press.

Campbell, A. J., Reinken, J., Allan, B. C., & Martinez, G. S. (1981). Falls in old age: A study of frequency and related clinical factors. *Age and Aging, 10,* 264.

Convertino, V., Hung, J., Goldwater, D., & DeBusk, R. (1983). Cardiovascular responses to exercise in middle-aged men after ten days of bedrest. *Circulation, 68*(2), 245-250.

Counte, M. A., Bieliauskas, L. A. & Pavlou, M. (1983). Stress and personal attitudes in chronic illnesses. *Archives of Physical Medicine and Rehabilitation, 64*(6), 272–275.

Dunlop, B. D. (1980). Expanded home-based care for the elderly: Solution or pipe dream? *American Journal of Public Health, 70,* 514–519.

Emerson, D. L. (1981). Facing loss of vision: The response of adults to visual impairment. *Journal of Visual Impairment and Blindness, 75*(2), 41–45.

Fatigue: The hidden disability. (1984). *National Arthritis News, 5*(2), 8.

Gordon, M. (1987). *Nursing diagnosis: Process and application* (2nd ed.). New York: McGraw-Hill.

Hathaway, G. (1984). The child with sickle cell anemia: Implications and management. *Nurse Practitioner, 9,* 16–20.

Hughes, S. L., Cordray, D. S., & Spiker, V. A. (1982). Evaluation of a long term home care program. *Working Paper #62.* Evanston, IL: Northwestern University.

Kim, M. J., McFarland, G. K., & McFarlane, A. M. (1987). *Pocket guide to nursing diagnosis* (2nd ed.). St. Louis: Mosby.

Liang, M. H., Partridge, A. J., Larson, M., & Gall, V. (1982). An evaluation of stepped-up rehabilitation for homebound elderly with musculoskeletal disability: A preliminary report. *Clinical Research, 30,* 302A.

Liang, M., Partridge, A. S., Larson, M. G., Gall, V., Taylor, J., Berkman, C., Master, R., Feltin, M., & Taylor, J. (1984). Evaluation of comprehensive rehabilitation services for elderly homebound patients with arthritis and orthopedic disability. *Arthritis and Rheumatism, 27*(3), 258–266.

Liang, M., Philips, E., Scamman, M., Lurye, C. A., Keith, A., Cohen, L., & Taylor, G. (1981). Evaluation of a pilot program for rheumatic disability in an urban community. *Arthritis and Rheumatism, 24,* 937–943.

McDonald, G., & Hudson, L. (1982). Important aspects of pulmonary rehabilitation. *Geriatrics, 37*(3), 12.

Mentzer, W. M., & Wang, W. (1980). Sickle cell disease: Pathophysiology and diagnosis, *Pediatric Annals, 9,* 287.

Report to the Chairman of the Committee on Labor and Human Resources, United States Senate (1982). *The elderly should benefit from expanded home health care but increasing these services will not insure cost reduction. GAO/IPE-83-1,* Gaithersburg, MD.

Rieser, J. J., Guth, D. A., & Hill, E. W. (1982). Mental processes mediating independent travel: Implications for orientation and mobility. *Journal of Visual Impairment and Blindness, 75*(5), 213–218.

Rubenstein, L. Z., Robbins, A. S., Shulman, B. N. L., Rosado, J., Osterweil, D., & Josephson, A. R. (1988). Falls and instability in the elderly. *Journal of the American Geriatric Society, 36,* 266–278.

Vinchinsky, E., & Lulen, B. (1980). Sickle cell anemia. *Pediatric Clinics of North America, 27*(2), 429–445.

Weissert, W., Wan, T., Livieratos, B., Katz, S., & Pellegrino, I. (1980). Cost-effectiveness of homemaker services for the chronically ill. *Inquiry, 17,* 230–243.

Wild, D., Nayak, U. S. L., & Isaac, B. (1981). Prognosis of falls in old people at home. *Journal of Epidemiology and Community Health, 35,* 200.

CHAPTER 7

Chronic Pain

Ilene Lubkin

Introduction

Experiencing pain is a major reason for seeking health care. Acute pain serves as a protective physiological mechanism that informs us that something is wrong with our bodies (Bonica, 1985) or prevents additional damage to tissue by limiting movement in injured parts. Pain occurs when tissue damage stimulates pain-sensitive neural receptors or if there is damage to the pain transmission system itself. Pain can also be chronic in nature and is a major cause of disability (Osterweis et al., 1987).

Melzack (1973) notes that pain is "a highly personal experience depending on cultural learning, the meaning of the situation, and other factors that are unique to each individual" (p. 22). In other words, pain is a subjective experience. McCaffery (1979) notes that pain cannot be measured and can be validated only by the person in pain. Acute pain presents with autonomic nervous system or behavioral responses and is time limited (minutes to weeks). It subsides when healing occurs and can usually be controlled by medications. Even when acute pain is severe, the client will sometimes tolerate it, knowing it is temporary.

When an individual has chronic pain the body has adapted physiologically and autonomic responses are absent. Chronic pain can be con-tinuous, intractable, intermittent, or recurrent. Even when mild, it can be so pervasive that it becomes a condition unto itself. Current terminology differentiates chronic pain as *malignant,* associated with progressive terminal illness, or *nonmalignant,* not associated with terminal illness but not adequately responsive to treatment to be relieved. Chronic nonmalignant pain is also known as *chronic benign pain* or *intractable pain.*

There is limited knowledge about the specific mechanism for transmission and perception of pain. However, several theories have been proposed as explanations, some of which are noted here.

The *specificity theory* is one of the oldest theories that serve to explain pain transmission. Based on the concept that there is always a relationship between cause and effect, it proposes that specific pain receptors (nociceptors) project impulses over specific neural pain pathways (A-delta and C fibers) via the spinal cord to the brain.

The *pattern theory* evolved when it was demonstrated that nociceptors respond to stimuli like pressure and temperature and not just to pain. This theory suggests that there are no nociceptors specific to pain, and that pain occurs from a combination of stimulus intensity and the central summation pattern of impulses in the dorsal horn of the spinal cord.

The theory used widely in clinical practice today is the *gate control theory* proposed by Melzack and Wall (1965), even though it is not fully supported by incontrovertible experimental evidence. According to this theory, a gating mechanism in the dorsal horn of the spinal cord permits or inhibits the transmission of pain impulses. It assumes that peripheral nerve fibers synapse in the gray matter of the dorsal horn, and this area serves as a gate. When the gate is closed, pain impulses are prevented from reaching the brain. This theory proposes that pain must reach a conscious awareness before it is perceived, and if awareness can be prevented, the perception is decreased or eliminated.

Although chronically ill individuals can be subjected to either acute or chronic pain, it is the ever present nature of chronic pain that controls so much of their lives. This chapter will look at some of the problems they face and provide general guidelines for some useful interventions. No effort is made to cover the myriad of problems that arise from chronic nonmalignant pain, nor are all possible interventions included. Focus is on information that the health professional with a basic education can use to help clients who suffer from chronic pain.

Problems and Issues

Thirty percent of our population suffers from chronic pain (Rosomoff & Steele-Rosomoff, 1988). The many diverse types of chronic nonmalignant pain states can involve any area of the body and vary in intensity from mild to excruciating. Individuals with chronic pain often find themselves in a "no-win" situation, since their pain no longer serves the purpose of acute pain nor does it respond adequately to conventional medical treatment. The pain itself becomes a chronic condition that requires daily management.

Chronic pain is the major cause of disability in the United States (Osterweis et al., 1987). About one-third of all those with chronic pain suffer from low back pain (Rosomoff & Steele-Rosomoff, 1988), making it the most prevalent cause of disability. A large number of these claimants have no demonstrable physiological basis for their pain (Flor & Turk, 1984). Some of these individuals are felt to be malingerers (Leavitt & Sweet, 1986), even though no evidence exists that they exaggerate their chronic pain or are more psychologically disturbed than people who are not receiving compensation (Mendelsohn, 1986; Labbe et al., 1988).

Undertreatment by Professionals

Pain relief is not as high a priority among health professionals as controlling the client's *expression* of pain (Fagerhaugh & Strauss, 1977). The clinical focus is on identifying and treating the underlying condition that is causing the pain. Many health care providers have a poor understanding of pain assessment and management, and are often frustrated with clients who either do not manifest symptoms of their pain state or do not respond well to ordered treatment.

The need for narcotics is often clearly indicated, yet undertreatment continues to be a pattern in health care. As many as 85 to 90 percent of patients with acute or prolonged pain from end-stage disease could be kept comfortable if narcotics were properly used (McCaffery & Beebe, 1989).

Physicians underprescribe either by ordering doses of analgesics that are less than effective or by ordering longer intervals between doses than the medication's duration of action warrants (Grossman & Sheidler, 1985; Angell, 1982; Marks & Sacher, 1973). Nurses tend to administer pain medication very conservatively and often lengthen the interval allowed or give less than or the minimum amount ordered (Fox, 1982; Marks & Sacher, 1973). To complicate matters, medications are administered inconsistently, so that relief is not continuous or adequate (Fagerhaugh & Strauss, 1977). Some clients contribute to the inadequate use of narcotics by not requesting medications or by refusing to take them if offered (Cleeland, 1987; Sriwatanakul et al., 1983).

The negative stereotypes of individuals with chronic pain held by many professionals contribute to the discounting of their pain complaints. This lack of validity only compounds the client's frustration and anguish. Professionals do not always give credence to pain complaints unless there is some identifiable pathology or the client demonstrates autonomic or behavioral responses (McCaffery, 1988). Nurses assume that all clients have the same pain perception threshold and therefore perceive the same intensity of pain from the same stimuli (Hardy et al., 1943). Many nurses have become desensitized to the pain experience and rate pain as less important than do clients (Fagerhaugh & Strauss, 1977). Professionals often assume that the depression found among chronic pain clients leads to decreased effectiveness of pain relief measures (Taylor et al., 1984).

When placebos work, the assumption is made that the pain is psychogenic, even though research shows that placebo analgesia may be due to an increase in endorphins (Greevert, et al., 1983). Many professionals believe chronic pain is not as intense as acute pain, especially if there is no sign of pathology. Research has shown that the opposite is true. Pain that continues for years results in a decrease in the client's internal narcotic, endorphins, resulting in the perception of even greater pain from the same stimuli (Koster & Kleber, 1987). Unfortunately, many health professionals tend to "put the blame on the victim" if cure is not possible (Flor & Turk, 1984).

Addiction Health professionals are afraid of addicting clients to narcotics (Angell, 1982; Trotter et al., 1981) based on behaviors seen among hospitalized clients that are erroneously interpreted as addiction (see Table 7-1). Addiction, which can be defined as "behavior of overwhelming involvement with obtaining and using a drug for its psychic effects, not for approved medical reasons" (McCaffery & Beebe, 1989), does not apply to the person in pain. Addicts do not use drugs to relieve pain, but use them for *psychological* reasons. They are compulsive in seeking drugs and tend to relapse even after they have undergone physical withdrawal.

Addiction among people taking narcotics for pain relief is rare. The person in pain who is using narcotics appropriately will stop taking the drug once the pain is relieved. In one study of nearly 12,000 medical inpatients receiving at least one narcotic, only four could be documented as addicts (Porter & Jick, 1980). In another study, less than 1 percent of inpatients receiving meperidine regularly became addicts

(Marks & Sacher, 1973). The need to continue drugs indicates that relief from pain has not been obtained and that medication is still necessary. What health professionals confuse with addiction is either physical dependence or drug tolerance.

Physical Dependence Physical dependence is not a sign of addiction, but is a *physiological response* of the body to repeated doses of a narcotic. If the narcotic is abruptly stopped, withdrawal symptoms will occur. During the first 6 to 12 hours after the narcotic is discontinued, the client may manifest anxiety, rhinorrhea, diaphoresis, shaking chills, anorexia, nausea, vomiting, and abdominal cramps. By the second to third day the client may show excitation, restlessness, insomnia, muscle spasms, low back pain, elevated blood pressure, tachycardia, dehydration, ketosis, and leukocytosis. Not everyone goes through demonstrable withdrawal, and increased doses of narcotics do not increase the severity of withdrawal (Hodding et al., 1980). Withdrawal symptoms can be avoided if narcotics are gradually discontinued—a common occurrence as pain subsides.

Drug Tolerance Drug tolerance is an *involuntary physiological behavior* that occurs when a narcotic begins to lose its effectiveness after repeated administration. Consequently, to gain adequate pain relief more narcotic is required (Foley & Rogers, 1981). Health professionals feel that each narcotic has a maximum dose that can be taken and are therefore concerned about inadequate pain relief should more medication be needed at a later time. They also fear that increased amounts of narcotics will result in respiratory depression or oversedation. What they should remember is that a concurrent tolerance to respiratory depression and sedation occurs as a person's body becomes tolerant to a narcotic (Martinson et al., 1982; Flor & Turk, 1984; McCaffery, 1981; Wright, 1981).

Mental and Emotional Effects of Unrelieved Pain

The individual with chronic pain may undergo a change from being someone with many roles (worker, friend, family member, and so forth) to

TABLE 7-1. Misconceptions about indications of addiction

Misconceptions	Comments/Corrections
1. Prolonged use of narcotics	1. Some pain is prolonged or lasts longer than expected. Length of time on narcotics does not increase likelihood of addiction.
2. Clock watching	2. This usually results from inadequate pain relief. Some narcotics are short acting; some patients metabolize narcotics rapidly. The pain returns before the designated interval elapses.
3. Prefers "needle" to the pill	3. This can be the result of not applying equianalgesic dosages when the route of narcotic is switched from injections to PO. The result is often undermedication. The effectiveness of a dose given IM may be 2 to 6 times greater than the same dose given PO.
4. "Enjoys his Demerol" (or other narcotic)	4. Why not? If a person has been in pain, he will probably be happy to get relief.
5. Knows the name and dose of narcotic	5. This knowledge should be encouraged. It can be helpful information in assessing effective analgesics at a future time.
6. "Orders" narcotic in anticipation of pain	6. This can be an indication that the interval between doses is not timed correctly for his individual pain. Reassess the pain and evaluate the interval; or, the patient may have been instructed appropriately in the use of a preventive approach.
7. Requires higher and higher doses given more frequently	7. The underlying reason for the pain could be advancing, e.g., cancer metastasis. The other possibility is the development of tolerance.

SOURCE: Reproduced by permission from McCaffery, M., & Beebe, A. (1989). *Pain: Clinical manual for nursing practice.* St. Louis: The C. V. Mosby Company.

someone who identifies only with pain. Because pain is invisible, clients may feel a need to explain or defend the pain in an effort to be believed. When faced with scepticism, they may even begin to question their pain experience (Finer & Melander, 1985).

Although many individuals with chronic pain manage to go on with other aspects of their lives, others have limited repertoires for coping with their illness and find the only safe way to respond to symptoms is to call the physician. These people's lives revolve around their pain, and every aspect of their lives is controlled by their response to it (Egan & Kanton, 1987).

The disturbed sleep seen in many clients with chronic pain indicates that there is either a psychological disturbance or poor pain relief (Finer & Melander, 1985). Clients sometimes experience a vicious cycle of poor sleep, which leads to musculoskeletal pain and depression, which in turn has a negative impact on sleep. After a night of inadequate rest, the following day is often filled with increased pain, increased fatigue, and hangovers from medication. Treating the sleep disturbance may be beneficial in easing both physical and emotional symptoms (Pilowsky et al., 1985).

Exhaustion can occur because pain requires increased energy to do even simple things. Poor sleep, medications, and inadequate physical and mental activities also lead to fatigue. Fatigue makes concentration difficult, leading to restlessness and boredom (Finer & Melander, 1985).

When persistent pain is coupled with fatigue, the client may limit movement, which increases dependency on family and friends. Increasing dependency creates a cyclic response in the client: fear of abandonment and impotence; a feeling of self-contempt; and a sense of being a burden on others, someone who is always receiving and never giving. Aggression shown toward others under these circumstances is poorly tolerated and may lead to withdrawal from the client. As negative feelings grow, the client may feel worthless or unfit and can show self-destructive behavior (Finer & Melander, 1985).

Body image can be altered when the painful part is seen as uninviting or less attractive or if the entire body feels ugly or repulsive (see Chapter 13, on body image). There may be an oversensitivity about body contact for fear of causing pain, and this can negatively impact on marital or sexual relationships, further isolating the person (Finer & Melander, 1985).

Life-Cycle Differences

Chronic pain in both children and the elderly is undermanaged more than in other age groups. It is not uncommon for those in these two categories to receive lower than therapeutic doses, causing them to have moderate to severe pain needlessly.

Inadequate pain control, common especially in the treatment of very young children, may result more from a lack of knowledge than a lack of concern. Many myths abound about pain in children that have no basis in fact (Jeans & Johnston, 1985; McCaffery & Beebe, 1989). It is believed that young children, especially neonates and infants, feel little if any pain; that young children do not experience pain to the same degree as adults; that they tolerate pain better than adults; and that they recover more quickly. It is also believed that the potential side effects of narcotics make such medication too dangerous for use with small children; that when narcotics are used with adolescents it will lead to addiction; that pain is not life-threatening to the young; and that young children do not remember pain.

McCaffery and Beebe (1989) note a number of studies that rebut many of these myths. Younger children may perceive a greater intensity of pain than older children (Fowler-Kerry & Lander, 1987; Haslam, 1969; Katz et al., 1982). Terminally ill children aged one to four require higher doses of intravenous fentanyl for procedural pain than do older children (Billmire et al., 1985; Maunuksela et al., 1986). In an article in the *New England Journal of Medicine,* Anand and Hickey (1987) listed 201 references pertaining to pain in the human neonate.

Jeans and Johnston (1985) note that children demonstrate pain regardless of age. They point out that neonates and infants show facial responses to pain and have distinct cries when in pain. Even though no systematic studies have been done with toddlers, nonverbal behaviors, such as lip clenching, a wide-eyed look, rocking, rubbing, agitation, or aggression are seen. Once language skills are present in preschoolers, more credence is given to the expression of pain.

As is the case with children, there are misconceptions about pain in the elderly (McCaffery & Beebe, 1989). Study of the special needs regarding pain in this population has been neglected. It is believed that pain is a natural outcome of growing old, that the potential side effects of narcotics make them too dangerous for use with the elderly, that pain perception decreases with age, and that the lack of pain behaviors indicates a lack or limited degree of pain. It is also believed that the elderly person is depressed if there is an absence of a known cause for the pain, and that the pain will subside when the cause is identified and the depression is treated.

McCaffery and Beebe (1989) note studies that refute these misconceptions. It has been shown that pain is not inevitable in the aged and its presence necessitates assessment and treatment (Butler & Gastel, 1980); the elderly have a greater number of disorders that can cause pain (Rowe & Bresdine, 1982), including a number of less common but painful problems (Butler & Gastel, 1980). Portenoy (1987) showed that close evaluation and knowledge of pharmacokinetics make the use of narcotics safe in this population. Other studies have failed to conclusively report age-related differences in sensitivity to pain (Clark & Mehl, 1971; Harkins et al., 1986; Harkins & Chapman, 1976). Where the elderly may differ is in atypical presentations of clinical pain (Clinch et al., 1984; MacDonald, 1984), but this cannot be generalized to all conditions.

Interventions for Dealing with Chronic Pain

Managing pain requires that a relationship of trust evolve between health provider and client.

Communication, which is always present, can be positive or negative (Twycross, 1985). If negative, it can lead to an adversarial position, which should be avoided. The professional should believe the client's statements of pain or at least give the client the benefit of the doubt. Not to believe these complaints, in effect, means the client is being called a liar, which is both an unethical and an unprofessional response. In addition, clients who feel that their providers are sincere are more likely to continue to seek methods that will help.

Problem-Solving Process

The goals of managing nonmalignant pain are to decrease the pain intensity as much as possible and to optimize the client's quality of life and level of function. Problem solving requires that assessment and diagnosis precede the development and implementation of any treatment plan, and that evaluation be done as a final step to determine the effectiveness of the plan. The steps involved from assessment through evaluation are frequently overlapping rather than sequential. The problem-solving process used by nurses is called *the nursing process.*

Initial assessment covers history taking, observation, and physical examination. Both objective findings, if they are present, and subjective factors, such as the client's perceptions and responses to the pain, need to be identified. Care must be taken to consider differences that exist in children and the elderly. The tool for pain assessment (Figure 7–1) is practical to any setting, easily adapted to the client's needs, and useful for any kind of pain. It may be duplicated for clinical use with permission of the author. Table 7–2 briefly discusses each section of this tool.

The analysis of collected data allows a diagnosis to be reached. Determination of appropriate outcomes and interventions, as well as how they should be attained, should be made jointly by the client and professional.

Interventions for managing nonmalignant pain are more numerous than the ones presented in this chapter. Those selected here are useful to the clinical practitioner without requiring extensive additional education or training. Much of the included material is drawn from McCaffery

and Beebe (1989). When other resources are used, they are so indicated. The guidelines and general principles covered here are for pharmacological management and a number of non-invasive measures that diminish, resolve, or prevent the recurrence of the pain state. Also included is information on pain management programs.

Most studies on pain management focus on the client; therefore, little is known about the impact of family dynamics. Studies on family involvement in treatment indicate that behavioral methods show promise. The reinforcement of pain expression and behavior by family members (Fordyce, 1976) needs to be changed to reinforcement of well-behavior. When well-behavior is reinforced, clients often show improvement in the areas of returning to work, increasing activity levels, and utilizing the health care system (Anderson et al., 1977).

Because of the strong influence a family can have on a client, some authors feel that family systems should be assessed along with other factors (Flor et al., 1987). It is suggested that family therapy might be helpful if the pain problem is exacerbated by family conflicts or if stress is caused by familial developmental milestones (Clarkin et al., 1979). However, there are no controlled outcome studies involving families in therapy, nor are there any criteria to indicate if therapy would be helpful.

Pharmacological Management of Pain[1]

Pharmacological control of pain is the responsibility of the entire health care team, including the client.

The goal of such management is to maintain the best possible pain control with the fewest side effects. Achieving this goal requires that the professionals be knowledgeable about pharmacological parameters of drugs, use effective communication skills, and provide research and

---

[1]Content on pharmacological management and noninvasive methods is drawn from McCaffery, M., & Beebe, A. (1989). *Pain: Clinical manual for the nursing practice.* St. Louis: The C. V. Mosby Company. When other sources are used, they are so noted.

Date_____

Patient's Name_____ Age_____ Room_____

Diagnosis_____ Physician_____

I. LOCATION: Patient or nurse mark drawing.

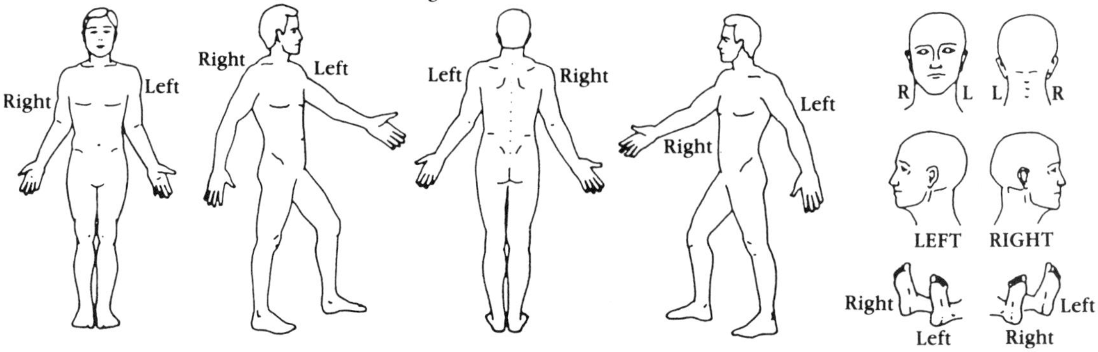

Nurse_____

II. INTENSITY: Patient rates the pain. Scale used_____

    Present:_____

    Worst pain gets:_____

    Best pain gets:_____

    Acceptable level of pain:_____

III. QUALITY: (Use patient's own words, e.g. prick, ache, burn, throb, pull, sharp)_____

_____

IV. ONSET, DURATION VARIATIONS, RHYTHMS:_____

_____

V. MANNER OF EXPRESSING PAIN:_____

_____

_____

VI. WHAT RELIEVES THE PAIN?_____

_____

_____

VII. WHAT CAUSES OR INCREASES THE PAIN?____ _____

_____

_____

VIII. EFFECTS OF PAIN: (Note decreased function, decreased quality of life.)

    Accompanying symptoms (e.g. nausea)_____

    Sleep_____

    Appetite_____

    Physical activity_____

    Relationship with others (e.g. irritability)_____

    Emotions (e.g. anger, suicidal, crying)_____

    Concentration_____

    Other_____

IX. OTHER COMMENTS:_____

_____

X. PLAN:_____

_____

FIGURE 7-1. Initial Pain Assessment Tool

SOURCE: Reproduced by permission from McCaffery, M., & Beebe, A. (1989). *Pain: Clinical manual for nursing practice.* St. Louis: The C. V. Mosby Company.

TABLE 7-2. Sections of the initial pain assessment tool

I.	Location	The site(s) where pain exists can be marked on the figures. If the client is unable to mark the figures, others can do so if the client points to painful areas on his or her body.
II.	Intensity	Translate pain intensity into numbers or words to objectify a subjective experience as much as possible. Any scale used must make sense to the client, needs to be used consistently, and should be noted each time it is used.
	Numerical scales (0-5, 0-10, etc.)	Zero means no pain, and the top number indicates the worst pain possible. Noting what the client considers an acceptable amount of pain indicates pain tolerance. This level should be the initial goal for which to strive.
	Pain descriptive words	If the client cannot use a numerical scale for any reason, terms like "no pain," "a little pain," "a lot of pain," or "too much pain" can be used.
III.	Quality	Descriptions of the pain can help determine its origin and help implement effective measures for its control. Suggest descriptors if the client has difficulty describing the pain.
IV.	Onset, duration, variations, and rhythms	Ask other questions that will help clarify the pain, such as length of time pain has existed, any changes in intensity or quality, what precipitates it, when it is worse or better, and so forth.
V.	Manner of expressing pain	An especially important section for the client who is unable to communicate for any reason. Family members can provide cues of what to look for. If clients can communicate, these cues should serve only as indicators that pain is present.
VI.	What relieves the pain	Specific pain-relieving methods used by the client at home can be incorporated into his or her plan of care.
VII.	What causes or increases the pain	Planning can be done to avoid these activities or things.
VIII.	Effects of pain	Indicates what is interfering with daily life and what other symptoms may need to be controlled.
IX.	Other comments	Note any other information from the client relating to the pain.
X.	Plan	The initial plan for pain control should be listed. Modifications should be listed on the flow sheet (Figure 7-2).

other articles to document a point or back up a suggestion.

When drugs for pain management are considered, narcotics come to mind. However, medications that help control pain work not only by modifying central nervous system perception, but also by interrupting the mechanisms responsible for causing the pain, increasing the pain threshold, blocking peripheral nervous system input, or relieving anxiety or depression. Pain control can sometimes be achieved by nonnarcotics, adjuvant analgesics (antidepressants, anticonvulsants, muscle relaxants, corticosteroids, etc.), antibiotics, vasodilators, and so forth. Only general information about narcotics and nonnarcotics will be discussed in this section.

Key Concepts in Administering Narcotics/ Nonnarcotics for Pain Control There are three major concepts to keep in mind when administering pain medication: (1) use a preventive approach; (2) titrate to effect; and (3) give the client as much control as possible.

Using a *preventive approach* means giving medication before the onset or increase of pain. Prevention, may involve administering medication around the clock (ATC) or giving it "as needed" (PRN) as soon as the pain begins so it does not escalate. There are a number of benefits of a preventive approach. The client is in pain less of the time, lower doses of analgesics are needed, fewer side effects occur, anxiety about the return of pain is decreased, and the client experiences an overall increase in activities. Clients on PRN schedules should be taught to request pain medication as soon as the pain occurs or before it increases.

To *titrate to effect* requires that enough medication be given to attain the desired pain relief with the fewest side effects. Titrating is done by tailoring analgesics to client needs in the following ways: adjusting doses up or down, changing intervals between doses, modifying the route of administration, or selecting the drug that is most effective to achieve the result that is wanted.

Titrating requires an ongoing evaluation of client response to ensure that safe and effective results are achieved. *Too much medication* is being given if the client is oversedated or has any respiratory depression, and *too little* if relief is poor and pain recurs too soon. The *wrong medication* should be suspected if relief is poor but the client is sedated, and *inadequate frequency* occurs if relief is adequate but does not last long enough. A lack of knowledge of equianalgesic doses is a common cause of undermedication for those in pain (Foley, 1985). The use of an equianalgesic chart that can be found in any good pharmacology text can serve as a guide to the amount and route of drugs that are used for pain control. The chart should be prominently displayed, used routinely, and updated regularly.

Giving the client as much control as possible in managing his or her pain is the third key concept. *Patient-controlled analgesia* (PCA) can be defined as "the patient's self-administration of all forms of pain control by methods that consider safety, as well as the patient's ability and willingness to exercise control" (McCaffery & Beebe, 1989, p. 49).

Not all clients are candidates for PCA. Some cannot understand instructions, and others lack the necessary confidence to manage their own pain situation. Ideally, all clients are given the opportunity to make this decision. Minimally, clients should be allowed as much control as they feel they can handle.

Narcotics Health professionals are often more concerned with the number of milligrams of a narcotic they give for pain than with a person's response to that dose. This is unfortunate, since clients respond to medication differently. Individualizing the dose, time interval, route, and choice of drug, and then monitoring the person's response are all vital to effective use of analgesics. Undertreatment with narcotics needs to be avoided. As tolerance to a medication increases, the dose also needs to increase. Fortunately, the concurrent increase in respiratory tolerance eliminates the concern professionals feel regarding this side effect. If narcotic-induced respiratory depression does occur in a conscious person, breathing will continue if instructions to breathe are given (Jaffe & Martin, 1985).

A pain flow sheet (see Figure 7–2) provides a tool for doing an ongoing assessment of medication effectiveness in any setting. The flow sheet can be modified, but the following factors should be included: the time the assessment is done, the client's rating of the pain, what medication is being used (including dose, time, and route), and physiological responses (especially respiratory status). Preferably the other factors listed here also will be included: other parameters needing assessment and a place for noting other strategies that are used or could be used to improve pain control.

Health providers concerned about the safe administration of medications should use a flow sheet to reassure themselves that the client is not experiencing any adverse effects. Professionals have no difficulty decreasing medication when necessary, but they need to be comfortable with increasing doses, especially if greater than usual amounts are needed or if the client is not getting adequate relief. A flow sheet provides a quick and easy reference to any increases and decreases in medication that have been given, the client's response, and any supplemental methods that are used. Such reassurances can only enhance pain management.

Professionals may need reeducation to relieve their fear of addicting the client. As long as medication is being used to control pain, clients do not become addicts. Any decrease in the effectiveness of a given dose requiring greater amounts of medication reflects drug tolerance.

Patient_____ Date_____

*Pain rating scale used_____

Purpose: To evaluate the safety and effectiveness of the analgesic(s).

Analgesic(s) prescribed:_____

Time	Pain rating	Analgesic	R	P	BP	Level of arousal	Other†	Plan & comments

FIGURE 7-2. Flow Sheet—Pain

*Pain rating: A number of different scales may be used. Indicate which scale is used and use the same one each time. For example, 0-10 (0 = no pain, 10 = worst pain).

†Possibilities for other column: bowel function, activities, nausea and vomiting, other pain relief measures. Identify the side effects of greatest concern to patient, family, physician, nurses.

SOURCE: Reproduced by permission from McCaffery, M., & Beebe, A. (1989). *Pain: Clinical manual for nursing practice.* St. Louis: The C. V. Mosby Company.

Remember, the overwhelming majority of people stop taking narcotics when their pain stops.

Morphine, the standard strong narcotic for severe acute pain and chronic cancer pain (American Pain Society, 1987), is only one of four commonly used strong narcotics (morphine, hydromorphine, levorphanol, and methadone) that are equally capable of relieving pain. There are various reasons for selecting one or the other, including the client's prior pain experience, the number and severity of side effects the client has had, the concentration or volume of doses that are available, the need for rapid or slower absorption or onset, the drug's duration or cumulative characteristics, and so forth.

McCaffery and Beebe (1989) also point out that although meperidine (Demerol) is extensively used, it is not recommended because of potential problems (American Pain Society, 1987, p. 4; Foley & Inturrisi, 1987, p. 214). Meperidine is shorter acting than other narcotics (Beaver, 1980; Jaffe & Martin, 1985), especially in young people (Kaiko, 1980) and smokers (Jick, 1974). It can irritate tissue, resulting in possible muscle fibrosis (Beaver, 1980; Jaffe & Martin, 1985); can have neuropsychiatric effects (Miller & Jick, 1978); is more toxic because of an active metabolite (Kaiko et al., 1983); and inadequate doses are usually prescribed for oral administration, resulting in poor pain control when that route is used.

Nonnarcotic Analgesics Nonnarcotics referred to as nonsteroidal anti-inflammatory drugs (NSAIDs) are best known not only for their anti-inflammatory effect but also for their effectiveness in pain control. They work primarily at the peripheral nervous system level. The reader is referred to any good pharmacology text for information on the mechanisms by which various NSAIDs work.

The pain-relieving effects of NSAIDs are underestimated and underused; most lay people and professionals do not realize how effective these drugs are as analgesics. McCaffery and Beebe (1989) note studies that show their effectiveness in postoperative patients (Dionne & Cooper, 1978; Slavic-Svircev et al., 1984; Tejada, 1986; Reasbeck et al., 1982); for control of pain when used alone with some cancer patients (Kantor, 1984; Ventafridda et al., 1980); and in achieving a significant analgesia when combined with narcotics (Beaver, 1984). They are sometimes effective for low back pain (Kantor, 1982; Brena, 1983); can relieve or prophylactically prevent migraine headaches (Bernstein, 1982); and have relieved painful menstrual cramps (Amadio & Cummings, 1986; Dingfelder, 1981; Wenzloff & Shrimp, 1984). The degree of pain relief varies, since some individuals are more responsive to NSAIDs than others.

Selecting the appropriate NSAID is dependent on individual variations, such as efficacy, side effects, compliance, and so forth (Williams, 1986). Equianalgesic tables show that average doses of nonnarcotics can be as effective as low oral doses of narcotics. Over the counter nonnarcotics, such as aspirin or tylenol, can be used at home to effectively and safely enhance pain relief.

NSAIDs should be used first if pain stays in the mild to moderate range of intensity. If necessary, they should be given ATC. If narcotics are needed, the NSAID should be continued if possible. Combining narcotics and nonnarcotics is a safe and logical method of pain relief because they relieve pain in different ways and have different side effects, and giving them together poses no more danger than alternating them. Peak effect of the nonnarcotic will begin about two hours after it is given—the span of time the narcotics effectiveness tends to decrease if it was given intramuscularly. Nonnarcotics provide an additive effect when combined with narcotics, resulting in a decrease in the amount of narcotic needed as well as a concurrent decrease in the narcotic's side effects (Beaver, 1981).

If oral narcotics do not fully relieve pain, supplement them with ATC doses of a nonnarcotic. To obtain the optimal therapeutic doses of each medication in a combination drug, supplement it with an additional amount of the nonnarcotic, since these compounds contain less than optimal doses of the nonnarcotic. For a client receiving parenteral narcotics who can take oral medications, give a NSAID for ongoing pain or when the narcotic is used for incident pain. To serve as an advocate for the client, use an equianalgesic chart and provide research findings or other articles to support your recommendations.

Noninvasive Methods for Pain Control

There are many noninvasive methods available to help the client in chronic pain. *Physical methods* include counter-irritation, vibration, percussion, local heat and cold, nerve fatigue via repetitive stimulation, trigger points, physiotherapy, occupational therapy, and neuromodulation. *Central methods* enhance pain acceptance and include doctrines such as yoga or transcendental meditation, relaxation, psychotherapy, operant conditioning, and behavior modification. Methods using *suggestion* include the placebo response and hypnosis or guided imagery (Mehta, 1986).

Noninvasive methods require a trial-and-error approach to determine what works for a given client or in a particular situation. The health professional can combine any technique within each or among all of the modalities. The client who feels he or she is believed and that the professional is genuinely trying to help will cooperate until some positive results are obtained. Only a few of the myriad methods will be covered here, with the discussion focusing on those noted in McCaffery and Beebe's book. These methods appear to be effective, but there is a lack of adequate research, which makes it difficult at times to document or support their use. The reference section includes citations to support each of the methods discussed.

Cutaneous Stimulation This is simply stimulating the skin for the purpose of relieving pain, especially localized pain. What works for some people and their pain differs from what helps others. Although its exact mechanism is unknown, the gate control theory suggests that stimulation of the skin may activate the large-diameter fibers that close the gate to pain messages carried by small fibers. Other possible mechanisms that have been suggested include the belief that some forms of cutaneous stimulation increase endorphins or may cause decreased sensitivity to pain.

Even though these are physical modalities, there is little knowledge about which conditions are responsive to what methods, how long a method should be used, and so forth. Ideas about the use of heat, cold, or other methods are more likely to be derived from our culture and personal experience than from well-tested, scientific information.

Cutaneous stimulation is not curative. Its effects are variable and unpredictable, but generally it reduces the intensity of pain during or after stimulation. Some kinds of stimulation work best with acute localized pain; other methods seem effective with chronic pain. Little client participation or activity is required, making these methods appropriate for those with limited physical or mental energy. Potential benefits include a decreased intensity of pain, relief of muscle spasm that is secondary to underlying skeletal or joint pathology or nerve root irritation, and increased physical activity.

Selecting the right cutaneous stimulation for a given client is not always easy. Not only must the most appropriate type of stimulation be selected, but choices must be made about the site, duration, and frequency of use, and what modifications are necessary to achieve the greatest relief. Some types, such as heat and cold, can be used interchangeably unless there are contraindications. When selecting a type, factors that should be considered are availability of method, cost, amount of time required, safety, possible side effects, potential effectiveness, contraindications, and client acceptability. When possible, the client should be given a choice of available methods.

Not all types of cutaneous stimulation can be used without special education or training. Table 7-3 lists some that are easy to use in the clinical setting. The "how to" of implementing these methods is not included, and the reader is encouraged to seek sources that provide details before attempting to perform any of them.

Distraction Distraction from pain is achieved by focusing attention on stimuli other than the pain sensation. By increasing other sensory input or even by focusing on the less bothersome qualities of the pain sensation, such as pressure or warmth, the client does not focus completely on the pain itself, thereby making it less intense, more bearable, and more acceptable. This is true even when the pain is severe. Not only does distraction help ease pain, but focusing on pleasant things improves one's mood, which helps

TABLE 7-3. Pointers on selecting a method of cutaneous stimulation

• Massage.	Minimal side effects and contraindications. Backrubs or body massage can be time-consuming and may relieve only mild pain, but pain need not be localized and most patients enjoy it. Modest patients may object to touch or disrobing. Massage of feet and hands may be more accessible, acceptable, and even more effective.
• Pressure, sometimes with massage.	Massage/pressure to trigger points or acupuncture points may be very effective but is briefly uncomfortable. Initially it requires time to locate the points. But then patients can learn to work on some trigger points on their own.
• Vibration.	A more vigorous form of massage that may be more effective. Low risk of tissue damage. Check on availability or cost of a vibrator. May be used for trigger points. May be unacceptable due to noise or intensity of stimulation if vibrator is not adjustable. Sometimes this is a less expensive substitute for TENS.
• Heat and cold.	Probably works best for well-localized pain. Both may be done with a minimum of equipment and both should be applied at a comfortable level of intensity. Cold has more advantages than heat. Unwanted side effects (e.g., burns, and contraindications—bleeding and swelling) are more frequent with heating than with cooling. When cold relieves pain, it tends to be more effective than heat. However, patients usually prefer heat to cold, and use of cold often requires some persuasion.
• Ice application/massage.	A frozen substance applied to the skin is uncomfortable, but only for a few minutes before numbness occurs. Continous use for 10 minutes or less. Pain must be well localized. May relieve severe pain. Simple, low-risk technique for brief, painful procedures. Especially effective in obliterating needle stick pain. May be used on trigger points. Sometimes this is a very inexpensive substitute for TENS.
• Menthol.	Refers to menthol-containing substances for application to skin. Intensity increases with amount of menthol; may be uncomfortable at higher concentrations. Odor offensive to some people. Use influenced by culture; more restricted use by Americans than other cultures (e.g., Asians). Inexpensive. Once it is applied, it provides continuous stimulation without additional effort. Well suited for nighttime use.
• TENS.	Compared with above methods, much more expensive, less available, and more time needed to teach nurse and patient, but supported by more research and regarded by many as more "scientific."

SOURCE: Reproduced by permission from McCaffery, M., & Beebe, A. (1989). *Pain: Clinical manual for nursing practice.* St. Louis: The C. V. Mosby Company.

counteract depression and gives the client a sense of control over the painful experience.

Distraction is easy to learn and is effective as long as the distracting stimuli are present. These techniques are appropriate for procedures with brief episodes of pain that last for an hour or less, such as lumbar puncture, bone marrow aspiration, burn or wound debridement, dressing changes, painful injections, and so forth. Dis-

traction will relegate the pain to the periphery of awareness, but will not completely eliminate it. It is not a substitute for medications, but should be added as needed prior to or during a painful procedure.

Distraction should be used when the client can understand instructions and is willing to try the technique, has the physical ability and energy to perform the activities, can concentrate on the stimuli being presented, and desires some self-control over the painful experience. Most distraction techniques require time and energy and are inappropriate for long periods of time. They are also not effective for clients who are hypersensitive to stimuli, such as people with migraine headaches or meningitis.

To individualize distraction techniques, capitalize either on methods that the client has used in the past or on those that would be of interest to him or her. Decide on what technique(s) will be used before the need arises, and give the client an opportunity to practice.

Suggested techniques should be consistent with the client's energy level and ability to concentrate. When pain is increasing, the complexity of distraction should increase; with pain of high intensity, simple distraction is more in keeping with the client's energy level. Techniques can be subtracted as pain intensity decreases.

Distraction techniques work best when a combination of sensory modalities is used. Focusing visually on a stationary object can be combined with slow rhythmic breathing, comfortable rhythmic massage of some part of the body, or singing silently or aloud. Active listening to recorded music via a cassette allows the volume to be increased if pain increases and decreased when pain decreases. Having the client describe a picture combines visual, verbal, and auditory distraction. Interestingly, Cousins (1981) found that laughter lasting for at least 20 minutes was a form of distraction that had a carryover effect that relieved pain after the laughter stopped.

Clients with ongoing pain do not benefit from distraction. However, if they are deprived of their usual sensory input because of a boring or monotonous environment or an excessive input of meaningless stimuli, simple or practical approaches can be used to normalize daily sensory input so that pain is more tolerable. Some clients may be highly motivated to modify their environment, while others will be resistant. Boredom tends to lead to more boredom, so clients may become passive victims of the very problem that needs to be addressed.

Increasing sensory input is appropriate for clients who have the physical energy and ability to engage in activities similar to their prior ones, are willing or motivated to do so, want to regain some previous function or quality of life, and are aware of being adversely affected by the present environment. Pacing is also helpful for individuals who occasionally overexert themselves and thereby precipitate more pain.

Normalizing sensory input is inappropriate for those whose pain has produced almost complete disability, since these individuals may need a multidisciplinary approach. It is also not a good method for those who are withdrawn and may need to gain a feeling of control over their illness and treatment before participating in creating a more normal day for themselves.

To normalize boring days requires planning the whole day with activities similar to those typical of previous healthy days. A list should be made of all prior activities, and the client should identify those that were most important or enjoyable. This list serves as the basis for selecting activities that the client can perform independently with minimal effort or that can be carried out if some help is provided. Having a written schedule helps, and activities should be paced to avoid overexertion. The client needs to know that devising and carrying out such a plan can be a difficult task but can become easier with encouragement and repeated success. As mentioned previously, selected activities should combine as many sensory modalities as possible. For example, a gentle exercise program (kinesthetic) could be done with a friend (possibly verbal), using music (auditory) and written instructions or videotapes (visual). To avoid having the plan itself become boring, activities should be varied at regular intervals and the schedule changed daily.

The client should be encouraged to combine regulated sensory input with other pain relief methods (such as drugs). Combining pain relief measures in this manner allows more opportunity to be involved in normal activities. The professional should help the client obtain any special assistance that is needed.

Relaxation Relaxation should be used as an adjunct to other pain relief methods. It is not a substitute for medications or other methods, since it does not relieve pain directly. Relaxation helps the client by breaking the cycle of pain, muscle tension, and anxiety. A recent literature review showed that its use led to a significant reduction in pain plus some improvement in areas such as medication intake, activity, and mood (Linton, 1986). Pain specialists agree that it is probably a significant part of a management program for someone with chronic nonmalignant pain.

Relaxation is attained when the client is in a state of relative freedom from both anxiety and skeletal muscle tension. Ideally, the client achieves the relaxation response: decreased oxygen consumption, decreased respiratory and heart rates, decreased muscle tension, normal blood pressure, and an increase in the brain's alpha waves. Some methods, such as slow rhythmic breathing, are easy to learn. Others, such as yoga, require a training program to build skill. Not everyone responds to all relaxation techniques, so time is required to develop an effective one for a specific individual. Any method attempted should be individualized to the client and the situation. Clients, whether children or adults, are candidates for relaxation if they express a need or desire to use relaxation to cope with or control their pain, can understand the instructions, and can concentrate on the directions.

The client can be actively involved, or relaxation techniques can be used passively with the client who is unable to participate. Active relaxation, especially when used preventively, can improve the individual's sleep; reduce skeletal muscle tension (which in turn may reduce strain or pressure on pain-sensitive structures); decrease fatigue, leading to a more energized feeling; increase the effectiveness of other pain relief measures; lead to improved mood and decreased distress; and increase confidence along with a sense of self-control in coping with pain.

Passive techniques are appropriate for those who have limited physical or emotional energy; are very young or very old; are confused, agitated, undergoing sudden distress or pain; or are extremely fatigued or sedated. Family members can learn to use simple touch, massage, or warmth to help achieve relaxation in these clients.

There are various factors to consider in selecting a relaxation technique. Table 7-4 contains practical guidelines to use in matching technique to client. Table 7-5 contains a sample of available relaxation techniques that are easily used in the clinical setting.

Relaxation techniques should be used only with individuals who are willing to attempt them. Clients should be informed that any selected technique serves primarily to reduce the distress caused by pain and not the pain itself. Clients should also be informed that relaxation is not a substitute for other methods, but will only enhance them. Previously learned techniques can be integrated. To accomplish the highest degree of effectiveness, the health provider should be with the client when relaxation is being used. However, instructions can be tape-recorded and provided for the client or family when the provider's time or energy is at a premium.

Relaxation is best if used preventively. Demonstrate the selected technique to the client prior to its need, and provide an opportunity to practice it. A return demonstration serves to assure client and professional that the technique is both understood and effective. Practice done at least once a day improves performance and should be undertaken when the client is fairly free of pain and tension. Any selected technique can be individualized by integrating changes suggested by the client.

Evaluation can be done by using a Likert-type pain scale before, during, and after performing the technique. Biofeedback, which is not a relaxation technique itself but measures its effect, can also be used for evaluation by taking the pulse rate or gently moving body parts to identify signs of tension before, during, and after using any form of relaxation.

Imagery Imagery is not effective with all clients, nor are all health professionals able to teach it. When used as a form of distraction from pain, it increases tolerance; when used to produce relaxation, it decreases distress. Imagery can also produce an image of pain relief that decreases the perceived intensity of the pain. Visualization is a form of imagery that takes advantage of one's ability to understand and interpret reality in a symbolic manner (McKay et al., 1981). Hypnosis, which requires additional training on the part of

TABLE 7-4. Practical guidelines for matching relaxation techniques to patients and situations

1. Consider the *amount of time* the patient will experience pain vs. the time involved in teaching and using the technique. Usually:

   • Use the less time-consuming techniques for brief episodes of pain (e.g., jaw relaxation or slow rhythmic breathing for procedural or postoperative pain).

   • Be willing to invest more time for patients with chronic pain (e.g., peaceful past experiences or meditative relaxation for cancer pain or recurrent headaches).

   • Beware of introducing time-consuming techniques to patients who are already under considerable stress, even if they have chronic pain, since this may add another stressor.

2. Consider how pain, fatigue, anxiety, and other factors influence the *patient's general ability to learn or engage in an activity.* Usually:

   • Use brief, simple techniques or massage during severe pain, lack of concentration, or along with other pain relief measures (e.g., deep breath/tense, exhale/relax, yawn), when narcotic is given such as for renal colic.

   • Teach more time-consuming techniques when the patient is alert and comfortable (e.g., medi-

   tative relaxation when severe back pain is in remission).

   • Even if the patient says relaxation is not helpful during pain or the anticipated pain will be too severe for him to use relaxation, suggest he use it before and after pain.

3. Note if the patient has *energy that needs to be dissipated* (e.g., restless, "up-tight," or the "fight or flight" response—meaning that he has generated energy to fight or flee but has nowhere to go). Use a technique that releases energy, e.g., progressive relaxation.

4. For the *patient who misunderstands the purpose of relaxation,* use other terminology and suggest humor, peaceful past experiences, or passive recipient techniques such as a back rub.

5. *Consider whether the focus is inward on the body or outward on peaceful scenes.* An inward focus can increase distress about changes in body image or feelings of failure about physical limitations. Be cautious about using an exclusively inward body focus for patients who are distressed about changes in body appearance or function, severely depressed, or have difficulty maintaining contact with reality.

SOURCE: Reproduced by permission from McCaffery, M. & Beebe, A. (1989). *Pain: Clinical manual for nursing practice.* St. Louis: The C. V. Mosby Company.

the professional, often uses imagery as a technique. Like other noninvasive methods, imagery is not a substitute for other methods of pain control, but should be considered an adjunctive treatment for pain. No form of imagery should be used with a resistant client regardless of the good intentions of the health provider.

The use of imagery for pain relief is based in part on two interrelated beliefs. First, it provides partial control over body functions that are not controlled by conscious, rational thoughts. Second, the body reacts to images or memories in a manner similar to its functioning or response during the actual event. The latter requires that one imagine performing an activity rather than observing or desiring it (Jones & Johnson, 1980; Mast, 1986).

The effectiveness of imagery should not be underestimated. For example, the fear of speak-

ing before a group of people can cause physiological responses, such as trembling and a pounding heart. The desire or will to stop the physical response is not adequate to counteract the threat or danger imagined in relation to speaking in public. Imagination consistently wins over will.

When used for pain management, imagery allows one's imagination to develop sensory images that decrease the intensity of pain or change it to a pleasant, more acceptable, or nonpainful substitute, such as numbness or coolness. An individual can imagine something about the pain that will provide pain relief, rendering this activity therapeutic. In this sense imagery acts as an analgesic or anesthetic. When imagery is systematically developed or uses involved techniques for pain relief, it is referred to as *therapeutic guided imagery.*

TABLE 7-5. Characteristics of specific relaxation techniques and indications for use

Deep Breath/Tense, Exhale/ Relax, Yawn	This takes only a few seconds; is easily learned by patient; is appropriate to introduce when patient is already tense and in pain (e.g., during a procedure) or may be taught prior to brief painful procedures or preoperatively.
Humor	This takes very little of the nurse's time to suggest to patients; patients may spend as much time as they wish using it. It may be appropriate for patients who are elderly; who resist or misunderstand the idea of relaxation; who are depressed or easily lose contact with reality; who have little time or energy for learning the skill of relaxation; or who are from a different culture (assuming a tape from that culture can be obtained). It may be used to relieve boredom of prolonged pain under confining circumstances; also appropriate for brief procedural pain.
Heartbeat Breathing	The nurse may have to teach the patient how to find and count the radial pulse, and some patients may have difficulty with this. If not, it takes very little of the nurse's or patient's time. Heartbeat breathing has an internal focus but is used only briefly. It may relieve a sudden, sharp increase in fear or anxiety and may be used without others noticing. It may be very helpful to patients who are aware of a sudden increase in heart rate during stress.
Jaw Relaxation	This takes very little time for the nurse to teach or for the patient to use. It is considered an abbreviated form of progressive relaxation. Its effectiveness may be due to relaxation of one area of the body leading to relaxation of the rest of the body. Useful for brief moderate to severe pain (e.g., postoperative pain), especially if taught in the absence of severe pain and tension. Effective with elderly patients.
Slow Rhythmic Breathing	This takes very little of the nurse's time to teach. It is very adaptable, patient can use for 30 to 60 seconds (a few breaths without others noticing) or for up to 20 minutes. It is also a useful technique for initial relaxation prior to engaging in more complex relaxation techniques.
Peaceful Past Experiences	This may prove to be the best of all approaches to relaxation since it relies on what the patient has already found relaxing. It is usually an outward focus (i.e., not focused on the present body state). Recalling a peaceful experience is often a therapeutic process, and this approach may be the most appropriate for patients with chronic pain, particularly those with terminal illness. Remembering certain past experiences may serve many purposes (e.g., releasing or letting go of treasured events or reinforcing the conviction that a valued event will occur again). However, the sharing of a valued past experience may require a trusting relationship between the nurse and patient. This may take a considerable amount of the nurse's time, but not always. Give *priority* to this for terminally ill patients, and tape record it.

Imagery may be helpful for those who have pain of clearly defined physical origin. It may alter the physical cause of pain or be beneficial without actually affecting the physiological aspects of pain. Imagery techniques may lead to more confidence in and ability to control or heal the painful experience, increase the effectiveness of other pain relief measures, decrease the intensity of pain, reduce related distress, or change its sensation to one that is more acceptable.

More involved forms of imagery, such as meditative imagery, should be taught by professionals who have received specialized training, since there can be adverse effects. Lengthy imagery is *inappropriate* for those who do not want to try it; have severe emotional problems or a history of

TABLE 7-5. *Continued*

Meditative Relaxation Script	This usually takes a minimum of three contacts with the patient. The first two take about 15 minutes each. The second usually involves tape recording the script. The third is a follow-up and may take only a minute unless problems occur. The script is highly effective in producing relaxation in English-speaking, middle-class Americans. It is permissive enough that patients can individualize it on their own, and it combines an inward focus (breathing techniques and modified progressive relaxation) with an outward focus (peaceful place). Even when patients say that certain options in the script are not helpful to them, it is seldom necessary to rerecord the tape, since patients usually say they simply ignore what does not help them. Give *priority* to this (or peaceful past experiences or progressive relaxation) for patients with prolonged pain. It takes more time than you may have and it is not a miracle, but it often makes a significant difference.
Progressive Relaxation Script	This also usually takes a minimum of three contacts with the patient for a total of 35 minutes or more. The first two contacts take about 15 minutes. The second usually involves tape-recording the technique. The third is a follow-up and may take only a few minutes, unless problems have occurred. Its potential advantages are that it involves physical activity that gives a sense of "doing something" (e.g., muscle contraction, dissipates energy), is focused inward without the necessity of keeping the eyes closed, does not rely exclusively on mental activity, and easily gets the patients' attention by asking them to perform specific tasks. Give this *priority* for patients with prolonged pain who exhibit signs of moderate to severe anxiety or "fight or flight," especially if they cannot engage in their customary physical exercise. They need to get rid of that muscular energy. Later they may benefit from a more meditative approach.
Simple Touch, Massage, or Warmth	This may be done by the nurse or the patient's family or friends. It need not take much time and is indicated for patients who do not have time or energy to do for themselves whatever would produce relaxation. Loved ones who want to feel useful may benefit themselves and the patient by committing to body rubs of only three minutes (e.g., back, feet, hands). Help family and friends identify definite times for performing body rubs. This gives structure for the patient and the loved ones.

SOURCE: Reproduced by permission from McCaffery, M., and Beebe, A. (1989). *Pain: Clinical manual for nursing practice.* St. Louis: The C. V. Mosby Company.

psychiatric illness; report hallucinations for any reason, including drug reactions or sensory restriction; have no time or energy for lengthy imagery; or cannot concentrate.

For most health professionals, simple forms of imagery that are suggested in a casual manner can be used effectively with clients, who can then decide to continue following or reject these methods. These simpler forms tend to be effective, consume little time, are low risk, and do not require advanced knowledge or skills beyond basic education.

Subtle or conversational imagery, such as routine statements and questions, may already be part of the health professional's repertoire. For example, nurses commonly imply that anti-arrhythmics will "strengthen" the heart or that a well-balanced diet will help the body "resist" infection. There are ways of enhancing one's ability to use subtle images more naturally. First, when explaining specific pain relief measures, use words that paint a mental picture of relaxation or have tactile-kinesthetic feelings. Effective words include *floating, softer, healing, dissolving, lighter, releasing, letting go,* and so forth. Second, suggest an image of how the pain will subside or be relieved to balance the client's image of what causes the pain. Above all, the professional should use images or descriptors that feel natural to ensure ease and comfort with what is described.

Simple, brief symptom substitution is best when used as a possible alternative for relieving brief pain. It allows the client to imagine pain as being a more acceptable sensation for a period of time—that is, sensing pressure rather than aching. Words used by the client to denote greater acceptance or less discomfort should be used. When the situation involves pain not previously experienced, select descriptive words that are less unpleasant, such as "warm" rather than "burning." Another technique is to help the client focus on a substitute sensation, such as the cold and numbness felt when holding an ice cube, rather than the pain felt elsewhere in the body.

Standardized imagery techniques and *systematically individualized imagery* are more extensive and require at least a moderate amount of client involvement. Both techniques can be used for several minutes or more, both should have client approval of what is included, and both can be practiced regularly or used fairly often. Standardized techniques should be stated permissively enough to be used safely, quickly, and effectively. Since they tend to be vague ("see yourself breathing out the pain"), the client can individualize them in his or her own imagination. Systematically individualized imagery is a personalized image created by the client of what the pain is and how it can be relieved. It is developed in specific detail by the individual with guidance from the health professional. For example, an antibiotic can be developed into an elaborate image of soldiers that are successfully killing individual bacteria.

For either of these techniques the image used needs to make sense to the client as a means of pain relief. Selected images need not be biologically or medically correct. They can include any variety of things: a sound that gets quieter, a shape that becomes smaller, a vicious animal that becomes friendly, or something of a religious or spiritual nature. The client should get into a comfortable position, and interruptions should be prevented if possible. Concentrating on the se-

lected image is important and can be done with the eyes either closed or open. If concentration is difficult, counting with each breath may help. Spending more than 20 minutes at a time or more than 1 hour a day may indicate the need for more pain relief measures. Remember, imagery rarely leads to complete pain relief, and the technique should be used either to prevent regularly recurring pain or to help pain from increasing to an intense level.

Pain Management Programs

The growth in numbers and kinds of pain management programs occurred secondary to clients' poor response to the usual medical treatment for chronic pain. Pain programs help clients, many of whom feel hopeless, deal with their pain and regain some control of their lives. Programs seek to decrease pain intensity to a bearable level, decrease depression, and decrease use of the health care system and medications, and increase independence in activities of daily living, involvement with family, and social activities. Treatment concentrates on restoring functional capacity in all spheres of living (Osterweis, 1987).

Pain management programs are extremely varied. Pain *clinics* are outpatient facilities, and pain *centers* have both inpatient and outpatient facilities. They range in scope from small single-discipline or modality clinics (such as an anesthesiologist doing nerve blocks) to large multidisciplinary centers, many university based. Most programs fall somewhere between these two extremes (Lipton, 1986). The effectiveness of these programs is poorly known. Linton (1986) points out that there are a limited number of studies on pain programs and that many of them have methodological problems, such as poor designs or inadequate isolation of treatment components.

Programs at centers have multidisciplinary teams consisting of a variety of physicians, nurses, physical therapists, occupational therapists, and other consultants, as deemed necessary. There is a strong emphasis on all members of the team diagnosing and assessing the client's physical, mental, and psychosocial status, so that a coherent treatment plan can be developed (Rosomoff et al., 1980). The client is a member of the team and participates in all decision making, since he or she carries a great deal of the responsibility for treatment. However, the client should be cautioned not to expect miracles.

Multiple modalities are used to improve the client's status, including *physical therapy* (exercise, transcutaneous electrical nerve stimulation (TENS), joint mobilization, heat or cold packs, massage, hydrotherapy, ultrasound, traction), *behavior modification* (operant conditioning, relaxation methods, distraction, cognitive reframing), education, psychological and vocational rehabilitation, stress management, and so forth (Osterweis, 1987). In Japan, acupuncture is used in conjunction with other treatment (Hyodo, 1985).

When the client finds that pain has become the central focus of living, the special help provided by a pain management program is indicated. Often the client needs assistance in determining which of these programs will best suit his or her needs, and the health care professional may be called on to provide guidance in making a selection. Information about programs can be obtained in literature put out by the programs and in published articles, by visiting a program, or by speaking to others who have attended it. It is important to know the types of pain that are dealt with, the types of clients treated, the modalities used and services offered, the program's goals, and whether the client or program decides on these goals. Additional important information includes the program's credentials or accreditation, the length of time it has been in existence, and how long most of the staff have been there.

Summary and Conclusions

Unlike acute pain, chronic nonmalignant pain serves no useful purpose. Its omnipresent nature makes it an entity unto itself that needs daily managing to achieve an adequate measure of relief and gain an improved quality of life.

Many problems arise from these pain states. Some result from poor pain management on the part of the health provider, which only compounds the client's problems. Poor management can be secondary to negative stereotypes about

people with chronic pain, fear of adverse side effects, or concern about addicting the client to narcotics. Other problems arise from the mental and emotional effects of unrelieved pain, family dynamics, life-cycle differences, and so forth. Many problem areas, such as pain behavior, are not discussed in this chapter.

Managing chronic pain requires that the health provider believe the client so that a trusting relationship can develop. Trust is important in working out an effective plan, since not every intervention works with every individual, and many trial-and-error attempts may be necessary in order to achieve success. A problem-solving approach should be used that incorporates the joint efforts of health care professional and client from assessment through evaluation. Data should be noted on an assessment tool. Throughout the entire process, both client and professional should avoid becoming discouraged if early attempts fail.

Medications are a cornerstone of pain control. To use them effectively, the professional should have a thorough understanding of pharmacokinetics. When using narcotics or NSAIDs, a preventive approach is important. As clients develop drug tolerance, narcotics should be titrated to ensure pain relief. In addition, the client should be given as much control as possible. The use of a flow sheet serves to provide accurate data and assures the professional that the client is tolerating medications that are being used. An equianalgesic chart identifies equivalent doses of different medications, and it should be displayed prominently, used routinely, and updated regularly.

Among the many noninvasive methods available for enhancement of pain management, several methods of cutaneous stimulation, distraction, relaxation, and imagery can be used by the clinical practitioner who has a basic education. General information that can serve as guidelines is provided here, but before attempting any of them, more extensive "how-to" information should be gained from other detailed sources.

When pain becomes the central focus of a client's life and other pain relief methods are no longer successful, pain management programs may serve to help clients gain some control of their lives and increase function. The health provider may be called on to assist the client in selecting the most appropriate program. This can be done by gathering information about the program, its goals, and its effectiveness.

NURSING DIAGNOSIS

9.1.1.1 Chronic Pain

Definition: A state in which the individual experiences pain that continues for more than six months in duration.

Defining Characteristics:

Major: Verbal report or observed evidence of pain experienced for more than six months.

Minor: Fear of reinjury; physical and social withdrawal; altered ability to continue previous activities; anorexia; weight changes; changes in sleep patterns; facial mask; guarded movement.

Related Factors: Chronic physical/psychological disability.

Editor's Note: Most handbooks on nursing diagnosis in current use still list *Altered Comfort: Chronic Pain,* but the taxonomy simplifies this as noted above. The definition implies only continuous pain and should be expanded to include recurring or intermittent chronic pain. Note that the characteristics of this diagnostic category do not contain autonomic or behavioral responses, since the body has adapted.

The only related factor noted, chronic physical/psychosocial disability, is dealt with collaboratively with the physician to manage the pain state. However, there are a number of contributing or related factors that the nurse can manipulate independently. These include such factors as *anxiety or depression; drug tolerance to current doses of medication; lack of knowledge of pain treatment modalities; prior experiences with pain and/or pain management; social isolation.*

The reader should note the cyclic nature of pain and the factors that influence it. For example, pain causes anxiety, which leads to increased pain, and so forth. The nurse needs to intervene at some point to break the cycle.

There are other diagnostic categories that can be identified in which chronic nonmalignant pain is the related factor. Powerlessness (7.3.2) is an example that comes to mind. (Its definition, defining characteristics, and related factors are noted in Chapter 9, on quality of life.) By mastering or controlling aspects of the pain, the client feels in better control of the pain situation.

STUDY QUESTIONS

1. How do professionals undermine pain management?
2. Differentiate *addiction* from *drug tolerance* or *physical dependence.*
3. Identify the mental and emotional effects of unrelieved pain.
4. What misconceptions exist about pain in children and the elderly? How can these misconceptions be refuted?
5. Discuss the concepts that should be considered in the pharmacological management of pain with narcotics or nonnarcotics.
6. How can an assessment tool, flow sheet, and equianalgesic chart be used to enhance pain management?

7. Compare the following noninvasive methods of managing pain from the perspective of effectiveness, benefits to client, costs, and ease of implementation.
   a. Cutaneous stimulation
   b. Distraction
   c. Relaxation
   d. Imagery
8. What are the advantages and disadvantages of a pain management program? How can the health professional assist the client in selecting an appropriate program?

References

Amadio, P., & Cummings, D. M. (1986). Nonsteroidal anti-inflammatory agents: An update. *American Family Physician, 34,* 147-154.

American Pain Society (1987). *Principles of analgesic use in the treatment of acute pain and chronic cancer pain: A concise guide to medical practice.* Washington D.C.: American Pain Society.

Anand, K. J. S., & Hickey, P. R. (1987, November 17). Pain and its effects in the human neonate and fetus. *New England Journal of Medicine, 317,* 1321-1329.

Anderson, T. P., Cole, T. M., Gullickson, G., Hudgens, A., & Roberts, A. H. (1977). Behavior modification of chronic pain: A treatment program by a multidisciplinary team. *Clinical Orthopedics, 129,* 96-100.

Angell, J. (1982, January 14). The quality of mercy. *New England Journal of Medicine, 306,* 98-99.

Beaver, W. T. (1980, December 12). Management of cancer pain with parenteral medication. *Journal of the American Medical Association, 244,* 2653-2657.

———— (1981, February 23). Aspirin and acetaminophen as constituents of analgesic combinations. *Archives of Internal Medicine, 141,* 239-300.

———— (1984, September 10). Combination analgesics. *American Journal of Medicine, 77* (3A), 38-53.

Bernstein J. (1982, March). Anti-inflammatories for migraine. *Aches and Pains, 3,* 32-37.

Billmire, D. A., Neale, H. W., & Gregory, R. O. (1985). Use of IV fentanyl in the outpatient treatment of pediatric facial trauma. *Journal of Trauma, 25,* 1079-1080.

Bonica, J. J. (1985). Biology, pathology and treatment of acute pain. In S. Lipton & J. Miles (Eds.), *Persistent pain.* London: Harcourt Brace Jovanovich.

Brena, S. F. (1983). Drugs and pain: the use and misuse. In S. F. Brena & S. L. Chapman (Eds.). *Management of patient with chronic pain.* New York: Raven Press.

Butler, R. N., & Gastel, B. (1980). Care of the aged: perspectives on pain and discomfort. In L. K. Ng and J. Bonica (Eds.), *Pain, discomfort and humanitarian care.* New York: Elsevier North Holland.

Clark, W. D. & Mehl, L. (1971). Therman pain. *Journal of Abnormal Psychology, 78,* 202-212.

Clarkin, J. F., Allen, F. J., & Moodie, J. L. (1979). Selection criteria for family therapy. *Family Practice, 18* (4), 391-403.

Cleeland, C. S. (1987, April). Barriers to the management of cancer pain. *Oncology* (Suppl.) *1,* 19-26.

Clinch, D., Banerjee, A. K., & Ostick, G. (1984). Absence of abdominal pain in elderly patients with peptic ulcer disease. *Age Ageing, 133,* 120-123.

Cousins, N. (1981). *Anatomy of an illness as perceived by the patient.* New York: Bantam.

Dingfelder, J. R. (1981). Primary dysmenorrhea treatment with prostaglandin inhibitors: A review. *American Journal of Obstretric Gynecology, 140,* 874-879.

Dionne, R. A., & Cooper, S. A. (1978, June). Evaluation of preoperative ibuprofen for post-operative pain after removal of third molars. *Oral Surgery, 45,* 851-856.

Egan, K. J., & Kanton, W. J. (1987). Responses to illness and health in chronic pain patients and healthy adults. *Psychosomatic Medicine, 49,* 470-481.

Fagerhaugh, S. Y., & Strauss, A. L. (1977). *Politics of pain management: Staff-patient interaction.* Menlo Park, CA: Addison-Wesley.

Finer, B., & Melander, B. (1985). Living with chronic pain. In S. Lipton & J. Miles (Eds.), *Persistent pain.* London: Harcourt Brace Jovanovich.

Flor, H., & Turk, D. C. (1984). Etiological theories and treatment for chronic back pain. 1. Somatic models and interventions. *Pain, 19,* 105-121.

Flor, H., Turk, D. C., & Rudy, E. T. (1987). Pain and families II. Assessment and treatment. *Pain, 30,* 29-45.

Foley, K. M. (1985, July 11). The treatment of cancer pain. *New England Journal of Medicine, 313,* 84-95.

Foley, K. M., & Inturrisi, C. E. (1987, March). Analgesic drug therapy in cancer pain: Principles and practice. *Medical Clinics of North America, 71,* 207-232.

Foley, K. M., & Rogers, A. (1981). The rational use of analgesics in the management of cancer pain. In *The management of cancer pain* (vol. 2). Nutley, NJ: Hoffman-LaRoche.

Fordyce, W. E. (1976). *Behavioral methods for chronic pain and illness.* St. Louis: C. V. Mosby.

Fowler-Kerry, S., & Lander, J. R. (1987). Management of injection pain in children. *Pain, 30,* 169-175.

Fox, L. S. (1982). Pain management in the terminally ill cancer patient: An investigation of nurses' attitudes, knowledge, and clinical practice. *Military Medicine, 147,* 455-460.

Greevert, P., Albert, L. H., & Goldstein, A. (1983). Partial antagonism of placebo analgesia by naloxone. *Pain, 16,* 129-143.

Grossman, S. A., & Sheidler, V. R. (1985). Skills of medical students and house officers in prescribing narcotic medication. *Journal of Medical Education, 60,* 552-557.

Hardy, J. D., Wolff, H. G. & Goodell, H. (1943). Pain threshold in man. *Proceedings, Association for Research in Nervous and Mental Disease, 23,* 1.

Harkins, S. W., & Chapman, C. R. (1976). Detection and decision factors in pain perception in young and elderly men. *Pain, 2,* 253-264.

Harkins, S. W., Price, D. D., & Martelli, M. (1986). Effect of age on pain perception thermonociception. *Journal of Gerontology, 41,* 58-63.

Haslam, D. R. (1969). Age and the perception of pain. *Psychological Science, 15,* 86-87.

Hodding, G. D., Jann, M., & Ackerman, I. P. (1980). Drug withdrawal syndromes: A literature review. *Western Journal of Medicine, 133*(11), 383-391.

Hyodo, M. (1985). Modern scientific acupuncture as practiced in Japan. In S. Lipton & J. Miles (Eds.), *Persistent pain.* London: Harcourt Brace Jovanovich.

Jaffe, J. H., & Martin, W. R. (1985). Opioid analgesics and antagonists. In A. G. Gillman, L. S. Goodman, T. W. Rall, & F. Murad (Eds.), *The pharmacological basis of therapeutics.* New York: Macmillan.

Jeans, M. E., & Johnston, C. C. (1985). Pain in children: Assessment and management. In S. Lipton & J. Miles (Eds.), *Persistent pain.* London: Harcourt Brace Jovanovich.

Jick, H. (1974, March). Smoking and clinical drug effects. *Medical Clinics of North America, 71,* 207-232.

Jones, G. E., & Johnson, H. J. (1980). Heart rate and somatic concomitant of mental imagery. *Psychophysiology, 17,* 185-191.

Kaiko, R. F. (1980, December). Age and morphine analgesia in cancer patients with post-operative pain. *Clinical Pharmacological Therapy, 28,* 283-826.

Kaiko, R. F., Foley, K. M., Grakinski, P. Y., et al. (1983). Central nervous system excitatory effect of meperidine in cancer patients. *Annals of Neurology, 13,* 180-185.

Kantor, T. G. (1982). Anti-inflammatory drug therapy for low back pain. In M. Stanton-Hicks & R. Ross (Eds.), *Chronic low back pain.* New York: Raven Press.

———. (1984, Summer). Nonsteroidal anti-inflammatory analgesic agents in management of cancer pain. In *The management of cancer pain* (Monograph). Hospital Practice.

Katz, E. R., et al. (1982). Beta-endorphin immunoreactivity and acute behavioral distress in children with leukemia. *Journal of Nervous Mental Disease, 170,* 2077.

Koster, T. R., & Kleber, H. D. (1987). Pain in children: Assessment and management. In S. Lipton & J. Miles (Eds.), *Persistent pain.* London: Harcourt Brace Jovanovich.

Labbe, E., Fishbain, D., Goldberg, M., Steele-Rosomoff, R., & Rosomoff, H. (1988, May/June). Compensation and non-compensation pain patients. *Pain Management,* pp. 133-138.

Leavitt, F., & Sweet, J. J. (1986). Characteristics and frequency of malingering among patients with low back pain. *Pain, 25,* 357-364.

Linton, S. J. (1986). Behavioral remediation of chronic pain: A status report. *Pain, 24,* 125-141.

Marks, R. M., & Sacher, E. L. (1973, February). Undertreatment of medical patients with narcotic analgesics. *Annals of Internal Medicine, 78,* 173-181.

Martinson, I. M., Nixon, S., Creis, D., YaDeau, R., Nesbit, M., & Kerser, G. (1982). Nursing care of childhood cancer: Methadone. *American Journal of Nursing, 82* (3), 432-435.

Mast, D. E. (1986). Effects of imagery. *Image: The Journal of Nursing Scholarship, 18,* 118-120.

Maunuksela, E. L., Rajantie, J., & Silmes, M. A. (1986). Flunitrazepam-fentanyl-induced sedation and analgesia in bone marrow aspiration and needle biopsy in children. *Acta Anaesthesiol Scand, 30,* 409-411.

MacDonald, J. B. (1984). Presentation of acute myocardial infarction in the elderly. *Age Ageing, 13,* 196-200.

McCaffery, M. (1979). *Nursing management of the patient with pain.* Philadelphia: J. B. Lippincott.

———. (1981, December). Large doses are safer than you think. *Nursing Life, 1,* 41-42.

———. (1988). *Pain management in clinical practice* (syllabus used in her workshop). M. McCaffery, 1458 Berkeley St., Apt. 1, Santa Monica, CA 90404.

McCaffery, M., & Beebe, A. (1989). *Pain: Clinical manual for nursing practice.* St. Louis: C. V. Mosby.

McKay, M., Davis, M., & Fanning, P. (1981). *Thoughts and feelings.* Richmond, CA: New Harbinger.

Mehta, M. (1986). Current views on non-invasive methods in pain relief. In M. Swerdlow (Ed.), *The therapy of pain.* Lancaster, England: MTP Press Limited.

Melzack, R. (1973). *The puzzle of pain.* New York: Basic Books.

Melzack, R., & Wall, P. D. (1965). Pain mechanisms: A new theory. *Science, 150,* 971-979.

Mendelsohn, G. (1986, Summer). Chronic pain and compensation: A review. *Journal of Pain Symptom Management, 1,* 135-144.

Miller, R. R. & Jick, H. (1978, April). Clinical effects of meperidine in hospitalized medical patients. *Journal of Clinical Pharmacology, 18,* 180-189.

Osterweis, M. (1987). Illness behavior and experience of chronic pain. In M. Osterweis, A. Kleinman, & D. Mechanic (Eds.), *Pain and disability: Clinical behavior and public policy perspectives.* Washington, D.C.: National Academy Press.

Osterweis, M., Kleinman, A., & Mechanic, D. (Eds.) (1987). *Pain and disability: Clinical behavior and public policy perspectives.* Washington, D.C.: National Academy Press.

Pilowsky, I., Crettenden, I., & Townley, M. (1985). Sleep disturbance in pain clinic patients. *Pain, 23,* 27–33.

Portenoy, R. K. (1987). Optimal pain control in elderly cancer patients. *Geriatrics, 42,* 33–44.

Porter, J., & Jick, M. (1980). Addiction rare in patients treated with narcotics. *New England Journal of Medicine, 302,* 123.

Reasbeck, P. G., Rice, M. L., & Reasbeck, J. D. (1982). Double-blind controlled trial of indomethacin as an adjunct to narcotic analgesia after major abdominal surgery. *Lancet, 2,* 115–118.

Rosomoff, H., Green, C., & Silbert, M. (1980). The multidisciplinary team approach to the diagnosis and treatment of chronic low back pain. In J. D. Post (Ed.), *Radiographic evaluation of the spine.* New York: Masson Publishing.

Rosomoff, H., & Steele-Rosomoff, R. (1988, March). Pain management programs for low back disorders. *Miami Medicine,* pp. 25–26.

Rowe, J. W., & Bresdine, R. W. (Eds.) (1982). *Health and disease in old age.* Boston: Little, Brown.

Slavic-Svircev, V., Kaiko, G., Heinrich, R. F., & Rusy, B. F. (1984, July 13). Ibuprofen in the treatment of postoperative pain. *American Journal of Medicine, 77,* 84–86.

Sriwatanakul, K., Weis, O. F., Alloza, J. L., Kilver, W., Weintraub, M., & Lasagna, L. (1983). Analysis of narcotic analgesia usage in the treatment of postoperative pain. *Journal of the American Medical Association, 250,* 926–929.

Taylor, A. G., Skelton, J. A., & Butcher, J. (1984, Jan./Feb.). Duration of pain condition and physical pathology as determinants of nurses' assessment of patients in pain. *Nursing Research,* 334–338.

Tejada, I. M. (1986, May/June). Indocin suppository for control of pain in post-thoracic surgery patients. *Oncology Nursing Forum, 13,* 87.

Trotter, J. M., Scott, R., Macbeth, F. R. et al. (1981, January 10). Problems of the oncology outpatient: Roles of the liaison health visitor. *British Medical Journal, 282,* 122–124.

Twycross, R. G. (1985). Terminal cancer care. In S. Lipton & J. Miles (Eds.), *Persistent pain.* London: Harcourt Brace Jovanovich.

Ventafridda, V., Fochi, C., DeConno, D., et al. (1980). Use of nonsteroidal anti-inflammatory drugs in the treatment of pain in cancer. *British Journal of Clinical Pharmacology, 10,* 3435–3465.

Wenzloff, N. J., & Shrimp, L. (1984). Therapeutic management of primary dysmenorrhea. *Drug Intell Clinical Pharmacology, 18,* 22–26.

Williams, N. E. (1986). Current views on pharmacological management of pain. In M. Swerdlow (Ed.), *The therapy of pain.* Lancaster, England: MTP Press Limited.

Wright, A. (1981). From IV to PO: Titrating your patient's pain medication. *Nursing '81, 11*(7), 39–43.

Bibliography

Lipton, S. (1986). Current views of the management of a pain relief center. In M. Swerdlow (Ed.), *The therapy of pain.* Lancaster, England: MTP Press Limited.

Lipton, S., & Miles, J. (Eds.) (1985). *Persistent pain.* London: Harcourt Brace Jovanovich.

CHAPTER 8

Social Isolation

Diana Biordi

Introduction

Most of us actively seek human companionship or relationships. The rarities of hermits or of cloistered, solitary existences are extraordinary because they so vividly remind us that, usually, life is richer for the human contact we share. As substantial as life may be when we engage in a variety of relationships, solitude is also a necessary foil as we seek rest or contemplative opportunity in "our own space." The weaving together of individual possibilities for social engagement or solitude develops a certain uniqueness and texture in personal and community relationships. These distinctive personal configurations of engagement and disengagement are consequential to our work and social lives. It is critical, therefore, that health professionals understand how and what is valued about social engagement and solitude.

When Is Isolation a Problem?

Social isolation ranges from the voluntary isolate who seeks disengagement from social intercourse for a variety of reasons, to those whose isolation is involuntary or imposed by others. Being alone, if actively chosen, has the potential for re-creating or reconstructing the human psyche. On the other hand, involuntary social isolation is negatively viewed because the outcomes are the dissolution of social exchanges and the support they provide. For some, such as those with cognitive deficits, being involuntarily isolated may not be well understood, although their parent, spouse, or another significant person may understand that social isolation can have a negative and profound impact.

When social isolation is experienced negatively by an individual or his or her significant other, it becomes an important problem that needs to be managed. In fact, according to much of the literature, only physical functional disability ranks with social isolation in its impact on the client and the client's social support network (family, friends, fellow workers). Therefore, social isolation is one of the two most important aspects of chronic illness to be managed in the plan of care.

Distinctions of Social Isolation

Social isolation is viewed from the perspective of the numbers, frequency, and quality of contacts; the longevity or durability of these contacts; and the negativism attributed to the isolation felt by the individual involved. Social isolation has been the subject of the humanities for hundreds of years. Who has not heard of John Donne's exclamation, "No man is an island," or, conversely, the philosophy of existentialism—

that humans are ultimately alone? Yet the concept of social isolation has been systematically researched only during the past fifty years. Unlike existentialists and some social scientists, health care workers, with their problem-oriented, clinical approach, tend to regard social isolation as negative rather than positive.

The Nature of Isolation   Isolation can occur at four layers of the term "social." The outermost layer is *community,* where one feels integrated or isolated from the larger social structure. Next is the layer of *organization* (work, schools, churches), followed by a layer closer to the person, that is, *confidantes* (friends, family, significant others). Finally, the innermost layer is that of the *person,* who has the personality, the intellectual ability, or the senses with which to apprehend and interpret relationships (Lin, 1986).

In the health care literature, primary focus is on the clinical dyad, so the examination of social isolation tends to be confined to the levels of confidante and person and only extends to the organization and community for single clients, one at a time. Thus, for the health care worker, the most likely relationships are bound to expectations of individually centered reciprocity, mutuality, caring, and responsibility. On the other hand, health policy literature tends to focus on the reciprocity of community and organizations to populations of individuals, and so it deals with collective social isolation.

At the level of the dyad, four patterns of social isolation or interaction have been identified; while these were originally formulated with elders in mind, they can be analogized easily to younger persons by making them age relative:

1. Persons who have been integrated into social groups throughout their lifetime
2. The "early isolate"—someone who was isolated as an adult but is relatively active in old age
3. The "recent isolate"—someone who was active in early adulthood but is not in old age
4. The "lifelong isolate"—someone whose life is one of isolation

Feelings That Reflect Isolation   Social isolation can be characterized by feelings of boredom

and marginality or exclusion (Weiss, 1973). Boredom occurs because of the lack of validation of one's work or daily routines; therefore, these tasks become only busy work. Marginality is the sense of being excluded from desired networks or groups. Secondary to these feelings, socially isolated individuals are motivated to seek out others in order to share activities or be accepted by the group as a member.

Description/Characteristics of Social Isolation   The existence of social isolation increases our awareness of the need for humans to associate with each other in an authentic intimate relationship, whether characterized by caring or some other emotion, such as anger. When we speak of social isolation, we think first of the affected person; then we almost immediately consider that individual's relationships. This chapter will show that, as a process, social isolation may be a feature in a variety of illnesses and disabilities across the life cycle.

Social Isolation versus Similar States of Human Apartness   Social isolation has been treated as a distinct phenomenon, or it has been combined or equated with other states relating to human apartness. The literature is replete with a variety of definitions of social isolation, many of which are interrelated, substitutable, or even confused with other distinct but related phenomena.

Social Isolation and Alienation   Social isolation and alienation have been linked together or treated as synonymous in much of the health care literature, although they differ from one another. Alienation encompasses powerlessness, normlessness, isolation, self-estrangement, and meaninglessness (Seeman, 1959). Powerlessness refers to the belief held by an individual that one's own behaviors cannot elicit the results one desires or seeks. In normlessness, the individual has a strong belief that socially unapproved behaviors are necessary to achieve goals. Isolation means the inability to value highly held goals or beliefs that others usually value. Self-estrangement has come to mean the divorce of one's self from one's work or creative possibilities. Finally, meaninglessness is the sense that few significant predictions about the outcomes of behavior can be made. Thus, one can see that isolation is only one psychological state of alienation. However, authors frequently merge the finer points of one or more of the five dimensions of alienation and call the result *isolation*.

Social Isolation and Loneliness While social isolation is typically viewed today as a deprivation in social contacts, Peplau and Perlman (1986) suggest that it is loneliness, not social isolation, that occurs when an individual perceives her or his social relationships as not containing the desired quantity or quality of social contacts. In an even more subtle distinction, Hoeffer (1987) found that simply the *perception* of relative social isolation was more predictive of loneliness than actual isolation. Loneliness has been referred to as an alienation of the self and is sometimes seen as global, generalized, disagreeable, uncomfortable, and more terrible than anxiety (Austin, 1989). Loneliness differs from depression in that in loneliness one attempts to integrate oneself into new relationships, whereas in depression there is a surrendering of oneself to the distress (Weiss, 1973).

Nonetheless, loneliness does relate to social isolation. In fact, loneliness is the one concept most invoked when social isolation is considered (Dela Cruz, 1986; Hoeffer, 1987; Mullins & Dugan, 1990; Ryan & Patterson, 1987). However, to use social isolation and loneliness as interchangeable terms can be confusing. To maintain some clarity, loneliness should be considered the *subjective emotional affect* of the individual, while social isolation is *the objective state of deprivation* of social contact and content (Bennet, 1980). Thus, loneliness refers to the psychological state of the individual, whereas social isolation relates to the sociological status. While it is true that social isolation might lead to loneliness, loneliness is not, in itself, a necessary condition of social isolation. Both conditions can exist apart from each other.

Peplau and Perlman's view of loneliness might be confused with the nursing diagnosis, Impaired Social Interaction, defined in almost identical terms (NANDA, 1994). However, this diagnosis refers to a negative state of social exchanges where the quantity or quality of participation is dysfunctional or ineffective (Gordon, 1982; Tilden & Weinert, 1987). Impaired social interaction and social isolation feed into each other, since they have similar causes and the effects of each diagnosis overlap.

Social Isolation and Aloneness Tightly linked to social isolation is the need for social support. Social support is the social context or environment that facilitates the survival of human beings (Lin, 1986) by offering social, emotional, and material support needed and received by an individual. While social support literature has focused on the instrumental and material benefits of support, recent literature on social isolation relates isolation more to the negative feeling state of aloneness. This feeling is associated with deficits in social support networks, diminished participation in these networks or in social relationships, or feelings of rejection or withdrawal.

As the ill person becomes more aware of the constricting network and declining participation, he or she may feel sadness, anger, despair, or reduced self-esteem. These emotions factor into a changed social and personal identity, but are also issues in and of themselves for the chronically ill person. Moreover, depending on their own emotional and physical needs, friends and acquaintances may drop out of the social support system until only the most loyal remain (Tilden & Weinert, 1987). For instance, women with breast cancer find that social isolation is the rule, not the exception (Spiegel, 1990). Families, however, are likely to remain in the social network. As the social network realizes its limitations, it may itself become needy of interventions, such as respite care for the parents of a chronically ill child or support groups for the siblings of children with cancer (Heiney et al., 1990).

Nursing Diagnosis and Social Isolation

Social isolation is defined in the nursing literature as "aloneness experienced by the individual and perceived as imposed by others as a negative or threatening state" (NANDA, 1994). That is, despite a need or desire to do so, and because of circumstances imposed on them, individuals are unable to participate fully or meaningfully in social relationships that are important to them (Carpenito, 1993). Note that Carpenito does not include the caveat that the social isolation is imposed by others. It may be that, initially, the socially isolated have withdrawn from their social network or that others have withdrawn from the isolate. Regardless of who initiates it, the isolation frequently becomes reciprocal.

Three critical characteristics were originally described as necessary and sufficient conditions for the diagnosis: absence of supportive, significant others; verbalized feeling of aloneness imposed by others; and verbalized feeling of rejection (NANDA, 1994). Other characteristics have since been added to expand these conditions for diagnosis: apathy, seclusion, few contacts with peers, verbalized awareness of isolation, and the lack of absence of contacts with significant others or the community (Gordon, 1989).

At least 20 subjective and objective characteristics of social isolation have been identified by various nurses, most of which express rejection, alienation, or the absence of critical significant others. An important study of this nursing diagnosis was done in respect to the elderly (Lien-Gieschen, 1993). Eighteen defining characteristics of social isolation were identified, five specific to the elderly. However, the single major identifying characteristic with this population was the absence of supportive significant others. All other defining characteristics, including two of the original three critical definers, were confirmed only as "minor," or secondary characteristics. In this study, nurses validated only ages over 75 as characteristic of social isolation.

This single validation study of social isolation as a nursing diagnosis indicates that nurses typically focus on substantive characteristics of social isolation itself (Lien-Gieschen, 1993). As mentioned, the chief characteristic that was validated was lack of supportive others, but several more associated characteristics were identified that fell within broad categories of dull affect, preoccupation with one's own thoughts, loss of

meaning or purpose in life, lack of communication, a personal sense or act of apartness, or sensory deficits. As can be seen from the descriptors that have been identified, the nursing view of social isolation is rather holistic and resonates strongly with earlier dimensions of the concepts of alienation and loneliness.

Problems and Issues of Social Isolation

Regardless of how the social isolation occurs, the result is that basic needs for authentic intimacy remain unmet. Typically the loss of social integration is perceived as alienating or unpleasant, and the social isolation that occurs can lead to depression, loneliness, or other social and cognitive impairments that then exacerbate the isolation.

Several predisposing or etiologic reasons for social isolation have been proposed: status-altering physical disabilities or illnesses; frailties associated with advanced age or developmental delays; personality or neurological disorders; or environmental constraints, which often refer to physical surroundings but are also interpreted by some to include diminished personal or material resources (Tilden & Weinert, 1987).

Social Isolation and Social Roles

Any weakening or diminishment of relationships or social roles might produce social isolation for affected individuals or their significant others. Clients who lose family, friends, and associated position and power are inclined to feelings of rejection, worthlessness, and loss of self-esteem (Ravish, 1985). An example of this is the situation of the woman whose husband had Alzheimer's disease. The couple had been confined for more than two years in an apartment in a large city from which her confused husband frequently wandered. Her comment, "I'm not like a wife and not like a single person either," reflected their dwindling social network and her loss of wifely privileges, but not obligations. This ambiguity is common to many whose spouses are incapacitated. Moreover, after the spouse dies, the widow or widower often grieves as much for the loss of the role of a married person as for the loss of the spouse.

Thus, the loss of social roles can occur as a result of illness or disability, social changes throughout the life span (e.g., in school groups, with career moves, or in unaccepting communities), marital dissolution (through death or divorce), or secondary to ostracism incurred by membership in a "wrong" group. The loss of social roles and the resultant isolation of the individual have been useful analytical devices in the examination of issues of the aged, the widowed, and the physically impaired, or in psychopathology.

The Elderly and Social Isolation   Old age, with its many losses of physical health, social roles, and economic status, contributes to a decreasing social network and increasing isolation (Creecy, Berg, & Wright, 1985; Ryan & Patterson, 1987; Trout, 1980). The location of the home, access to transportation or buildings, and immobility have all been implicated in social isolation for this population. Strictly speaking, social isolation is not confined to a place: The socially isolated are not necessarily homebound or placebound, although that is more typically the case (Ryan & Patterson, 1987; Stephens & Bernstein, 1984; Watson, 1988). That being said, however, environments that are removed, such as rural locations, or those not conducive to safety, such as high-crime areas, can contribute to social isolation (Glassman-Feibusch, 1981; Kivett, 1979; Lyons, 1982). In these cases, elderly individuals cannot leave their homes for lack of transportation or for fear of assault, and so they increasingly isolate themselves from others. This situation is worse if the elderly have chronic illness compounding their constraints.

One objective of planned senior housing is to provide individuals with a ready-made social network within a community (Lawton, Greenbaum, & Liebowitz, 1980; Lawton, Kleban, & Carlson, 1973; Lawton, Moss, & Grimes, 1985), although this objective is not always met. Through such a social network, it was hoped that social isolation would be counteracted among the elderly living in these communities. However, the frail elderly were found to be less interactive with the more mobile, healthier elderly, possibly because healthier elderly have few extra resources to expend on others who may have even fewer resources, or they may have better health and networks that are incongruent with, and less likely to cross, those of the frail elderly (Heumann, 1988).

Nursing home residents with chronic illness or sensory impairments tend to be more isolated than others. For instance, in England, those in residential care who are ill or disabled are considered socially dead, impoverished by the inactive nature of institutionalization and unable to occupy any positive, valued role in the community (Watson, 1988). Stephens and Bernstein (1984) found, in another study, that older, sicker residents were more socially isolated than healthier residents, but, interestingly, at times of crisis (such as hospitalizations) healthier residents rallied to aid sicker ones. Moreover, the investigators found that family and longer-standing friendships served as better buffers to social isolation than did other residents.

Social isolation has been linked to confusion, particularly in elderly chronically ill individuals. But when the socially isolated are also immobilized, the combination of isolation and immobilization can lead to greater impairments such as perceptual and behavioral changes (e.g., noncompliance or time distortions) (Stewart, 1986). Physical barriers (such as physical plant designs) or architectural features (such as too-heavy doors) also contribute to social isolation or homeboundedness (DesRosier, Catanzaro, & Piller, 1992). All of these limits have been found to contribute to social isolation in ways that motivation alone cannot easily overcome.

Social Components of Social Isolation

Mere numbers of people surrounding someone do not cure negative social isolation; an individual can be socially isolated in a crowd if he or she loses his or her significant social network. This situation is true for such groups as those living or working in sheltered-care workshops, residents in long-term care facilities, or people in prisons. What is critical to social isolation as a diagnosis is that, because of situations imposed on them, individuals *perceive* themselves as disconnected from meaningful discourse with people important to them, irrespective of place or number of surrounding people.

Associated with social isolation is reciprocity or mutuality, that is, the amount of give and take that can occur between isolated individuals and their social networks. Throughout the years, much evidence has accumulated to indicate that informal networks of social support offer significant emotional assistance, information, and material resources for a number of different populations. These support systems appear to foster good health, help maintain appropriate behaviors, and alleviate stress (Cobb, 1979; DiMatteo & Hays, 1981; Stephens & Bernstein, 1984). One of the most consistent findings is that family members, regardless of ethnic group, are major providers of assistance (Stephens & Bernstein, 1984; Weeks & Cuellar, 1981).

Examining reciprocity in the relationships of social networks focuses not only on social roles and the content of the exchange but also on the level of agreement between the isolated person and his or her "others" in the network (Goodman, 1984). The incongruence between respondents in a social network regarding their exchanges can help alert the health care provider to the level of emotional or material need or exhaustion that exists in either respondent. For example, this author observed, during a visit by a nurse, that a homebound elderly woman complained that her children had done very little for her. However, it was discovered that the children visited every day, brought meals, shopped for their mother, and managed her financial affairs. In this case, the elderly mother felt isolated notwithstanding her children's visits and assistance.

Demographics and Social Isolation

Few studies focus directly on demographic variables and social isolation; typically this topic is embedded in other research questions across a variety of illnesses. Nevertheless, when these disparate studies are taken together, the impact of demographics on social isolation in the chronically ill is quite evident. Issues of gender, marital status, family position and context, and socioeco-

nomic standing (such as education or employment) have been shown to affect social isolation.

Socioeconomic Factors   Employment status is only one concern for the social network; for instance, parents worry about the potential for employment and insurance for their children who have chronic illnesses (Cohen, 1993). Lower income status, along with less education, negatively influences health status and is associated with both a limited social network and greater loneliness, which in turn, cyclicly, affects health status and social isolation (Cox et al., 1988; Williams & Bury, 1989). For instance, almost half of the head-injured clients in one study could not work, which then affected their family's economic status and increased their social isolation (Kinsella et al., 1989).

In addition to problems of employment potential, there are economic and social concerns over the costs incurred by health care, employment discrimination, subsequent inability to secure insurance, and loss of potential friendship networks at work—all of which are factors in increasing social isolation or reducing social interactions. In fact, economics exaggerates the costs of chronic illness and so adversely affects the isolation of the individual. People with disabilities suffer disproportionately in the labor market, which then affects their connections with family and community social networks (Christ, 1987).

General Family Factors   As chronic illness persists, and given the tasks that must be managed, relationships are drained, leaving individuals with chronic illnesses at high risk for social impairment or social isolation (Berkman, 1983; Tilden & Weinert, 1987). When isolation does occur, it can remain a long-term reality for the chronically ill and their families. However, where they have social support and involvement, chronically ill people are more likely to lean toward psychological well-being. Particularly important is the adequacy, more than the availability, of social relationships.

There is evidence that social isolation does not necessarily occur in every situation. In fact, the impact of social isolation on families with chronically ill children has been questioned. One study, which used a large community-based, random sample, found that families with chronically ill children did not experience a greater degree of social isolation than those with healthy children. That study also found that, contrary to clinical opinion, the families of chronically ill children did not function differently from families of healthy children, except for modest increases in maternal dysfunction (Cadman et al., 1991). Cadman and his associates argue that prior studies were subject to biases because the families in those studies were in the clinic populations of the hospital or agency. By definition, such populations were receiving care for illnesses or responses to illnesses and hence were suffering from an unusual aggregation of problems, which brought them to the clinic or hospital. Therefore, such families were not representative of the community at large, that is, families spread throughout a community. In another study, classroom teachers evaluated chronically ill children (cancer or sickle cell disease) with a matched sample of controls. The authors found that the chronically ill children were remarkably resilient in the classroom setting, although those who survived their brain tumors and could attend regular classes were perceived as more sensitive and isolated (Noll et al., 1992).

Similarly, some studies of elderly individuals also found that isolation did not always occur. Although childless elderly individuals tend to be more socially isolated than those with children, when adult children live nearby, older people frequently interact with at least one of them (Mullins & Dugan, 1990). Interestingly, older people tend to be less influenced by their children than by contacts with other relatives, friends, and associates (Berkman, 1983; Ryan & Patterson, 1987). In fact, one study found no relation between the elders' emotional well-being and the frequency of interaction with their children (Lee & Ellithorpe, 1982).

In *every* group from 30 to over 70 years of age, it was primarily those with the fewest social and community ties who were nearly three times as likely to die as those with more ties (Berkman, 1983). In other words, maintaining social contacts enhanced longevity. In a study of chronically ill elders living in the general community,

those who had fewer social contacts were more socially isolated than younger chronically ill individuals (Berkman, 1983). The major factor that led to isolation was that these individuals were widowers or widows and lacked membership in formal groups (Berkman, 1983), thereby limiting their social contacts. In another study, the elderly who lived in senior housing complexes showed little difference in friendship patterns and life satisfaction (Poulin, 1984). Both of these studies found that living alone, being single, or not having family does not necessarily imply social isolation. Rather, if older people have social networks, many developed throughout a lifetime, and if these networks remain available to them, they are provided with support when needed (Berkman, 1983).

Gender and Marital Status Typically, women have more extensive and varied social networks than men do (Antonucci, 1985). However, if one spouse is chronically ill, married couples spend more time together and less with networks and activities outside the home (DesRosier et al., 1992; Foxall, Eckberg, & Griffith, 1986). Although gender differences in caregiving occur (Miller, 1990; Tilden & Weinert, 1987), women caregivers indicate greater isolation, increased loneliness, and decreased life satisfaction than do men. Yet both genders show psychological improvement if social contacts, whether by telephone or in person, increase (Foxall et al., 1986).

While women caregivers may have professionals, community, and social networks to aid them in coping with their disabled spouses, over time they reduce their links to these potential supports. Physical work, social costs and barriers, preparation time for care and outings, and other demands of caregiving become so extreme that women curtail access to and use of support networks external to home. As these caregivers narrow their use of social networks, they unwittingly isolated their chronically ill spouse as well. Although women reported needing personal or psychological time alone for relief, the subject of their isolation, the chronically ill person, also became their greatest confidante as the pair struggle in their joint isolation (DesRosier et al., 1992).

Illness Factors and Social Isolation

Chronic illness is multidimensional, with several tasks that the chronically ill or their networks must assume: managing treatment regimens, controlling symptoms, preventing and managing crises, reordering time, managing the illness trajectory, dealing with health care professionals, normalizing life, preserving a reasonable self-image, keeping emotional balance, managing social isolation, funding the costs of health care, and preparing for an uncertain future (Strauss et al., 1984) (see Chapter 4, on illness roles). As people with chronic illnesses struggle to understand their body failure and maintain personal and social identities, they may become fatigued or sicker, or lose hope more readily. Should this happen, they may more easily withdraw from their social networks.

It has been suggested that isolation leads to depression and suicide (Lyons, 1982; Trout, 1980), particularly in the elderly (Frierson, 1991), and may impact on the individual's social network (Newman et al., 1989). Women whose illnesses required more physical demands on themselves and greater symptom management reported greater depression but no effect on their relationship with their partner. Women who have concerns about the meaning of their illness reported greater marital distress and lower satisfaction with their family network (Woods, Haberman, & Packard, 1993).

In the case of people with severe head injuries, it was not the chronic physical disability that disrupted family cohesion as much as the resulting social impairment (Kinsella, Ford, & Moran, 1989). The greatest burden identified was social isolation brought on by the impaired self-control of the head-injured and their inability to learn from social experience. However, the social isolation was particularly burdensome for the families because the head injury reduced the client's capacity for recognition of and reflection on the deficiencies in social relationships and precluded formation of new close relationships. Consequently, although friendships and employment possibilities were reduced for the client, the real impact was felt by the constrained family (Kinsella et al., 1989).

The Isolation Process

A typical course of isolation that evolves as the illness or disability becomes more apparent is the change in social network relationships. Friends or families begin to withdraw from the isolated individual or the individual from them. This process may be slow or subtle, as with individuals with arthritis, or it may be rapid, as with for example, the person with AIDS. Unfortunately, the process of isolation may not be based on accurate or rational information. One woman with cancer reported that, at a party, she was served her drink in a plastic cup while everyone else had glasses (Spiegel, 1990).

Individuals with serious chronic illnesses come to perceive themselves as different from others and outside the mainstream of ordinary life (Williams & Bury, 1989). This perception of differentness may be shared by others, who then reject them, their disability, and their differentness. At least part of this sense of being different stems from the ongoing demands of the illness. For example, as the demands of the illness continue, social relationships are interrupted because families and friends cannot adjust the erratic treatment and illness trajectory to acceptable social activities and their timing. From such real events, or from social perceptions, social isolation can occur, either as a process or as an outcome.

Chronically ill individuals often face their own mortality more explicitly than others. As they grapple with the meaning of life, they may withdraw from their networks or the networks may withdraw from them. For example, unmarried or younger cancer patients expressed a loss of meaning in life, suggested to be due to cancer's threat to their lives (Noyes et al., 1990; Weisman & Worden, 1976–1977; Woods, Haberman, & Packard, 1993).

Even if death does not frighten those who are chronically ill, it frequently frightens their social networks. This fright leads to guilt, which, in turn, leads to strained silences and withdrawal. In the case of individuals with cancer (Burnley, 1992; House, Landis, & Umberson, 1988; Reynolds & Kaplan, 1990), and heart disease (Kaplan et al., 1988; Orth-Gomer, Unden, &

Edwards, 1988) and in Type A personalities (Orth-Gomer & Unden, 1990), social support is significant to their survival. For those who lack this social support, then, social isolation is not merely a metaphor for death: It can hasten death.

Stigma Social isolation may occur as one effect of stigma: Many persons will risk anonymity rather than expose themselves to a critical and judgmental audience. Because chronic illnesses can be stigmatizing, the concern about the possibility of revealing a damaged or discredited self can slow or paralyze social interaction (see Chapter 5, on stigma). The chronically ill, or their families, grapple with how much information about themselves or their diagnoses they should share, with whom, and when (Gallo et al., 1991). If the illness is manageable or reasonably invisible, it is disguised or its presence is hidden from all but a select few, often for years. Parents of children with chronic illnesses were reported to manage stressful encounters and uncertainty by disguising, withholding, or limiting information to others (Cohen, 1993), an action that may have the added effect of tightening, or limiting, their social network. Jessop and Stein (1985) found that invisible illnesses of chronically ill children led to greater difficulty in social interactions because of the uncertainty of ambiguity (disagreement about revealing or passing, or what courses of action to take). For example, parents of a child with cystic fibrosis may tell a teacher that the child is taking pills with meals because of a digestive disease (Cohen, 1993).

As siblings of children with cancer dealt with the isolation of their brother or sister they became vulnerable to being socially isolated themselves (Bendor, 1990). Tamlyn and Arklie (1986) specifically address social isolation by arguing that nurses must explicitly plan for it in families with chronically ill children. Thus, social isolation is not only a burden for the chronically ill, it extends itself into family dynamics and requires the health professional to consider how the family manages the illness and the isolation.

Where the stigmatized disability is quite obvious, as in the visibility of burn scars or in the odor of colitis, the chronically ill person might venture only within small circles of understanding individuals (Gallo et al., 1991). Where employment is possible, it will often be work that does not require many social interactions, such as night work or jobs within isolated environments (sheltered workshops, home offices). Regardless of what serves as reminders of the disability, the disability is incorporated into the isolate's sense of self; that is, it becomes part of his or her social and personal identity. Consequently, isolates and their social networks must develop new strategies to incorporate or otherwise manage the disability—this new feature—in their management of self.

Health Care Perspectives

People with chronic illnesses struggle to understand their body failure and what it does to their activities and lives (Corbin & Strauss, 1987). In doing so they also struggle to maintain their sense of personal and social identity, often in the face of altered self-image and enormous financial, psychological, and social obstacles. If chronically ill people lose hope or become fatigued or otherwise incapacitated, they may withdraw from their social networks, isolating themselves and others important to them.

Frequently, this daily management of illness means working with health care professionals who often do not recognize the inconspicuous but daily struggles of the chronically ill person's confrontations with the realities of a "new" body, the issues of care, and the development of a new self-identity (Corbin & Strauss, 1987; Dropkin, 1989; Hopper, 1981).

In the last three decades, with the advent of high technology, the aging of the population, and changes in economics, chronic illness has begun to assume major proportions in the United States. Concomitantly, the literature has more articles describing various chronic illnesses, the strategies used to manage them, and issues of social and psychological well-being including social isolation.

The impact of prevailing paradigms of care interventions held by various constituencies is evident. For example, most health care professionals still see clients only episodically, usually using the medical model of "cure." But in the case of cancer in children, the child's perspective focuses on the meaning of impairment (which varies by age); the parents' perspective focuses first on the immediate concern with their child's longevity and cure and later on the impairment and long-term effects; the health professional's perspective focuses on client survival; the mental health professional's perspective focuses on identifying and minimizing impact, impairments, and social barriers; and the public's (third-party payers, employers, schoolmates, partners) perspective focuses on contributions and cost. All of these perspectives center on the interaction and exchange, as well as the specific responsibilities and obligations, incurred. These interactions are intensified by the potential withdrawal of any party from the network (Christ, 1987).

Given the variety of care-versus-cure paradigms, the real, but additive, daily micro-impositions of chronic illness on social identity and social networks are often lost. However, the compassion felt by health care professionals is evident in the increasing number of articles available and the attempts to present evidence of the isolation felt by clients and their networks. Nevertheless, the perspective of these articles may not be explicit, and therefore the proposed interventions for the isolate are unclear, irrelevant, or even discouraging. For example, when discussing facial disfigurement, one article noted that the health professional sought and expected evidence of the client's image integration as early as one week postsurgery (Dropkin, 1989). In that same article, suggested interventions were to reiterate that, although the surgery was necessary for removal of the cancer, the resulting *defect* [italics mine] was confined to a relatively small aspect of the anatomy and that the alteration in appearance or function did not change the person (Dropkin, 1989). Both the terminology and the interventions in this article focused on the acute postoperative period and did not (perhaps could not) take into account what disfigured clients were likely to feel later than one week postsurgery. However, the word "defect" gives a strong cue as to the understanding that the disfiguring surgery is obvious and emotionally charged toward the negative.

For a clearer view of the impact of such surgery from the perspective of the client, Gamba et al. (1992) asked postsurgical patients, grouped by extent of their facial disfigurement, about their self-image, relationship with their partner and social network, and overall impact of the therapy. Those with extensive disfigurement reported that it was "like putting up with something undesirable" (p. 221): Many were unable to touch or look at themselves (see Chapter 13, on body image). Patients with extensive disfigurement reported more social isolation, poor self-images, and/or a worsened sexual relationship with their partner but satisfactory relationships with their children. In another study reported in the Gamba article, half of the individuals who underwent hemimandibulectomy for head and neck cancers became social recluses, compared to 11 percent of patients who had laryngectomies (Gamba et al., 1992). Therefore, in more than one study respondents attached a negative meaning to their disfiguring surgery and its results.

Clients with ulcerative colitis had similar findings. Once home from acute-care environments, which managed the social and medical stigmatization and aftereffects of surgery, these clients ultimately left jobs and curtailed their social contacts. The acute-care environments, unlike the home, were better equipped to assist the client in the management of odor, illness, and frequency of visitors and social interruptions. At home, these aspects of the illness and its management became the sole responsibility of the client without the care and support of professionals "running interference." Consequently, clients often curtailed their social and work life (Reif, 1973).

Such findings take into account the client's personal meaning of illness and treatment and their effects on social isolation, meaning that is critical because the isolating treatment or illness (e.g., disfigurement) often is not associated with objective disability. In fact, others have found that the degree of isolation is *not* directly proportional to the extent of disability (Creed, 1990; Fitzpatrick et al., 1991; Maddox, 1985; Newman et al., 1989). Thus, health professionals cannot afford to ignore or discount the meaning of

illness to the client, regardless of their professional opinion about any objective disability or
the desirability of treatment.

Interventions: Counteracting Social Isolation

In social isolation, the interventions of choice
need to remain at the discretion of the client
or caregiver. As can be seen from this chapter,
writers focus largely on definitions and correlates of social isolation and relatively less on interventions. When interventions are reported they
often relate to the aggregate such as the policy-
related interventions of community housing. The
results of many of these larger-scale interventions
have been noted in this chapter. Other interventions are mentioned here, although the list is not
all inclusive.

Since each chronically ill person's situation
is unique, interventions can be expected to vary.
Nonetheless, certain techniques and strategies
are useful and generalizable, depending on the
substance of the illness or its effects such as using
existing day care centers for client placements.
Basically, these strategies require that a balance
of responsibilities be developed between the
health care professional and the client with the
aim of:

1. Increasing the moral autonomy or freedom
   of choice of the isolate
2. Increasing social interaction at a level acceptable to the client
3. Using repetitive and recognizable strategies
   that are validated with the client, which
   correlate to reducing particular isolating
   behaviors.

                              (Dela Cruz, 1986)

Another point to remember is that evaluation is a key principle in any problem-solving
system such as the nursing process. Throughout
the assessment and intervention phases, the
health professional should always, and explicitly,
consider how effective the intervention is or
was. The willingness and flexibility to change an
ineffective strategy is the mark of the competent
professional.

Assessment of Social Isolation

When social isolation does occur, a systematic
assessment can help determine proposed interventions. However, before action is taken, the
professional must validate potential interventions with the client. Guiding people versus forcing them to go along with interventions requires
the health professional to offer a rationale for
the proposed interventions. One must ask if one
is giving reasonable rationales, assurances, or
support.

The key to social isolation is to observe for
three differentiators: (1) *negativity* attached to
(2) *involuntary, other-imposed solitude*, and
(3) *declining quality and numbers within the
isolate's social networks*. Social isolation must
be distinguished from other conditions, such
as loneliness or depression. Both loneliness and
depression are often accompanied by anxiety,
desperation, self-pity, boredom, and signs of
attempts to fill a void, such as overeating,
substance abuse, excessive shopping, or klepto-
mania. In addition, loneliness is often associated
with losses, while depression is frequently regarded as anger turned inward. Since social isolation, loneliness, and depression can all be
destructive, the health professional must be re-
sourceful in assessing which issue predominates
at any particular point in time.

Properly conducted, an assessment yields its
own suggestions for responsive intervention. For
instance, the assessment may indicate that the
client is a lifelong isolate and that future isolation
is likely to be a continuation of a desired and
comfortable life-style. In this case, the professional's best intervention is to remain available
and observant but noninterfering. Pressing for
social involvement for such a person is not likely
to be welcomed. Intervention in this instance
would be an imposition on the client.

On the other hand, if the client is, in fact,
isolated and wants or needs relief, then the
intervention should be constructed along lines
consistent with current needs and history. For
example, if it is discovered that the support network is lax in calling or contacting the client,
then the provider can help the client and support
network rebuild bridges to each other. Are there
support groups to which those in the social net-

works can be referred for aid? On the other hand, if the network is overwhelmed, they may need to be informed of respite programs. Interventions such as these will help members of the social network maintain energy levels necessary to help their chronically ill relative or friend.

Assessment typically involves the clinical dyad of caregiver and client. Thus, it is at this level that assessment is critical to the development of appropriate and effective interventions. Without an adequate and sensitive assessment, interventions are likely to be ineffective or incomplete.

The case study about Will gives some idea about how this client was assessed, his unwanted isolation identified, and, with his knowledge, satisfactory supports contacted that met his needs.

Management of Self: Identity Development

Identity level is closely aligned with stigma, as individuals seek a level where they can overcome, avoid, or internalize stigma and, concomitantly, manage resulting social isolation. Managing various concerns requires chronically ill people to develop a new sense of self consistent with their disabilities. This "new" life is intertwined with the lives of members of their social networks, which may now include health caregivers and other chronically ill persons. Lessons must be learned to deal with new body demands and associated behaviors. Consequently, the chronically ill must redevelop an identity with norms different from previous ones.

The willingness to change to different and unknown norms is just a first step, one that often takes great courage and time. For instance, one study indicated that patients with pronounced physical, financial, and medical care problems following head and neck surgery exhibited prolonged social isolation one year postsurgery (Krouse, Krouse, & Fabian, 1989). Although no single study has indicated the time necessary in such identity transformations, anecdotal information suggests that it can last several years, and indeed, for some, it is a lifelong experience.

Identity Transformation Charmaz (1987), using mostly middle-aged women, has developed a framework of hierarchical identity transformations that the reader may find useful in diagnosing a chronically ill individual's proclivity to social networking and in discovering which social network might be the most appropriate audience. This hierarchy of identity takes into account a reconstruction toward a desired future self, based on past and present selves, and reflects the individual's relative difficulty in achieving specific aspirations. Charmaz's analysis progresses toward a "salvaged self" that retains a past identity based on important values or attributes while still acknowledging dependency. She reports several levels of preferred identities.

Initially, the individual takes on a *supernormal identity,* which assumes functioning success values, social acclamation, struggle, and competition. At this identity level the chronically ill attempt to participate more intensely than those in a nonimpaired world, despite the limitations of their illness. The next identity level that the chronically ill person moves to is the *restored self*—that is, the expectation of returning to the previous self, despite the chronic illness or its severity. Health care workers might identify this self with the psychological state of denial, but in terms of identity, the individual has simply assumed that there is no discontinuation with a former self. Then, at the *contingent personal identity* level, one defines oneself in terms of potential risk and failure, indicating the individual still has not come to terms with a future self but has begun to realize that the supernormal identity will no longer be viable. Finally, the level of the *salvaged self* is reached, where the individual attempts to define the self as worthwhile, despite recognizing that present circumstances invalidate any previous identity (Charmaz, 1987).

Social isolation not only develops from stigma, but can develop as an individual loses hope of sustaining unrealistic aspirations for a normal or supernormal self. As chronically ill persons act out regret, disappointment, and anger, their significant others and health providers may react in kind, perpetuating a downward spiral of loss, anger, and subsequent social isola-

CASE STUDY

Social Isolation

Will, a 76-year-old childless widower, continued to live alone in his own single-story, urban-area home following the death of his wife, Hazel, three years ago. At the time of her death, he had moderately limited physical mobility from his arthritis, was slightly deaf, and his eyesight, while not severely impaired, was diminishing. Hazel's death had been sudden and unexpected following complications of treatment for illness. They had been very dependent upon each other for material and social support, had lived quietly but interacted to a limited degree with their friends and neighbors, two of whom had lost spouses within the past few years. Although they maintained relationships with family peers about their ages, they interacted with them only rarely. Will described his small social network as follows: "We didn't need for anything and we kept to ourselves."

In the first year following Hazel's death, Will deeply grieved her loss, withdrawing even more from friends and family. During the second year, he was less despairing but began giving away dishes, silverware, and other items, saying "I won't need these anymore." Over this time span, his physical mobility, vision, and hearing became more limiting, so that he found trips outside the home exhausting and logistically difficult. Consequently, he avoided grocery shopping, going to the barber, worship activities, or any social activities. He used the telephone to contact friends only when he became too lonely, but for the most part rarely initiated such contacts.

It was now nearly three years since Hazel's death. Because of his slowly deteriorating health status, he had been referred to the visiting nurse association. In Will's case, the visiting nurse came by twice a month for assessment and treatment of Will's arthritis, deafness, and vision difficulties, as well as his psychological state. He expressed to Ms. B., the visiting nurse, that he sorely missed his wife, rarely saw even the few family members he had, didn't have many friends left, and could not easily leave his home, even to obtain necessities such as food and medicine. Increasingly homebound, Will, a lifelong isolate, had joined the many for whom social isolation becomes problematic or undesirable.

Ms. B., in developing a plan of care, examined the elements of Will's isolation and the levels of identity characterizing Will. She worked with Will to determine the best way to manage the course of his care. In this way, he came to "own" the management of care, that is, the goals of the plan.

First, the nurse *diagnosed* Will as moderately to severely socially isolated, based on his loneliness and unwanted and unpleasant homebound isolation from others in his limited but existing social network. Then Ms. B. acknowledged the *value differentiation* that existed between the two of them. For example, the idea of family was much more important to Ms. B. than to Will. Next, she considered and prioritized relationships and their *meaning* to Will, that is, the relationships that were significant to Will as an individual. The meaning of Will's current situation was defined by him as lonely, unpleasant, confining, and cumbersome.

Moving to the level of *confidante,* she explored his social relationships and their importance to him. In Will's case, the most significant person in his life had been his wife; following in importance were close friends, neighbors, and then some family members. Given that Hazel was no longer part of his social network, the nurse considered which of Will's significant others remained viable alternatives to isolation. Since friends who were also neighbors were available and willing to visit, Ms. B. encouraged Will to accept their overtures of friendship. They then began to visit about every two weeks or telephoned every week. Knowing that age mates within the family were also part of Will's limited social network, she helped Will reach out to them. Will later invited a male cousin, who accepted, to come by for a card game about every ten days. Still, none of these individuals could help Will drive to other places, since they themselves were somewhat debilitated or could not help move Will easily in and out of their vehicles.

Ms. B. sought ways of expanding Will's horizons, mentally and spiritually. The local community library rented large-print books and magazines, which were sent to Will on a periodic basis. She also contacted Will's place of worship, and members of his faith made arrangements to visit Will regularly and to transport him to worship services. Gradually, Will was reconnected in some respects to his organizations in addition to his small social network.

Finally, at the level of *community,* Ms. B. considered widening Will's network. To do this, she considered his *physical limitations, needs,* and *barriers.* The nurse not only contacted community social agencies to provide Will with transportation for grocery shopping and to get his medications; she also arranged for a neighbor to telephone or look in on Will at least once a day. When the neighbor protested that such a schedule was too demanding, the nurse solicited two other neighbors to develop a rotation scheme so that Will was assured assistance in the event of a fall or some pressing need. In addition, she contacted the postal person to observe for mail or newspapers cluttering the driveway, indicating Will was not able to pick them up when he should. Once motivated, Will noted that remote beepers could be used to notify the local hospital or fire department: He made arrangements to obtain such support.

The nurse decided that Will was moving into a *salvaged* identity, although elements of previous identity stages were still present. At no point in the plan was there an attempt to move Will, a lifelong social isolate, into more social activity than he could comfortably manage. Importantly, throughout the development of his diagnosis and plan of care, the nurse and client together validated and negotiated each arrangement. At each new intervention, the nurse evaluated the outcome. For instance: How did Will feel after the visits of the members of his network? Did he go to worship services? Was the nurse hurrying Will into more than he could handle at the time? Ultimately, the desired *outcome* was reached: Will was able to accommodate each step of the plan according to his temperament and resources. This accommodation was verified by Will's ability to articulate whether he felt less isolated than at the beginning of the interventions and whether his social network had, indeed, expanded.

tion. The idea of identity hierarchies thus alerts the caregiver to a process in which shifts in identity are expected.

Not only are reactions, health advice, and the experiences of the chronically ill taken into account in managing that particular identity, but various factors that help shape it are considered. Both the social network (audience) and adapted norms now available to the chronically ill person play a role at each stage in identity transformation. For example, in Charmaz's study, certain referral sources pooled at particular identity levels. Thus, at the supernormal identity level, chronically ill individuals were in only limited contact with health care professionals but presumably in greater contact with healthier individuals who acted as their referents; at the level of the salvaged self, a home health agency typically was used (Charmaz, 1987).

Clarifying how networks form and function is a significant contribution to the management of the struggles of the chronically ill and isolated client. The perceptive health care worker should know that much of the management done by the chronically ill and their networks is not seen or well understood by health care professionals today (Corbin & Strauss, 1987). However, we can use Charmaz's findings to point us to markers of the likely identity level of the individual as we try to understand potential withdrawal or actual isolation.

Respite

The need for respite has been cited as one of the greatest necessities for the elderly isolated ill and their caregivers, many of whom are themselves elderly (Miller, 1990; Subcommittee on Human Services, 1987). Respite involves four elements: purpose, time, activities, and place. The purpose of respite is to relieve caregivers for a period of time so that they may engage in activities that help sustain them or their loved ones, including the care recipient. The time may be in short blocks or for a longer (but still short-term) period, both of which temporarily relieve the caregiver of responsibility. Activities may be practical, such as grocery shopping; psychological, such as the need for self-replenishment or re-creation; or physical, such as rest or medical/

nursing attention. Respite may occur in the home or elsewhere, such as senior centers, day care centers, or long-term care facilities. Senior centers usually accommodate persons who are more independent and flexible, often offering social gathering places and events, meals, and health assessment/exercise/maintenance activities. Day care centers typically host individuals with more diminished functioning. Other places, such as long-term care facilities, manage clients with even greater inabilities to function.

And, finally, respite may be delivered by paid or unpaid persons, who may be friends, professionals, family, employees, or neighbors. Although many care recipients welcome relief from their caregiver, some may fear abandonment. The caregiver and professional must work together to assure the care recipient that he or she will not be abandoned (Biordi, 1993). Therefore, the professional has a great deal of latitude in using the four elements to devise interventions tailored to the flexible needs of an isolated caregiver and care recipient.

Support Groups and Other Mutual Aid

Support groups have been identified for a wide variety of chronic illnesses and conditions, such as cancer (Reach to Recovery), bereavement (Widow to Widow), and alcoholism (Alcoholics Anonymous), or for other illnesses such as multiple sclerosis or blindness. These groups assist individuals in coping with their illness and the changes in identities and social roles that illnesses may incur for clients. They can help enhance one's self-esteem, provide alternative meanings of the illness, suggest ways to cope, assist in specific hints or interventions that have helped others, or offer services or care for the isolate or caregiver (Matteson & McConnell, 1988).

In almost every large city or county are lists of resources that can be accessed: health departments, social work centers, schools, and libraries; even the telephone book's yellow pages can assist in finding support groups or other resources. Some resources list group entry requirements or qualifications. Because of their variety and number, support groups are not always available in every community, and so health professionals may find themselves in the position of developing a group. Therefore, as part of a community assessment, the health professional should not only mark the groups currently available, but identify someone who might be willing to develop a needed group. The health professional also may have to help find a meeting place, refer clients to the group, assist clients in discussing barriers to their care, and, if necessary, develop structured activities (such as exercise regimens for arthritic individuals). In addition, the use of motivational devices, such as pictures, videos, audio recordings, reminiscence, or games may be helpful in developing discussion. Demonstrations of specific illness-related regimens, such as exercises, clothing aids, or body mechanics, are also useful to support groups.

Professionals should be alert to problems the isolate may have in integrating into groups, such as resistance to meeting new people; low self-esteem; apprehension over participation in new activities; or the real problems of transportation, building access, and inconvenient meeting times (Matteson & McConnell, 1988).

Social activity groups are one way of integrating isolated institutionalized individuals or of reversing hospital-induced confusion; such groups could be recreational therapy groups or those developed particularly to address a special interest (e.g., parents facing the imminent death of a child). Given the limited resources typical of most chronically ill persons, support groups that are not costly to the chronically ill or their families are more likely to be welcomed.

Spiritual Well-being

For many an individual, religious or spiritual beliefs offer an important social connection and give great meaning to one's life. Religious groups range from formal gatherings to church-aided social groups. Spiritual well-being typically affirms the unity of the person with his or her environment, often expressed in a oneness with his or her god(s) (Matteson & McConnell, 1988). Consequently, assuring isolates some means of connection to their religious support may help them find newer meaning in life or illness and provide them with other people with whom to share that meaning. The health professional should assess the meaning of religion to the individual, the kind of spiritual meeting place he or she finds most comforting, and the types of religious support available in the community.

Frequently, churches or temples have outreach or social groups that will make visits, arrange for social outings, or develop pen pals or other means of human connectedness. The nurse or other health professional may have to initiate contact with these groups to assist in developing the necessary outreach between them and the isolate.

Rebuilding Family Networks

Keeping, or rebuilding, family networks has much to offer. However, families that are disintegrated may have a history of fragile relationships. The health professional must assess these groups carefully to develop truly effective interventions.

The professional must also take into account the client's type of isolation (lifelong versus recent) and the wishes of the isolate: With whom (if anyone) in the family does the isolate wish contact? How often? What members of the family exist or care about the isolate? What is their relationship to the isolate—parent, sibling, child, friend-as-family, other relative? The professional can then make contact with the individuals indicated to be most accommodating to the isolate, explain the situation, make future plans to bring them and the isolate together, and afterward assess the outcome. However, it may not be possible to bring disinterested family members back into the isolate's social network.

For family members who are interested and willing, rebuilding networks means the professional must take into account the location or proximity of family members to the isolate. If they live near each other, and since needing a "space of one's own" is a critical human response, a balance of territorial and personal needs must be managed if they are to be reintegrated. Should the isolate and family agree to live together, the family's physical environment will require assessment for safety, access, and territo-

rial space. Not only are factors such as sleeping space and heat and ventilation important, but personal space and having one's own possessions are as important to the family members as they are to the ill person. Teaching the family and isolate how to respect each other's privacy (such as by getting permission to enter a room or to look through personal belongings, speaking directly to one another, and so forth) is a way to help them bridge their differences.

Understanding Family Relationships   Finally, the nature of the relationship between family and isolate must be understood. The family's meanings and actions attached to love, power, and conflict, and observations of the frequency of controlling strategies by various individuals will inform the professional of potential interventions. For example, the elderly woman's use of guilt with an otherwise accommodating family (cited earlier) informed the nurse about interventions most likely to succeed.

In some families, love is thought to indicate close togetherness, while in other families, love is thought to provide members with independence. Power and hierarchy can be developed and thought of either as a pyramidical (top-down) set of relationships or as an equalitarian circle. Conflict may be a means of connection or of distance and expressed in shouting and insults or in quiet assertion.

Community Resources to Keep Families Together   Using community resources, such as support groups, is a way to help keep a family together. Families draw on each other's experiences as models and lessons. For example, families in which there is a child with cancer find ways to help their child cope with the isolation induced by chemotherapy. When necessary, the health professional may wish to refer the isolate and family to psychiatric or specialty nurses, counselors, psychiatrists, or social workers to help them overcome their disintegration. Successful implementation of the wide range of family-related interventions requires sensitive perceptions of the needs not only of the isolate but of the various family members with whom that individual must interact.

Touch   Families and professionals must learn the comfort of touch. Studies indicate that the elderly are the least likely group to be touched, and yet they find touch very comforting. Pets may be useful as an alternative to human touch and human interaction. Feeling loved and having it demonstrated through touch can do much to reduce isolation and its often concommitant lowered self-esteem. Since some individuals find touch uncomfortable, professionals must assess (by simply asking or observing flinching, grimacing, or resignation) the family's or isolate's responsiveness to touch.

Behavior Modification

Behavior modification is a technique that is best used by skilled professionals. It involves the systematic analysis of responses and their antecedent cues and consequences; the use of cognitive therapy to change awareness, perceptions, and behaviors; and the specification of realistic, measurable goals or actual behaviors. Also, reward structures and understanding support persons are necessary in the definition of the problem and its solution. Consistency is needed to develop stable patterns of responses. The time frame of such modification can vary with the problem.

Behavior modification is particularly useful in discrete problems, for example, the isolate who is fearful of going outside the house. It is also an important intervention when the environment can be held stable, such as in an institutional setting. Matteson and McConnell (1988) note that where groups are small or the motivation intense, successful behavioral interventions have been instituted for the socially isolated in institutions as well as in the home.

Telephones

The telephone is another method used to counteract the effects of place-boundedness. However, in one study it had equivocal findings (Kivett, 1979; Praderas & MacDonald, 1986). Still, the telephone is considered almost a necessity in reducing the isolation of a place-bound individual.

Summary and Conclusions

Social isolation, as a concept, is not always clearly defined in the literature, frequently being confused with loneliness, alienation, aloneness, and, at times, impaired social interactions. Social isolation may be either positive, as in the re-creation of the human psyche, or negative. Where it is involuntary and perceived as negative, and where the social network is shrinking in quality or quantity of contacts, it is defined as social isolation.

Where social isolation exists, it becomes a concern for isolates, their social networks, and their health care providers. Care should be taken to avoid stereotypical judgments of its existence or intensity. On the other hand, systematic observations of clinical populations argue that social isolation does, in truth, exist and to the detriment of the isolate. This is particularly so in the case of chronic illness. Across various conditions (cancer, heart disease, neurological disease, trauma, and so forth), and across the life span with its social activities and roles, social isolation contributes to greater risk for mortality and morbidity. Regardless of whether individuals are constrained at the level of the person, his or her confidantes, the organization, or the community, the potential exists for social isolation.

The quality of interactions is the most important variable in reintegrating the isolate. The health professional needs to help manage the client's illness trajectory and its effects on physical and emotional stamina, which requires that the professional recognize the meaning of social isolation to the isolate as well as to the isolate's social network. Furthermore, the professional needs to understand the meaning that chronic illness and isolation have on the identity of the isolate.

All of these issues need to be taken into account and each considered. Assessments of the client always require validation, and strategies need ongoing evaluation by the health professional. Such action takes the isolated client or social network into an equalitarian relationship that offers full opportunity to exercise moral agency and authority. Since the perception of isolation varies, the health professional must remain vigilant to symptoms and flexible in attempting interventions.

Wherever possible, the health professional must recognize that the isolate need not exist in a vacuum, but should consider the impact of the person's social network. As social networks deplete their emotional, material, and financial resources, the health professional should consider means to support them.

Finally, social isolation is a model of human disconnectedness. Its systematic examination, therefore, will allow the health professional to develop purposeful interventions to reduce the misery of unwanted social isolation.

NURSING DIAGNOSIS

Editor's Note: As is apparent from this chapter, interventions for social isolation are not adequately researched and are therefore dependent on the interpretation of secondary sources. The reader is encouraged to consider other handbooks, such as Carpenito (1993), when dealing with this diagnosis or with impaired social interaction in planning interventions.

3.1.2 Social Isolation

Definition: Aloneness experienced by the individual and perceived as imposed by others and as a negative and threatening state.

Defining Characteristics:[1]

Objective: *Absence of supportive other(s) (family, friends, group); sad dull affect; inappropriate or immature interests/activities for development age/stage; uncommunicative, withdrawn, no eye contact; preoccupation with own thoughts, repetitive meaningless actions; projects hostility in voice, behavior; seeks to be alone or exists in a subculture; evidence of physical/mental handicap or altered state of wellness; shows behavior unaccepted by dominant cultural group.

Subjective: *Expresses feelings of aloneness imposed by others; *expresses feelings of rejection; experiences feelings of difference from others; inadequacy in or absence of significant purpose in life; inability to meet ex-

pectations of others; insecurity in public; expresses values acceptable to the subculture but unacceptable to the dominant cultural group; expresses interests inappropriate to the developmental age/stage.

Related Factors: Factors contributing to the absence of satisfying personal relationships, such as delay in accomplishing developmental tasks, immature interests; alterations in physical appearance or mental status; unaccepted social behavior or social values; altered state of wellness; inadequate personal resources; inability to engage in satisfying personal relationships.

Editor's Note: When considering the possibility of isolation of a client, the nurse must also consider the related nursing diagnosis of impaired social interaction.

3.1.1 Impaired Social Interaction

Definition: The state in which an individual participates in an insufficient or excessive quantity or ineffective quality of social exchange.

Defining Characteristics:

Major: Verbalized or observed discomfort in social situations; verbalized or observed inability to receive or communicate a satisfying sense of belonging, caring, interest, or shared history; observed use of unsuccessful social interaction behaviors; dysfunctional interaction with peers, family and/or others.

Minor: Family report of change of style or pattern of interaction.

---

[1]The asterisk denotes critical defining characteristics.

Related Factors: Knowledge/skill deficit about ways to enhance mutuality; communication barriers; self-concept disturbance; absence of available significant others or peers; limited physical mobility; therapeutic isolation; sociocultural dissonance; environmental barriers; altered thought processes.

STUDY QUESTIONS

1. Is loneliness the same thing as social isolation? Why or why not?
2. How might the distance that a manually powered or an electrically powered wheelchair goes relate to social isolation?
3. List six characteristics that might incline a client to social isolation. What criteria did you use to develop these characteristics?
4. Suppose another health professional said about a very new client: "Oh, we must make certain that Mrs. Jones has company. She's a widow, you know." With regard to social isolation, what arguments could you make, pro or con, about this statement?
5. Develop at least five questions you could adapt to assess and validate social isolation in a client. Consider how you might approach identity levels, actual isolation, network assessment, and feelings of the isolate. Add other priorities as you wish, but offer rationales for each of them.
6. Name three community resources you could use to reduce the social isolation of clients.
7. What two principles should guide a health professional when developing any intervention with an isolated client? Why are these important?
8. If a client said to you: "I have had arthritis in my fingers and hands for a long time now. I simply can't do what I used to do. I now have new handles for my kitchen cabinets because the knobs hurt my hands, and new clothes especially made for people like me who can't work buttons. My daughter was shopping and she saw them and told me about them. Now I feel better when I get together with them to see my grandchildren." At what stage of identity might you expect this client to be? Why? Is this person an isolate? Explain your answer.
9. A gay teenager is your client. He has recently "come out" and is now depressed because his schoolmates shun him, his parents are going through a grief reaction to his announcement, and he has few other friends who share his interests or sexual preference. Is he at risk for social isolation? How would you assess his social network? What interventions, if any, would you recommend? Explain your answers.

References

Antonucci, T. (1985). Social support. Theoretical advances, recent findings and pressing issues. In I. G. Sarason & B. R. Sarason (Eds.), *Social support: Theory, research and application.* Boston: Martinus Nyhoff.

Austin, D. (1989). Becoming immune to loneliness: Helping the elderly fill a void. *Journal of Gerontological Nursing, 15*(9), 25–28.

Bendor, S. (1990). Anxiety and isolation in siblings of pediatric cancer patients: The need for prevention. *Social Work in Health Care, 14*(3), 17–35.

Bennet, R. (1980). *Aging, isolation, and resocialization* (Chapters 1, 2). New York: Van Nostrand Reinhold.

Berkman, L. (1983). The assessment of social networks and social support in the elderly. *American Geriatric Society Journal, 31*(12), 743–749.

Biordi, D. (primary investigator) (1993). In-home care and respite care as self-care (Grant # NRO2021-0183). Washington, D.C.: National Institute of Nursing Research.

Burnley, I. H. (1992). Mortality from selected cancers in NSW and Sydney, Australia. *Social Science and Medicine, 35*(2), 195–208.

Cadman, D., Rosenbaum, P., Boyle, M., & Offord, D. (1991). Children with chronic illness: Family and parent demographic characteristics and psychosocial adjustment. *Pediatrics, 87*(6), 884–889.

Carpenito, L. J. (1993). *Nursing diagnosis: Application to clinical practice.* Philadelphia: J. B. Lippincott.

Charmaz, K. (1987). Struggling for a self: Identity levels of the chronically ill. In J. Roth & P. Conrad (Eds.), *Research in the sociology of health care.* Greenwich, CT: JAI Press.

Christ, G. (1987). Social consequences of the cancer experience. *The American Journal of Pediatric Hematology/Oncology, 9*(1), 84-88.

Cobb, S. (1979). Social support and health through the life course. In M. W. Riley (Ed.), *Aging from birth to death.* Boulder, CO: Westview Press.

Cohen, M. (1993). The unknown and the unknowable—managing sustained uncertainty. *Western Journal of Nursing Research, 15*(1), 77-96.

Corbin, J., & Strauss, A. (1987). Accompaniments of chronic illness: Changes in body, self, biography and biographical time. In J. Roth and P. Conrad (Eds.), *Research in the sociology of health care.* Greenwich, CT: JAI Press.

Cox, C., Spiro, M., & Sullivan, J. (1988). Social risk factors: Impact on elders' perceived health status. *Journal of Community Health Nursing, 5*(1), 59-73.

Creecy, R., Berg, W., & Wright, Jr. (1985). Loneliness among the elderly: A causal approach. *Journal of Gerontology, 40*(4), 487-493.

Creed, F. (1990). Psychological disorders in rheumatoid arthritis: A growing consensus? *Annual Rheumatic Disorders, 49,* 808-812.

Dela Cruz, L. (1986). On loneliness and the elderly. *Journal of Gerontological Nursing, 12*(11), 22-27.

DesRosier, M., Catanzaro, M., & Piller, J. (1992). Living with chronic illness: Social support and the well spouse perspective. *Rehabilitation Nursing, 17*(2), 87-91.

DiMatteo, M. R., & Hays, R. (1981). Social support and serious illness. In B. H. Gottlieb (Ed.), *Social networks and social support.* Beverly Hills, CA: Sage.

Dropkin, M. (1989). Coping with disfigurement and dysfunction. *Seminars in Oncology Nursing, 5*(3), 213-219.

Fitzpatrick, R., Newman, R., Archer, R., & Shipley, M. (1991). Social support, disability, and depression: A longitudinal study of rheumatoid arthritis. *Social Science and Medicine, 33*(5), 605-611.

Foxall, M., Eckberg, J., & Griffith, N. (1986). Spousal adjustment to chronic illness. *Rehabilitation Nursing, 11,* 13-16.

Frierson, R. L. (1991). Suicide attempts by the old and the very old. *Archives of Internal Medicine, 151*(1), 141-144.

Gallo, A. M., Breitmayer, B. J., Knafl, K. A., & Zoeller, L. H. (1991). Stigma in childhood chronic illness: A well sibling perspective. *Pediatric Nursing, 17*(1), 21-25.

Gamba, A., Romano, M. Grosso, I., Tamburini, M., Cantu, G., Molinari, R., & Ventafridda, V. (1992). Psychosocial adjustment of patients surgically treated for head and neck cancer. *Head and Neck,* 218-223.

Glassman-Feibusch, B. (1981). The socially isolated elderly. *Geriatric Nursing, 2*(1), 28-31.

Goodman, C. (1984). Natural helping among older adults. *The Gerontologist, 24*(2), 138-143.

Gordon, M. (1982). *Nursing diagnosis: Process and application.* New York: McGraw-Hill.

———— (1989). Social isolation. *Manual of nursing diagnosis.* St. Louis: C. V. Mosby.

Heiney, S., Goon-Johnson, K., Ettinger, R., & Ettinger, S. (1990). The effects of group therapy on siblings of pediatric oncology patients. *Journal of Pediatric Oncology Nursing, 7*(3), 95-100.

Heumann, L. (1988). Assisting the frail elderly living in subsidized housing for the independent elderly: A profile of the management and its support priorities. *The Gerontologist, 28,* 625-631.

Hoeffer, B. (1987). A causal model of loneliness among older single women. *Archives of Psychiatric Nursing, 1*(5), 366-373.

Hopper, S. (1981). Diabetes as a stigmatized condition: The case of low income clinic patients in the United States. *Social Science and Medicine, 15B,* 11-19.

House, J., Landis, K., & Umberson, D. (1988). Social relationships and health. *Science, 241,* 540-544.

Jessop, D., & Stein, R. (1985). Uncertainty and its relation to the psychological and social correlates of chronic illness in children. *Social Science and Medicine, 20*(10), 993-999.

Kaplan, G., Salonen, J., Cohen, R., Brand, R., Syme, S., & Puska, P. (1988). Social connections and mortality from all causes and from cardiovascular disease: Prospective evidence from Eastern Finland. *American Journal of Epidemiology, 128*(2), 370-380.

Kinsella, G., Ford, B., & Moran, C. (1989). Survival of social relationships following head injury. *International Disability Studies, 11*(1), 9-14.

Kivett, V. (1979). Discriminators of loneliness among the rural elderly: Implications for interventions. *The Gerontologist, 19*(1), 108-115.

Krouse, J., Krouse, H., & Fabian, R. (1989). Adaptation to surgery for head and neck cancer. *Laryngoscope, 99,* 789-794.

Lawton, M., Greenbaum, M., & Liebowitz, B. (1980). The lifespan of housing environments for the aging. *The Gerontologist, 20,* 56-64.

Lawton, M., Kleban, M., & Carlson, D. (1973, Winter). The inner-city resident: To move or not to move. *The Gerontologist,* 443-448.

Lawton, M., Moss, M., & Grimes, M. (1985). The changing service need of older tenants in planned housing. *The Gerontologist, 25,* 258-264.

Lee, G. R., & Ellithorpe, E. (1982). Intergenerational exchange and subjective well-being among the elderly. *Journal of Marriage and the Family, 44,* 217-224.

Lien-Gieschen, T. (1993). Validation of social isolation related to maturational age: Elderly. *Nursing Diagnosis, 4*(1), 37-43.

Lin, N. (1986). Conceptualizing social support. In N. Lin, A. Dean, & W. Ensel (Eds.), *Social support, life events, and depression.* New York: Academic Press.

Lyons, M. J. (1982). Psychological concomitants of the environment influencing suicidal behavior in middle and later life. *Dissertation Abstracts International, 43,* 1620B.

Maddox, G. L. (1985). Intervention strategies to enhance well-being in later life: The status and prospect of guided change. *Health Services Research, 19,* 1007-1032.

Matteson, M. A., & McConnell, E. S. (1988). Gerontological nursing: Concepts and practice. Philadelphia: W. B. Saunders.

Miller, B. (1990). Gender differences in spouse caregiver strain: Socialization and role explanations. *Journal of Marriage and the Family, 52,* 311-322.

Mullins, L., & Dugan, E. (1990). The influence of depression, and family and friendship relations, on residents' loneliness in congregate housing. *The Gerontologist, 30*(3), 377-384.

NANDA (1994). *Nursing diagnoses: Definitions and classification.* St. Louis: NANDA.

Newman, S. P., Fitzpatrick, R., Lamb, R., & Shipley, M. (1989). The origins of depressed mood in rheumatoid arthritis. *The Journal of Rheumatology, 16*(6), 740-744.

Noll, R., Ris, M. D., Davies, W. H., Burkowski, W., & Koontz, K. (1992). Social interactions between children with cancer or sickle cell disease and their peers: Teacher ratings. *Developmental and Behavioral Pediatrics, 13*(3), 187-193.

Noyes, R., Kathol, R., Debelius-Enemark, P., Williams, J., Mutgi, A., Suelzer, M., & Clamon, G. (1990). Distress associated with cancer as measured by the illness distress scale. *Psychosomatics, 31*(3), 321-330.

Orth-Gomer, K., & Unden, A. (1990). Type A behavior, social support and coronary risk: Interaction and significance for mortality in cardiac patients. *Psychosomatic Medicine, 52*(1), 59-72.

Orth-Gomer, K., Unden, A., & Edwards, M. (1988). Social isolation and mortality in ischemic heart disease: A 10-year follow-up study of 150 middle aged men. *Acta Med Scan, 224*(3), 205-215.

Peplau, L. A., & Perlman, D. (Eds.) (1986). *Loneliness: A sourcebook of current theory, research, and therapy.* New York: John Wiley & Sons.

Poulin, J. (1984). Age segregation and the interpersonal involvement and morale of the aged. *The Gerontologist, 24*(3), 266-269.

Praderas, K., & MacDonald, M. (1986). Telephone conversational skills training with socially isolated, impaired nursing home residents. *Journal of Applied Behavior Analysis, 19*(4), 337-348.

Ravish, T. (1985). Prevent isolation before it starts. *Journal of Gerontological Nursing, 11*(10), 10-13.

Reif, L. (1973). Managing a life with chronic disease. *American Journal of Nursing, 73*(2), 261-264.

Reynolds, P., & Kaplan, G. (1990). Social connections and risk for cancer: Prospective evidence from the Alameda County study. *Behavioral Medicine, 16*(3), 101-110.

Ryan, M., & Patterson, J. (1987). Loneliness in the elderly. *Journal of Gerontological Nursing, 13*(5), 6-12.

Seeman, M. (1959). On the meaning of alienation. *American Sociological Review, 24,* 783-791.

Spiegel, D. (1990). Facilitating emotional coping during treatment. *Cancer, 66,* 1422-1426.

Stephens, M., & Bernstein, M. (1984). Social support and well-being among residents of planned housing. *The Gerontologist, 24,* 144-148.

Stewart, N. (1986). Perceptual and behavioral effects of immobility and social isolation in hospitalized orthopedic patients. *Nursing Papers/Perspectives in Nursing, 18*(3), 59-74.

Strauss, A., Corbin, J., Fagerhaugh, S., Glaser, B., Maines, D., Suzek, B., & Wiener, C. (1984). *Chronic illness and the quality of life* (2nd ed.). St. Louis: C. V. Mosby.

Subcommittee on Human Services of the Select Committee on Aging: U.S. House of Representatives (1987). *Exploding the myths: Caregiving in America* (Committee print: No. 99-611). Washington, D.C.: Government Printing Office.

Tamlyn, D., & Arklie, M. (1986). A theoretical framework for standard care plans: A nursing approach for working with chronically ill children and their families. *Issues in Comprehensive Pediatric Nursing, 9,* 39-45.

Tilden, V., & Weinert, C. (1987). Social support and the chronically ill individual. *Nursing Clinics of North America, 22*(3), 613-620.

Trout, D. (1980). The role of social isolation in suicide. *Suicide and Life Threatening Behavior, 10,* 10-22.

Watson, E. (1988). Dead to the world. *Nursing Times, 84*(21), 52-54.

Weeks, J. R., & Cuellar, J. P. (1981). The role of family members in the helping networks of older people. *The Gerontologist, 21,* 388-394.

Weisman, A. D., & Worden, J. W. (1976-1977). The existential plight in cancer: Significance of the first 100 days. *International Journal of Psychiatry in Medicine, 7,* 1-15.

Weiss, R. S. (1973). *Loneliness: The experience of emotional and social isolation.* Cambridge, MA: Massachusetts Institute of Technology Press.

Williams, S., & Bury, M. (1989). Impairment, disability, and handicap in chronic respiratory illness. *Social Science and Medicine, 29*(5), 609-616.

Woods, N., Haberman, M., & Packard, N. (1993). Demands of illness and individual, dyadic, and family adaption in chronic illness. *Western Journal of Nursing Research, 15*(1), 10-30.

Bibliography

Bell, D. (1959). The rediscovery of alienation: Some notes along the quest for the historical Marx. *Journal of Philosophy, 56,* 933-952.

Holmen, K., Ericsson, K., Anderson, L., & Winblad, B. (1992). Loneliness among elderly people living in Stockholm: A population study. *Journal of Advanced Nursing, 17,* 43-51.

Kornhauser, W. (1959). *The politics of mass society.* New York: The Free Press.

Shanas, E. (1968). *Old people in three societies.* New York: Atherton Press.

Shils, E. (1963). The theory of mass society. In P. Olson (Ed.), *America as a mass society.* New York: The Free Press.

PART II

Impact on Client and Family

CHAPTER 9

Quality of Life

Elizabeth Johnson-Taylor •
Patricia Jones • Margaret Burns

CASE STUDY

C. F. was a 50-year-old career woman who started having difficulty with voluntary movement. She went to her personal physician, who was not too alarmed. While attending a conference, she noticed more changes, such as not being able to control her walking all the time. She was alarmed enough to see a neurologist who, after testing, indicated she might have myasthenia gravis. However, further testing revealed that she had ALS (Lou Gehrig's disease).

Following the initial shock of the diagnosis, she made some decisions about how the rest of her life would be lived. She traveled with a longtime friend to Europe after selling her home and moving closer to a sister. On her return she spent time with old friends. She also decided that she did not want any life-sustaining methods instituted as she deteriorated. She died at her home with her sister and other family members by her side within a year after her diagnosis was confirmed. During this time, she had made choices that influenced the quality of her remaining life.

Introduction

C. F. was a woman comfortable with herself and her decisions. Even though she knew she was dying, she maintained the quality of her life. She remained independent and through her friends and family was able to do those activities that enhanced her life. Not all clients are able to retain such quality, and it would behoove health professionals to become aware of the factors that affect the quality of chronically ill individuals' lives.

Acknowledgment: The authors wish to thank the following individuals who provided information for the case studies: Roy Tanabe, volunteer, AIDS project, Los Angeles, California; and Chris Haynal of College Place, Washington.

Analgesic advertisements that tout pain relief in the face of ongoing diseases, such as cancer, illustrate the emphasis currently placed on maintaining a positive quality of life amidst chronic illness. Indeed, any chronic illness that changes and challenges an individual's quality of life needs to be addressed by health care providers and care recipients alike. The purpose of this chapter is to discuss the physical, psychological, spiritual, sociocultural, and economic changes and challenges that chronically ill individuals experience, and how health practitioners can provide care that improves this quality of life.

Nurses and other health providers typically assume that a chronic illness brings only negative qualities such as pain, suffering, deficit, and loss. However, there is evidence that, for some, chronic illness brings positive side effects such as release from disliked roles, increased attention, or sympathy. For others, the chronic illness experience leads to the development of positive coping strategies to maintain or improve their quality of life (Calman, 1984; Padilla et al., 1990; Cella, 1991). To illustrate, many patients develop cognitive strategies or spiritual resources that bring them satisfaction and a sense of well-being that compensate for their physical losses. Thus, although quality of life may be changed, it does not necessarily decrease for some individuals.

The growing recognition of quality-of-life issues parallels increasing medical knowledge and technology, which, of course, contribute to increasing cure rates for various diseases. Many diseases that were fatal in the past, such as end-stage renal disease, are now chronic in nature. In addition, the improved longevity of the population as a whole leads to the increased likelihood that more and more persons will develop chronic illnesses. Thus, when the *quantity* of life is extended, *quality* of life becomes particularly pertinent.

The acquired immune deficiency syndrome (AIDS) epidemic illustrates this phenomenon. Not long ago, a diagnosis of AIDS meant imminent death. It is now treated with multiple experimental therapies, and those with the virus are living longer and longer. In addition, many comorbid conditions that often killed people with AIDS, are now controlled by various pharmacological interventions. Many of these individuals employ health-promoting diets, positive ways of thinking, and activities to enhance and, possibly, prolong their lives. Going from a fatal to a chronic state contributes to various quality-of-life concerns such as, How can I function socially with a stigmatized illness? How can I pay for needed care? How do I live for an unknown length of time knowing that premature death is on my horizon?

The case study of living with AIDS illustrates how a fatal illness can become chronic and how quality-of-life issues can arise incrementally over time. This case also depicts the ethical, psychosocial, and spiritual dimensions of living with chronicity and tells how living with imminent death is a part of living with any one of several chronic illnesses.

Another factor that has contributed to quality-of-life issues is the patients' rights movement (Aaronson, 1988), which has given individuals the right to participate in making decisions that affect their health. Many care recipients now demand to know how treatments and sequelae will affect the quality of their lives. For instance, they want to know if the positive outcomes of their treatment (such as symptom control or prolonged life) will be greater than the negative effects (including financial drain, anxiety, or disrupted life-style). To satisfy clients' right to an information-based decision, health care professionals must attend to how chronic disease treatments relate to quality of life.

Defining the Concept

Because nurses and other health care professionals are interested in the influences that health and illness have on quality of life, the phrase "health-related quality of life" is preferred (Aaronson, 1988). Padilla and colleagues (1990) viewed quality of life as "a subjective evaluation of the positiveness or negativeness of attributes that characterize one's life." Ferrans (1985) defined it as "a person's sense of well-being that stems from satisfaction or dissatisfaction with the areas of life that are important to him/her."

Some researchers recognize that the care recipient's past and future contribute to how quality of life is perceived in the present. Calman (1984) asserted that health-related quality of life "depends on present lifestyle, past experience, hopes for the future, dreams and ambitions." Cella (1991) acknowledged that health-related quality of life refers to clients' "appraisal of and satisfaction with their current level of functioning as compared to what they perceive to be possible or ideal." Thus, a good quality of life is attained when the gap between a patient's aspirations and hopes and actual experience is narrow.

All researchers agree that quality of life can be determined only by the care recipient. Among the numerous definitions that have evolved, two recurrent themes emerge: multidimensionality and subjectivity (Cella, 1991; Padilla et al., 1990; Aaronson, 1988; Calman, 1984).

CASE STUDY
Living with AIDS

Ben and David were a homosexual couple deeply committed to each other. Two years before he died, Ben was diagnosed with acquired immune deficiency syndrome (AIDS). David, who was HIV negative, accompanied Ben during his illness journey.

As his illness progressed, Ben experienced significant pain from treatment-related neuropathy, which was controlled with morphine. However, he feared the other physical sequelae his AIDS or its treatment might bring: incontinence, nausea, anemia, and fatigue.

After many thoughtful conversations, Ben and David decided that a life of quality meant not suffering any of the endstage effects of AIDS. They agreed that Ben should not have to experience what for them would have been the ultimate assault of AIDS: dementia. They both wanted David to be able to remember Ben as a healthy, caring individual.

Thus, together they contacted the Hemlock Society and obtained information about euthanasia. They set a date. For them a "good" death for Ben would include no discomfort, playing Chopin nocturnes in the background, and having only David present. This allowed Ben to maintain control, self-respect, and meaning even at his death.

The meaningfulness of life and death were nurtured for Ben by regular visits to his synagogue and to support group meetings. Although Ben's family had broken off their relations with him when he announced his homosexuality, David's family's love enriched Ben's life.

Although the illness forced Ben to stop teaching, he was able to assist David in his real estate business and thereby "earn his keep" and maintain his self-worth. Ben also found satisfaction during his last two years of life by organizing and distributing "leftover" AIDS medications to South Americans.

Multidimensionality   There are many dimensions to quality of life that vary from author to author in regard to labeling and content (Padilla et al., 1990; Aaronson, 1986; Cella, 1991). This chapter's discussion of problems and issues associated with health-related quality of life treats the four dimensions of physical, psychological, social, and spiritual well-being created by Donovan et al. (1989) and Ferrell and associates (1992). In addition, because chronic illness can change or challenge the financial situation of an individual or family, the economic impact of illness on quality of life will be discussed (Given et al., 1992).

Subjectivity   From interviews with persons with cancer, numerous subjective attributes that influenced their physical, psychological, and interpersonal well-being were identified (Padilla et al., 1990). Attributes that diminished physical well-being included feeling sick; slow or poor functioning; feeling dependent and burdensome; not being able to work; and feeling weak, fatigued, or in pain. Those attributes that diminished psychological well-being included not enjoying life, being unable to concentrate, feeling

insecure, having a negative mental attitude, and having questions and fears about the disease. Indicators of lessening interpersonal well-being included nonsupportive relationships, perceptions of making others unhappy, and the sense of not fulfilling family roles.

Theoretical Framework

Promoting quality of life for chronically ill individuals is enhanced when practice is guided by frameworks that explain some of the personal and interpersonal challenges these individuals face. Both sociological and nursing frameworks are helpful.

Sociological Frameworks   Two sociological frameworks that best apply to quality-of-life issues are Mead's symbolic interactionism and Strauss and others' trajectory. Both are briefly described here.

Symbolic Interactionism   Symbolic interaction theory, synthesized by George Herbert Mead (1934), proposes three major concepts as a basis for understanding human behavior: mind,

CASE STUDY

Changing Roles: Ms. A. G.

Ms. A. G., a single, 40-year-old woman lives in the southwest. Her parents retired some years earlier on the east coast and decided that they wanted to be closer to her, so they moved within an hour's drive from her. She subsequently became the caregiver for her parents before she was prepared to take on this role.

Her father had a chronic cardiac condition that was poorly controlled. However, her mother's physical health, although frail, appeared to be intact. Because they were less able to manage their own care, they let her take on the parental role. This was an uncomfortable role reversal for her. A couple of years after moving, her father's cardiac condition changed for the worse. She consulted with her sister, who lived in another state, and they decided that her parents should move to a smaller home within walking distance of where she lived. Her sister served as an important part of her support network as she made decisions about their parents.

With the changes in living space and physicians, her father stabilized, but her mother became increasingly forgetful and was diagnosed as having Alzheimer's disease. The demands placed on A. G. impacted her ability to maintain quality of life, both for herself and her parents.

Her mother's mental deterioration worsened and her father became increasingly weak, again requiring realignment of family roles in an attempt to maintain quality of life for all concerned. Her support network increased in importance to her and helped her find resources that enabled her to cope with her parents' changing health status.

---

self, and society. The human being, Mead explained, interacts with the environment subjectively, communicating and interpreting meaning through the use of symbols. Because of the role played by symbols in influencing interaction, Mead called the theory *symbolic interactionism,* since it encompassed both the interpretation of and response to symbols in human interactions.

In interaction theory, the *mind* is defined as the process of thinking, assessing, anticipating, and defining a situation, and then constructing a course of action. This process emerges through efforts of individuals to adjust to their social world. Utilizing the processes of the mind, human beings develop feelings and attitudes toward the *self* and construct responses to the self based on their interactions with others. As individuals interact, each takes on a particular role that further influences development of the self in relation to others.

Society represents the constantly changing, but somewhat coordinated and patterned, interactions among individuals. It arises out of the individual's attempts to adjust to environmental challenges. Mead described the mind and self, basic to interactions and role development, as the basis of society. Thus, *self* and *society* develop together.

Illness Trajectory Strauss (1975), Glaser and Strauss (1978), and Corbin and Strauss (1988) developed theoretical concepts grounded in the experiences of chronically ill individuals and their families. The central concept, *trajectory,* focuses on the role people play in shaping the experience of unfolding physiological changes. Each person's view of the trajectory is individualistic and uncertain. In the course of a trajectory, efforts are made at *normalizing,* that is, attempting to live as normally as possible despite symptoms and a possible downward course (see Chapter 3, on illness trajectory).

Changes in the body's ability to perform affect one's perception of self and may be perceived as a failure or loss of self. As the individual, family members, and others interact, each aligns and realigns his or her roles in order to manage the situation and all the work involved. The case study of Ms. A. G. demonstrates how roles change as the physical self changes.

As various phases of the trajectory are experienced and the demands associated with them are faced, *balancing* of energy, efforts, and resources is required for quality of life to be preserved. The way in which one manages these challenges significantly influences the quality of life experienced.

Nursing Frameworks   Concern for the quality of life of individuals, with and without health problems, is inherent in nursing's commitment to caring as its reason for being (see Chapter 19, on nursing ethics). This concern is either explicit or implicit in a number of nursing theories. For example, in Parse's theory of human becoming (1981), "quality of life" is the explicit goal of nursing, with *quality* being defined by each individual or family.

In Watson's theory of human care (1985) nursing aims at helping individuals find meaning in their existence, particularly in the face of disharmony and suffering. Increased awareness of one's potential as a spiritual being opens up possibilities for becoming more fully human, transcending physical limitations, and preserving meaning and quality in living.

Orem's self-care model (1990) is also useful in both guiding nursing practice with the chronically ill and improving the quality of existence. Since functional status is closely related to quality of life (Cowan, et al., 1992), maintaining or restoring the person's ability to perform self-care will contribute to meaning and satisfaction in life.

Benner and Wrubel (1989) feel that the sense of well-being comes from the freedom to choose actions, outcomes, meanings, and relationships. Living with an illness does not mean that one's life is dominated by it, that one tries to conquer it, or that it can be mastered. Rather, the human being goes forward and reaches the highest level of outcome possible by finding meaning and harmony in existence, even with chronic illness. Thus, meaning, harmony, and attaining the highest level of well-being possible can constitute quality of life.

Problems and Issues of the Chronically Ill

As noted earlier, problems associated with quality of life can be physical, psychological, socio-cultural, spiritual, or economic. Although these dimensions overlap and interact, they provide organization for a discussion of the issues that an individual living with a chronic illness may confront.

Physical Issues

Functional Status   The perception of quality of life is affected by the ability of chronically ill persons, whether children or adults, to continue functioning in daily activities, such as self-care, school, work, or creative outlets, as a means of avoiding lessened self-esteem and autonomy. For instance, in elderly individuals functional status and autonomy are closely related to morale and quality of life (Clark, 1988); the elderly are adversely affected by such things as hospitalization, anesthesia, and invasive surgical or diagnostic procedures. Functional status was also found to affect the perceived quality of life in clients with cancer (Cowan, Graham, & Cochrane, 1992).

Symptoms   Chronically ill individuals not only experience symptoms associated with their disease, but are subjected to side effects from the treatments they undergo. Since these symptoms are multiple and vary with each disease, a discussion of each symptom is well beyond the scope of this chapter. Instead, general observations about responses to symptoms will be discussed.

Significance of Symptoms   Symptoms are metaphors of illness that characteristically indicate that disease is present or advancing. Typically, it is a physical symptom that prompts an individual to seek professional help—for example, weakness and incoordination in the individual with multiple sclerosis or excessive thirst and frequent urination in a person with diabetes. A new pain can send a cancer patient back to the oncologist.

Symptoms are often symbols of many things for those living with chronic illness. For example, three levels of meaning for pain were found among cancer patients, their family caregivers, and their home care nurses. On a basic level, informants stated that pain signified disease and served as a reminder of eventual death. On a more abstract level, pain meant a variety of psychosocial losses and changes, such as power-lessness, grief, fear, and challenge. Finally, the meaning of pain was described on a cognitive and spiritual level; these informants presented a variety of meanings, or ultimate causes, for why the pain occurred, such as fate or God's will (Ferrell et al., 1993).

The meaning assigned to a symptom will influence how a care recipient responds to that symptom. If individuals view their symptoms as inevitable or necessary, they passively accept them. On the other hand, if symptoms are viewed as challenges or enemies, clients will likely engage in active battle against them. Bark-well (1991) observed that specific meanings given to cancer pain were indeed related to specific outcomes. Subjects who perceived pain as a challenge had significantly less pain and depression and coped better than did those who perceived their cancer pain as inevitable or as punishment.

Physically distressing symptoms affect not only the physical but the psychosocial and spiritual aspects of quality of life. For example, reported dyspnea contributed to decreased health-related quality of life among elderly persons with chronic lung diseases (Scrier, Dekker, & Kaptein, 1990). Likewise, symptom distress had a positive correlation with mood disturbance among lung cancer patients (McCorkle & Quint-Benoliel, 1983). Patients with recurrent cancer reported less purpose in life with increased symptom distress (Taylor, 1993).

Pain symbolizes the multidimensionality of symptoms. Persons living with chronic pain frequently are depressed (France, 1987; McCaffery & Beebe, 1989). Those with chronic low back pain often search for a causal explanation for their pain. For these individuals, the pain effects a sense of struggle, loss of control, despair, and helplessness—especially when it is accepted as no longer being temporary (Bowman, 1991). Furthermore, unrelieved pain, at least among cancer patients, has been identified as a factor that increases the likelihood of suicide and requests for physician-assisted suicide (Foley, 1991).

Symptom Distress: Care Recipient versus Care Giver Clients and their caregivers interpret symptom distress differently. In one study, health care professionals felt that the cancer patients they were caring for were significantly more angry, hostile, and depressed than the patients felt themselves to be, even when patients' denial was statistically controlled (Jennings & Muhlen-kamp, 1981; Ferrell et al., 1993). Similarly, family caregivers of cancer patients having pain gave their loved one a higher pain score than did the respective patient (Ferrell, 1991).

Symptom control perspectives also differ among individuals, their significant others, and health care professionals. For example, a client may want to take analgesics, the spouse may advocate folk remedies, and the physician may recommend surgical intervention. Similarly, a hypertensive patient may choose to use only relaxation, exercise, and diet as treatment, but caregivers encourage a medication regimen.

Psychological Issues

Psychological well-being, an essential component of health-related quality of life, influences overall adjustment to chronic illness. For example, a general level of discomfort was found to be negatively associated with life satisfaction and perceived coping ability among individuals with multiple sclerosis (Counte, Bieliauskas, & Pavlou, 1983). On the other hand, the presence of a positive attitude toward challenge was related to good adaptation to diabetes (Pollock, 1986).

Several psychologists have theorized how persons cope or adapt to an illness in an attempt to maintain well-being (Weiner, 1986; Lazarus & Folkman, 1984; Nerenz & Leventhal, 1983; Taylor, 1983; Rothbaum, Weisz, & Snyder, 1982). Taylor (1983) theorized that people adapt to life-threatening illnesses in three ways: by searching for meaning, by cognitively controlling events, and by enhancing self-esteem.

Searching for Meaning The search for meaning involves making sense of negative or unexpected events, finding some purpose for these events, or placing them within a larger context (Thompson & Janigian, 1988). Often this search includes asking any of three questions: Why did this happen? Why did it happen to me? and What or who is responsible for letting it happen?

(Thompson, 1991). Several researchers have observed that this search for meaning is a response to a variety of chronic illness situations, including stroke, cancer, and spinal cord injury (Thompson, 1991; O'Conner, Wicker, & Germino, 1990; Taylor, 1993; Ferrell et al., 1993; Bulman & Wortman, 1977).

However, not all ill persons actively search for meaning, especially if their assumptions about the world are not shattered (Wortman & Silver 1992). To illustrate, people who believe that they were genetically predisposed to an illness may never question why it happened to them. However, nonsmoking individuals who now have lung cancer may question why if they believe that not smoking should have prevented the disease.

Various meanings have been ascribed to illness situations. For example, spinal-cord–injured subjects reported six reasons for their disabling accident: God had a reason ("God knows what He's doing; maybe it was to increase my faith in Him"); chance ("I just wasn't lucky"); predetermination ("It was intended that this should happen to me"); a good reason ("This illness has drawn my family closer together"); probability ("There was a 1-percent chance of this happening, and I was the 1 percent"); and it was deserved ("I was a workaholic and really stressed out") (Bulman & Wortman, 1977). These reasons can be generalized to other chronic conditions.

Control   Persons with chronic illness may use a variety of strategies for maintaining control in order to create quality of life psychologically. Approaches to control, and perceptions of personal control, vary from patient to patient and circumstance to circumstance.

Cognitive adaptation can be achieved by gaining a sense of mastery, or personal control. Gaining mastery implies that individuals perceive a contingency between what they do and what happens as a result. Persons can have *primary control,* that is, they change their world to meet their desires or, if that fails, change themselves to "go with the flow" of their world (Rothbaum, Weisz, & Snyder, 1982). For instance, a young woman with sickle cell anemia may attempt to control what happens to her by avoiding stressors that she feels bring about

sickle cell crises. When she fails at avoiding these crises, she may regain control by predicting when they will occur.

This illustration demonstrates that there are several types of personal control that can improve quality of life. *Processual control* allows the ill person to participate in the process of health caring; *contingency control* allows the person to believe that personal actions influence outcomes; *cognitive control* consists of intellectual management of events so they are perceived as less threatening; *behavioral control* involves the individual acting or behaving to directly change the situation; and *existential control* implies creating meaning and purpose for a negative event so that it becomes endurable (Lewis, 1987).

Whereas the concept of control has been discussed historically in terms of internal and external locus of control, the concept is now accepted as more complex. Rock, Meyerowitz, Maisto, and Wallston's (1987) findings suggest that there are several types of control profiles when the categories of internal control, external (or "powerful other") control, and chance are combined in different ways. That is, persons with a "pure internal" locus of control profile have a strong sense of internal control and a low sense of external or chance control. They believe they can influence their health a great deal. In contrast, persons with "double external" profiles reflect low degrees of internal control, but highly attribute control to powerful others and chance. These persons feel there is little they can do to affect their health, because they perceive it controlled mostly by external factors and/or chance. Similarly, persons with a "pure chance" profile ascribe much control to chance and little control to internal or powerful other sources. The labels "yea sayers" and "nay sayers" describe individuals who assign a great deal of control to all three sources or little control to these sources, respectively. "Believers in control" have a high sense of external and internal control, but think chance has little control. Thus, persons with chronic illness can reflect a variety of views about what forces control their lives.

Self-enhancement   Psychological well-being during a chronic illness requires that a person be able to view the self in a positive manner, that is, have self-esteem. Imagine the patient whose chronic illness interferes with independence, sexual function, or body image. What may have provided self-esteem in the past may now be gone—the ability to work and earn an income, the ability to please a sexual partner, or the ability to be physically attractive.

One method for self-enhancement frequently observed in chronically ill persons is "downward social comparison," which occurs when "persons can increase their subjective well-being through comparison with a less fortunate other" (Wills, 1981). Downward social comparison becomes psychologically necessary when there has been a decrease in one's subjective sense of well-being.

This form of social comparison allows individuals to distance themselves from a negative threat or challenge and thereby find security as well as self-worth. For example, a hemiplegic may say, "That poor quadriplegic; he can't even wheel himself around like I can—thank God I am not like that!" Or the emphysema patient may think, "I am so fortunate that I did not have to live with a disease all my life as people with asthma do." Nurses often hear patients say, "It could be worse!" Indeed, this expression is comforting to patients. Although studies have described the use of this cognitive strategy among persons with chronic illness (e.g., Taylor, 1983), there is no research investigating its efficacy as an intervention.

Another cognitive strategy used by patients that contributes to their well-being is illusion (Taylor & Brown, 1988). Although it has often been argued that mental health is dependent on contact with reality, people normally exaggerate the positive evaluations they give themselves, and they often possess an unrealistic sense of control, mastery, or optimism (Taylor & Brown, 1988). Thus, when chronically ill persons receive bad news, they may assign it a meaning that is less threatening than it is realistic. Living with a degree of illusion frees persons from some fear and anxiety, thereby allowing them to pursue activities that bring quality of life. For example, terminally ill patients who are told of their grave condition, but who remain optimistic that they will live longer than expected, are likely to be more active, cheerier, and less depressed than those realistically embracing imminent death (Taylor & Brown, 1988).

Sociocultural Issues

Chronic illness frequently affects the quality of clients' social relationships and roles; at the same time, clients' social support impacts their quality of life. Likewise, individuals' sociocultural backgrounds and relationships influence their response to illness and notions of quality of life. There can also be a significant impact on a client's family. The effect of chronic illness on one's social quality of life is illustrated in the case study of Jill, about living with Type I diabetes. The case study also illustrates that social support is usually provided by immediate family members, although it can also be provided by friends and health care workers.

The Significance of Social Support Social support has been identified as a contributor to health-related quality of life. In one study, a patient support group, one form of social support, reinforced self-worth and promoted adaptation among women with breast cancer (Rice & Szopa, 1988). In another study, affect, affirmation, and reciprocity from spouses and family members of women with a variety of chronic illnesses correlated with less depression and improved marriage and family functioning (Primomo, Yates, & Woods, 1990). Cancer patients who did not expect much social support had greater emotional distress during the first 100 days after diagnosis (Weisman & Worden, 1976).

Social support contributes to quality of life in a variety of ways. It influences how meaning is ascribed to illness, alters the coping strategies used to manage stress, augments motivation to employ adaptive behaviors, promotes self-esteem, and protects individuals from the negative effects of stress by altering their mood (Wortman, 1984). Indeed, most people know the positive effect of having "moral support" and companionship at times of difficulty.

Impact on Family For families with a chronically ill member, the goal is often "normalization."

CASE STUDY
Living with Juvenile-Onset Diabetes Mellitus

Jill was 3 years old when diagnosed with diabetes mellitus. Now at 13, she, her parents, and her older sister have learned much about living with an endless illness. Since Jill's brittle diabetes is impossible to control, her mother says that "things have never been normal."

The struggles of living with a diabetic child are innumerable: blood glucose monitoring five or more times a day and injecting appropriate insulin doses; frequent trips to endocrinologists and family doctors; occasional infections that can keep Jill in bed and cause her to miss school; paying the 25 percent medical insurance deductible for all medical expenses; planning and providing an appropriate diet; awkwardness about what

Jill should eat when dining out or when invited to friends' homes for dinner; having to live close to urban areas where Jill can receive health care; remaining calm and collected when Jill "passes out" in a diabetic crisis; wondering if the sibling conflicts that arise are normal sibling rivalry or illness-related tension; not being able to go camping as a family because of the distance from emergency services; experiencing frustration when friends, family, and even health care professionals condemn choices or decisions made; asking "Why?" and trying to accept the injustice of suffering. Of course, many other personal struggles exist for each member of the family.

Knafl and Deatrick (1986) reviewed several studies that describe how parents of chronically ill children normalize—behaviors that can be applied to other family-illness contexts as well. Behaviors that families use so they are perceived as normal by others include engaging in activities that a normal family would, limiting contacts with persons who are similarly disabled or ill, making the ill member appear normal, avoiding embarrassing situations, and controlling the amount of illness information shared with others.

Any illness affecting a patient will inherently affect the patient's family and their quality of life. Factors that affect family quality of life include family structure and interaction patterns; the availability of social networks or support resources; the potential for adaptation; family philosophy such as beliefs, attitudes, values, and perceived stressors; and impact of illness (Jassak & Knafl, 1990).

Cultural Perspectives Perceived quality of life is greatly influenced by individuals' ideas of what constitutes well-being, which, in turn, are shaped by cultural interpretations of health and illness. Thus, perceptions of quality of life vary greatly across cultures (Marshall, 1990). Although measuring this variable by survey instru-

ments is very difficult, interview data that focus on understanding the meaning of symptoms, patterns and interactions in a cultural group can describe perceived quality of life with at least some degree of validity, and contribute significantly to the planning of nursing interventions. The difficulties inherent in measuring quality of life cross-culturally support the need for more studies from different cultural perspectives. A few of the studies contained in the literature are noted here.

In one study, the meaning of comfort in immigrant Hispanic patients with cancer was explored. The two characteristics of comfort described most frequently were (1) feeling integrated, and (2) being nurtured. Feeling integrated was interpreted as a complex sense of inner peace and wholeness beyond the physical dimension. Being nurtured referred to care provided with patience and reciprocity by family or caregivers. Quality of life, one of six categories of comfort needs identified as important, was described as having things meaningful to them. *Amino,* another category of identified need, was described as having a positive mental disposition, drive, or energy to face what one is going through. While the term is specific to Spanish-speaking clients, those who reported this need indicated that it is fundamental to being human (Arruda, Larson, & Meleis, 1992).

The relationship between ethnicity, chronic pain, and satisfaction with active life roles was investigated in a sample of Mediterranean (Italian and Portuguese) and Canadian Anglo-Saxon patients (Baptiste, 1988). The Mediterranean group indicated more observable, overt emotional reactions during the interviews and scored higher on satisfaction with life, particularly satisfaction with the spiritual self.

In another study examining differences in how mental illness is viewed by mental health professionals and minority groups, the professionals were more likely to interpret problem behaviors as mental illness and recommend illness-related management, whereas the minority groups viewed the behaviors (and appropriate management) from a broader perspective that encompassed spiritual, moral, somatic, psychological, and metaphysical components (Flaskerus, 1984).

The impact of antihypertensive medications on quality of life was investigated in a sample of black, low-income, elderly women. No significance was found in the quality-of-life indicators examined (depression, general health) according to type of medication. Instead, symptoms that were reported correlated with the effectiveness of blood pressure control. It is possible that the tools used to measure quality of life were inappropriate for this group or that the patients were giving socially desirable answers (Glik et al., 1990).

Spirituality Issues

Spirituality has been defined as the "life principle that pervades a person's entire being and that integrates and transcends one's biologic and psychosocial nature" (Kim, McFarland, & McFarlane, 1984). Reed (1992) expanded this definition of spirituality by stating that it involves transcendence: intra-, inter-, and transpersonal connectedness. Spirituality is clearly a core dimension and critical determinant of health-related quality of life. Indeed, it has been referred to as the "will to wellness" (Kloss, 1988).

Definitions of spirituality distinguish it from religiosity (Emblen, 1992). While *spirituality* is an innate, universal, human phenomenon, *religiosity* usually refers to a system or codification of beliefs and behaviors that reflect one's spirituality. Although many definitions of religion and spirituality include reference to "God," they also often recognize that God is defined differently by each person.

When spirituality is discussed in the nursing literature, it is typically described in terms of needs or distress. Indeed, "spiritual distress" is an accepted nursing diagnosis (NANDA, 1994). However, spiritual distress, or need, can be related to a multitude of factors. For example, one researcher placed spiritual needs in one of four categories: the need for hope and creativity, the need for meaning and purpose, the need to give love, and the need to receive love (Highfield & Cason, 1983).

Meaning of Chronic Illness As discussed earlier, before interventions that promote well-being can be developed, there must be an assessment of the meaning of the chronic illness from the care recipient's viewpoint. Indeed, when care recipients provide answers to questions of meaning, they are offering the hearer a glimpse through a window to their "soul," the label often assigned to the seat of one's spirituality.

Foley (1988) reviewed the various meanings found in our society for suffering and categorized them into 11 "interpretations of suffering." Foley's categories are punishment (such as for sins); testing (such as loyalty to God); bad luck (negative odds); submission to the laws of nature (nature taking her course); resignation to the will of God (accepting what happened without knowing why); acceptance of the human condition (including suffering and pain); personal growth (becoming a better person as a result of the suffering); defensiveness and denial (not thinking about it); minimalization (downplaying the severity or significance of suffering); divine perspective (transcending personal perspective); and redemption (finding joy in suffering).

Not only is it apparent that spiritual status influences quality of life, but it has received empirical support as well. For instance, Granstrom (1987) found that spiritual well-being was inversely correlated with both frequency and amount of pain among 210 cancer patients. Miller

(1992) observed that loneliness and spiritual well-being were negatively correlated among a sample of chronically ill patients. Similarly, Taylor (1993) observed that as cancer recurred, patients' sense of purpose decreased over time, adversely affecting their psychosocial adjustment to illness. Thus, nursing care for the chronically ill that promotes quality of life must include attention to the spiritual components of individuals.

Economic Issues

Although the economic impact of chronic illness on patients and their families has received scant attention in nursing literature, chronic illness often has a significant effect on care recipients' finances and economic resources. Typically, this effect is negative; that is, the illness causes a financial burden and drains the individual's or family's financial resources (see Chapter 22, on financial impact).

The reasons for financial strain and its effects vary. Frequently, a chronic illness requires individuals to decrease, suspend, or end their work, leading to a reduction or loss of income. Furthermore, if the client requires much assistance or supervision, the primary family caregiver also may have to terminate employment. Thus, a family with one chronically ill member may sustain the financial burden resulting from two members' unemployment.

Persons living with chronic illness also suffer financially due to the additional expenses that are incurred, such as increased medical insurance rates or out-of-pocket expenses for items not covered by insurance, assuming there is insurance. For example, the cost of transportation to medical or treatment appointments or the extra cost incurred for special diet foods can add up. The desperately ill person who has found little benefit from traditional therapies may spend large amounts of money on folk or alternative forms of treatment in an effort toward improvement (Cassileth et al., 1991).

The combined effect of decreased income and increased expenses on quality of life may not appear obvious, but nurses must be aware of how this financial burden may contribute to decreased quality of life (Arzouman et al., 1991). For example, clients may take fewer medications because they cannot afford to take the prescribed amount. Or the family caregiver may be overtaxed by the burden of care-giving because the family cannot afford assistance (see Chapter 12, on family caregivers). If care recipients are economically stressed, nurses can play a pivotal role in linking them to community resources that provide services (Tehan, 1991).

Ethical Issues

There are three principal ethical issues that apply to health-related quality of life. These are the conflict between sanctity of life and quality of life; the contention between individual good and aggregate good; and the struggle between respect for autonomy and beneficence, when expressed as paternalism (Dean, 1990).

The sanctity of life ethic prompts people to want to preserve life at any expense. Indeed, high technology makes this an option and a reality. However, it is this extension of life in the presence of deteriorating chronic illness that typically threatens the quality of a person's life. For example, persons with endstage renal disease may live longer when they receive dialysis three times every week, yet may perceive that the limitations imposed by the chronic illness make life unsatisfactory (Motes, 1989).

Contentions between individual good and aggregate good exist when what is good for a family or society is bad for an individual patient or, vice versa, when what is best for an individual may cause adversity for a larger group of individuals. For example, there are circumstances when terminally ill patients receive medical interventions that prolong life, but at the expense of others. These "expenses" might be direct, such as finances, time, and energy spent, or indirect, such as life-saving technologies that deplete funds and personal or societal resources that could be allocated for things like education directed at maintaining health.

Likewise, the struggle between respect for autonomy and beneficence occurs when health professionals make decisions for patients that are "in their best interest" rather than respect care recipients' rights to self-determination. These ethical issues are summarized in the questions Dean (1990) asks:

Whose quality of life is at issue? Who defines the quality of life? What happens when the patient's view of quality of life differs from that of the family, the health care professional, the policy-makers? Who measures quality of life? And, for what purpose is quality of life to be used? Will quality of life be used as a means to justify limiting treatment options for individuals? Will quality of life be used as a means for forcing treatment on someone who refuses?

Interventions for Improving Quality of Life

The above discussion of physical, psychological, social, spiritual, and economic dimensions that influence health-related quality of life implies that there are interventions that can promote improved quality of life. However, a complete discussion of all possible interventions is beyond the scope of this chapter, although a cursory overview of many of them is in order.

Goal Setting

The ultimate goal of any health professional committed to improving quality of life is to promote physical, psychological, sociocultural, and spiritual well-being satisfactory to the client or care recipient. Yet it is the care recipient, not the professional, who determines what is satisfactory and who knows whether these proposed goals are appropriate, desirable, or valued. Thus, it is essential when goals for quality of life are established that they be determined with clients and their families.

There needs to be a balance between clients having complete control over decisions about their health and the paternalistic approach used by some health care providers (Gadow, 1990). What is required is assistance for care recipients to "authentically exercise their freedom of self-determination." However, clients exhibit a variety of preferences about their involvement in decision making that range from complete relinquishment of control to physicians or others, to various joint or collaborative decision-making

approaches, to maintaining complete control (Degner & Russell, 1988).

Goals should be set collaboratively with care recipients (Steckel, 1982). These goals can be subdivided into manageable increments that the care recipient perceives as achievable. Rewards for each goal or subgoal can be determined at a planning session; whenever a care recipient fulfills a subgoal, a reward can be enjoyed. In this way, motivation to pursue the next subgoal is created. These goals, and the steps for achieving them, should be documented and appreciated as a contract.

Physical Interventions

The importance of assessing and treating functional ability and symptom distress is indisputable. Part of assessment is identifying the meaning and the degree of distress involved.

Cella (1991) proposed a four-step hierarchical framework for interventions that improve quality of life. First, the disease needs to be treated and the underlying cause addressed. If cure is possible, health professionals and patients alike will usually be willing to suffer any negative side effects of treatment. Second, symptoms of the illness and side effects of treatment must be dealt with. If the chronic disease is not treatable, then palliation should be undertaken. Third, communication needs to be enhanced between care recipients and providers of health care. Although open communication is always necessary for quality health care, it becomes more critical at times when both curative and palliative care treatments appear ineffective. The fourth step involves the reframing of attitudes toward suffering. "Helping patients and loved ones to reframe their thinking and adjust their expectations can convert an untreatable disease into a treatable person" (Cella, 1991).

Cella's (1991) framework suggests how practitioners should prioritize their care for the chronically ill. That is, by addressing patients' curable pathologies or incurable symptoms and by fostering open communication and cognitive adaptation to a chronic illness, practitioners are promoting quality of life. However, although addressing disease and its symptoms is the first priority of care, open communication and cognitive adaptation are to be equally valued.

Enhancing Functional Status A nursing intervention based on Orem's self-care framework was applied to the functional status of hospitalized elderly medical patients (Wanich et al., 1992). The intervention included (1) orientation to time and place; (2) mobilization; (3) modification of the environment to maintain sensory input; (4) frequent family contact; (5) monitoring of medications for central nervous system side effects; and (6) regular discharge planning by a team composed of the primary nurse, a social worker, a discharge planning nurse, physical and occupational therapists, and a nutritionist. Patients receiving the intervention showed significant improvement in functional status at discharge compared with their status on admission and compared with patients who did not receive the intervention. The investigators concluded that activities aimed at maintaining normalcy through mobilization, social interaction, and prevention of hazards were successful in improving functional status, ultimately contributing to quality of life.

Symptom Control Effective and appropriate symptom control requires that both care recipients' and caregivers' interpretations of symptoms be considered. When decisions are made about the management of symptoms, the care recipients' values and beliefs should be assessed, as well as the values and beliefs of the caregiver (Ferrell et al., 1993; Cella, 1991).

Psychological Interventions

Having a sense of control, self-esteem, and meaning are necessary for psychological adaptation to illness and maintaining quality of life. Again, it is important to assess the presence and efficacy of patients' cognitive strategies so that they can then be facilitated. For example, encouraging patients to participate in decision making about their health care can promote a sense of control. Offering honest compliments to patients for their use of adaptive coping strategies can enhance their self-esteem and reinforce adaptive behavior.

Other recommendations for improving psychological quality of life were made by Belcher (1990) and apply to any chronic illness circumstance. These practical recommendations include staying with the client or caregivers during difficult times, answering questions openly and willingly, providing opportunities for care recipients to talk about their desires and fears, allowing care recipients to do as much as possible or desired, and teaching family caregivers how to keep clients comfortable.

Many of these strategies for promoting psychological quality of life are illustrated in the case study of Jill, the diabetic adolescent mentioned earlier. Jill's story also demonstrates how a chronic illness can stress a family and put a strain on social relations even outside the family. Jill's family make a concerted effort to understand their responses to her illness (e.g., mother spends time alone with each member). They also make sure life is still filled with pleasurable experiences (e.g., music, frozen yogurt).

Social Support

Nurses can do much to facilitate social support, which is critical to quality of life for chronically ill persons. Support groups can be suggested that would be appropriate for patients and their family caregivers among the numerous community and nationally and internationally based groups that exist. For example, there are groups for persons with a variety of chronic illness conditions such as chronic fatigue syndrome, breast cancer, ostomies, alcoholism, and so forth. Suggestions can also be made on how to maintain social relations amidst chronic illness, such as how to conserve strength for socializing or how to decrease others' anxieties about the illness (Wortman & Dunkel-Schetter, 1979).

When chronic illness affects an individual, it also affects that individual's family system. Thus, the family must be assessed, be it a nuclear family, a homosexual couple, or any other configuration. Once assessment is done, the family needs to learn how to evaluate the impact of the chronic illness on their system. Family members need to increase their awareness of altered or dysfunctional family dynamics. Families also benefit from

---

CASE STUDY

Living with Diabetes, Part II: The Story of Jill

Jill's family uses a variety of strategies to promote quality in their lives. For example, Jill's mother takes Jill on weekly walks to the corner store to buy sugar-free frozen yogurt and talk about things of interest to them. Her parents go on weekly dates "to the cheapest place we can find" in order to nurture their marriage. They were alarmed when they learned that 90 percent of parents with chronically ill children get divorced. They also undergo counseling and belong to a support group.

Pursuing a life with quality forces Jill and her family to take risks. For example, even though sending Jill to a camp for diabetic children has the potential of her being more sick than before she goes, her parents think the psychosocial bene-fits outweigh any possible physical cost. Similarly, they believe that Jill's joy from learning to play a double bass outweighs the risk of finger infections and calouses.

Jill's mother also described how nurses have contributed to Jill's and the family's quality of life. "What really makes a difference is when a nurse always listens and is noncondemning," she stated. "It is reassuring when a nurse lets you know that you can call her anytime and even gives out her home phone number. And it is important when they return your phone calls, or even call spontaneously to just check up on Jill. And now that Jill is getting older, I think it is nice when doctors and nurses talk to *her*."

---

learning how to develop open, healing communication between family members (Craig, 1983). Nurses should refer families with complex problems to other professionals, such as marriage and family counselors, when that is appropriate.

Spiritual Interventions

Numerous interventions promote spiritual well-being, including referral to a chaplain or clergy; facilitating religious rituals, prayer, meditation, and relaxation; providing spiritual music or art work; active listening; dialogue about spiritual matters; recommending spiritual reading material; and being therapeutically present—that is, trusting, loving, vulnerable, empathic, and humble (Taylor et al., 1995; Millison & Dudley, 1992; Carson, 1989). Because of the significant impact of meaning on quality of life, discussion of spiritual care interventions will be limited to those related to the promotion of meaning and purpose.

Health professionals can promote a healthy sense of meaning by facilitating experiences that are known to create a sense of meaning. There are three ways in which people can find meaning: (1) by giving of themselves; (2) by undertaking creative, aesthetic, meaningful experiences for themselves, such as watching a sunset or listening to beautiful music; and (3) by choosing a redeeming attitude in the face of suffering (Frankl, 1984).

The health provider can encourage a variety of "secular activities" that provide a sense of meaning. *Altruism* allows one to leave the world a better place, while *dedication to a cause* involves commitment to a political, religious, or social crusade. *Creativity* leads to generating something new, artistic, or scientific, and *hedonism* allows appreciation of life to the fullest. *Self-actualization* encourages one to develop the self's fullest potential, and *self-transcendence* allows the individual to place his or her focus away from the self (Yalom, 1980).

There are a number of activities that create meaning for chronically ill patients that should be encouraged by health providers. These include producing written or oral histories that could also be a legacy, continuing with old hobbies or pursuing new ones, and helping others. Particularly for persons who feel they are a burden to others, helping others may decrease the imbalance between giving and receiving love. Even homebound individuals can write cards to persons needing care or make telephone calls to raise funds for a charity (Taylor, 1993).

Economic Interventions

Although nurses are not trained financial planners, they can introduce care recipients to available resources. These resources may be free or discounted services from a charity organization, hospital, or business corporation. Nurses also can teach time and energy conservation and decision-making skills, both areas that influence economic well-being.

Research and Education

As discussed above, health-related quality of life for the chronically ill continues to need a clear definition. Subjective aspects as well as objective considerations are necessary parts of defining the meaning of quality of life. Many areas exist that would benefit from further study, including evaluating the impact of age on health-related quality of life among those who are chronically ill; identifying key variables that influence the quality of life for these individuals; and determining specific interventions that can improve their quality of life (see Chapter 17, on research). Clarifying these areas will better equip health care professionals to assist chronically ill individuals in maintaining an improved quality of life. Additionally, other research areas to be addressed are methodological and cultural issues (Dimond & Jones, 1983; Gilmer et al., 1993; Souder, 1992; West et al., 1991).

Education needs to focus on teaching students how to promote the client's quality of life as well as to appreciate the care recipient's perspective. It becomes important that students grow to understand the meanings and values of their own lives and how these values impact on the care they give. In addition, exposing students to how chronically ill individuals cope with their disease process enables students, as caregivers, to help these individuals cope more effectively. Because of the many components that influence chronically ill individuals, increased awareness of these factors allows the nurse to more effectively intervene (Anderson & Bauwens, 1981; Dimond & Jones, 1983; Forsyth, Delaney, & Greshan 1984; Pender & Pender, 1986).

Summary and Conclusions

This chapter has pointed out the multidimensionality and subjectivity of quality of life as it applies to the chronically ill individual. Various frameworks, both sociological and nursing, that allow health care workers to focus on quality of life issues were briefly discussed. Factors influencing the quality of life for the chronically ill were identified, and specific issues related to these factors were examined. A number of interventions that promote health-related quality of life for the chronically ill were introduced.

Of continuing concern, while not addressed in this chapter, is the effect of health policy on quality of life for the chronically ill. With the current changes in health care, a vital question becomes: How will the chronically ill maintain quality of life? As technology increases the length of life, quality-of-life issues will expand. Thus, the health professional faces a challenge in seeking to promote care that continues to place emphasis on an individual's quality of life.

NURSING DIAGNOSIS

Editor's Note: There are three nursing diagnoses that must be considered when dealing with a client's quality of life: spiritual distress, decisional conflict, and powerlessness. In addition, there are several others that should be considered, and they are therefore noted here.

4.1.1. Spiritual Distress (distress of the human spirit)

Definition: Disruption in the life principle that pervades a person's entire being and that integrates and transcends one's biological and psychosocial nature.

Defining Characteristics: Expresses concern with meaning of life/death and/or belief systems; anger toward God; questions meaning of suffering; verbalizes inner conflict about beliefs; verbalizes concern about relationship with deity; questions meaning of own existence; unable to participate in usual religious practices; seeks spiritual assistance; questions moral/ethical implications of therapeutic regimen; gallows humor; displacement of anger toward religious representatives; description of nightmares/sleep disturbances; alteration in behavior/mood evidenced by anger, crying, withdrawal, preoccupation, anxiety, hostility, apathy, and so forth.

Related Factors: Separation from religious/cultural ties; challenged belief and value system, e.g., due to moral/ethical implications of therapy, due to intense suffering.

5.3.1.1. Decisional Conflict (specify)

Definition: The state of uncertainty about course of action to be taken when choice among competing actions involves risk, loss, or challenge to personal life values.

Defining Characteristics:

Major: Verbalized uncertainty about choices; verbalization of undesired consequences of alternative actions being considered; vacillation between alternative choices; delayed decision making.

Minor: Verbalized feeling of distress while attempting a decision; self-focusing; physical signs of distress or tension (increased heart rate, increased muscle tension, restlessness, etc.); questioning personal values and beliefs while attempting a decision.

Related Factors: Unclear personal values/beliefs; perceived threat to value system; lack of experience or interference with decision making; lack of relevant information; support system deficit; multiple or divergent sources of information.

7.3.2. Powerlessness

Definition: Perception that one's own actions will not significantly affect an outcome; a perceived lack of control over a current situation or immediate happening.

Defining Characteristics:

Severe: Verbal expression of having no control or influence over situation; verbal expression of having no control or influence over outcome; verbal expression of having no control over self-care; depression over physical deterioration that occurs despite patient compliance with regimens; apathy.

Moderate: Nonparticipation in care or decision-making when opportunities are provided; expression of dissatisfaction and frustration over inability to perform previous tasks and/or activities; does not monitor progress; expression of doubt regarding role performance; reluctance to express true feelings; fearing alienation from caregivers; passivity; inability to seek information regarding care; dependence on others that may result in irritability, resentment, anger, and guilt; does not defend self-care practices when challenged.

Low: Expressions of uncertainty about fluctuating energy levels; passivity.

Related Factors: Health care environment; interpersonal interactions; illness-related regimen; life-style of helplessness.

3.1.1. Impaired Social Interaction

See chapter 8, on social isolation for definition, defining characteristics, and related factors.

3.1.2. Social Isolation

See chapter 8, on social isolation for definition, defining characteristics, and related factors.

STUDY QUESTIONS

1. Using a broad definition, how does quality of life relate to the chronically ill individual?
2. Identify a framework that would be useful in dealing with some of the quality-of-life issues you can identify. Discuss how this framework would be useful.
3. Why is the term "health-related quality of life" preferred over just "quality of life"?
4. What significance does symptom control have in influencing quality of life for the chronically ill individual or the individual's family?
5. What interventions can health professionals employ to promote health-related quality of life? Discuss them.
6. Why is it essential to understand the care recipient's definitions of quality of life and meanings of illness?

References

Aaronson, N. K. (1986). Methodological issues in psychosocial oncology with special reference to clinical trials. In V. Ventafridda, F. S. A. M. van Dam, R. Yancik, & M. Tamburini (Eds.), *Assessment of quality of life and cancer treatment* (pp. 29-42). Amsterdam: Elsevier.

——— (1988). Quality of life: What is it? How should it be measured? *Oncology, 2*(5), 69-74.

Anderson, S. V., & Bauwens, E. E. (1981). *Chronic health problems: Concepts and application.* St. Louis: C. V. Mosby.

Arruda, E. N., Larson, P. J., & Meleis, A. I. (1992). Comfort: Immigrant Hispanic cancer patients' views. *Cancer Nursing, 15*(6), 387-394.

Arzouman, J. M. R., Dudas, S., Ferrans, C. E., & Holm, K. (1991). Quality of life of patients with sarcoma postchemotherapy. *Oncology Nursing Forum, 18,* 889-894.

Baptiste, S. (1988). Muriel Driver Memorial Lecture: Chronic pain, activity and culture. *Canadian Journal of Occupational Therapy, 55*(4), 179-184.

Barkwell, D. (1991). Ascribed meaning: A critical factor in coping and pain attenuation in patients with cancer-related pain. *Journal of Palliative Care, 7*(3), 5-14.

Belcher, A. E. (1990). Nursing aspects of quality of life enhancement in cancer patients. *Oncology, 4*(5), 197-199.

Benner, P., & Wrubel, J. (1989). *The primacy of caring.* Menlo Park, CA: Addison-Wesley.

Bowman, J. M. (1991). The meaning of chronic low back pain. *Journal of the American Association of Occupational Health Nurses, 39*(8), 381-384.

Bulman, R. J., & Wortman, C. B. (1977). Attributions of blame and coping in the "real world": Severe accident victims react to their lot. *Journal of Personality and Social Psychology, 35,* 351-363.

Calman, K. C. (1984). Quality of life in cancer patients—An hypothesis. *Journal of Medical Ethics, 10,* 124-127.

Carson, V. B. (1989). *Spiritual dimensions of nursing practice.* Philadelphia: W. B. Saunders.

Cassileth, B. R., Lusk, E. J., Guerry, D., Blake, A. D., Walsh, W. P., Kascius, L., & Schultz, D. J. (1991). Survival and quality of life among patients receiving unproven as compared with conventional cancer therapy. *New England Journal of Medicine, 314,* 1180-1185.

Cella, D. (1991). Functional status and quality of life: Current views on measurement and intervention. In *Functional status and quality of life in persons with cancer* (pp. 1-12). Atlanta: American Cancer Society.

Clark, P. G. (1988). Autonomy, personal empowerment and quality of life. *The Journal of Applied Gerontology, 7*(3), 279-297.

Corbin, J. M., & Strauss, A. (1988). *Unending work and care: Managing chronic illness at home.* San Francisco: Jossey-Bass.

Cowan, M. J., Graham, K. Y., & Cochrane, B. L. (1992). Comparison of a theory of quality of life between myocardial infarction and malignant melanoma. A pilot study. *Progress in Cardiovascular Nursing, 7*(1), 18-28.

Counte, M. A., Bieliauskas, L. A., & Pavlou, M. (1983). Stress and personal attitudes in chronic illness. *Archives of Physical Medicine and Rehabilitation, 64,* 272-275.

Craig, H. M. (1983). Adaptation in chronic illness: An eclectic model for nurses. *Journal of Advanced Nursing, 8,* 397-404.

Dean, H. E. (1990). Political and ethical implications of using quality of life as an outcome measure. *Seminars in Oncology Nursing, 6,* 303-308.

Degner, L. F., & Russell, C. A. (1988). Preferences for treatment control among adults with cancer. *Research in Nursing and Health, 11,* 367-374.

Dimond, J., & Jones, S. L. (1983). *Chronic Illness across the life span.* Norwalk, CT: Appleton-Century-Crofts.

Donovan, K., Sanson-Fisher, R. W., & Redman, S. (1989). Measuring quality of life in cancer patients. *Journal of Clinical Oncology, 7,* 959-968.

Emblen, J. D. (1992). Religion and spirituality defined according to current use in nursing literature. *Journal of Professional Nursing, 8*(1), 41-47.

Ferrans, C. (1985). *Psychometric assessment of a quality of life index for hemodialysis patients.* Dissertation, University of Illinois, Chicago.

Ferrell, B. R. (1991, September). Quality of life issues and the family. Lecture presented at conference "Maintaining Quality of Life for Home Care Patients," at California Polytechnic University, Pomona, CA. (Sponsored by United Way, Inc., and the City of Hope National Medical Center).

Ferrell, B. R., Ferrell, B. A., Rhiner, M., & Grant, M. (1991). Family factors influencing pain management. *Postgraduate Medical Journal, 67,* 564-569.

Ferrell, B., Grant, M., Rhiner, M., & Padilla, G. (1992). Home care: Maintaining quality of life for patient and family. *Oncology, 6*(2 Suppl), 136-140.

Ferrell, B. R., Taylor, E. J., Sattler, G. R., Fowler, M., & Cheyney, B. L. (1993). Searching for the meaning of pain: Cancer patients', caregivers', and nurses' perspectives. *Cancer Practice, 1*(3), 185-194.

Flaskerus, J. J. (1984). A comparison of perceptions of problematic behavior by six minority groups and mental health professionals. *Nursing Research, 33*(4), 190-197.

Foley, K. M. (1991). The relationship of pain and symptom management to patient requests for physician-assisted suicide. *Journal of Pain and Symptom Management, 6,* 289-297.

Foley, D. P. (1988). Eleven interpretations of personal suffering. *Journal of Religion and Health, 27,* 321-328.

Forsyth, G., Delaney, K., & Greshan, M. (1984). Vying for a winning position: Management style of the chronically ill. *Research in Nursing and Health, 7,* 181-188.

France, R. D. (1987). Chronic pain and depression. *Journal of Pain and Symptom Management, 2*(4), 234-236.

Frankl, V. (1984). *Man's search for meaning.* New York: Washington Square Press.

Gadow, S. (1990). Existential advocacy: Philosophical foundations of nursing. In T. Pence & J. Cantrall (Eds.), *Ethics in nursing: An anthology* (pp. 41-51) (Pub. no. 20-2294). New York: National League for Nursing.

Gilmer, J. S., et al. (1993). Instrument format issues in assessing the elderly: the Iowa self-assessment inventory. *Nursing Research. 42*(5), 297-299.

Given, C. W., Given, B., Stommel, M., Collins, C., King, S., & Franklin, S. (1992). The caregiver reaction assessment (CRA) for caregivers to persons with chronic physical and mental impairments. *Research in Nursing and Health, 15,* 271-283.

Glaser, B., & Strauss, A. (1978) *Chronic illness and the quality of life.* St. Louis: C. V. Mosby.

Glik, D. C., Steadman, S., Michels, P. L., & Malin R. (1990). Antihypertensive regimen and quality of life in a disadvantaged population. *The Journal of Family Practice, 30*(2), 143-152.

Granstrom, S. (1987). *A comparative study of loneliness, Buberian religiosity and spiritual well-being in cancer patients.* Doctoral dissertation, Rush University, Chicago.

Grant, M., Padilla, G. V., Ferrell, B. R., & Rhiner, M. (1990). Assessment of quality of life with a single instrument. *Seminars in Oncology Nursing, 6*(4), 260-270.

Highfield, M. F., & Cason, C. (1983). Spiritual needs of patients: Are they recognized? *Cancer Nursing, 6,* 187-192.

Jassak, P. F., & Knafl, K. A. (1990). Quality of family life: Exploration of a concept. *Seminars in Oncology Nursing, 6,* 298-302.

Jennings, B. M., & Muhlenkamp, A. F. (1981). Systematic misperception: Oncology patients' self-reported affective states and their caregivers' perceptions. *Cancer Nursing, 4,* 485-489.

Kim, M. J., McFarland, G. K., & McFarlane, A. M. (1984). *Classification of Nursing Diagnoses: Proceedings of the Fifth National Conference.* St. Louis: Mosby.

Kloss, W. E. (1988). Spirituality—The will to wellness. *The Harding Journal of Religion and Psychiatry, 7*(1), 3-8.

Knafl, K. A., & Deatrick, J. A. (1986). How families manage chronic conditions: An analysis of the concept of normalization. *Research in Nursing and Health, 9,* 215-222.

Lazarus, R. S., & Folkman, S. (1984). *Stress, appraisal, and coping.* New York: Springer.

Lewis, F. M. (1987). The concept of control: A typology and health-related variables. *Advances in Health Education and Promotion, 2,* 277-309.

Marshall, P. S. (1990). Cultural influences on perceived quality of life. *Seminars in Oncology Nursing, 6*(4), 278-284.

McCaffery, M., & Beebe, A. (1989). *Pain: Clinical manual for nursing practice*. St. Louis: C. V. Mosby.

McCorkle, R., & Quint-Benoliel, J. (1983). Symptom distress, current concerns and mood disturbance after diagnosis of life-threatening disease. *Social Science Medicine, 17,* 431-438.

Mead, G. H. (1934). *Mind, self, and society.* Chicago: The University of Chicago Press.

Miller, J. F. (1992). *Coping with chronic illness: Overcoming powerlessness* (2nd ed). Philadelphia: F. A. Davis.

Millison, M., & Dudley, J. R. (1992). Providing spiritual support: A job for all hospice professionals. *The Hospice Journal, 8*(4), 49-66.

Motes, C. E. (1989). Discontinuation of dialysis. *ANNA Journal, 16*(6), 413-415.

NANDA (1994). *Nursing Diagnoses: Definitions and classification.* Philadelphia: North American Nursing Diagnosis Association.

Nerenz, D. R., & Leventhal, H. (1983). Self-regulation theory in chronic illness. In T. C. Burish and L. A. Bradley (Eds.), *Coping with chronic disease: Research and applications* (pp. 13-37). New York: Academic Press.

O'Conner, A. P., Wicker, C. A., & Germino, B. B. (1990). Understanding the cancer patient's search for meaning. *Cancer Nursing, 13*(3), 167-175.

Orem, D. (1990). *Nursing: Concepts of practice.* St. Louis: Mosby.

Padilla, G. V., Ferrell, B., Grant, M. M., & Rhiner, M. (1990). Defining the content domain of quality of life for cancer patients with pain. *Cancer Nursing, 13*(2), 108-115.

Parse, R. (1981). *Man-living-health. A theory of nursing.* New York: John Wiley and Sons.

Pender N., & Pender, A. (1986). Attitudes, subjective norms, and intentions to engage in health behaviors. *Nursing Research, 35,* 15-18.

Pollock, S. E. (1986). Human responses to chronic illness: Physiologic and psychosocial adaptation. *Nursing Research, 35*(2), 90-95.

Primomo, J., Yates, B. C., & Woods, N. F. (1990). Social support for women during chronic illness: The relationship among sources and types to adjustment. *Research in Nursing and Health, 13*(3), 153-161.

Reed, P. G. (1992). An emerging paradigm for the investigation of spirituality in nursing. *Research in Nursing and Health, 15,* 349-357.

Rice, M. A., & Szopa, T. J. (1988). Group intervention for reinforcing self-worth following mastectomy. *Oncology Nursing Forum, 15,* 33-37.

Rock, D. L., Meyerowitz, B. E., Maisto, S. A., & Wallston, K. A. (1987). The derivation and validation of six multidimensional health locus of control scale clusters. *Research in Nursing and Health, 10,* 185-195.

Rothbaum, F., Weisz, J. R., and Snyder, S. S. (1982). Changing the world and changing the self: A two-process model of perceived control. *Journal of Personality and Social Psychology, 42,* 5.

Scrier, A. C., Dekker, F. W., & Kaptein, A. A. (1990). Quality of life in elderly patients with chronic non-specific lung disease seen in family practice. *Chest, 98,* 894-899.

Souder, J. E. (1992). The consumer approach to recruitment of elder subjects. *Nursing Research, 41*(5), 314-316.

Steckel, S. B. (1982). *Patient contracting.* Norwalk, CT: Appleton-Century-Crofts.

Strauss, A. (1975). *Chronic illness and the quality of life.* St. Louis: C. V. Mosby.

Taylor, E. J. (1993). Factors associated with sense of meaning among people with recurrent cancer. *Oncology Nursing Forum, 20,* 1399-1407.

Taylor, E. J., Amenta, M. O., & Highfield, M. F. (1995, January). Spiritual care practices of oncology nursing. *Oncology Nursing Forum.*

Taylor, S. (1983). Adjustment to life threatening events: A theory of cognitive adaptation. *American Psychologist, 38,* 1161-1173.

Taylor, S. E., & Brown, J. D. (1988). Illusion and well-being: A social psychological perspective on mental health. *Psychological Bulletin, 103*(2), 193-210.

Tehan, C. (1991). The cost of caring for patients with HIV infection in hospice. *Hospice Journal, 7,* 41-59.

Thompson, S. (1991). The search for meaning following a stroke. *Basic and Applied Social Psychology, 12*(1), 81-96.

Thompson, S. C., & Janigian, A. S. (1988). Life schemes: A framework for understanding the search for meaning. *Journal of Social and Clinical Psychology, 7,* 260-280.

Wanich, C. K., Sullivan-Marx, E. M., Gottlieb, G. L., & Johnson, J. C. (1992). Functional status outcomes of a nursing intervention in hospitalized elderly. *Image: The Journal of Nursing Scholarship, 24*(3), 201-207.

Watson, J. (1985). *Nursing: Human science and human care. A theory of nursing.* Norwalk, CT: Appleton-Century-Crofts.

Weiner, B. (1986). *An attributional theory of motivation and emotion.* New York: Springer-Verlag.

Weisman, A. D., & Worden, J. W. (1976). The existential plight in cancer: Significance of the first 100 days. *International Journal of Psychiatry in Medicine, 7*(1), 1-15.

West, M., Bondy, E., Hutchinson, S. (1991). Interviewing institutionalized elders: Threats to validity. *Image: The Journal of Nursing Scholarship, 23*(3), 171-176.

Wills, T. A. (1981). Downward comparison principles in social psychology. *Psychological Bulletin, 90*(2), 245-271.

Wortman, C. B. (1984, May 15). Social support and the cancer patient: Conceptual and methodological issues. *Cancer* (Suppl), pp. 2339-2362.

Wortman, C. B., & Dunkel-Schetter, C. (1979). Interpersonal relationships and cancer: A theoretical analysis. *Journal of Social Issues, 35*(1), 120-155.

Wortman, C. B., & Silver, R. C. (1992). Reconsidering assumptions about coping with loss: An overview of current research. In L. Montada et al. (Eds.), *Life crises and experiences of loss in adulthood* (p. 341). Hillsdale, NJ: Lawrence Erlbaum Associates.

Yalom, I. D. (1980). *Existential psychotherapy.* New York: Basic Books.

Bibliography

Derogatis, L. R., & Lopez, M. C. (1983). *PAIS & PAIS-SR administration, scoring, & procedures manual.* Baltimore: Johns Hopkins University Schoool of Medicine.

Ferrell, B. R., Eberts, M. T., McCaffery, M., et al. (1991). Clinical decision making and pain. *Cancer Nursing, 14,* 289-297.

Karnofsky, D. A., & Buchenal, J. H. (1949). The clinical evaluation of chemotherapeutic agents in cancer. In C. M. Mackad (Ed.), *Evaluation of chemotherapeutic agents* (pp. 191-205). New York: Columbia University Press.

Miller, J. F. (1989). Hope-inspiring strategies of the critically ill. *Applied Nursing Research, 2*(1), 23-29.

Moos, R. H. (1977). *Coping with physical illness.* New York: Plenum Medical Book Company.

Pruyser, P. (1976). *The minister as diagnostician: Personal problems in pastoral perspective.* Philadelphia: Westminster Press.

Romano, J. M., & Turner, J. A. (1985). Chronic pain and depression: Does the evidence support a relationship? *Psychological Bulletin, 18-34.*

Thompson, S. C. (1985). Finding positive meaning in a stressful event. *Basic and Applied Social Psychology, 6,* 279-295.

Thornburg, K. (1982). Coping: Implications for health practitioners. *Patient Counseling and Health Education, 4,* 3-9.

Whedon, M. B. (1992). Physical well-being. *Quality of life: A Nursing Challenge, 1*(1), iii-iv (L. L. Powel, Ed.). Philadelphia: Meniscus Health Care Communications.

CHAPTER 10

Compliance

Dorothy Blevins • Ilene Lubkin

Introduction

Tradition and scientific knowledge support the belief that a client's well-being increases when health care behavior is in accord with health providers' recommendations. Such compliance is often a stated goal of client–provider interactions, whether health care delivery is preventive, curative, or restorative. This traditional perspective places the major responsibility for enhancing compliance on the provider and overlooks mutuality.

The lack of agreement between health care recommendations and client behavior has received extensive study. Several theories and models have been developed to guide further research. Health care providers can apply these theories, models, and research findings as they work with clients who have chronic illnesses, even though the current state of knowledge has not resolved the many issues and problems influencing compliance.

Compliance and Chronic Illness

The predominant pattern of illness has changed from acute illness to chronic illness as science and technology have advanced. Treatment regimens have become more complex and, at the same time, have frequently required unsuper-

vised implementation by the client or family caregivers in the home.

Client responsibility for managing chronic conditions has grown. For example, an individual having insulin-dependent diabetes mellitus (IDDM) may have a computerized insulin pump and a computerized or manual blood testing device, and may, at some point, be a candidate for hemodialysis or renal transplant. All these modalities of treatment require compliant behaviors to effect therapeutic outcomes that ensure maximal benefit and minimal harm to the client.

Attention has focused not only on the study of compliance but on the development of strategies to increase desired behaviors. The evaluation of new technological and therapeutic measures for chronic diseases must take into account compliance when determining efficiency of these measures in achieving therapeutic outcomes. Practitioners must also be concerned with the extent to which clients comply when designing plans of treatment or evaluating client responses to treatment measures.

Definition of Terms

Compliance is an umbrella term for all behavior consistent with health care recommendations. It is "the extent to which a person's behavior coincides with medical or health advice" (Haynes, 1979). *Noncompliance* denotes behaviors that are not consistent with such rec-ommendations. These two terms are used with an acknowledgment of concerns expressed about their appropriateness for describing client responses. These concerns focus on the notion that compliance implies that the client is passive and lacks autonomy and that the health professional is coercive and paternalistic. This chapter attaches no such meaning to these words. We agree with Connelly (1984), who laments that concerns about these words are unfortunate, since they arise from inaccurate and unfavorable connotations associated with the concept of compliance, whereas ethical issues really center on the ethics of strategies to promote effective self-care.

Adherence and *nonadherence* are generally used as synonyms for compliance and noncompliance. One notable exception in the meaning of these words is presented by Barofsky (1978), who proposed a continuum of self-care with three levels of client response to health care recommendations: compliance, adherence, and therapeutic alliance. In this model, compliance is linked to coercion; adherence, to conformity; and self-care, to a therapeutic alliance with provider–client interactions.

Components of Compliance

The relevance of compliance to the total well-ness–illness continuum was described by Marston in 1970, who considered compliance as self-care behaviors that individuals undertake to promote health, to prevent illness, or to follow recommendations for treatment and rehabilitation in diagnosed illnesses. When compliance is viewed as self-care, the agent of compliance is the client.

However, it may be more helpful to consider compliance as more than self-care behaviors—as behavior that is often shared, since clients cannot always implement their medical regimens without the participation of family members. The delineation of responsibilities is not always clear when there is a change in the dependence/independence status of the client, as with the teenager who assumes greater responsibility for management of his or her health care regimen

or the older client who now requires more supervision by family members.

Strauss and associates (1984) noted that family members often take on assisting or controlling roles in influencing clients to adhere to medical regimens. Further study of how couples managed chronic disease revealed that coordination and collaboration between the couple was necessary to carry out the work of the medical regimen (Corbin & Strauss, 1984). Given this shared responsibility, it seems reasonable to conclude that compliance-increasing strategies should be directed toward all individuals who are involved in implementing medical regimens.

The *act* of compliance may be analyzed by examining the frequency, occurrence, and variation of behaviors undertaken in response to health care recommendations. Compliance behaviors are often categorized by type: general (commission, omission, or modification) and specific (keeping appointments, taking medications, abstaining from alcohol). Several role conceptions reflect differences in clients' perceptions of their health status and the purposes for which health-related behavior is undertaken. Dimond and Jones (1983) summarize these role behaviors as follows:

- *Health behavior:* Any activity undertaken by a person believing himself to be healthy for the purpose of preventing disease or detecting it in an asymptomatic state (Kasl & Cobb, 1966).
- *Illness behavior:* Any activity undertaken by a person who feels ill to define the state of health and to discover a suitable remedy (Kasl, 1974; Baric, 1969).
- *Sick role behavior:* Any activity undertaken by a person who is considered ill by self and others for the purpose of getting well (Kasl, 1974; Baric, 1969).

These role conceptions are inadequate when the agent of compliance is managing chronic rather than acute illness (Baric, 1969). With chronic illness, even though the illness continues, there may be no subjective feelings of being ill during asymptomatic periods. In addition, the chronically ill client no longer expects a cure or a return to prior health. Parsons's original presentation of the sick role (1951) related only to illnesses that lasted for relatively short periods, identified that the client was granted privileges and exemptions from responsibilities and duties during those periods, and noted that the health care practitioner was directed to take responsibility for cure-focused care (see Chapter 4, on illness roles).

Prevalence of Noncompliance

Several reviewers of the vast compliance literature concur that, on the average, one-third to one-half of clients in study populations are noncompliant with health care recommendations in some way (Marston, 1970; Sackett & Snow, 1979; Gillam & Barsky, 1974). Marston noted the wide variation in published rates of compliance, ranging from 4 to 100 percent. She also emphasized the difficulties intrinsic to comparing compliance and noncompliance rates because of the variations in conceptual and methodological designs. For example, Marston cites two studies, both using urine tests to detect the presence of antituberculin medications, that show disparity in criteria used to distinguish compliance from noncompliance. In one study (Morrow & Rabin, 1966), those characterized as noncompliant had 50 percent or higher negative urine test results; the other study (Nymm-Williams & Arris, 1958) characterized individuals as noncompliant if they had one negative test result. It becomes readily apparent that a "compliant" subject in the former study might exhibit more noncompliant behavior than a "compliant" subject would in the latter study.

Compliance studies are typically disease-specific; that is, the study population is defined by the presence of a specific disease. These studies show the high rates of noncompliance noted throughout the literature. For example, in their review of compliance studies related to diabetes mellitus, Becker and Janz (1985) describe alarming rates of noncompliance in this client population:

- Dietary noncompliance was reported at 73 percent (Korhonen et al., 1983), 65 percent

(Christensen et al., 1983), and 35 percent (Cerkoney & Hart, 1980).
- Noncompliance rates for testing urine in an acceptable manner were reported as 67 percent (Watkins et al., 1967), 70 percent (Korhonen et al., 1983), and 43 percent (Cerkoney & Hart, 1980).

The reviewers also noted that although Cerkoney and Hart reported comparatively low noncompliance rates for specific types of compliance behavior, only 4 percent of the study population were found to comply with all components of the diabetic treatment regimen.

Although ascertaining the true picture of noncompliance in chronic illness is very difficult, one is impressed by the consistency with which high noncompliance rates are reported and must conclude that noncompliance is a major problem in the delivery of health care.

Problems and Issues

For more than 30 years, numerous studies have demonstrated that large numbers of people having acute and chronic illnesses do not follow health care recommendations thoroughly, indicating that noncompliance is an endemic phenomenon. Although noncompliance is increasingly recognized as a problem in health care delivery, there is less consensus about appropriate or effective methods to decrease it. Some of the difficulty lies in the inadequacies of research on compliance, some lies in differing role expectations of clients and providers, some relates to motivation, and some relates to conflict in values. These difficulties often underlie questions and concerns about compliance-increasing strategies. As health care providers prescribe, teach, and counsel clients about medical regimens, they must be cautious in making assumptions about compliance or noncompliance in a given situation before imposing any one strategy on the client. Understanding phenomena that adversely affect compliance is a preliminary to efforts to achieve more positive outcomes.

Barriers to the Study of Compliance

Although a comprehensive discussion of research and compliance is not appropriate to this chapter, some of the barriers that plague investigators and limit the confidence with which researchers or practitioners can use reported findings of specific studies can be indicated. As we shall see, the methodological and conceptual problems in the study of compliance, and the lack of consistent results, lead one to the conclusion that there is no well-founded knowledge base for selecting and using compliance-increasing strategies.

Methodological Barriers Numerous methodological problems characterize compliance research (Gordis, 1979; Haynes, 1979). Sackett and Snow (1979) highlight the inadequacies of research design in their review of 537 original articles on compliance, which revealed only 40 studies meeting the methodological standards established for the review. They noted deficiencies in study design, specification of the illness or condition, compliance measurement, description of the therapeutic regimen, and definition of compliance. On the basis of these findings, Haynes (1979) proposed four specific suggestions for priorities in future research on compliance:

1. Studies should use inception cohorts rather than cross-sectional samples. These samples would follow all clients who were started on a therapeutic regimen, and the study would encompass the least compliant individuals who "drop out."
2. Complete compliance distributions of all study patients would be published to reveal determinants of variance in distributions.
3. Description of the relationship between compliance levels and the achievement of treatment goals should be included.
4. The study design should be precisely described.

Sampling errors can cause a distorted description of the extent and nature of noncompliance. For example, studies of compliance with antihypertensive medications that use a cross-sectional sample generate a population of the most compliant individuals (Sackett & Snow, 1979). In contrast, a longitudinal study using an inception cohort as the study population would follow all clients who were prescribed medication and thus present a more representative sample. The advantage of inception cohorts is apparent when one considers that many clients who have hypertension never begin treatment and others discontinue treatment within the first year (Steckel & Swain, 1981).

Research designs in compliance studies that focus on specific diseases or treatment modalities, such as those on hypertension mentioned previously, allow researchers to consider the special characteristics of the disease and its treatment. Although such designs avoid the potential of some confounding variables, they limit applicability of results to the general population of persons having chronic illnesses or to the many clients who have multiple diseases and receive many treatment measures (Hulka et al., 1976; Kasl, 1978).

Measurement is another area presenting inherent methodological problems. Measurements may be either direct or indirect; direct measures of health-related behavior are more costly and difficult to implement, but yield more reliable data. For example, urine or blood samples are direct measures used to evaluate medication taking, while indirect measures used for the same purpose include client reports, prescription-filling, pill counts, and interviews of client and physician. It is generally believed that the more frequently used indirect measures yield compliance rates that exceed the actual level of compliance (Marston, 1970; Hulka et al., 1976).

Although direct measures are considered more reliable, differences in time spans of chronic illness make drawing accurate conclusions difficult when such measures are used. For example, testing a single sample of blood or urine for drug presence reveals only whether medication was taken during the preceding hours or days. Accurate inferences about medication use over months or years are obviously difficult to draw from such a limited measurement. The development of the glycosated hemoglobin test in diabetes mellitus exemplifies technological advances that provide better measures of compliance. This test gives information about the level of blood glucose over a 6- to 12-week period and thus is superior to a single blood glucose test.

Accuracy of findings may also be adversely affected by the presence of an investigator or by the client's knowledge of planned compliance measures. Studies have shown that the introduction of an observer into the home can increase compliance behavior (Marston, 1970). The primary writer has been impressed with the frequency with which individuals with diabetes mellitus have described more compliant behavior on days immediately preceding their checkup visits.

Conceptual Barriers   Not only do methodological problems serve as barriers because of contradictory or inconclusive findings (Marston, 1970; Dracup & Meleis, 1982), but inadequate conceptualization of the phenomenon of compliance has led to the lack of consistent findings. For example, Sackett and Snow (1979) note the failure of many investigators to define compliance and noncompliance carefully, an inadequacy limiting the use of replication studies.

Theories and Models   Theoretical frameworks can provide direction for health care providers by guiding the focus and dimensions of assessment and providing structure to the interaction of client and provider. A model or theory alerts the practitioner to attend to specific factors known to influence compliance.

Several authors point out the lack of a unifying theoretical framework in studies that address the phenomenon of compliance (Becker & Maiman, 1978; Dracup & Meleis, 1982; Connelly, 1984). The most popular theories and models do not take into account important variables, nor do they emphasize the interactive and communication processes considered increasingly important by many researchers (Dracup & Meleis, 1982; Connelly, 1984; Anderson, 1985; Hulka et al., 1976). Dracup and Meleis (1982) analyzed the medical model, the health belief model, the locus of control construct, and social learning theory, all of which are frequently used in compliance research, and felt that all contained conceptual inadequacies.

At this point it would be helpful to distinguish theories from models (Fawcett, 1984):

> The primary distinction between a conceptual model and a theory is the level of abstraction. A conceptual model is a highly abstract system of global concepts and linking statements. A theory, in contrast, deals with one or more specific, concrete concepts and propositions. Conceptual models are only general guides, which must be specified further by relevant and logically congruent theories before action can occur . . . . A conceptual model cannot be tested directly because its concepts are not operationally defined, nor are the relationships among concepts observable. More specific concepts and propositions have to be derived from the conceptual model, that is, a theory must be formulated.

International Model   Dracup and Meleis (1982) proposed a theoretical approach of mutual participation of clients and physicians, drawn from role theory and based on the health transaction model (initially introduced by Stone in 1979). The advantages of role theory as a framework are that it emphasizes interaction and communicating processes and addresses the multiple compliance-related variables that have been identified. Using this model, one would expect that communication would focus on compliance expectations of both client and provider and that there would be attempts to resolve conflicts about different expectancies of behavior and outcomes. Essential propositions of this framework include the following:

1. To the extent a client demonstrates knowledge and competency in enacting a proposed role, a higher level of health regimen compliance is expected. The relationship is mediated through the level of complexity and duration of the medical regimen.
2. Compliance is maximized when there is evidence that the sick or at-risk roles have been incorporated into the self-concept of the client.
3. Compliance is enhanced when relevant other roles are congruent and/or complementary with client roles.

4. Compliance is enhanced if the compliance role is reinforced by significant others and other reference groups.
5. The level and extent of the client's compliance with a health care regimen depend on the degree to which behaviors of compliance are judged valuable by the client and are validated by significant others (Dracup & Meleis, 1982).

Variables of Noncompliance

Investigators of compliance have focused primarily on the relation of compliance to individual variables such as characteristics of clients, providers, disease, and regimen, or to client–provider interactions (Dracup & Meleis, 1982). Although correlations are found, studies of particular variables without attention to interrelatedness among them have contributed to contradictory or inconclusive findings and to the scarcity of studies that can be generalized to other populations (Dracup & Meleis, 1982; Becker & Maiman, 1975). One reason for this situation is the complexity of the phenomenon of compliance and of the relationships between compliance and the variables studied (Dracup & Meleis, 1982; Becker & Maiman, 1975).

Single Variables of Compliance Compliance has been shown to be poorly related to severity of illness, pain, disability, or threat to life (Hingson et al., 1981). No study showed that severity of symptoms encouraged compliance, although four studies reported that lower compliance was present when there were more symptoms (Haynes, 1979). Few client characteristics were shown to be influential in studies of noncompliance (Haynes, 1979). Those that were influential include the following:

1. Extremes of age in medication taking (Becker & Maiman, 1975)
2. Some mental illnesses, particularly schizophrenia, paranoia, and personality disorders (Haynes, 1979)
3. Denial in clients with coronary artery disease (Craig, Shapiro, & Levine, 1971).

Complexity of the medical regimen was the characteristic most often found to interfere with compliance in medication taking (Marston, 1970). Complexity has two components: frequency of dose and number of drugs prescribed (Blackwell, 1979). The degree of behavioral change required by the regimen and the duration of the regimen were also associated with noncompliance (Hellenbrandt, 1983).

Variables Related to Life Span There are particular issues of compliance related to specific age groups. These issues are associated with developmental processes rather than chronological age.

Children and Adolescents In children, developmental issues that are factors in compliance include adolescence, gender, family support, perceived severity of illness, duration of treatment, and parents' concerns about the child (Cohen et al., 1991). For children and adolescents, clear accountability and family communication about health care responsibilities are important, as are conflict negotiation and cooperative problem solving (Wysocki & Wayne, 1992).

For the child with a chronic illness, one of the developmental tasks to be accomplished within the family is the gradual assumption of self-care by the child. The transfer of responsibility is particularly difficult when nonadherence brings the risk of acute illness to the child, anxiety and increased cost of remedial action to the parent, and increased conflict between parents and child. If increases in responsibility are taken on too early, there is a risk of treatment errors; if the increases are long delayed, the child or adolescent may develop problems of overdependence, diminished initiative, and decreased self-confidence (Wysocki & Wayne, 1992).

In adolescence, compliance with health care regimens often loses to the many competing demands for teenagers' attention. Adolescents typically are self-focused, self-conscious, and concerned about peer reactions. They engage in risk taking even when concerned about personal health patterns (Whatley, 1991), and they strive for greater autonomy in relation to authority figures. Adolescents also increase their social experimentation and involvement of peer support (Smith & Schreiner, 1993). It is small wonder, then, that compliance rates typically are lower during these years.

Young Adults With their busy lives, many young adults find compliance difficult. Jones, Jones, and Katz (1988) found that the 18-to-29-year age group had the lowest compliance rates when it came to making and keeping referral appointments. However, higher compliance rates were found in those with chronic diseases, those who were currently or previously married, and those who had knowledge of the disease.

Older Adults A decrease in functional ability is only one indicator of possible noncompliance in the elderly. Other identified risk factors were complicated regimens, cost and inconvenience of medicine taking, lack of supervised practice, and inadequate labeling of medicine containers (Cargill, 1992). When taking medications, there was less compliance if there was a decrease in physical strength, coordination, visual acuity, or comprehension of medications and doses (Cargill, 1992). The noncompliance in this study group was frequently that of underuse, with many reporting a belief that they were being overmedicated.

Socio-Cultural-Economic Factors

It has long been known that economics, sociocultural factors, and family support are associated with compliant behavior (Jones, Jones, & Katz, 1988). Therefore, it is necessary to assess pertinent sociocultural beliefs, attitudes, and health behaviors if barriers to compliance are to be identified. In addition, providers need to develop sensitivity to these factors in order to devise compliance strategies.

Economic Factors Poverty, inadequate English-language proficiency, and limited access to health care are known predictors of noncompliance with recommended health care behaviors (Gonzalez, 1990). The burdens of financial costs alone may serve as a barrier to obtaining health care services, supplies, or medications needed to manage chronic illness. Another major barrier to compliance is a lack of resources, including inadequate or difficult transportation, inade-

quate availability of child care, loss of time from low-paying jobs, and little job security.

Some barriers to compliance are clearly related to an ineffective "health care system" for chronic disease management. For instance, a large number of persons who come to emergency departments for nonurgent care related to chronic illness have limited access to primary care services that would be more appropriate for chronic disease management (Jones, Jones, & Katz, 1987, 1988). Hellenbrandt (1983) noted that inefficient and inconvenient clinics serving the poor have long waiting lines and tend not to provide long-term relationships with the same provider. Well known is the decreased availability of primary care services, particularly in inner cities and rural areas, and to groups such as migrant workers, new immigrants, the homeless, and those with AIDS. In addition, the maze of governmental and third-party payers' policies and regulations often deny provider reimbursement for preventive or educational services, making these services less available to clients (See Chapters 22 and 23, on financial impact and social policy, respectively.)

Anderson, Blue, and Lau (1993) argue that poverty and class membership are more important than ethnic or cultural background in how people manage chronic illness. These researchers found multiple barriers to compliance for newly immigrated, poor Chinese women. Poverty, lack of personal resources (literacy, language, financial, and so forth), and the demands of survival in a new land were some of the factors that contributed to their noncompliance.

Cultural Aspects More attention is being given to the ways culture influences health behaviors and the interactions of clients with health care providers. Cultural influences affect the way adults and children experience, interpret, and respond to illness and its treatment (Munet-Villaro & Vessey, 1990). Newly immigrated persons also may lack financial and social support from an extended family, a major resource in many non-Western cultures (Kleinman, Eisenberg, & Good, 1988).

For effective interaction with persons of a different culture, "cultural translation" is needed (Murphy et al., 1993). One requisite for a cultural translator is learning about the historic rituals and norms of the particular group that relate to health. Another requisite is examining health behaviors in the cultural context to determine competing priorities, environmental obstacles, or degree of knowledge and skills (Murphy et al., 1993).

The provider needs to recognize that his or her belief system, values, and attitudes toward health care management also are culturally determined and may be responsible for the inability of providers to recognize that the source of noncompliance might be ideological or philosophical. The emphasis on self-care in Western medical systems is ideologically quite consistent with the value of individual enterprise in Western cultures (Anderson, Blue, & Lau, 1993). Persons of other cultures may find this value for self-care very foreign. For example, the stereotypical image of the Latino[1] culture is of a hierarchical family structure with male domination. Current research disputes this image (Friedman, 1990). Some Hispanics believe there is no need to attempt to prevent disease since actions do not matter. Novello, previous Surgeon General of the U.S. Public Health Service, notes that notions of prevention and maintenance of health by self-care measures are not consistent with their fatalistic view and that some Hispanics feel "what causes a disease, and its impact on you and your family, does not hold much weight when your sole purpose is just to live and, when God wills it, to die" (Ingle, 1993, p. 45).

Knowing only an ethnic label is inadequate for understanding a particular individual's or group's beliefs (Friedman, 1990). Other cultural aspects that need to be assessed include whether traditional, folk, or alternative remedies are being used by the client; if ordered prescriptions interfere with important cultural practices; and what rituals, restrictions, meanings, and norms are associated with cultural use of items such as food.

Family communication and authority patterns are also influenced by culture. For African Americans, role obligations are seen as mandatory and family rights as strong. Therefore, family-centered care is more appropriate than the usual individual-centered approach seen in Western practice (Friedman, 1990). Black family patterns include strong kinship systems within the extended family; values for family, church and religious life; active involvement of both parents in parenting; and assistance with child care by the maternal grandparent (Friedman, 1990).

Client-Provider Interactions

From a traditional medical perspective, the client is considered passive and poorly informed about the prevention and treatment of disease. Since treatment is directed toward the disease, any noncompliance indicates that the client is the problem (Anderson, 1985). Here, three specific aspects of client-provider interactions are examined: expectations about interactions, feelings about personal control, and perspectives of the client.

Of the variables associated with compliance, provider-patient interactions are the most consistent (Jones, Jones, & Katz, 1988). Hellenbrandt (1983) identified these variables in client-physician interactions that adversely influence compliance:

1. Inadequate supervision
2. Client dissatisfaction
3. No explanation of illness given to the client
4. Physician disagreement with the client
5. Formality toward or rejection of the client

Differing Expectations An issue of importance to providers and clients centers on the question of how much active client participation is appropriate to interactions with providers. The question is framed in such a way that one must acknowledge that both providers and clients have expectations about the appropriate level of participation. Both make judgments based on these expectations about suitable behavior in various roles—expectations that are formed in large part from previous socialization experiences.

Providers and clients have, by and large, been socialized to expect the client to exhibit sick role behaviors and the provider to use com-

[1]*Latino:* People living in the United States who are of Mexican, Central or South American, or Caribbean ancestry. Often used as a synonym for Hispanic.

plementary role behaviors (Parsons, 1951). In the sick role, clients are expected to try to get well by seeking help and cooperating with the prescribed regimen (see Chapter 4, on illness roles). The complementary role of the provider is that of dominance as the professional expert and manager of the condition. Parsons's view served to underline the asymmetry in doctor–client relationships (Hingson et al., 1981) and described an authority-to-subordinate relationship.

Alternative interactional roles characterized by more mutuality of responsibility and decision making have been noted in the literature. Szasz and Hollander (1956) described a mutual participation model that is more appropriate to chronic illness because clients have management roles in implementing their treatment regimens. The following are features of this model: (1) the physician's role is to help clients help themselves; (2) clients are in partnership with the provider; and (3) clients are users of expert help. The complementary roles presented in this model are that of a provider who offers guidance to the client and a client who cooperates with the provider.

Sometimes decisions not to comply are rational when viewed from the client's perspective. Thorne (1990) identified two themes for noncompliance: self-protection and maintenance of services. Reasons for willful noncompliance included troublesome side effects of medications, disbelief in recommendations, and the necessity of juggling conflicting recommendations from different physicians. Often, clients misled health care professionals about their intentions, since they wanted to maintain relationships with the health providers for other needed services. Thorne suggests that health care professionals consider the chronically ill individual as the expert and aim for credibility in the role of consultant rather than assume expertise and moral authority.

Although further research is needed to test the relationship of complementary roles and compliance, it seems logical to assume that communication between provider and client might well include discussing the expectations each holds about the participation expected of the client and the assistance to be offered by the provider. Providers might become more effective in their communication and interaction with clients if they viewed clients as occupying various positions on a passivity-to-autonomy continuum, rather than focusing on a preconceived notion of expected client behavior. The result would be increased sensitivity to each client's requirements for autonomy, guidance, and direction. Instead of a question about the extent of participation clients should have in interactions, a more appropriate question would be, What is the optimal kind of participation for a particular client? The answer can only evolve through the provider–client dyad as they communicate about expectations, goals, and perceived problems.

Feelings about Personal Control The locus-of-control construct has been used to study client choices of self-care behavior; it focuses on individual expectancies about outcomes (rewards, reinforcements) and the perceived efficacy of behavior to modify outcomes. According to this construct, persons are at different positions on an internality–externality continuum of orientation to perceived control. Internals believe in personal influence on future events, and externals attribute influence to others. The health locus-of-control construct modifies this generalized expectancy to specific expectancies of health and illness outcomes and health behaviors (Rotter, 1966; Wallston et al., 1976).

Research findings have been contradictory about the relationship of locus of control to compliance (Wallston, Wallston, & DeVellis, 1978; Dimond & Jones, 1983). Oberle (1991) describes externals as more compliant with treatment and less active in seeking information, whereas internals actively seek knowledge and manipulate treatment regimens.

Some researchers have suggested that treatment programs should reflect the differing characteristics and learning styles of internals and externals (Wallston, Wallston, & DeVellis, 1978). Approaches for externals would be most appropriate if they included an authority-to-subordinate interpersonal relationship, support of a positive self-concept, and structured teaching plans. Approaches for internals would be appropriately tailored if they included multiple options, participation in decision making, and emphasis on personal responsibility and accountability for treatment outcomes (Schroeder & Miller, 1983).

Internality may be increased through educational programs that emphasize personal responsibility. However, Dimond and Jones (1983) point out that the inculcation of personal responsibility is stressful and not without danger. These authors caution:

> It would be foolish if not dangerous to attempt to make the orientation of all clients internal. Personal control can be so stress-producing as to outweigh the benefits . . . attempts to control uncontrollable conditions are likely to induce self-blame, depression, or despair.

Perspectives of the Client   Clients and providers are likely to hold different perspectives of chronic illness, its treatment, and the relative merits of compliant behavior. The client lives with the disease, and treatment is only one aspect of that individual's life. Living with treatment consequences is vastly different from offering advice, counsel, education, or exhortation about health care recommendations. Clients rarely, if ever, seek help from health care providers because they want to comply. Rather, they ask for help for a variety of reasons: They feel ill, they are worried, they are responding to others' recommendations, they need evidence to validate claims for entitlement benefits, and so forth. Providers, on the other hand, are very much concerned about compliance, which may be seen as the desired outcome of the interaction (Anderson, 1985).

Anderson points out two important ways in which clients' perspectives of chronic illness—in this case, diabetes mellitus—differ from those of providers. First, there is a relative difference in understanding of the treatment regimen, not just on the level of specificity, rationale, and consequences, but with respect to the sources of problems; clients may see treatment as part of the problem of having diabetes, whereas providers see treatment as a solution. Second, clients are more concerned about the "here and now" experience, in contrast to providers' concern over a problem that places future health at risk.

For example, clients express more concerns about preventing hypoglycemic reactions than about managing higher than normal blood glucose levels. Providers, on the other hand, express more concern about the importance of achieving close to normal blood glucose levels because of their perceptions of serious long-term consequences if control of blood glucose levels is not achieved (Anderson, 1985).

The client's perspective of chronic illness, its treatment, and compliance is also influenced by the demands of living, of time and energy, and of the talents required by life conditions (Strauss et al., 1984). Other commitments and demands compete with those of the treatment regimen, so that treatment benefits may be viewed as less valuable than the costs that are incurred. According to Strauss and associates (1984), whether the client adheres to regimens of treatment depends on certain conditions, including these:

1. There is an initial or continuing trust in the physician or whoever else prescribes the regimen.
2. No rival supersedes the physician in his or her legitimating.
3. There is evidence that the regimen works to control either the symptoms or the disease itself, or both.
4. No distressing, frightening side effects appear.
5. The side effects are outweighed by symptom relief or by sufficient fear of the disease itself.
6. There is a relative noninterference with important daily activities, either of the client or of people around him or her.
7. The regimen's perceived good effects are not outweighed by a negative impact on the client's sense of identity.

Motivation

In the traditional medical model, noncompliance is often attributed to poor motivation and not to an inadequacy of communication between client and provider. The provider attributes mastery of and continuation with the prescribed regimen as a result of high motivation and iden-

CASE STUDY
Mrs. J.

Mrs. J., a 52-year-old matron of Eastern European descent, seemed not to listen to or understand the dietician's explanation of a 1,400-calorie diet prescribed for newly diagnosed non-insulin–dependent diabetes mellitus. Educational level and learning abilities were rated as above average. The nurse noted that Mrs. J.'s conversations concerned her daughter's wedding, which was to occur in two weeks and had been planned for two years. According to Mrs. J., this wedding was to be the "biggest event of my life," and one in which her status as a good mother, future mother-in-law, and member of a newly extended family would be affirmed. It would be "unthinkable for me not to join in the festivities . . . in which eating and drinking would last hours and hours." It was not until the dietician offered to work with Mrs. J. to plan this day's food intake, negotiating with her some compromise between the ideal of 1,400 calories/24 hours and Mrs. J.'s ideal of feasting, that Mrs. J. showed some willingness to engage in learning to incorporate the diet into her daily life pattern.

---

tifies the lack of motivation as an obstacle to compliance.

Most current models of motivation of health care decisions and behavior are derived from psychological cognitive theories that focus on attitudes, beliefs, intentions, and perceptions of the client's ability to initiate and maintain recommended health behavior (Fleury, 1992). These models views individual motivation as related to beliefs and values held by the client about the outcome to be achieved, the client's intentions, and the client's perceived ability to initiate and maintain behavioral change.

Client's Life Perspective   Differing levels of motivation for health care behaviors are more understandable when the client's perspective of life is taken into account. Complying with a provider-recommended treatment regimen may compete with other valued tasks, roles, or relationships. Chronically ill clients must continue to manage their daily existence under specific sets of financial and social conditions (Strauss et al., 1984). Consequently, the strength of motivation to carry out health care behaviors may vary with perceptions of current life demands.

The case studies of Mrs. J. above and Mr. M. on page 233 illustrate the necessity of learning the client's life perspective in order to understand apparent low-level motivation for assuming recommended health care behavior. They demonstrate the need to consider the client's primary motivating forces at a given time and to determine the way these forces affect the strength of motivation for specific health care behavior.

Labeling a client as poorly motivated without considering that person's perspective impedes the process of helping and offers no suggestions as to how to intervene in an effective manner. However, taking the client's perspective into account can assist the health care provider in gaining clues about barriers to compliance perceived by the client. Clients may be more motivated to learn when their perspective is considered and they are involved in planning, allowing them to achieve more complete compliance over longer time periods.

Health Belief Model   Motivation is clearly related to beliefs and attitudes held by an individual. The health belief model (HBM), developed by Hochman, Leventhal, Kegles, and Rosenstock to explain preventive health behavior, contains a cluster of pertinent beliefs and attitudes (Becker & Maiman, 1975). It was modified to include a general health motivation (Becker, 1976) (see Figure 10–1) and was again modified for sick role behaviors. Figure 10–2 shows modifying and enabling factors that reflect the individual's readiness to undertake sick role behaviors that influence the likelihood of compliance in chronic illness. The HBM's major proposition is that the likelihood of an individual taking recommended health actions is increased by two

INDIVIDUAL
PERCEPTIONS

MODIFYING
FACTORS

LIKELIHOOD OF
ACTION

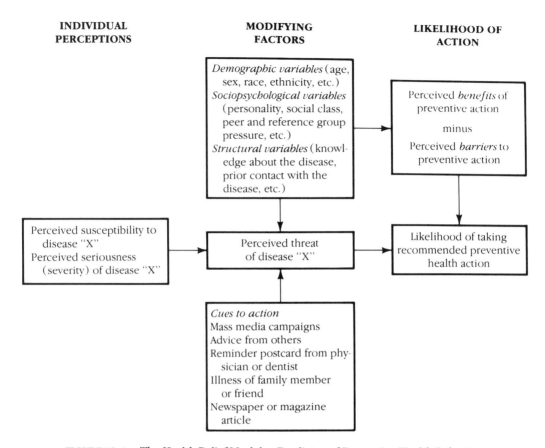

FIGURE 10-1.   The Health Belief Model as Predictor of Preventive Health Behavior

SOURCE: From Becker, M. H. (1974a). A new approach to explaining sick-role behavior in low-income populations. *American Journal of Public Health, 64,* 205–216.

variables: (1) the value placed by the individual on a particular goal, and (2) the individual's estimate of the likelihood that a specific action will achieve that goal (Becker & Janz, 1985).

The HBM remains the dominant explanation of the relationships of attitudes and behaviors to compliance; research using this model has generally produced more predictability than has research using other models (Cargill, 1992). Even so, a recent meta-analysis of studies of the HBM showed that conceptual and methodological issues are still problematic in research reports of the HBM (Harrison, Mullen, & Green, 1992).

The HBM is less effective in explaining noncompliance and compliance in curative situations than in preventive situations (Kasl, 1978), yet findings of many studies have generally supported the HBM as useful in discerning the relationship of client beliefs to compliance (Becker, 1976). Research using the HBM shows that perceptions of susceptibility, severity, and benefits are positively correlated with a variety of desirable health behaviors: taking medications, following dietary restrictions, observing exercise prescriptions, and keeping clinic appointments (Hallel, 1975; Becker & Janz, 1985).

It is believed that perceptions and beliefs can be altered by "corrective factual information, motive-arousing appeals . . . recommendations from other sources of information that have greater credibility to the patient" (Becker & Janz, 1985). Yet in an education program for self-management, although subjects did increase their

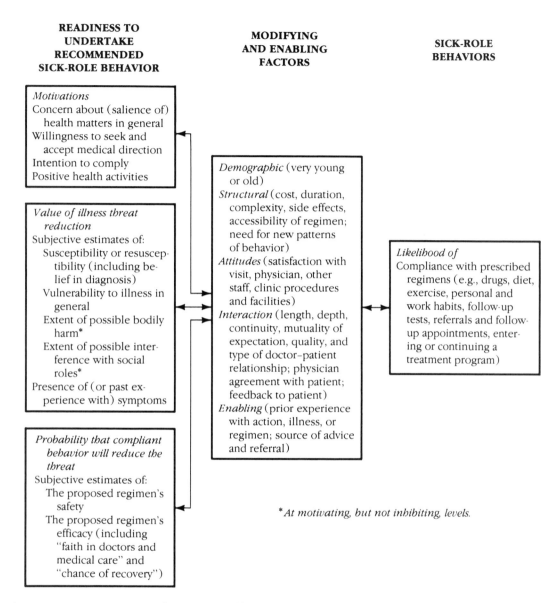

READINESS TO
UNDERTAKE
RECOMMENDED
SICK-ROLE BEHAVIOR

MODIFYING
AND ENABLING
FACTORS

SICK-ROLE
BEHAVIORS

Motivations
Concern about (salience of)
  health matters in general
Willingness to seek and
  accept medical direction
Intention to comply
Positive health activities

*Value of illness threat
reduction*
Subjective estimates of:
  Susceptibility or rescep-
    tibility (including be-
    lief in diagnosis)
  Vulnerability to illness in
    general
  Extent of possible bodily
    harm*
  Extent of possible inter-
    ference with social
    roles*
  Presence of (or past ex-
    perience with) symptoms

*Probability that compliant
behavior will reduce the
threat*
Subjective estimates of:
  The proposed regimen's
    safety
  The proposed regimen's
    efficacy (including
    "faith in doctors and
    medical care" and
    "chance of recovery")

Demographic (very young
  or old)
Structural (cost, duration,
  complexity, side effects,
  accessibility of regimen;
  need for new patterns
  of behavior)
Attitudes (satisfaction with
  visit, physician, other
  staff, clinic procedures
  and facilities)
Interaction (length, depth,
  continuity, mutuality of
  expectation, quality, and
  type of doctor–patient
  relationship; physician
  agreement with patient;
  feedback to patient)
Enabling (prior experience
  with action, illness, or
  regimen; source of advice
  and referral)

Likelihood of
Compliance with prescribed
  regimens (e.g., drugs, diet,
  exercise, personal and
  work habits, follow-up
  tests, referrals and follow-
  up appointments, enter-
  ing or continuing a
  treatment program)

At motivating, but not inhibiting, levels.

FIGURE 10-2.   Summary Health Belief Model for Predicting and Explaining
Sick-Role Behaviors

SOURCE: From Becker, M. H. (1974b). The health belief model and sick-role behavior. *Health Education Monograph, 2,* 409–419.

beliefs of perceived severity and self-efficacy, they did not report higher adherence levels (Wooldridge et al., 1992). Wooldridge and colleagues felt that lack of change in adherence might be related to the increased costs (financial, time use) of the recommended health behaviors in the program. In the Jones, Jones, and Katz study of appointment keeping (1988), an educational intervention based on the HBM did result in increased compliance.

Self-Efficacy A recent addition to the evolving HBM is the construct of self-efficacy, defined as the client's expectations or confidence in his or her *ability* to perform a recommended action. These perceptions of ability "affect behavior, level of motivation, thought patterns, and emotional reactions in response to potentially threatening situations" (Fleury, 1992). Self-efficacy is a predictor of health status, preventive self-care, and disease self-management (Gonzalez, 1990). High self-efficacy has been related to the enactment of behaviors useful in anxiety disorders, depression, pain, smoking cessation, eating disorders, pulmonary disease, and prevention of postoperative complications (Black, 1992).

Health Promotion Model The HBM has been extended by focusing on health promotion and including determinants of health-promoting behavior (Pender, 1987; Fleury, 1992). There are three components to this model. First, the primary predictors of health-promoting behavior are cognitive/perceptual factors: the importance of health, perceived control of health and self-efficacy, definition of health, perceived health status, and perceived benefits and barriers to health-promoting behaviors (see Figure 10–3). Second, the HPM consists of factors that modify the beliefs and perceptions that influence health-promoting behaviors. And third, the likelihood of engaging in action is dependent on internal or external cues to actions.

The HPM has been given credence by research findings that explain and predict a variety of health-promoting activities, including self-actualization, health responsibility, exercise, nutrition, interpersonal support, and stress management (Fleury, 1992).

Ethical Issues in Compliance

Noncompliance in chronic illness can contribute to more costly hospitalizations and to more extensive and expensive treatments should severe illness result (Connelly, 1984). Ethical issues center on reciprocal rights and responsibilities of caregivers and clients, use of paternalism and coercion by caregivers, autonomy of the client, relative risks and benefits of proposed regimens, and the costs to society of noncompliance.

Compliance or noncompliance with recommendations for health behavior is an increasingly important ethical issue in health care cost containment, since conflicts arise when health care resources are limited and decisions about the best use of time, money, and the energy of providers must be made. However, economic and ethical issues differ. Whereas economic issues concern the most efficient distribution of resources, ethical issues concern the most equitable distribution (Barry, 1982). Connelly (1984) believes that strategies that promote and improve client's active and effective self-care are both ethically and economically significant (see Chapter 19, on nursing ethics).

Sackett (1976) described three preconditions for ethical practice that must precede strategies to change client behavior toward increased compliance. These preconditions mandate the use of informed consent and the development of a partnership with responsibility for compliance equally shared.

1. The diagnosis must be correct.
2. Therapy must provide more benefit than harm.
3. The client who accepts the treatment regimen must be a partner in strategies used to increase compliance.

Jonsen (1979) added a fourth condition, the importance of client consent to the regimen, and emphasized that the ethics of compliance are based on freedom, mutual understanding, and mutual responsibility. Connelly (1984) incorporated both Sackett's and Jonsen's conditions in an ethical approach to compliance that has three phases:

1. Developing client competencies and reinforcing and supporting the client's self-care ability.
2. Evolving a consensual regimen and outcome goals through a client–provider interaction based on mutuality.
3. Focusing compliance-increasing strategies on joint exploration of problems and negotiation of conflicts in goals or implementation.

Threats, pressure, and inappropriate fear-arousal tactics are not ethical (Jonsen, 1979; Con-

COGNITIVE/PERCEPTUAL
FACTORS

MODIFYING
FACTORS

PARTICIPATION IN
HEALTH-PROMOTING
BEHAVIOR

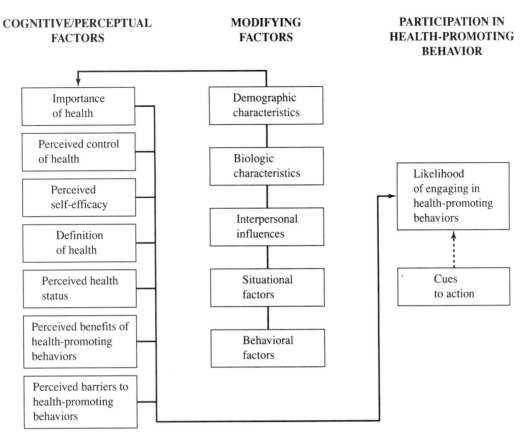

FIGURE 10-3.   Health Promotion Model

SOURCE: From Pender, N. J. (1987). *Health promotion in nursing practice* (2nd ed.) (p. 58). Norwalk, CT: Appleton-Century-Crofts. Used with permission.

nelly, 1984). Punitive responses that can be implemented by the provider for revealed or suspected noncompliance include decreased time and attention from the provider, less availability for crisis management, and limited access to services, resources, or supplies. The high incidence of noncompliance, and the provider's frequent inability to differentiate clients who comply from those who do not, presents an argument against the withdrawal or diminution of services to clients who disclose noncompliance. If others may be equally noncompliant, punitive responses only to those who are honest about noncompliance constitute inequality of care, which is an issue of social justice.

If the client has been informed and understands that the consequence of noncompliance will be withdrawal by the provider, then termination of the relationship may be the right of the provider. If economic or social conditions preclude access to other caregivers, this termination raises serious questions about the ethical nature of withdrawing and abandoning the client. Assisting the client in finding another caregiver is "ethically preferable to unilateral and abrupt termination" (Jonsen, 1979).

Interventions to Attain Compliance

The complexity of the problems involved in noncompliance should not deter the health practitioner from working with the client to achieve maximum possible integration of optimal health recommendations, given the client's needs, demands, and lifestyle. To accomplish maximum compliance, those who use compliance-increasing strategies have a responsibility to ensure the client's safety and comprehension. For the nurse, often working as liaison between client and physician, communicating with either or both is often necessary before matters are clear enough to select and begin specific compliance-increasing strategies.

Assessment Factors

Before any one intervention can be selected to assist a client in adhering to a proposed medical regimen, a careful assessment is necessary to distinguish those situational and personal factors that can and will be modified from those that cannot or will not be modified. In addition, assessment will help determine the relative harm or benefit expected from a regimen implemented under the client's current conditions. The client and family should be included in the assessment process.

A systematic assessment of the client should include sociocultural and economic factors, knowledge level, beliefs, attitudes, and current understanding of the proposed regimen. Attention should also be given to the client's perceptions of illness threat and the efficacy of recommendations and the client's ability to carry out these recommendations. The importance of not perceiving an illness threat was illustrated in a study of persons with severe and persistent schizophrenia. The majority of patients were noncompliant with medications, did not believe they needed medication, and denied they were ill (Mulaik, 1992).

There should be a determination of the "rightness" of the prescriptions for the particular client, including an estimation of relative harm or benefit that is expected. The outcome of assessment will allow the nurse to determine which aspects of the regimen management (1) are most unlikely to achieve compliant behavior, (2) are most important in attaining therapeutic goals, and (3) require the most learning to attain desired behavioral change.

Hingson et al. (1981) suggest that the following questions be asked in a compliance-oriented history:

1. Have you been taking anything for this problem already?
2. Does anything worry you about the illness?
3. What can happen if the recommended regimen is not followed?
4. How likely is that to occur?
5. How effective do you feel the regimen will be in treating the disorder?
6. Can you think of any problems you might have in following the regimen?
7. Do you have any questions about the regimen or how to follow it?

Mrs. Z.'s case study illustrates many of the factors that interact and result in decisions and actions that lead to compliance or noncompliance. This case example also demonstrates the importance of properly identifying the sources of noncompliance as well as using guidelines for analysis of a situation involving apparent noncompliance.

First, we should recognize that health care providers are not infallible and that errors can occur in prescribing, in dispensing, in communicating with the client and family caregiver, or in maintaining updated written records, especially in clinics where health care is provided by different physicians and nurses. A second consideration is that the client/caregiver simply may not understand, or remember, instructions. Hulka and associates (1976) emphasize that lack of comprehension is different from volitional noncompliance and may be responsible for considerable errors in medication taking. In the Hulka and associates study, when clients were informed of the behavior expected of them and understood it, more than 85 percent of the time behavior conformed to that expectation.

Third, it is important to be aware of a tendency among care providers to see compliant behavior as positive, admirable, and wise on the part of "good patients" and noncompliant behavior as negative, deplorable, and unintelligible on the part of "problem patients." Noncompliance, from this view, is considered a rejection of advice, a negation of professional expertise, or an obstruction to the helping process. It seems

CASE STUDY
Mrs. Z.: An Appearance of Noncompliance

Mrs. Z., who was caregiver to her father, Mr. A., received from the pharmacist a vial of antibiotic medicine. The label on the vial was incorrect; instead of the prescribed "once a day" (q.d.), the label read "four times a day" (q.i.d.). Mrs. Z. remembered that six months previously the dosage of this antibiotic had been prescribed once a day. She decided that four times a day was too often and administered it twice a day. After a few days she decreased it to once a day and finally stopped giving it when her father became confused. Because her father attributed confusion to a prescribed vasodilator, she also stopped giving that.

She could not recall what she had been told about the dosage when she last saw the physician, nor did she recall receiving written directions. With her father's previous physician, Mrs. Z. had been comfortable about calling with questions about her father's care. That physician had stopped practicing because of his own sudden illness. The new physician seemed competent enough, but Mrs. Z. "did not know him well enough to call him." She readily accepted the home health care nurse's offer to call the physician to clarify the prescription, to report the onset of confusion, and to let him know about the omission of prescribed medications.

---

probable that health professionals who have this view would be less likely to search out barriers to noncompliance that might include their own actions or nonactions.

A fourth guideline in analyzing a situation involving apparent noncompliance is to be cautious in attributing causation of noncompliance or in making predictions about levels of compliance based on any one characteristic of a client. Compliance is poorly related to sociodemographic characteristics or stable personality traits (Kasl, 1978).

Insufficient knowledge may undermine the purpose of the recommendation made by the prescriber; sometimes previous experience was negative because of incorrect use of treatment remedies. For example, one client having an acute exacerbation of eczema (duration 35 years) was told to take prednisone in decreasing amounts (five times, four times, three times, two times, and then one time on five succeeding days). His initial resistance became understandable when it was learned that he had developed "terrible stomach pain and a personality change" during past use of this medication. Exploration revealed that he had taken all the required number of pills at one time each day. Suggestions to space the pills and to use antacids were accepted; he later reported no side effects. This same person, for the first time, complied with directions to wear gloves at night following appli-

cation of ointment to his hands, after he learned that gloves increased absorption of the medicine: "Never before has anyone told me . . . that makes sense."

Assessment should also lead to a determination of the proper focus of compliance-increasing strategies. It was said earlier that the notion of compliance as self-care may be too restrictive for situations in which compliance with medical regimens cannot be achieved without the assistance of others. The combination of marked disability and chronic illness makes the conceptualization of compliance as a self-care ability inappropriate if the major concern is congruence of the client's treatment with provider recommendations.

Strauss and others (1984) describe two roles of family members in relation to compliance: controlling (commanding, manipulating, shaming, reminding) and assisting. This conceptualization of family roles retains the primary focus on the client as the agent of compliance and may be adequate in situations in which the client's disabilities are not marked. When abilities are markedly diminished, family members may be the most important agents of compliance and should become the focus of compliance-increasing strategies.

Additional case data about Mrs. Z. and her father illustrate the multiple factors that influence compliance with a treatment regimen for a frail, elderly person. Before describing the problem this family has in managing the treatment regimen, two other aspects of a family's involvement need to be mentioned. One is the obvious fact that families have many goals, concerns, and conditions besides managing the illness of one member. The second is that managing the medically prescribed treatment regimen is only part of the work involved in caring for a client. Supervision, assistance, persuasion to eat and move about, hygiene, diversional activities, and so on, are some of the obvious tasks (see Chapter 3, on illness trajectory).

Mrs. Z.'s case demonstrates the complexity and the reality of barriers to compliance when client and family members are sharing the work of implementing the regimen. Compliance is affected by the multiple and competing demands and commitments of family members, as well as by family-member–client interactions. The case also demonstrates the need to focus compliance strategies on all those involved in management of regimens.

Education

There is wide support for education strategies in prevention and treatment of noncompliance among individuals interested in the ethical implications of compliance behavior (Jonsen, 1979) and researchers studying compliance (Green, 1979). For example, the overwhelming suggestion offered by nurses in an opinion survey related to improving client compliance with medication taking was "Teach, teach, teach" (Moree, 1984).

Sadly, knowledge about illness and treatment in itself does not ensure desired results. However, without knowledge, clearly, compliance cannot occur (Sackett, 1976; Becker & Janz, 1985). For example, taking medication has been the focus of a large number of compliance studies. Reported results indicate that knowledge of drug function has been correlated with both decreased error rates and improved compliance (Hulka et al., 1976). In one study, using a sample of chronically ill elderly individuals, inaccurate knowledge about drugs was associated with a 20-percent error factor and occurred among 41 percent of clients (Schwartz et al., 1962).

Kasl (1978) described the complexity of the relationship of knowledge to compliance and cited the following studies as support:

- Knowledge of the regimen is helpful (Kirscht & Rosenstock, 1979), but may have dubious value when the regimen is relatively simple and not exceedingly demanding (Taylor et al., 1978).
- Knowledge of the disease seems to have little impact on compliance of those subjects who have a rich experience with their illness, treatment management, and the medical-care system (Tagliacozzo & Irma, 1970).

There is contradictory evidence about the impact of information giving on compliance (Steckel & Swain, 1981). One conceptual issue in the relation of education to compliance deals with the difference between information giving by the provider and a planned program of education designed to achieve specified cognitive, psychomotor, and affective health behaviors. This difference is not always appreciated in studies on compliance. To be effective, client education must include both an accurate assessment of learning needs and abilities as well as barriers, and a plan designed and executed to maximize the potential for learning how to incorporate health care behavior into daily life (see Chapter 16, on teaching).

Anderson (1985) describes an educational approach that has a different basic assumption from that of the medical model. This approach uses teaching as a means of persuading clients to comply. In this model the problem is viewed from the client's perspective, and the practitioner must understand and work through the client's frame of reference. In other words, clients are accepted as capable and responsible for managing their own lives and are allowed to define and meet their own needs.

Educational goals must be broader than solely the acquisition of knowledge if compliance is to result. Abilities beyond knowledge and comprehension are required. It follows that the outcome of compliance depends on participation of the learner beyond that of listening, reading, or assimilating information.

CASE STUDY

Mrs. Z., Part II: Managing a Therapeutic Regimen

Mr. A. moved to his daughter's home more than a year ago, after a month's stay in the hospital for treatment of a life-threatening urinary infection with sepsis. At the time of discharge, he weighed 98 pounds, but now he weighs 115 pounds. Given his 5-foot, 11-inch frame, he still appears emaciated. He spends most of his time in bed because of weakness. Although alert and communicative, he often asks his daughter, Mrs. Z., to fully interpret conversations between the home health nurse and himself. On rare occasions, he has unpredictable episodes of confusion.

The physician's prescriptions have consisted of daily Lasix, antibiotics that have varied from once to four times a day, and Tylenol with codeine that is to be taken as necessary. Ordered diet is low-salt, regular. There is daily catheter care, including catheter irrigations, plus monthly change of the in-dwelling catheter by the nurse.

Mrs. Z., 46, describes her father as stubborn: He had insisted on living alone after the death of her mother. Because he had managed chronic urinary incontinence by self-catheterization for three years, he was distressed by the need for an in-dwelling catheter. She acknowledges that he is not happy about being "forced" to move from his old neighborhood because he misses his independence and the opportunity to visit with friends at the senior citizens' club. Mrs. Z. describes her husband as being good to her and her father. She works at her husband's shop, where they are very busy, and she does most of her own housework. She goes to great lengths to prevent her husband from knowing the extent of work involved in the care of her father.

Mrs. Z. takes responsibility for administering medications ("I can't trust him"), preparing the diet, and handling some of the catheter management, as well as other aspects of care. On occasion her father does not receive one or more doses because she forgets or finds him asleep when they are due. When he is confused, she has to argue to persuade him to take the pills. She is unable to manage a four-times-a-day routine with her work schedule at the shop, so she gives him medicine three times a day. She was uncomfortable having a health aide in the house when she was not there and finds that her father often neglects to take the noon pill she leaves for him unless she calls from the shop to remind him.

Managing the low-salt diet is not difficult for Mrs. Z. because she already used salt minimally in food preparation. Mr. A. has gained nearly twenty pounds since coming to his daughter's home. At first he was served meals in bed, but now is expected to eat at the table, which he enjoys. There are a snack and water at the bedside for the hours when she is away.

Managing the catheter has been very difficult for both father and daughter. Mr. A. considers the catheter painful, a major handicap, and continually frustrating. He has cut it and removed it twice. A trial self-catheterization was negotiated with the physician, but this lasted only three months until infection recurred. Daily catheter care, which involves cleaning and inspecting the penis and catheter, is stressful for Mrs. Z. Initially she felt she could not look at her father "there," but seemed more comfortable about the irrigations, although she occasionally forgets them. She reluctantly asked her husband to do the daily catheter care until her father gained the ability to manage it himself. She prefers to avoid involving her husband because she does not want him to know the amount of time actually involved in caregiving.

For Mrs. Z., the shifting of roles between assisting and control agent occurs at her father's transitions between confusion and alertness and between varying states of dependency. The organization of time and effort for management of the regimen falls on Mrs. Z. She values her ability to provide care for her father in addition to her commitment to her marriage, home management, and success in the family business.

In a review of compliance studies, Hogue (1979) observed that facilitating participation of clients in their own care (including education) may be more effective in achieving compliance than disseminating information. In studies cited by Hogue (1979), participation in learning included the following:

1. Using knowledge to increase one's level of wellness (Davis, 1976)

2. Contracting with the nurse to change behavior (Sheridan & Smith, 1975)
3. Discussing health, structure, and functioning of the family in relation to experience and abilities for health behavior (Fink, 1969)
4. Receiving social support designed to increase competence and motivation to adhere (Caplan, 1976; Hogue, 1978)
5. Discussing ways to achieve congruence between the regimen and clients' life-styles (Hecht, 1974)

Principles of adult education as defined by Knowles (1970) emphasize the necessity of involvement of adult patients in decisions about what to learn, when to learn, and how to learn. Adults learn best what is clearly relevant and pertinent to them, not to the health care provider. Educative efforts need to be directed to showing the association between recommended behaviors and desired effects that are not obvious or immediate, including those associated with complex regimens (Cohen et al., 1991).

Communication with the child needs to be developmentally appropriate (see Chapter 2, on growth and development). Helping parents learn how to incorporate play into regimens of treatment may promote compliance in children. Instilling fun in therapeutic activities can encourage more participation by the child, since therapeutic play can provide children with an emotional outlet while they learn about their bodies, medical conditions, and treatment protocols (Vessey & Mahon, 1990). For example, developmentally appropriate play can be incorporated into respiratory exercises by tickling or laughing for the infant, blowing whistles for toddlers, blowing bubbles for preschoolers, or playing cotton ball "tetherball" for school-age children.

Recognition that the client's family patterns of communication may differ from the provider's is important for effective interactions. For example, in Hispanic culture "children's autonomy is not encouraged and parent and children do not openly discuss difficult issues" (Kleinman, Eisenberg, & Good, 1988). Nurses, therefore, should teach parents and children from this culture separately and assist the parent in developing explanations that can be more comfortably shared with children. Hispanic women have an important role in controlling health care information and its use in the family; clearly the wife and/or mother needs to be included in compliance-increasing strategies (Ingle, 1993).

Nursing Diagnosis

One of the nursing diagnoses accepted by the North American Nursing Diagnosis Association is *noncompliance.* Carpenito (1993) notes that this diagnosis should be used only with a client who desires to comply and not if assessment reveals a client who has made an informed autonomous decision not to comply. *At risk for noncompliance* is the diagnostic label that can be used if risk factors for noncompliance are present (Carpenito, 1993).

Thus, noncompliance is most appropriate as a diagnosis when the client is not following a treatment regimen because of a lack of resources (personal, material, or social) or because of competing demands (other needs, goals, or concerns) of the client or family. Such demands, commitments, and concerns may compete with those posed by the regimen, as the case study of Mr. M. illustrates. When the client or family caregiver is encouraged to describe daily activities, living conditions, and present concerns, it is more likely that these and other situational factors related to compliance will be identified. For example, the increasing number of aged persons make it likely that a particular caregiver will be more concerned about a loved one's chronic illness than about his or her own health.

There continues to be controversy over the validity of noncompliance as a nursing diagnosis (Whitley, 1991). One concern about this diagnosis is the lack of cultural sensitivity on the provider's part when the client's culture is different and the provider has insufficient understanding of that culture (Geissler, 1991). This concern reflects the major objection to using this diagnosis: possible interference with the right of a client to make informed decisions not to comply.

Encouraging Client Participation

It is generally believed that compliance is increased when clients actively participate in

CASE STUDY

Mr. M.: Competing Demands and Concerns

Mr. M., a 70-year-old business executive, was newly diagnosed with non-insulin–dependent diabetes mellitus (NIDDM). He was educated, alert, and able to solve problems, and he attended classes on diabetes education so he "could learn why and how to follow his regimen." He decided to do home blood glucose monitoring instead of urine testing, but he showed no interest in being compliant about diet and indicated little enthusiasm for changing food intake habits except to omit concentrated sugars.

Only when asked specific questions about his daily schedule, living conditions, and present concerns did he reveal that his attention, energy, and time were completely devoted to his business and to his respirator-dependent wife. His business took most of his daytime hours and he provided direct care to his wife seven nights and four evenings each week. Since her sudden respiratory failure six months earlier, he had learned to manage medicines and respirator and oxygen equipment and to perform other specific therapeutic tasks. He described the dinner hour as "precious time when we can talk about something besides sickness."

Mr. M. identified a number of factors that influenced his noncompliance with diet. First, breakfast was sometimes missed if he slept late. Second, it was difficult to be more consistent in eating lunch at the same time each day because his schedule revolved around his customer's needs, which led to missing this meal frequently. Third, dinner with his wife was the only time either could focus on family matters without interruption, and he did not want to be thinking about what he should be eating at that time. Fourth, he considered his wife's illness and care as more serious and having more immediacy than his own; consequences from his diabetes were seen somewhere in the future, making it easy not to focus on his own care needs. Finally, it was determined that he received little reinforcement from the presence of symptoms or from his physician contact, which was scheduled every three months.

---

learning and deciding how to implement prescribed regimens. However, insistence by the health care provider on a preconceived or stereotyped notion of the most desirable level of participation may be inappropriate. A mismatch between an authoritarian provider and an assertive, active learner may result in poor communication and may influence compliance adversely. On the other hand, a passive and nonactive learner can be overwhelmed by the provider who expects active involvement in the learning and communication processes. Some studies using the locus-of-control construct support different approaches to "externals" and "internals" (see the section "Feelings about Personal Control" earlier in this chapter) and suggest that increasing active participation for "externals" may not be appropriate.

Tailoring The minimal outcome of client participation with the nurse in developing a compliance strategy should be tailoring the treatment to the client's daily behaviors, since this process may help to cue compliance (Haynes, 1979). Integrating treatment activities so that they coincide with routine activities, called rituals, is an important way of individualizing and enhancing the treatment plan. The daily schedule of eating, arising and retiring, hygiene, favorite television program, and so on, identifies rituals that may be used to incorporate health behaviors into daily life.

Simplifying the Regimen As a result of discussion between client and nurse, it may become apparent that the client is unable to manage the complexity of the prescribed regimen. Negotiation with the prescribing source may result in better compliance if this barrier is cleared and the regimen is simplified. As a general rule, the number of times medications are taken and the number of pills should be held to a minimum.

Providing Reminders The use of memory aids should not be overlooked. With the high level of illiteracy in the United States today, the ability to read, tell time, and understand numbers must be assessed before such aids are suggested. Calendars, clocks, and individually prepared posters with medication and food reminders can be very helpful. Separating a day's supply of medications can also help the person who has difficulty remembering if a particular dose was taken.

The health care provider can reinforce the importance of compliance at episodic visits. Such reinforcement may involve pill counting or attention to client diaries or to other reports of behavior and self-monitoring, these are all methods that remind the client of the value of compliance and that elicit participation.

Telephone calls can be useful in reminding patients about health care recommendations, in encouraging compliance with medications in the elderly (Cargill, 1992), and as an effective intervention in enhancing compliance with making and keeping follow-up appointments after referral from emergency departments (Jones, Jones, & Katz, 1987). Telephone calls take less time (about 10 minutes), and when compared with the longer clinical nurse–patient interaction (25 minutes), they make the cost/benefit ratio an important difference (Jones, Jones, & Katz, 1987).

Enhancing Coping The nurse should be very sensitive to clues from individual clients suggesting emotional responses that interfere with learning optimal health behaviors. Situational anxiety, marked depression, and denial are associated with low levels of compliance. These three emotional responses should be interpreted as signals that the client's coping skills are inadequate and that a modification in approach may be more effective. Mrs. T.'s case study illustrates the influence of inadequate coping on compliance.

Contracting Contracting can be viewed as an educational strategy that engages clients' commitment to learn, to make changes, and to be accountable for their own behavior (see Chapter 15, on change agents, and Chapter 16, on teaching). Contracting involves the nurse and client in a collaboratively developed written contract with specified goals and methods and explicitly

identified incentives. Based on principles of behavioral modification, contracting uses reinforcements to establish and maintain new or changed behaviors. Contracting has been successfully used as a strategy to increase compliance in various settings and with different types of behavior (Steckel & Swain, 1981).

Social Support

It is commonly believed that social support—by significant others or support networks—helps clients cope with chronic illness and reinforces compliant behavior. The increase in self-help groups reflects this belief, as does the current practice of referring people to such groups. In spite of this trend, it is unclear from the literature whether these groups increase compliance behaviors.

Clients do not always want tangible help from others. In one study, more subjects reported *receiving* help than *wanting* help with self-care activities (Connell, 1991). Providing unwanted support may result in negative outcomes. Assessment of the relationship between potential support providers and recipients may determine whether support is perceived to be helpful or unhelpful (Connell, 1991).

Parents are often seen as the primary social support for the ill child; receiving social support from others enables parents to continuously provide needed care for the child (Cohen et al., 1991). It is also useful to have elderly clients identify others to assist them. "Forgetting" was the most common reason for missed doses among community-dwelling older adults, with more than half reporting that the tendency to forget medications was counteracted by assistance from others (Conn, Taylor, & Stineman, 1992).

Social isolation is associated with low compliance; a supportive family, with high compliance (Haynes, 1979) (see Chapter 8, on social isolation). Elderly women with social supports were found to adhere to medical regimens; assessing the strengths and weaknesses of the individual client's supportive networks is therefore important (Chang et al., 1985). The findings of these authors did not support the stereotype that

CASE STUDY
Client Participation

Mrs. T., a 51-year-old practical nurse, was referred to a diabetic education program because she had been unable to manage her weight, then over 200 pounds, and because she needed insulin therapy. She cried as she expressed feelings of failure and shame. She agreed to share information about her living conditions so a plan could be developed to attain two goals: weight reduction and better control of blood glucose levels. An interview revealed the following:

1. She experienced feelings of discomfort ("feeling panic") when visiting the physician.
2. She had had feelings of anxiety and stress since her husband's heart attack two years earlier. She had performed cardiopulmonary resuscitation at home at that time.
3. She needed to "keep busy" so she did not have time to worry about her husband. She did this by working twelve-hour night shifts on weekends and maintaining a busy social schedule and housework during the week. Even though she did not have to work for the income it provided, she noted that the activity kept her from worrying: "I'm so afraid to be alone with my husband in case he has another cardiac arrest."
4. She had an excellent knowledge level of calorie and nutrient content of foods and could perform blood glucose monitoring and insulin injections.
5. She actively sought information and help: participation in many weight reduction programs over the years with successful loss of weight each time.
6. She recognized that maintenance of weight loss was a problem and that she had not learned effective strategies to achieve weight control.

Several situational factors were identified. First, daily insulin therapy was a hazard, given Mrs. T.'s day-and-night schedule. Her schedule also violated the need for consistency in daily activities that were essential in helping her achieve better control. The nurse's planning with the client and physician resulted in these strategies:

1. continued involvement in the diabetic education program to integrate needed changes into her life
2. supportive counseling to help her gain coping skills via referral to a mental health center
3. a month's leave of absence from work as a trial period of consistent daily activities
4. discussion by client and physician of the helping relationship desired by both

The client followed through on these plans. Six weeks later, the physician reported that Mrs. T. had better control of blood glucose, had shown some weight loss, and was asking for a permanent change in work schedule. It was clear that these outcomes were achieved because Mrs. T. was able to implement changes in her life.

widowed and single people have fewer supportive networks than married persons.

For some persons, support groups promotes better understanding of medical regimens and better compliance, but their efficacy in enhancing compliance is unclear. In one study the support group was an adjunct to an educational program, which may have facilitated behaviors thought to evolve in support groups: individual self-disclosure, mutual comparison, interpersonal feedback, and so forth (Maxwell, Hunt, & Bush, 1992).

Summary and Conclusions

Compliance in chronic illness is an important area of consideration for researchers and practitioners. Several issues and problems relevant to the development and ethical use of effective compliance strategies have been discussed: barriers to the study of compliance, variables affecting compliance, the state of current knowledge about compliance, the impact of differences in expectations of clients and providers, motivation, and ethical issues. Research in compliance is currently focusing on models that explain and, to some degree, predict compliance: health beliefs, self-efficacy, reasoned behavior, and health promotion. Several of these models and theoretical frameworks were presented to provide guidance.

The chapter has proposed that assessment include the client's and family's living conditions, demands, commitments, and concerns in order to gain the client's perspective of living with chronic illness and implementing health care recommendations. In this way the provider can more effectively engage the client in problem solving. Assessment and interactions may be directed to the individual client; when assistance is needed or disabilities are marked, family members must be the focus.

The importance of various strategies that increase client participation has been noted: tailoring, simplifying the regimen, providing reminders, enhancing coping skills, education, contracting, and social support. An important concern for client and provider is determining the optimal level of compliance appropriate to the situation.

Given the increasing numbers of chronically ill individuals, the importance of adherence to necessary regimens becomes obvious. Responsibility for management falls to the client or family on a day-to-day basis. The provider is responsible for ensuring that the client or family has the needed knowledge, motivation, and skills. Another provider responsibility is helping the client to find ways to make compliance more feasible. Through research, assessment, and strategies that are presented in a nonjudgmental way, the effective performance of compliant behavior can be accomplished.

NURSING DIAGNOSIS

5.2.1.1. Noncompliance (specify)

Definition: A person's informed decision not to adhere to a therapeutic recommendation.

Defining Characteristics: *Behavior[2] indicative of failure to adhere (by direct observation or by statements of patient or significant others); objective tests (physiological measures, detection or markers); evidence of development of complications; evidence of exacerbation of symptoms; failure to keep appointments; failure to progress.

Related Factors: Patient value system; health beliefs, cultural influences, spiritual values; client-provider relationships

Editor's Note: The definition noted above for this nursing diagnosis has remained unchanged since 1973 when the diagnosis became part of the original NANDA taxonomy. It continues to be fraught with problems, since every client has a right not

to adhere to a therapeutic recommendation. To negate this right is not supportable ethically even if the health provider does not agree with that decision. The key word to consider is that the client be *informed.*

Carpenito's definition (1993) of noncompliance is "The state in which an individual or group *desires to comply but is prevented from doing so by factors that deter adherence* to health-related advice given by health professionals (p. 498). She also notes that this category should be used only when a client desires to comply, but cannot because of factors that prevent him or her from doing so. Only if the desire to comply exists can the nurse intervene ethically. (Emphasis is that of the editor.)

Carpenito also adds the following as a major defining characteristic, which she feels must be present: "Verbalization of noncompliance or nonparticipation or confusion about therapy and/or direct observation of behavior indicating compliance" (p 498). She also suggests the following as etiologies or related factors: anxiety, negative side effects of prescribed treatment, and unknown etiology. Although the last is not nurse treatable, the rest of Carpenito's changes seem appropriate and should be considered by NANDA.

---

[2]The asterisk denotes critical defining characteristics.

STUDY QUESTIONS

1. Why is trying to increase compliant behaviors important for clients who are chronically ill?
2. What factors are involved in compliance? Discuss them.
3. Do you agree that *compliance* and *noncompliance* are terms as acceptable as *adherence* and *nonadherence?* Why?
4. How prevalent is noncompliance? What are the problems of trying to determine the extent of noncompliance?
5. What are the methodological barriers to the study of compliance? What is the relationship of single variables to compliance? What conceptual barriers exist?
6. If you were given a choice, which conceptual model would you prefer to provide support for a study on noncompliance? Explain your preference, citing examples to defend it.
7. How do clients and providers differ in their expectations about participation? Discuss different models that are useful for client participation.
8. What is the difference between internal and external locus of control? How does this difference affect compliance?
9. What are the differences in client and provider perspectives of the facets involved in managing medical regimens?
10. What ethical issues arise when a provider tries to increase a client's compliance? Discuss an ethical approach.
11. Using your own or a client's culture, identify how norms, rituals, and practices affect compliance with health care recommendations.
12. How does motivation influence compliance? How does the health belief model affect a client's motivation?
13. What are the strengths and weaknesses of education as a means of increasing compliance?
14. Given a client situation, what factors would you assess to gain a thorough picture of potential compliance or noncompliance? Discuss assessment from this perspective.
15. What are the factors that allow you to use the nursing diagnosis of noncompliance?
16. How can you encourage client participation to increase compliance? Discuss tailoring, simplifying the regimen, and reminders.
17. How can you enhance coping to increase compliance?
18. What are the advantages and disadvantages of contracting? of support groups?

References

Anderson, J. M., Blue, C., & Lau, A. (1993). Women's perspectives on chronic illness: Ethnicity, ideology and restructuring of life. *Diabetes Spectrum, 6*(2), 102-115.

Anderson, R. M. (1985). Is the problem of noncompliance all in our head? *Diabetes Educator, 11,* 31-34.

AAN Expert Panel on Culturally Competent Nursing Care (1992). Culturally competent nursing care. *Nursing Outlook, 40*(6), 277-283.

Baric, L. (1969). Recognition of the "at-risk" role: A means to influence health behavior. *International Journal of Health Education, 12,* 24-34.

Barofsky, I. (1978). Compliance, adherence, and the therapeutic alliance: Steps in the development of self-care. *Social Science and Medicine, 12,* 369-376.

Barry, V. (1982). *Moral aspects of health care.* Belmont, CA: Wadsworth.

Becker. M. H. (1974a). A new approach to explaining sick-role behavior in low-income populations. *American Journal of Public Health, 64,* 205-216.

———— (1974b). The health belief model and sick-role behavior. *Health Education Monograph, 2,* 409-419.

———— (1976). Socio-behavioral determinants of compliance. In D. L. Sackett, & R. Haynes (Eds.), *Compliance with therapeutic regimens.* Baltimore: Johns Hopkins University Press.

Becker, M. H. & Janz, N. K. (1985). The health belief model applied to understanding diabetes regimen compliance. *Diabetes Educator, 11,* 41-47.

Becker, M. H., & Maiman, L. A. (1975). Sociobehavioral determinants of compliance with health and medical care recommendations. *Medical Care, 13,* 10-24.

———— (1978). Models of health-related behavior (pp. 539-566). In D. Mechanic (Ed.), *Medical sociology* (2nd ed.). New York: Free Press.

Black, S. (1992). Preoperative self-efficacy and postoperative behaviors. *Applied Nursing Research, 5*(3), 134-139.

Blackwell, B. (1979). The drug regimen and treatment compliance. In R. B. Haynes, D. W. Taylor, & D. L. Sackett, (Eds.), *Compliance in Health Care* (pp. 144-156). Baltimore: Johns Hopkins University Press.

Cargill, J. M. (1992). Medication compliance in elderly people: Influencing variables and interventions. *Journal of Advanced Nursing, 17*(4), 422-426.

Carpenito, L. J. (1993). *Nursing diagnosis: Application to clinical practice* (5th ed.). Philadelphia: J. B. Lippincott.

Chang, L., Uman, G., Linn, L., Ware, J., & Kane, R. (1985). Adherence to health care regimens among elderly women. *Nursing Research, 34,* 27-31.

Cohen, B., Kagan, L., Richter, B., Topor, M., & Saveedra, M. (1991). Children's compliance to dialysis. *Pediatric Nursing 17*(4), 359-368.

Conn, V., Taylor, S. G., & Stineman, A. (1992). Medication management by recently hospitalized older adults. *Journal of Community Health Nursing, 9*(1), 1-11.

Connell, C. M. (1991) Psychosocial contexts of diabetes and older adulthood: Reciprocal effects. *The Diabetes Educator, 17*(5) 364-371.

Connelly, C. E. (1984). Economic and ethical issues in patient compliance. *Nursing Economics, 2,* 342-347.

Corbin, J. M., & Strauss, A. L. (1984). Collaboration: Couples working to manage chronic illness, *Image: The Journal of Nursing Scholarhip 16*(4), 109-115.

Dimond, M., & Jones, S. L. (1983). *Chronic illness across the life span.* Norwalk, CT: Appleton-Century-Crofts.

Dracup, K. A., & Meleis, A. I. (1982). Compliance: An interactionist approach. *Nursing Research, 31,* 32-35.

Fawcett, J. (1984). *Analysis and evaluation of conceptual models of nursing.* Philadelphia: F. A. Davis.

Fleury, J. (1992). The application of motivational theory to cardiovascular risk reduction. *Image: The Journal of Nursing Scholarship, 24*(3), 229-239.

Friedman, M. (1990). Transcultural family nursing: Application to Latino and Black Families. *Journal of Pediatric Nursing, 5*(3), 214-221.

Geissler, E. M. (1991). Transcultural nursing and nursing diagnoses. *Nursing and Health Care, 12*(4), 190-192.

Gillam, R. F. & Barsky, A. J. (1974). Diagnosis and management of patient noncompliance. *Journal of the American Medical Association, 228,* 1563-1567.

Gonzalez, J. (1990). Factors relating to frequency among low-income Mexican American women: Implications for nursing practice. *Cancer Nursing, 13,* 134-142.

Gordis, L. (1979). Conceptual and methodologic problems in measuring patient compliance. In R. B. Haynes, D. W. Taylor, & D. L. Sackett, (Eds.), *Compliance in health care* (pp. 23-48). Baltimore: Johns Hopkins University Press.

Green, L. W. (1979). Educational strategies to improve compliance with therapeutic and preventive regimens: The recent evidence. In R. B. Haynes, D. W. Taylor, & D. L. Sackett (Eds.), *Compliance in health care* (pp. 157-173). Baltimore: Johns Hopkins University Press.

Hallel, J. (1975). The relationship of health beliefs, health locus of control, and self concept to the practice of breast self-examination in adult women. *Nursing Research, 31,* 137-142.

Harrison, J. S., Mullen, P. D., & Green, L. W. (1992). A meta-analysis of studies of the Health Belief Model with adults. *Health-Education-Research, 4*(1), 107-116.

Haynes, R. B. (1979). Determinants of compliance: The disease and the mechanics of treatment. In R. B. Haynes, D. W. Taylor, & D. L. Sackett (Eds.). *Compliance in health care* (pp. 49-62). Baltimore: Johns Hopkins University Press.

Hellenbrandt, D. (1983). An analysis of compliance behavior: A response to powerlessness. In J. F. Miller (Ed.), *Coping with chronic illness* (pp. 215-243). Philadelphia: F. A. Davis.

Hingson, R., Scotch, N., Sorenson, J., and Swazey, J. (1981). *In sickness and in health.* St. Louis: C. V. Mosby.

Hogue, C. C. (1979). Nursing and compliance. In R. B. Haynes, D. W. Taylor, & D. L. Sackett (Eds.), *Compliance in health care* (pp. 247-259). Baltimore: Johns Hopkins University Press.

Hulka, B. S., Cassel, J. C., Kupper, L. L., & Burdette, J. A. (1976). Communication, compliance, and concordance between physicians and patients with prescribed medications. *American Journal of Public Health, 66,* 847-853.

Ingle, K. L. (1993, July). Surgeon General broadcasts diabetes message to Hispanics. *Diabetes Forecast, 15*(8), 44-46.

Jones, P. K., Jones, S. L., & Katz, J. (1987, September). Improving follow-up among hypertensive patients using a health belief model intervention. *Archives of Internal Medicine, 147,* 1557-1560.

——— (1988). Health Belief Model intervention to increase compliance with emergency department patients. *Medical Care, 26*(12), 1172-1183.

Jonsen, A. R. (1979). Ethical issues in compliance. In R. B. Haynes, D. W. Taylor, & D. L. Sackett, (Eds.), *Compliance in health care* (pp. 113-120). Baltimore: Johns Hopkins University Press.

Kasl, S. V. (1974). The health belief model and behavior related to chronic illness. *Health Education Monograph, 2,* 433-454.

Kasl, S. V., & Cobb, S. (1966). Health behavior, illness behavior, and sick role behavior. *Archives of Environmental Health, 12,* 246-266.

Kasl, S. V. (1978). Social and psychological factors affecting the course of disease. In D. Mechanic (Ed.), *Medical sociology* (2nd ed.). New York: Free Press.

Kleinman, A., Eisenberg, L., & Good, B. (1988). Culture, illness, and care. *Annals of Internal Medicine, 88*(2), 251-258.

Knowles, M. S. (1970). *The modern practice of adult education.* New York: Association Press.

Marston, M. V. (1970). Compliance with medical regimens: A review of the literature. *Nursing Research, 19,* 312-323.

Maxwell, A. E., Hunt. I., & Bush, M. A. (1992). Effects of a social support group as an adjunct to diabetes training on metabolic control and psychosocial outcomes. *The Diabetes Educator, 18*(4), 303-309.

Moree, N. A. (1984). Nurses speak out on patients and drug regimens. *American Journal of Nursing, 85,* 51-54.

Mulaik, J. S. (1992). Noncompliance with medication regimens in severely and persistently mentally ill schizophrenic patients. *Issues in Mental Health Nursing, 13*(3), 219-237.

Munet-Villaro, F., & Vessey, J. A. (1990). Children's explanation of leukemia. *Journal of Pediatric Nursing, 5*(4), 274-282.

Murphy, K. G., Anderson, R. M., & Lyns, A. E. (1993). Diabetes educators as cultural translators. *The Diabetes Educator, 19*(2), 113-118.

Oberle, K. (1991). A decade of research in locus of control: What have we learned? *Journal of Advanced Nursing, 16*(7), 800-806.

Parsons, T. (1951). *The social system.* New York: Free Press.

Pender, N. J. (1987). *Health promotion in nursing practice* (2nd ed.). Norwalk: Appleton-Century-Crofts.

Rotter, J. B. (1966). Generalized expectancies for internal versus external control of reinforcement. *Psychological Monographs, 80,* 1-28.

Sackett, D. L. (1976). Introduction. In D. L. Sackett & R. B. Haynes (Eds.). *Compliance with therapeutic regimens* (pp. 1-6). Baltimore: Johns Hopkins University Press.

Sackett, D. L., & Snow, J. C. (1979). The magnitude of compliance and noncompliance. In R. B. Haynes, D. W. Taylor, & D. L. Sackett (Eds.), *Compliance in health care* (pp. 11-22). Baltimore: Johns Hopkins University Press.

Schroeder, P. S., & Miller, J. F. (1983). Qualitative study of locus of control in patients with peripheral vascular disease. In J. F. Miller, (Ed.), *Coping with chronic illness,* Philadelphia: F. A. Davis.

Schwartz, D., Wang, M., Zettz, L., & Goss, M. E. (1962). Medication errors made by elderly, chronically ill patients. *American Journal of Public Health, 52,* 2018-2029.

Smith, K. E., & Schreiner, B. (1993). Teaching assertive communication skills to adolescents with diabetes: Evaluation of a camp curriculum. *The Diabetes Educator, 19*(2), 136-141.

Steckel, S. B., & Swain, M. A. (1981). Contracting with patients to improve compliance. *Hospitals: Journal of American Hospital Association, 51,* 81-84.

Stone, G. C. (1979). Patient compliance and the role of the expert. *Journal of Social Issues, 35,* 34-59.

Strauss, A. L., Corbin, J., Fagerhaugh, S., Glaser, B., Maines, D., Suczek, B., & Wiener, C. (1984). *Chronic illness and the quality of life* (2nd ed.). St. Louis: C. V. Mosby.

Szasz, T. S., & Hollander, M. H. (1956). A contribution in the philosophy of medicine. *Archives of Internal Medicine, 97,* 585-592.

Thorne, S. E. (1990, October). Constructive noncompliance in chronic illness. *Holistic Nursing Practice, 5*(1), 62-69.

Vessey, J. A., & Mahon, B. B. (1990). Therapeutic play and the hospitalized child. *Journal of Pediatric Nursing, 5*(5), 332-339.

Wallston, B., Wallston, K., Kaplan, G., & Maides, S. (1976). Development and validation of the health care locus of control scale. *Journal of Consulting and Clinical Psychology, 44,* 580-585.

Wallston, K., Wallston, B., & DeVellis, R. (1978). Development of the multidimensional health locus of control (MHLC) scales. *Health Education Monograph, 6,* 160-170.

Whatley, J. H. (1991). Effects of health locus of control and social network on adolescent risk taking. *Pediatric Nursing, 17*(2).

Whitley, G. G. (1991). Noncompliance: An update. *Issues in Mental-Health Nursing, 12*(3), 229-238.

Wooldridge, K. L., Wallston, K. A., Graber, A. L., Brown, A. W., & Davidson, P. (1992). The relationship between health beliefs, adherence and metabolic control of diabetes. *The Diabetes Educator, 18*(6), 495-500.

Wysocki, T., & Wayne, W. (1992). Childhood diabetes and the family. *Practical Diabetology, 11*(2), 29-32.

Bibliography

Ajzen, L. (1985). From intention to action: A theory of planned behavior. In J. Kuhl & J. Beckman (Eds.), *Action control: From cognition to behavior.* Heidelberg: Springer.

Anderson, J., & Kirk, L. M. (1982). Methods of improving patient compliance in chronic disease states. *Archives of Internal Medicine, 142,* 1673-1675.

Anderson, R., Fitzgerald, J. T., & Oh, M. S. (1993). The relationship between diabetes-related attitudes and patient's self-reported adherence. *The Diabetes Educator 19*(4), 287-292.

Blackwell, B. (1976). Treatment adherence: A contemporary overview, *Psychosomatics, 20,* 27-35.

Bloom, B. S. (1971). *Taxonomy of educational objectives: Cognitive domain,* New York: David McKay.

Bushy, A. (1992). Cultural considerations for primary health care: Where do self-care and folk medicine fit? *Holistic Nursing Practice, 6*(3), 10-18.

Fink, D. L. (1976). Tailoring the consensual regimen. In D. L. Sackett, & R. R. Haynes (Eds.), *Compliance with therapeutic regimens* (pp. 110-118). Baltimore: Johns Hopkins University Press.

Fink, D., Malloy, M. J., Cohen, M., Greycould, M. A., & Martin, F. (1979). Effective patient care in the pediatric ambulatory setting: A study of acute care clinic. *Pediatrics, 43,* 927-935.

Gordon, M. (1989). *Manual of nursing diagnosis.* St. Louis: C. V. Mosby.

Levine S., & Kozlaff, M. (1978). The sick role: Assessment and overview. *Annual Review of Sociology, 4,* 317.

Mechanic, D., & Voikart, E. (1961). Stress, illness behavior, and the sick role. *American Sociological Review, 26,* 51-58.

Sackett, D. L. (1979). Methods for compliance research. In R. B. Haynes, D. W., Taylor, & D. L. Sackett (Eds.), *Compliance in health care* (pp. 323-333). Baltimore: Johns Hopkins University Press.

Simons, M. R. (1992). Interventions related to compliance. *Nursing Clinics of North America, 27*(2), 477-492.

Vincent, P. (1971). Factors influencing patient noncompliance: A theoretical approach. *Nursing Research, 20,* 509-670.

CHAPTER 11

Coping with Fear and Grieving

Arlene Miller Kahn

Introduction

The onset of chronic illness is a major life crisis that not only poses a formidable challenge to a previously workable adaptation to life (Feldman, 1974) but also provides little possibility of complete return to the pre-illness state. Because of the illness's long-term nature, major changes must be made in the way life is conducted. Both client and family have to incorporate multiple tasks into their daily living style, including carrying out medical regimens, controlling symptoms, preventing medical crises, learning how to normalize interactions with others despite the intrusive aspects of the illness, preventing or adjusting to social isolation, and managing the financial burdens imposed by the illness (Strauss, 1984). This implies life-style changes for clients and their significant others and requires adoption of other coping skills than those needed for acute or limited illness.

An understanding of the concept of coping and how it manifests itself in a given client is crucial to appropriate health care. Such an understanding makes it possible to accurately assess the client's needs and help the client manage both the stress and the illness more effectively.

Definitions of Coping

People cope in all situations and under all conditions, not just when they are ill, so any definition must be broad based. Unfortunately, because of underlying theoretical differences, there is significant disagreement regarding the parameters to be used in defining coping. One school of thought restricts coping to those conscious and overt behaviors that foster adaptation. (Meyers et al., 1977). Others believe that the inclusion of unconscious intrapsychic processes—for example, defense mechanisms—as part of the coping process is appropriate because they take the unmanageable threat out of the illness situation until the individual can deal with it realistically (Moos & Tsu, 1977).

A review of the coping literature led Lazarus (1966) to conclude that coping should be viewed as a general term; he felt that defense mechanisms describe a process in which anticipation of harm is dealt with through psychological means rather than directly. The client deceives himself or herself somewhat about the actual reality, producing a benign appraisal of reality rather than a threatening one.

A definition of coping, originally offered by Lazarus and Launier (1978), has been adopted for use here:

> . . . efforts, both action-oriented and intrapsychic, to manage (i.e. master, tolerate, reduce, minimize) environmental and internal demands and conflicts among them which tax or exceed a person's resources (p. 311).

Applying this definition to the chronically ill person, one could say that coping constitutes all ways that are used to minimize threats to personal integrity and emotional equilibrium while simultaneously maximizing body function. One could say that if a diagnosis of chronic illness is perceived as being a significant threat to one's self-concept and life-style, the client may take direct action to reduce the threat and/or automatically use defense mechanisms that reduce the emotional effects of the threat, deny the actual condition, or deny its importance.

Factors Affecting Coping

The coping abilities of clients and their significant others are affected by premorbid personality and adjustment, current developmental stage, the meaning of the illness, and available social support resources. Each of these factors will be addressed in relation to their influence on the client's and family's adaptation to chronic illness.

Premorbid Personality and Adjustment During the course of living, all persons develop unique but characteristic modes of managing life stresses, which constitute their premorbid personality and adjustment. These can be either socially and personally adequate or unsatisfactory. In their efforts to adjust to the onset of chronic illness, individuals invoke previously successful patterns of adaptation or resort to familiar but maladaptive patterns. The more maladjusted the premorbid personality, the more pathological will be the reaction to disease (Parets, 1967). The shy and somewhat withdrawn child may become even more withdrawn and isolated in relationships with others. The very suspicious adult may show a heightening of projection even to the extent that severe distortion of reality occurs. The significance of premorbid personality and adjustment speaks to the oft-quoted statement that it is more important to know what kind of patient has the disease than what kind of disease the patient has (Coleman, 1973).

The family unit's premorbid adjustment is also significant in adapting to one of its member's chronic illness. A family that is reasonably stable is more likely to meet the crisis of chronic illness in an adaptive manner. Conversely, families with a history of poor premorbid adjustment will have more difficulty making a good adaptation (Steinhauer et al., 1974). In his study of cancer patients, Weisman (1976) found that those who coped poorly had histories of pessimism, regrets about the past, and a tendency to feel worthless and destructive. In addition, they came from families with many problems and reported a number of current marital problems.

Developmental Stage Erikson (1963) posited the existence of sequentially unfolding stages for human development, each characterized by a central conflict and the need to master key developmental tasks to move on to further personal growth (see Chapter 2, on growth and development). The manner in which this conflict is resolved influences the individual's future development, adaptation to internal and external demands, and self-evaluation.

The chronically ill client's developmental stage has a significant impact on his or her ability to cope with the stresses of the illness (Larkin, 1987). In addition, illness can impair the client's ability to master tasks required of present and future developmental stages, leaving the client with specific vulnerabilities. Illness can also cause the client to invoke coping strategies used during prior, unresolved developmental stage conflicts. When this happens, behavior is seen that appears to be quite uncharacteristic.

Chronic illness often restricts important physical activities necessary for successful resolution of specific stage conflicts. The child who is just learning to walk is affected by a chronic illness that curtails movement or makes movement painful. Such impediments to mastery are particularly significant for the child because specific skills need to be mastered in relatively short periods of time (National Institutes of Health, 1982). Loss of these opportunities may slow or even distort current and future development.

Parental overprotection can prevent the child from developing a real sense of independence. If children are seen and treated as "normal" there is decreased likelihood that a developmental stage will be impaired (Steinhauer et al., 1974). To enhance development, parents should maintain normal discipline, provide a sense of social acceptability, set appropriate boundaries to the child's behavior, and provide emotional support. Health professionals can help parents with these tasks by stressing the similarity of their child to normal children (Moos & Tsu, 1977).

It is not always easy to specify how to help the chronically ill without interfering with developmental stages. For example, a chronically ill middle-aged adult male may be unable to provide parental responsibility or financial support for himself or his family, both necessary for successful resolution of conflicts inherent in the developmental stage of generativity. The client's family may have to assume these roles, leading to consequent loss of his self-esteem and resulting in his regression to self-absorption and stagnation. The task of balancing reality with illness needs, while encouraging normal developmental functioning, is a very difficult one.

The presence within a family unit of someone with a chronic illness may interfere with other members' mastery of their own developmental tasks, as well as making it difficult for them to provide an environment to meet the client's developmental needs (Eisenberg et al., 1984). For example, the demands of caring for a 50-year-old woman with Alzheimer's disease can be so great as to preclude her caregiver husband's mastery of tasks associated with his stage of generativity.

Both illness needs and developmental needs must be considered to achieve the most constructive balance between them. Assessment must include both the impact a developmental stage has on the client and family's ability to cope with a chronic illness and the impact the illness has on the ability to master a developmental stage. Failure to show behaviors appropriate to each person's respective developmental stage can indicate maladaptive coping. In the case of the Alzheimer's client cited above, suggestions might be made to use respite care and encourage other family members to relieve the primary caregiver, giving him time to participate in the activities necessary to master his developmental stage.

Meaning of the Illness   The significance and implications of illness differ with each person and family and affect coping behavior. A relatively benign chronic illness may be interpreted by a client or family as very threatening. Conversely, a serious chronic illness may be minimized by either client or family or both. In either case, coping behaviors will be partially based on interpretations of the illness's significance.

It is not the stress of illness that is of uppermost importance but rather the individual's cognitive appraisal of it (Lazarus, 1974). If the illness is viewed as significant, heightened anxiety and depression are more likely to manifest themselves in an attempt to cope; if the illness is viewed as insignificant, the client will feel less personally threatened and will have greater energy for dealing with the problems presented by the illness (Miller, 1992). For some clients, an illness may provide desired relief from other roles or an opportunity to receive service or attention that may otherwise be absent or perceived as absent.

Health professionals need to remain highly aware of their own perceptions of various chronic illnesses, since personal biases can cause a lack of awareness of inadequate evaluation of the stresses being experienced by the client. The health provider may see hypertension as an easily treatable condition with a good prognosis, while the client may feel it implies a severe and depressing decline in bodily functioning (see Chapter 3, on illness trajectory). An accurate evaluation of the client's perception enhances the therapeutic relationship and the health provider's ability to develop with the client a realistic perception of the illness and appropriate means of coping.

Some clients or families bring to any illness long-standing misconceptions of its nature, prognosis, and cause. Different cultures have different mythologies concerning various illnesses, their significance, and their outcomes, which can lead to anxieties. To be effective, the health professional should understand what the illness is like for the client and family, so that needed corrective information can be supplied if necessary.

Social Support   The terms *social network* and *social support* are sometimes used interchangeably in the coping literature and elsewhere. These terms can be differentiated by the following definitions: *social networks* are the interpersonal ties of family, friends, neighbors, coworkers, health professionals, and others who provide support to the person in need; *social support* refers to the actual psychosocial and tangible aid provided by the social network (Tilden & Weinert, 1987).

Chronic illness can significantly affect both the social network and the quality of social support normally received by a person. Some illnesses severely deplete the energy reserves an individual ordinarily uses to maintain a social network. Other illnesses reduce the time available for social contacts because of the need to control symptoms and to carry out illness-related regimens. Chronic illnesses that cause mobility problems can lead to social isolation.

Social support can exert a major influence on a client's ability to cope with a chronic illness. An individual's coping responses during crises are influenced not only by his or her ego strength, but also by the quality of service and emotional support provided by the social network. Social support buffers the stresses of chronic illness and increases the client's ability to deal effectively with them.

Social support takes many forms (Tilden & Weinert, 1987) and can provide a client with emotional support through love, caring, and general affirmation of self-worth. It can offer informational support through useful suggestions and knowledge needed to solve many of the problems generated by a chronic illness. It can provide tangible goods and task-oriented assistance.

The perceived stigma of an illness (see Chapter 5, on stigma) can prevent some clients from seeking support from the very persons who can help them reaffirm their worth as valued human beings. Family members and friends may feel excluded from the care process and may not realize how important they can be in helping the client to adapt. They need both information and assistance to realize how they can be an extension of the clinical team. Family members can provide support for adaptive coping, encourage compliance with medical regimens, and support behaviors that are consistent with minimizing the effects of the illness (Burish & Bradley, 1983).

The support network may have difficulty coping with the burdens inherent in the illness situation. Emotionally, it is painful to see a loved one experience so many losses. Personality changes in the client, such as the expression of unexpected anger, make social interaction and the provision of supportive care a difficult task. The severe physical and financial demands imposed by chronic illness and the personal difficulties some have coping with it may also cause the social network to withdraw. These problems have to be addressed before members of the social network are able to provide essential support to the client.

When the realities of an illness dictate that the client adjust to having fewer social interactions, new modified sources for social support will have to be discovered along with the types of support each can provide (Tilden & Weinert, 1987).

There are at least two significant reasons for clients to provide whatever support they can. First, social networks are reciprocal systems, making it important for the client to participate both as a "giver" and a "receiver" to keep the network intact. Second, "giving back" enhances self-esteem by automatically validating the client's worth even as a "damaged" person.

Every opportunity should be provided to help clients preserve existing relationships with friends and family members who help satisfy their physical and emotional needs. In addition, opportunity should be available to foster the development of new relationships if appropriate. When evaluating the support system needs of a client, consideration should be given to such preexisting resources as religious organizations, self-help groups, and health care agencies.

Adaptive versus Maladaptive Coping

Controversy exists in differentiating adaptive from maladaptive coping strategies, given the enormous variations possible in individual coping styles and responses to illness and treatment demands (McGrath, 1970). What proves effective in one situation may be ineffective or maladaptive for the same individual in another. Similarly, coping strategies that are effective in the short run may become maladaptive if used for too long or exclusively. Finally, what might be effective coping for one individual can be ineffective or maladaptive for another.

Some judge coping to be effective if it protects the individual from overwhelming psychological stresses, even if it is socially or medically undesirable (Meyers et al., 1977). Yet great harm can come to the individual in complete denial who does not obtain appropriate and needed medical help. Others judge coping behavior in terms of the individual's ability to carry out socially or medically desirable goals irrespective of any psychological distress the client may experience.

The health provider's personal value judgment regarding what constitutes "correct coping" is another consideration in evaluating the adaptive merits of any coping strategy (Garland & Bush, 1982). Such personalization hinders the health professional from assessing the total impact of a client's coping method on his or her actual well-being. The compliant patient is seen as a "good client" who is "coping correctly" because no immediate management problems are posed. However, this client may be so internally stressed that adaptation to the illness is only superficial and it could eventually have an adverse impact on overall improvement (Weisman, 1976).

Coping is described as effective when it:

1. Resolves the disturbed affect associated with threat and loss

2. Preserves the physical integrity of the client.
3. Helps to maintain relationships and life roles.
4. Preserves a positive self-concept.

While such criteria help clarify the adaptive end of the coping continuum, the health provider needs to determine when a coping strategy ceases to be adaptive and becomes an impediment to further development (Miller, 1992).

Coping responses become maladaptive when any of the following conditions are present:

1. Essential treatment is not sought by the client or is impeded by virtue of the client's emotional state.
2. Attempts at coping cause more client stress than does the disease itself.
3. The coping response impedes activities of everyday living or causes the abandonment of the client's usual sources of personal gratification.
4. The coping responses give rise to psychiatric symptoms, such as severe distortion of reality or clinically significant depression (Senescu, 1963).

Understanding the criteria at the extreme ends of the coping continuum allows the health professional to make sound judgments as to whether coping responses will have adaptive or maladaptive consequences for each client. Accurate assessment determines if a given coping response should be reinforced and supported or if another intervention is needed to help the client cope.

Emotional Reactions to Chronic Illness

The psychological impact of chronic illness is largely underrated by the health care team, clients, and society (Lambert & Lambert, 1987), even though chronic illnesses produce profound psychological effects that dramatically tax the client's and family's resources (Strauss, 1984; Miller, 1992). While most clients will acknowledge the physical effects of a chronic illness, perception of its emotional sequelae is far less frequently accepted (Green, 1985). Emotional effects that are acknowledged by health professionals are treated as transient and unusual events not worthy of attention or follow-up.

Emotional responses to chronic illness vary with different phases of illness and treatment. Many chronic illnesses are episodic in nature, with acute flare-ups giving rise to such feelings as fear, profound sadness, and anger. Unfortunately, these emotional states often go unrecognized until they complicate the treatment process, a situation commonly seen when depression becomes so severe that the client becomes neglectful of needed treatment or creates a negative feedback loop that results in psychological deterioration (Green, 1985).

The two major responses to be covered in this chapter are fear and grieving. Although the content is presented largely from the client's point of view, many of these same responses are also experienced by the client's significant others. In spite of a commonality of emotional responses to chronic illness, a multitude of factors converge in the minds of clients that cause them to perceive, evaluate, and defend against loss of health in an extremely subjective manner (Green, 1985). Because each client forms a unique understanding of his or her illness, the following discussion should be viewed only as a general guide to assessing emotional responses to chronic illness.

Fear

Fear is activated when a person is physically or psychologically exposed to a threatening situation that can be identified and described (Stuart & Sundeen, 1991). Fear is a major psychological response of chronic illness (Parets, 1967; Strain, 1979) based on fact and reality, such as frequent hospitalizations, painful treatment, or repeated surgery (Steinhauer et al., 1974). The chronically ill are faced with potential threats that tax their ability to carry out even routine activities. Many chronic illnesses are characterized by an exacerbation of symptoms that can have serious consequences on the life-style of

the client. Both the anticipation and the reality of an exacerbation can generate fear.

Fear can be either adaptive or maladaptive. As an adaptive mechanism fear, (1) alerts the client to seek medical attention when new symptoms or exacerbations occur, (2) helps the client anticipate the stressors of chronic illness, and (3) mobilizes problem solving and other strategies to cope with the identified stressors.

Fear becomes maladaptive when it is more intense or of greater duration than is warranted by a particular stress (Green, 1985). In such a circumstance, fear no longer serves the purpose of alerting the client; it actually causes a decline in adaptive functioning. Preoccupation with the illness occurs, or great significance is given to even minor or transient sensations. The client can even place so much emphasis on inconsequential events that the ability to give a useful and accurate medical history is impaired (Green, 1985).

Fear can generate its own physical symptoms, so that separating fear-based symptoms from illness-derived symptoms can be a difficult task. Symptoms based on fear can give rise to several unfortunate consequences, including initiation of inappropriate medical treatments, the worsening of illness symptoms, and the development of new psychological disturbances. Fear can become so pathological that it results in such excessive demands for support and services that relationships with significant others and health professionals are affected (Green, 1985).

Death Many clients with chronic illness fear death (Parets, 1967). For the family, the possible death of one of its members has multiple economic, personal, and social implications that can cause grave concern. The fear of a member's death can lead other family members to modify their relationship with the ill person, resulting in a pattern of mutual withdrawal, a decreased quantity of interactions, and a lessening of the supportive quality of these interactions.

Loss of Body Parts or Function Chronically ill clients also fear the loss of body parts or function (Strain, 1979). The potential for such loss attacks the very identity of clients and has marked implications for their ability to fulfill role expectations and partake in social interactions in the future. For some clients, fear of being incapacitated transcends their fear of death.

Loss of Love and Approval The chronically ill individual is concerned that incapacity and physical dependence will cause resentment among family members, who may subsequently withdraw emotionally (Miller, 1992). This concern underlies the fear of loss of love and approval. The client also fears that friends will withdraw support to avoid the depressing and threatening experience of seeing an ill friend.

Pain Clients fear pain because of its detrimental effects on their coping resources (Strain, 1979). With chronic or recurrent pain, the client may come to doubt the ability of the medical community to control or relieve the pain, and may conclude that intolerable levels of pain will have to be endured. Such conclusions may generate profound depression, with significant implications for treatment. The fear of pain cuts across other fears and may never be fully overcome (Strain, 1979). The client remains aware that even if the pain is eased, it will recur.

Strangers Hospitalization gives rise to fear of strangers providing care (Strain, 1979). Given that the chronically ill are knowledgeable about the interplay between regimen and their own unique body reactions (Strauss, 1984), they may have severe doubts about the ability of unknown health care workers to provide needed care. They are particularly alert to changes in medication times, routines, or anything else that affects continuity of care. Fears concerning the competence of strangers to provide the correct care tends to keep the client in a hyper-alert state, ever watchful for potential mistakes.

Grief

In addition to fear, grief is common to all chronic illness and takes place at the time of the initial diagnosis or when an exacerbation occurs. Uncomplicated grief is a healthy and natural process that allows the client and family to accept an illness and all its implications. Ideally, at the end of the normal grief process the client and family will stabilize at a level of functioning that is optimal for their particular situation.

For a myriad of reasons, some clients and families are unable to effectively grieve for the losses incurred by a chronic illness. Essentially, the client or family becomes fixated at a particular stage of the grief process, thereby preventing emotional resolution regarding the loss of health (Green, 1985). To better understand the adaptive and maladaptive consequences of the grief response, one must examine the sequential stages of denial, anger, mourning, and acceptance.

Denial In response to the many fears associated with a chronic illness, various defense mechanisms are activated to protect the client from being overwhelmed by the reality of the situation. Denial is the most important and most frequently used, since it protects from emotional disorganization by allowing a disregard of certain threatening facts of the illness situation. For example, the client may disregard factual evidence that a given chronic illness carries with it certain serious complications. Denial also allows the client to isolate or dissociate painful emotions associated with the illness (Moos & Tsu, 1977). Evidence of denial is readily apparent when clients discuss their illness and its impact in a clinically detached manner.

Feelings such as fear, anger, and profound sadness are normal responses to a chronic illness, and an absence of such feelings suggests that denial is operating. Steinhauer and associates (1974) believe that all clients and families react with some degree of denial to the fears generated by a chronic illness. Clients with chronic illness are more prone to the use of denial than are patients with acute conditions. This is especially true of clients with cancer, those who have had a myocardial infarction, and those who are receiving hemodialysis (Kiening, 1978).

Denial protects clients by providing them with the time needed to assimilate the impact of the illness. Threats associated with the illness are allowed to reach conscious awareness in increments that are tolerable to the client. The client also gains time to marshal coping strategies needed to deal with these threats. For most clients, the use of denial will gradually diminish as they slowly come to terms with threats imposed by the illness. However, denial is never completely abandoned, as it is needed to some degree to maintain the client's hope for a relatively normal productive life (Steinhauer et al., 1974).

Most experts in the study of chronic illness agree that prolonged and extensive denial in the face of obvious illness indicates that the client has inadequate internal resources to cope with the threats imposed by illness (Steinhauer et al., 1974; Moos & Tsu, 1977; Green, 1985). Prolonged and massive denial leads patients to miss clinic appointments, fail to carry out prescribed treatment, disregard or selectively attend to symptoms, and resist health professionals' best efforts to establish helping relationships with them.

Persistent denial can have a direct impact on symptoms. In a study of chronic pain patients, those who could not accept the chronic nature of their pain tended to be less active, had more pain, and were more impaired in their daily activities than were patients who accepted the truth about their condition (Shutty, 1988).

Fortunately, clinical experience indicates that the use of prolonged and complete denial by the chronically ill individual is a rare occurrence (Kaplan et al., 1977). Clients may actively block out painful thoughts and feelings associated with their illness, but they rarely deny themselves necessary medical treatment. The most common way of denying an illness appears to be disregarding only certain aspects of it. This process can be called partial denial, and while it may have an adverse impact on a client's treatment compliance, it presents fewer problems than those resulting from total denial.

As denial is gradually relinquished, the threats imposed by chronic illness are evaluated as to their impact on daily living and self-concept. This phase is characterized by numerous approach–avoidance cycles (Carlson, 1978). The client begins to confront the painful realities of the illness, but still retreats into denial when the threat is too great or psychological readiness is not yet present. As the client begins to focus on what has been lost and other realities, painful emotions, especially anger and profound sadness, will be experienced.

Anger   Anger is an expected and normal reaction to chronic illness that arises when the client realizes that certain needs, wishes, and plans for the future can no longer be fulfilled because of limitations imposed by an illness. An intense feeling of unfairness subsequently leads to feelings of frustration and anger. The manifestation of anger varies considerably from client to client, depending on the stress imposed by the illness. It is frequently not possible to detect the underlying threat causing the anger, since this feeling is often displaced onto sources other than the actual one.

Covert expressions of anger are particularly difficult to identify. The only indicators of inner turmoil may be facial expression, bodily posture, and emotional withdrawal (Kiening, 1978). Covert expression is frequently the only option available to chronically ill clients who feel they cannot express anger directly to family members or health professionals for fear of alienating the very people upon whom they are dependent (Shekleton, 1987).

Overt expressions of anger include verbal accusations or attacks and aggressive or destructive behavior. Anger may be directed at various persons or objects, or the target may be a specific person or object (Lambert & Lambert, 1987). In the hospital setting, displacement of anger is often directed toward the nursing staff. Patients become demanding, accusatory, and continually find fault with the care provided. Most of these individuals are rarely angry at the targets of their displaced feelings, but rather are largely distressed by the attributes they represent, such as wellness, purpose, vitality, freedom, mobility, and the ability to control one's life (Lambert & Lambert, 1987).

Some people simply cannot accept the loss of health and consequently cannot move beyond the anger phase of the grief process (Green, 1985). Their preoccupation with the unfairness of life inhibits daily functioning and affects family life, social relationships, and work responsibilities.

Anger is maladaptive when it is prolonged or when its expression is likely to elicit counter-hostility from significant others, alienating the very people the client is dependent on for support and health care. Clients may feel guilty about their angry behavior, which fosters feelings of anxiety and loss of self-esteem (Potter & Perry, 1991). Some clients fear the consequences of anger and are unable or reluctant to express this feeling directly, a situation that can lead to more anger and finally despair (Shekleton, 1987). Anger expressed inwardly to the self rather than outwardly to the environment eventually gives rise to depression. Repressed anger also gives rise to various somatic symptoms, such as headaches, backaches, and stomach problems, and can even aggravate symptoms associated with the chronic illness itself (Pitzele, 1985).

The anger phase of grief is one of the most difficult experiences a client can live through (Pitzele, 1985). It keeps the client from truly confronting the profound sadness associated with the loss of health and requires both time and effort for an individual to learn more appropriate ways to express the anger. Only with the onset of mourning, are these painful feelings acknowledged and expressed.

Mourning Mourning is a prelude to making the necessary changes in living required by the disease (Moos & Tsu, 1977). The client begins to reminisce about what has been lost and acknowledges the feelings related to that loss. The expression of sadness is an integral part of this phase and allows the client to "let go" of what can no longer be. In describing her own grief, Pitzele (1985) stated,

> We grieve for ourselves. We are sad because of what we have lost, including our health, our normal routines, and the future opportunities that will never be. I grieved for the loss of control of my body, my sense of wellbeing, and all those things which I might no longer be able to do. (p. 28)

Mourning is generally an intermittent process, with periods of emotional stability giving way to profound sadness and episodes of crying. It extends over a long period of time— approximately six months to a year. Mourners feel empty, isolated, despairing, and helpless, with little interest in social or vocational activi-

ties (Green, 1985). They may also have difficulty in sleeping, disinterest in eating, impaired concentration, decreased libido, and increased fatigue.

At this time, chronically ill clients often feel a significant lowering of self-esteem, coupled with the view that their useful lives are over. As time passes, the intensity of the initial reaction decreases, sadness lessens, and a more realistic perspective occurs (Stuart & Sundeen, 1991). The end of mourning is evident when the client begins to take stock of what remains rather than fixating on what is lost (Pitzele, 1985). This change leads to a more balanced sense of what one can and cannot do and the setting of new personal goals.

Clients and families who cannot accept the chronic illness and its implications may find their lives dominated by unresolved depression. In mourning there is an acknowledgement of the loss, whereas the depressed client seeks to deny the loss. Depression is a prolonged, over-elaboration of sadness and mourning that can range from mild to severe states that have psychotic features (Stuart & Sundeen, 1991). While mourning leads to emotional growth, depression interferes profoundly with normal functioning and leads to stagnation. Even though the depressed client appears sorrowful, the need to engage in the mourning process is denied.

Five factors have been identified that can inhibit the process of mourning and put the client at risk for depression (Stuart & Sundeen, 1991). First, the mourner is immersed in the practical and necessary tasks that accompany a chronic illness, preventing the emotional significance of the loss from reaching conscious awareness. Second, mourning is inhibited if it is not allowed or supported by the client's significant others, leading to the adoption of feeling states that are contrary to the client's true feelings of anger and sadness. Third, early social learning can lead to controlling feelings, since overt expressions of sadness are considered a sign of weakness. Fourth, there is the belief that one's feelings of overwhelming sadness are unique and cannot be communicated or understood. And fifth, the widespread use of tranquilizers and antidepressant medications may chemically suppress normal reactions.

A recent review of the literature shows that depression is common among clients with medical illness (Davis & Jensen, 1988). This is a major concern because clients who are depressed do not cope as well with chronic illness as do those who are not depressed. Research shows that chronic illness results in statistically significant increases in morbidity and mortality when the client is depressed (Green, 1985). Various psychological and physiological hypotheses have been suggested to explain the above findings. Some researchers point to the decreased immunological response found in depressed individuals, while others stress the profound lowering of self-esteem in depressed clients, which can lead to a neglect of self-care needs (Green, 1985).

Depression among medically ill clients is largely unrecognized and hence untreated by health care personnel (Stuart & Sundeen, 1991). This finding is particularly significant, since depression can progress and become a greater threat to the client than the physical illness (Green, 1985). Depression must be treated if the client is to successfully complete the stage of mourning and progress to acceptance, the final stage of grieving.

Acceptance Once the intensity of feelings about the losses imposed by chronic illness has diminished, clients accept the fact that even though many choices in life are eliminated, many satisfying and fulfilling ones remain. A more balanced view of personal strengths and weaknesses leads to the formation of new life goals. The performing musician with rheumatoid arthritis, for example, may discover that composing and teaching music can provide a truly satisfying vocation.

At the stage of acceptance, there is a renewed interest in life. Energy returns, social relationships once again become a source of pleasure, and activities that are still within the client's level of functioning are resumed or developed anew. Daily behavior becomes more routine, and the physiological problems that plagued the client during earlier phases become normalized. At the end of the grieving process, chronically ill clients accept that life is forever different, but they recognize that they have strength and an ability to carry on and even enjoy future happiness (Green, 1985).

Interventions

The establishment of good and comfortable communication between health provider and client/family is probably the single most important underlying skill for the later delivery of specific interventions. An identification needs to be made of a client's full range of coping behaviors and their consequences to client and family. Information should be gathered concerning pre-illness coping styles to provide clues of coping strengths and limitations. Tactful, open-ended questions yield pertinent information about coping skills and resources. Based on this assessment, judgments can be made regarding the adaptiveness of the client's and family's behaviors.

Health professionals should not let statistics determine their beliefs and attitudes (Siegel, 1986). Statistics address groups of people, not individuals, so a setback in a chronic illness should not be seen as a defeat. Current knowledge concerning chronic illness is incomplete, and researchers continue to look for new solutions (Beland, 1980). Nor is chronic illness synonymous with a decline in quality of life. There is always a margin that allows life to be lived with meaning and joy despite illness (Cousins, 1981).

Intervening with the Fearful Client

Diagnosis or exacerbation of a chronic illness often precipitates a crisis for client and family. The resulting intense fear must be dealt with and reduced, or it may aggravate existing physical symptoms as well as create new psychological problems. During intense emotional reactivity, clients will frequently need reassurance that their feelings and concerns are normal, and actions taken must be supportive and protective. A calm presence in the face of obvious distress also provides a source of reassurance for them.

Such contacts should be especially frequent during the crisis period.

Initially, active listening should be used and the client encouraged to express these fears. The health professional's verbal and nonverbal communications should convey an awareness and acceptance of the client's feelings. The discussion must be unhurried and occur in a setting that ensures privacy, so that feelings and concerns can be disclosed without embarrassment. Including significant others in the discussion may provide immediate support for the client and assist in later recall of important information.

While these fears are based on reality, they may also be the product of inadequate knowledge and lack of understanding of available options. What is heard and understood may differ considerably from what has been said. Clients and family members frequently seek supplementary information or interpretation of the physician's communication (National Institutes of Health, 1982). Consequently, it is essential that the client's knowledge of the illness be thoroughly assessed (Craig & Edwards, 1983) so that fears due to lack of knowledge can be eliminated and the door opened for future discussions.

Many clients want only knowledge specific to their *current* needs (Forsyth et al., 1984). The health professional must remain sensitive to these needs lest education be carried too far, resulting in aggravation rather than amelioration of the client's fears. When communicating relevant information, words should be used that the client will understand and that avoid unwarranted optimism or excessive pessimism. Questions should be encouraged and answered when possible, and reassurance given that future questions will be answered as they arise. Clients should be encouraged to write down questions, as this activity gives permission to ask questions and provides relevant direction for subsequent interactions with health professionals.

In some situations, clients may not want all available or pertinent information, since too much information may interfere with their retention of hope, morale, and involvement with daily living (Burhardt, 1987). Health professionals need to be sensitive to these clients to determine if more information is wanted. According to Burhardt (1987), "the belief that more information is always best for all patients under all circumstances is not documented by current research" (p. 545).

Extending hope appropriate to the circumstances can be very reassuring to fearful clients and acts to reinforce their confidence in the care and support they receive (National Institutes of Health, 1982). Health professionals who despair over chronic illness may be robbing clients of the very courage needed to cope with their disease. Klagsbrun's study (1977) found that staff nurses on a cancer research unit tended to view their patients as "walking dead," an attitude manifested in covert rejection of the patient's emotional needs. To improve morale on the unit, group sessions with a psychiatrist were instituted so the staff could see patients as functioning and productive human beings. A radical experiment in self-care was begun, allowing patients to take more responsibility for their own care. This experiment resulted in diminished patient fear and demands for nursing attention and a visible increase in happiness. In addition, the nurses started offering patients support before a crisis situation developed that would require their presence.

Intervening with the Patient in Denial

Denial that protects clients and families from the crisis generated by diagnosis or exacerbation of an illness is adaptive. It remains so unless it becomes overused and seriously interferes with the treatment process. The presence of denial indicates that a client is too threatened by the illness to face it directly. Attempts to confront denial can cause alienation and even harm to the client (Green, 1985). When prematurely forced to face reality, some clients emotionally and physically regress; others, to restore emotional equilibrium, may leave treatment (Green, 1985).

Although clients need to be allowed to deny the threatening aspects of their illness, care must be taken not to reinforce such denial by agreeing with the clients' inaccurate perceptions. To do so would support an unrealistic appraisal

CASE STUDY
Mr. K.

Mr. K., age 55, was admitted to the coronary care unit following a myocardial infarction. He was quite anxious and demanding. The nurse's assessment revealed a self-sufficient person who had held positions of leadership in the community and had his own successful small business. The logical hypothesis she reached was that he felt threatened by his perceived dependency and lack of control in his present situation and that he feared the possible loss of autonomous function in the future.

To reduce this threat, he was given as many opportunities as possible to make decisions about his care. The nursing staff's conversations with him focused on his areas of expertise, competency, and accomplishments. During these conversations, he grew increasing aware that he was more than just someone with a myocardial infarction, that he was still unique and competent. As he improved, he was sent from the CCU unit to the post-coronary unit at the hospital. The nurses there continued the intervention. Prior to discharge, he began planning realistically about how he could adapt his life-style and work. The staff made a point of answering questions he asked and clarifying misperceptions.

(Craig & Edwards, 1983). For example, a client who has recently become a quadriplegic may strongly assert that he will walk again. While the health professional cannot agree with this perception, it is possible to support his hope for a future that will bring medical breakthroughs, since there may be medical advances for his particular condition. At other times the appropriate response to a denying client is a simple statement of fact. Kiening (1978) describes a situation where the mother of a dying child repeatedly commented that her daughter would get well. The nurse's response to these comments was the simple statement, "She is very, very sick" (p. 222). In this manner a frontal attack on the denial was avoided, while the unrealistic perception was not reinforced.

The best way to decrease a client's need for denial is to determine the threat underlying the denial and to intervene therapeutically to reduce that threat. Identifying the nature of the threat requires consideration of the client's values and beliefs and how these are apt to be affected. How significant others perceive the client's illness is also important in the identification of the nature of the threat. Although the hypothesis eventually formulated may not be correct, intervention will either reduce the client's denial or indicate a need for further assessment. In these interactions clarification may be needed regarding any misperceptions about the impact of the illness on life-style. If the threat underlying the denial has been successfully identified and treated, then a reduction in both fear and denial will occur. The case study of Mr. K. demonstrates successful assessment and intervention.

Establishing a therapeutic relationship is crucial for the patient in denial. The client must see the health professional as an interested and helpful person who can be trusted. Careful listening is necessary to identify cues that indicate client readiness to talk about fears underlying the denial. Continual assessment of the client's anxiety level is also needed to determine when painful realities are such that the client needs to be allowed to escape from them temporarily.

The client's use of denial will vary from day to day, and health professionals should not become discouraged by a temporary increase in denial. For the vast majority of clients there will be a gradual reduction of denial over time, with some denial being retained in order to maintain hope.

Persistent and extensive denial is a serious concern, however, as it tends to block important learning and often results in noncompliance with treatment recommendations. Clients who are severely impaired by denial will generally need the assistance of a skilled expert to help them overcome their emotional impasse or to provide continuing support if the denying behavior is static and ingrained (Green, 1985).

Intervening with the Angry Client

As clients begin to relinquish denial they realize that certain needs, wishes, and plans for the future will not be fulfilled because of limitations imposed by the illness. Although anger is an expected and normal response to the losses experienced, angry clients are often labeled as problems by health professionals, which greatly limits effectiveness in giving them care. To be effective with angry clients, there must first be awareness of one's own angry feelings, the characteristic ways by which such feelings are handled, and those situations that tend to evoke anger.

Remaining unaware of one's own feelings of anger leads to three characteristic and nontherapeutic responses toward angry clients (Thomas, 1984). *Counter-anger* generally escalates the anger of provider and client. *Defensive responses* tend to personalize the client's anger; the resulting tendency to explain, defend, or justify the situation either blocks or escalates the client's expression of anger. *Avoidance* leads to a decrease in the amount of time spent with the client or a refusal to recognize or deal with the client's feelings.

Because of fear of rejection, it is often difficult to approach a client who looks angry. However, the professional must assume responsibility for initiating the interaction, or the client will remain withdrawn (McElvain, 1986). Often the best way to begin is to share with the client observations concerning his or her behavior and inquire if something has happened. Simple recognition of the appearance of trouble conveys concern and a willingness to help (Kiening, 1978). However, care must be taken not to push the client into revealing feelings of anger that are not yet ready for expression, as this will increase anxiety. Often the client needs time to develop trust in the caregiver before a productive working through of feelings can take place (Kiening, 1978).

Clients' overt expressions of anger may be sarcastic, abusive, argumentative, demanding, or fault-finding (Kiening, 1978). It is difficult not to take these expressions of anger personally, especially when they emerge as an attack on one's competency. The health professional must remember that overtly angry clients want to be listened to and understood. The use of paraphrasing or restating the feeling and content of what has been communicated can achieve the desired outcome (McElvain, 1986). For example, the client says, "these medications are not helping my pain at all. Don't you people have any answers?" An effective reply might be, "I see how upset you are about your situation and that you feel that we don't take your pain seriously." This nondefensive and empathic response allows for open discussion on the part of the client. In communicating empathy, one's tone of voice should be light and matter-of-fact rather than intense and authoritarian. Maintaining eye contact during a client's expression of anger indicates that these strong feelings can be tolerated and accepted.

Acceptance of the client does not mean that professionals should give up their role as limit setters when this becomes necessary. Occasionally, the free expression of anger may stimulate the client to further agitation rather than relieve his or her emotional distress (Kiening, 1978). It can even aggravate the client's physiological status, for example, by increasing respiratory symptoms among COPD clients (Shekleton, 1987). Limit setting in such situations can be very reassuring to clients and also helps preserve their dignity and self-respect.

Clients also benefit from interventions that reduce hostility-provoking stimuli in the environment that merely add to their overall reactivity. Contending with feelings of anger is difficult enough without being exposed to additional irritations from health professionals and the health care environment.

Intervening with the Client Who Is Mourning

As anger diminishes, the client begins to emotionally confront losses associated with chronic illness and experiences the profound sadness of mourning. The function of mourning is to achieve acknowledgment of the loss, allowing a return of energy for reinvestment in everyday life and for coping with the changes required by the illness.

The health professional can encourage clients to express significant feelings by discussing the nature of the illness and eliciting perceptions of how it impacts on their life-style and self-concept. Another method is to suggest how the client might be feeling or to indicate how others might feel (Stuart & Sundeen, 1991). During the period of mourning, much support is needed from significant others; it may be up to the health professional to mobilize these support systems to help open expressions of grief between them and the client.

Crying is an important emotional release, but many clients feel embarrassed by what they perceive as a loss of control or weakness. Acceptance of a client's need to cry can be achieved by silent companionship and the judicious use of touch. Because of the intensity of their emotions, clients will frequently need reassurance that their feelings are normal. As Pitzele (1985) poignantly states in describing her own illness:

> No one explained to us that our feelings of loss and pain were normal. Not only were we supposed to hurt, but acknowledging our losses would have been one of the healthiest activities we could have done for ourselves and for each other. (p. 30)

She further states that helping clients and their significant others understand all the stages of grief makes it easier for them to bear the painful feelings encountered during the process.

As the intensity of mourning waxes and wanes clients will seem emotionally stable one moment and have intense grief sweep over them the next. Such emotional lability can be particularly painful and psychologically draining to health providers who must share their bereaved clients' grief work (Stuart & Sundeen, 1991). Health professionals need to develop support systems of their own that will allow the venting of their feelings and help them continue to provide supportive work to mourning clients.

Tranquilizers and antidepressants should be avoided during normal mourning because they inhibit the expression of feelings and prolong the mourning process. There is also concern that medical suppression of grief-related feelings can push the client into the maladaptive response of depression (Stuart & Sundeen, 1991).

Unlike mourning, which involves a free flow of feeling and is time limited, depression tends to persist and causes significant interference with effective day-to-day functioning (Burns, 1980). Early symptoms of depression need to be recognized, and appropriate interventions need to be instituted. These interventions focus on four major areas of client function: affective, cognitive, behavioral, and social.

Affective interventions are a continuation of those interventions begun in the mourning phase that enable the client to express feelings of loss, anger, and sadness (see Stuart & Sundeen, 1991).

Cognitive interventions focus on modifying maladaptive thinking patterns. Distorted perceptions arise when the sense of loss that accompanies chronic illness pervades individuals' thoughts of themselves, their world, and their future. The outcome is a view of themselves as inadequate and the adoption of strongly pessimistic views of their present situation and the future. Cognitive approaches help clients interpret illness-related events in an adaptive, health-promoting fashion and to resist interpretations that are maladaptive and that produce stress (McEntee & Peddicord, 1987).

Many negative thinking patterns lie outside the client's awareness. Consequently, the first step is to help clients identify perceptions that are self-defeating. Much guidance is needed to examine the accuracy of assumptions and conclusions inherent in negative thinking. As clients become aware of errors of belief, they are assisted in examining illness-related stressors from a more realistic and positive framework (Goldfarb et al., 1986). For example, at the time of diagnosis some hypertensive clients may be so consumed by the loss of health and its impact on their self-esteem that they no longer see themselves as vital individuals. Cognitive reframing can help such clients to redefine the problem as an opportunity to develop a healthy life-style that can improve their overall health and well-being (McEntee & Peddicord, 1987). People can become so skilled in their use of cognitive reframing that they view their chronic illness as having only beneficial effects on their development as a person.

Cognitive interventions also focus on self-derogatory statements, which contribute greatly to a client's depression. Initially, clients must learn about the harmful effects of negative self-talk upon self-esteem. Next their self-derogatory statements are presented to them for examination of accuracy. Once there is recognition of the irrationality of a statement, substitute statements can be taught that are both accurate and positive (Miller, 1992). Additionally, they are encouraged to increase their positive thinking by reviewing personal assets, strengths, and accomplishments (Stuart & Sundeen, 1991).

Behavioral interventions focus on one of the most destructive aspects of depression, its inhibitory effect on activity. Clients are frequently unaware of the significant relationship of inactivity and depression. Consequently, they accomplish very little when depressed and begin to feel increasingly worse (Burns, 1980). Behavioral interventions entail a structured daily program of activity to help them overcome their lethargy. Working together, the health professional and client schedule activities that are realistic enough to ensure successful completion and rewarding enough to promote interest in further activities. To increase awareness of those activities that yield a sense of accomplishment or pleasure, Burns (1980) suggests that clients label each completed activity with the letter *M* for mastery or the letter *P* for pleasure. He further suggests that clients estimate the actual amount of pleasure or mastery derived from a completed activity by using a zero-to-five rating. Clients may not be able to carry out successfully all activities on their list and need to be reminded that trying to fulfill the plan is the most important stop.

Social interventions counteract the social factors that play a significant role in the causation and maintenance of depression (Stuart & Sundeen, 1991). The many limitations imposed by chronic illness can lead to the loss or disruption of social relationships and thus place the client at risk for depression. Interventions that increase socialization can act to reduce the experience of depression by directly decreasing opportunities for withdrawal and by increasing self-esteem through social reinforcement (Stuart & Sundeen, 1991). Clients need to be told of the benefits of successful social interaction as a means of moderating their depression.

Social experiences of a positive nature have the greatest potential to reinforce the client's sense of self-worth. Often, professionals can use themselves as a means of initiating social interaction with depressed clients. The professional can then serve as a powerful social reinforcer and facilitator, enabling clients to accept and partake additional outside social contacts. Eventually, clients may need to explore ways of reaching out to others to further increase their level of social interactions.

Unlike clients who are experiencing normal mourning, depressed clients may need the assistance of antidepressant medications. Such clients will need to know that generally the therapeutic effects of these medications begin after two to six weeks of adherence to the medical regimen. Clients who are not informed of this lag time can lose all hope and become further depressed because they do not experience rapid relief.

Intervening with the Client in Acknowledgment

During the acknowledgment stage of the grief process, clients take stock of what remains rather than fixate on what is lost, and begin to set new goals for their life (Pitzele, 1985). It is a time when clients are particularly motivated to learn about the limitations set by the illness and to determine how they want to function within those limits. Interventions that emphasize client control are particularly useful, as they encourage the highest level of function possible and enhance a sense of self-worth. Research has shown that the most significant predictor of quality of life for chronically ill clients is their sense of personal control (Lewis, 1982). Interventions that foster such control include increasing knowledge, teaching self-management skills, setting realistic goals, and modifying the environment.

Increasing Knowledge Clients need to know about their illness so they can make appropriate decisions concerning its management. Chronically ill clients are not receptive to standard patient education formats, but seek information specific to their individualized needs (Forsyth et al., 1984). Thus, in addition to general information being given, areas of special concern must be identified and the client allowed to prioritize them. The client must not be overwhelmed with information, as this can lead to frustration and a failure to internalize the information appropriately. Education may be more effective if it includes the problem-solving process, which can increase the client's ability to manage and control the many unique issues that will arise in the course of coping with chronic illness (Armstrong, 1987).

Self-Management Skills Providing clients with adaptive coping strategies for dealing with illness-related problems is the aim of self-management skills. Cognitive interventions, daily activity schedules, and problem-solving skills are methods that have been discussed and continue to be important sources of intervention for the client at this time.

Relaxation procedures are among the most common and most effective forms of self-management taught to chronically ill clients. These procedures can significantly reduce the fear and anxiety associated with chronic illness and have a direct impact on the illness itself—for example, the lowering of blood pressure in hypertensive clients. An additional benefit of relaxation training for hypertensive clients is a significant increase in perceived control over health (Pender, 1985).

Encouraging the client to keep a log of daily activities, feelings, and symptoms is another self-management technique that facilitates a sense of control. An analysis of this data can help the client to determine which activities and feeling states tend to exacerbate symptoms. The client can then institute appropriate action to reduce these stressors whenever possible.

Setting Realistic Goals Goals that fulfill needs are essential to health and happiness (McKay et al., 1981). Clients should receive necessary help to develop realistic health goals and strategies appropriate to their individual life-style. Although client goals may seem inappropriate or undesirable, the health professional must not impose his or her own goals on clients. Rather, the client's behavior and its consequences should be reflected back to them (Stuart & Sundeen, 1991). Once agreed upon, goals should be stated as positive statements and be as specific as possible. Finally, a realistic plan should be developed for achieving these goals. Often clients will need reassurance that they do have the strengths needed to successfully assume the responsibilities for managing their own health care.

Modifying the Environment During hospitalization the professional should take responsibility for needed environmental modifications to lessen client stress, such as placing the call light where it can be easily reached and keeping frequently used items available and nearby. Prior to discharge, realistic changes in the home or work environment should be discussed. Modifications can be a means for clients to increase control over their illness (Miller, 1992). Changes, such as grab bars by the bathtub and toilet, installation of ramps rather than steps, conveniently placed telephones, and so forth, will enable clients to function autonomously and more comfortably as well as foster their self-esteem.

Summary

An understanding of the concept of coping and how it manifests itself in chronically ill clients is crucial to appropriate health care. Such an understanding makes it possible to accurately assess clients' needs and to provide interventions that enable them to manage both the stress and the illness more effectively.

The coping abilities of clients and their significant others are greatly affected by pre-existing factors. First is the client's premorbid personality and adjustment, which corresponds with subsequent adaptation to a chronic illness. Second, the client's developmental stage has a reciprocal relationship with chronic illness. Consequently, one needs to assess not only what impact illness has on mastering stages of development but also what impact the developmental stage has on the ability to cope. Third, the meaning of the illness to the client determines which coping behaviors he or she will select. And finally, the amount and kind of social support can greatly facilitate the coping process by affirming worth and providing tangible goods and task-oriented assistance.

Chronic illnesses produce profound psychological effects, which vary with the different phases of illness and treatment. Primary among these is fear, which occurs in response to the many perceived or realistic threats inherent in the illness situation. As an adaptive response, fear alerts clients to the symptoms of illness and mobilizes coping behaviors. Maladaptive fear can cause a preoccupation with illness and an aggravation of symptomatology.

Grief, common to all chronic illnesses, occurs at the time of diagnosis and following an exacerbation. The process of grieving consists of four sequential stages: denial, anger, mourning, and acceptance. Denial protects clients from emotional disorganization and gives clients time to assimilate the impact of the illness and marshal coping strategies that are needed to deal with the threats imposed by the illness. Prolonged and extensive denial is considered maladaptive and can have an adverse impact on compliance with treatment regimens.

Anger and frustration occur as denial is gradually relinquished and the client becomes aware of what has been lost. Some clients remain in the stage of anger and become preoccupied with the unfairness of life, leading to a decline in daily functioning and family relationships. Only when anger is resolved can the client begin to confront the profound sadness associated with the loss of health.

Mourning allows the client to finally "let go" of what can no longer be. The end of mourning is evident when the client begins to take stock of what remains rather than fixate on what has been lost. Clients who cannot accept the illness and its implications may find their lives dominated by unresolved depression. This type of depression may pose a greater threat to the client than does the physical illness.

When clients reach the final stage of acceptance they have achieved a more balanced view of what they can and cannot do and begin to formulate new life goals in keeping with their limitations. As energy returns, everyday activities and relationships once again become a source of interest and pleasure.

Successful intervention in chronic illness depends on the effectiveness of the health professional's communication skills. Good communication between health provider and client facilitates a working relationship and fosters adaptive coping. With fearful clients, communication involves active listening and encouraging clients to express their fears. Corrective information should be provided in keeping with the client's needs and wants. A realistic but hopeful perspective should be conveyed. Angry clients also benefit from communication that facilitates the expression of feelings. To feel understood, they require responses that are both nondefensive and empathic. Clients who are mourning need the active support of the health professional to face the many painful losses associated with chronic illness.

Health professionals facilitate adaptive coping by teaching clients self-management techniques, thereby increasing perceived control. Clients should also be helped to develop realistic health goals and master strategies to achieve successful life management.

NURSING DIAGNOSIS

9.3.2 Fear

Definition: Feeling of dread related to an identifiable source which the person validates.

Defining Characteristics: Ability to identify object of fear.

Related Factors: To be developed.

Editor's Note: Fear can be an adaptive response, since it alerts the client to seek assistance or directs the client to find solutions. The defining characteristic noted above is not a cue that explains how fear can be identified. Defining characteristics of maladaptive fear discussed in this chapter include preoccupation with the disease process, the occurrence of new symptoms or a worsening of disease symptoms, decreased ability to give useful or accurate medical history, initiation of inappropriate treatment, excessive demands for support and services.

It would be helpful if the category were listed as "Fear (specify)" to identify the specific problem faced by the patient. Several fears are discussed in this chapter: fear of death, fear of loss of body part/function, fear of loss of love and approval, fear of pain, and fear of strangers.

9.2.1.1 Dysfunctional Grieving

Definition: None noted.

Defining Characteristics: Verbal expression of distress at loss; denial of loss; expression of guilt; expression of unresolved issues; anger; sadness; crying; difficulty in expressing loss; alterations in eating habits, sleep patterns, dress patterns, activity level, libido; idealization of lost object; reliving of past experiences; interference with life functioning; developmental regression; labile affect; alterations in concentration and/or pursuit of tasks.

Related Factors: Actual or perceived object loss (object loss is used in the broadest sense); objects may include people, possessions, a job, status, home, ideals, parts and processes of the body.

9.2.1.2 Anticipatory Grieving

Definition: None noted.

Defining Characteristics: Potential loss of significant object; expression of distress at potential loss; denial of potential loss; guilt; anger; sorrow, choked feelings; change in eating habits; alterations in sleep patterns, alterations in activity level; altered libido; altered communication patterns.

Related Factors: To be developed.

Editor's Note: Content provided in this chapter fits either of the grieving diagnostic categories. The presence of definitions would help differentiate them. Defining characteristics do not differentiate the two sufficiently from each other. The potential loss of any significant object is more a *related factor* for anticipatory grieving than a characteristic. Some of the defining characteristics are appropriate to specific stages of the grieving process.

Anticipatory grieving is more appropriately used prior to or during the loss process, and dysfunctional grieving when the loss is not resolved within six months to a year. Unfortunately, actual grieving is considered a "normal" process and is not in the taxonomy, even though nurses intervene to help clients or families cope with it.

STUDY QUESTIONS

1. What four pre-existing factors affect a client's ability to cope with chronic illness?
2. How is adaptive coping differentiated from maladaptive coping?
3. How can fear facilitate or hinder the coping process?
4. What common fears are associated with chronic illness?
5. How can denial facilitate or hinder the coping process?
6. How does the anger stage of the grief process lead to interpersonal repercussions?
7. What five factors can inhibit mourning?
8. Without threatening the client, how can the health professional avoid reinforcing denial?
9. Describe cognitive, behavioral, and social interventions for helping depressed clients.

References

Armstrong, N. (1987). Coping with Diabetes. *The Nursing Clinics of North America, 22,* 559-568.

Beland, J. A. (1980). Nursing and the concept of hope. In J. A. Werner-Beland, (Ed.), *Grief responses to long-term illness and disability.* Reston, VA: Reston.

Burhardt, C. S. (1987). Coping strategies of the chronically ill. *The Nursing Clinics of North America, 22,* 543-550.

Burish, T. G., & Bradley, L. A. (1983). *Coping with chronic disease.* New York: Academic Press.

Burns, D. D. (1980). *Feeling good: The new mood therapy.* New York: Signet.

Carlson, C. E. (1978). Grief. In C. E. Carlson & B. Blackwell (Eds.), *Behavioral concepts and nursing intervention.* Philadelphia: J. B. Lippincott.

Coleman, J. C. (1973). Life stress and maladaptive behavior. *American Journal of Occupational Therapy, 27,* 169-180.

Cousins, N. (1981). *Anatomy of an illness as perceived by the patient.* New York: Bantam.

Craig, H. M., & Edwards, J. E. (1983). Adaption and chronic illness: An eclectic model for nurses. *Journal of Advanced Nursing, 8,* 397-404.

Davis, T., & Jensen, L. (1988). Identifying depression in medical patients. *Image: The Journal of Nursing Scholarship, 20,* 191-195.

Eisenberg, M. G., Sutkin, L. C., & Jansen, M. A. (1984). *Chronic Illness and disability through the life span.* New York: Springe.

Erikson, E. (1963). *Childhood and society.* New York: Norton.

Feldman, D. J. (1974). Chronic disabling illness: A holistic view, *Journal of Chronic Disease, 27,* 287-291.

Forsyth, G. L., Delaney, K. D., & Gresham, M. L. (1984). Vying for a winning position: Management style of the chronically ill. *Research in Nursing and Health, 7,* 181-188.

Garland, L. M., & Bush, C. T. (1982). *Coping behaviors and nursing.* Reston, VA: Reston.

Goldfarb, L. A., Brotherson, M. J., Summers, M. J., & Turnbell, A. (1986). *Meeting the challenge of disability or chronic illness: A family guide.* Baltimore: Brookes.

Green, S. A. (1985). *Mind and body: The psychology of physical illness.* Washington D.C.: American Psychiatric Press.

Haan, N., (1977). *Coping and defending: Process of self-environment organization.* New York: Academic Press.

Kaplan, D. M., Smith, A., Grobstein, R., & Fischman, S. E. (1977). Family mediation of stress. In R. H. Moos (Ed.), *Coping with physical illness.* New York: Plenum.

Kiening, M. M. (1978). Denial of illness. In C. E. Carlson & B. Blackwell (Eds.), *Behavioral concepts and nursing intervention.* Philadelphia: J. B. Lippincott.

Klagsbrun, S. C. (1977). Cancer, emotions, and nurses. In R. H. Moos (Ed.), *Coping with physical illness.* New York: Plenum.

Krantz, D. S., & Deckel, A. W. (1983). Coping with coronary artery disease. In T. G. Burish, & L. A. Bradley (Eds.), *Coping with chronic disease.* New York: Academic Press.

Lambert, C. E., & Lambert, V. A. (1987). Psychosocial impacts created by chronic illness. *The Nursing Clinics of North America, 22,* 527-533.

Larkin, J. (1987). Factors influencing one's ability to adapt to chronic illness. *The Nursing Clinics of North America, 22,* 535-542.

Lazarus, R. S. (1966). *Psychological stress and the coping process.* New York: McGraw-Hill.

——— (1974). Psychological stress and coping in adaptation and illness. *International Journal of Psychiatry in Medicine, 5,* 321-333.

Lazarus, R. S., & Launier, R. (1978). Stress-related transactions between person and environment. In L. A. Pervin & M. Lewis (Eds.), *Perspectives in interactional psychology.* New York: Plenum Press.

Lewis, F. M. (1982). Experienced personal control and quality of life in late stage cancer patient. *Nursing Research, 31,* 113-118.

Lipowski, Z. J. (1969). Psychological aspects of disease. *Annals of Internal Medicine, 71,* 1197.

McElvain, M. S. (1986). Suspicious, hostile and aggressive behavior. In B. S. Johnson (Ed.), *Psychiatric-mental health nursing.* Philadelphia: J. B. Lippincott.

McEntee, M. A., & Peddicord, K. (1987). Coping with hypertension. *The Nursing Clinics of North America, 22,* 583-592.

McGrath, J. E. (1970). *Social and psychological factors in stress.* Altanta: Rinehart & Winston.

McKay, M., Davis, M., & Fanning, P. (1981). *Thoughts and feelings: the Art of cognitive stress intervention.* Richmond, CA: Harbinger.

Meyers, B. A., Friedman, S. B., & Weiner, I. B. (1977). Coping with a chronic disability: Psychosocial observations of girls with scoliosis. In R. H. Moos (Ed.), *Coping with physical illness.* New York: Plenum.

Miller, J. F. (1992). *Coping with chronic illness: Overcoming powerlessness.* Philadelphia: F. A. Davis.

Moos, R. H., & Tsu, V. D. (1977). The crisis of physical illness: An overview. In R. H. Moos (Ed.), *Coping with physical illness.* New York: Plenum.

National Institutes of Health (1982). *Coping with cancer* (pub. no. 82-2080). Bethesda, MD: National Cancer Institute.

Parets, A. D. (1967). Emotional reactions to chronic physical illness. *Medical Clinics of North America, 51,* 1399-1407.

Pender, N. J. (1985). Effects of progressive muscle relaxation training on anxiety and health locus of control among hypertensive adults. *Research in Nursing and Health, 8,* 67-72.

Pitzele, S. K. (1985). *We are not alone: Learning to live with chronic illness.* New York: Thompson.

Potter, P. A., & Perry, A. G. (1991). *Fundamentals of nursing.* St. Louis: C. V. Mosby.

Senescu, R. A. (1963). The development of emotional complications in the patient with cancer. *Journal of Chronic Diseases, 16,* 813-832.

Shekleton, M. E. (1987). Coping with chronic respiratory difficulty. *The Nursing Clinics of North America, 22,* 569-581.

Shutty, M. S. (1988, December). When truth doesn't hurt. *Psychology Today,* p. 11.

Siegel, B. S. (1986). *Love, medicine, and miracles.* New York: Harper & Row.

Steinhauer, P. D., Musin, D. N., & Grant, Q. R. (1974) Psychological aspects of chronic illness. *Pediatric Clinics of North America, 21,* 825-839.

Strain, J. J. (1979). Psychological reactions to chronic illness. *Psychiatric Quarterly, 51,* 173-181.

Strauss, A. L. (1984). *Chronic illness and the quality of life.* St. Louis: C. V. Mosby.

Stuart, G. W., & Sundeen, S. J. (1991). *Principles and practice of psychiatric nursing.* St. Louis: C. V. Mosby.

Tilden, V. P., & Weinert, C. (1987). Social support and the chronically ill individual. *The Nursing Clinics of North America, 22,* 613-620.

Thomas, S. L. (1984). Anger. In C. M. Beck, R. P. Rawlins, & S. R. Williams (Eds.), *Mental health-psychiatric nursing.* St. Louis: C. V. Mosby.

Weisman, A. D. (1976). Early diagnosis of vulnerability in cancer patients. *The American Journal of the Medical Sciences, 271,* 187-196.

CHAPTER 12

Family Caregivers

Mary Elizabeth Payne • *Ilene Lubkin*

Introduction

With improved medical technology we find more and more clients surviving acute illnesses. Many of these individuals live with chronic conditions requiring ongoing assistance and care in managing or performing activities of daily living (ADLs), but they do not need continuous supervision or input from health professionals. Although predominantly an older population, there is an ever-increasing number of younger chronically ill people. Most of these individuals are cared for by family, friends, or neighbors. It is this group of caregivers that we will be addressing in this chapter.

There are both common experiences and unique problems among family caregivers often dependent on characteristics of the client, such as cognitively impaired adults, chronically ill children, or those dying at home. One also finds differences by type of family composite or socio-cultural group. We will look primarily at problems shared by family caregivers as a whole, but will identify some areas where selected client populations present specialized concerns for their caregivers.

A "family caregiver" is a social status, that is, a position in society with obligations, specific behavioral and attitudinal expectations, responsibilities, and anticipated rewards (Suitor & Pil-

lemer, 1990). Society assumes that caregivers of older adults will provide emotional and physical support with a minimum of resentment (George, 1987). Even when clients use multiple caregivers, there is usually one person may who serves as the main or primary caregiver (Sankar, 1991).

Advantages of Home Caregiving

As compared with institutional care, the very setting of home care is beneficial for chronically ill clients, since it enhances the quality of their lives and that of their families (Birren et al., 1991). For instance, older adults have strong emotional attachments to where they live (Carp, 1987); remaining in the home setting allows them to maintain a sense of identity, autonomy, and purpose, which institutionalization threatens (Rubinstein, 1989; O'Brien, 1989) and which most adults have a strong aversion to (Pastalan, 1983).

Providing care to another can enhance the caregiver's sense of efficacy and contribute to a positive self-image as a nurturing person (Shumaker & Brownell, 1984). In-depth interviews of families of chronically ill clients, ranging from children to older adults, found that families who cared for their loved ones at home maintained a "semblance of normality" even when the client was dying (Sankar, 1991; Thorne, 1993). This semblance of normality was found to enhance the quality of life for both client *and* family despite the ever present demands of caring for the client.

Cost of Providing Care

A number of studies have examined cost-effectiveness of community-based home services to groups of individuals at risk of nursing home use (Miller, 1987; Shapiro & Tate, 1988; Thornton et al., 1988; Weissert & Cready, 1989; Weissert, Gooch, & Cready, 1989). Examining only the service program level showed insufficient savings to offset the cost of provided services. Factors that influence program cost-effectiveness include the type of service given, its price per unit, the client's individual risk level for nursing home placement, the difference between the cost of providing community program services and the cost of a nursing home, and the individual client's responsiveness to specific services (Greene et al., 1993). Not taken into account were care given to less frail individuals not in danger of institutionalization, gains to *specific* clients, and improvement in the quality of clients' lives. Also not considered were the indirect costs of unpaid informal help provided by caregivers in the home (Weissert et al., 1989). When all of these variables are taken into account, community-based services become more effective than nursing home care in terms of expected long-term costs and reducing the risk of institutionalization (Greene et al., 1993).

Studies have shown that the family is an important source of emotional and social support for clients at any age. Of noninstitutionalized older disabled people, three-fourths rely exclusively on informal help and the remainder rely on either formal (paid) help alone or a combination of formal and informal help (Coward, Cutler, & Mullens, 1990).

Characteristics of Family Caregivers

Frail elders rely first on a spouse, then on children and other family members, and finally on outside sources (USDHHS, 1990; Stoller & Cutler, 1993). Older adults with disabilities turn to out-side support only when their needs for assistance exceed their family resources. Factors most influential in a family's decision to use paid help rather than rely exclusively on family assistance are the older adult's household income (Stoller & Cutler, 1993) and level of frailty (Tennstedt, Crawford, & McKinlay, 1993). Other factors that predict the use of paid help among older adults are availability of informal help; whether the older adult lives alone or with others; and types of tasks requiring assistance, e.g., heavy yard work or daily personal care (Stoller & Cutler, 1993).

Gender and Family Differences   "Caregiver" is an inexact term, and studies do not clearly define it (Spitze & Logan, 1990). *Caregiver* refers to a host of persons and associated activities, from individuals who help a parent or other relative in any area to those who provide full-time intensive assistance to a frail elderly person (Spitze & Logan, 1990).

Married Individuals If married, the disabled older adult is most likely to depend on his or her spouse for assistance. Since older men are much more likely to have a surviving spouse, wives provide over half of the care received by elderly men (Soldo & Agree, 1988; USDHHS, 1990). Spouses are found to provide more emotional, tangible, and informational support to clients than either close friends or other family members (Revenson, 1990).

Widowed or Divorced Individuals When a spouse is unavailable, the primary caregiver of an older individual is often an adult child. Unmarried adult children have fewer family responsibilities that might interfere with parent-caring roles than their married siblings (Silverstein & Litwak, 1993). Factors that present barriers for both married and unmarried adult children in parent caregiving include geographical distance, cost to the child, and differences in norms and needs that motivate their performance as caregivers (Silverstein & Litwak, 1993).

Single older parents who are disabled and live alone are viewed as "vulnerable," which elicits household support from their adult children (Silverstein & Litwak, 1993). If these elderly parents have declining health, they are more likely to move in with their adult children, depending on various factors such as the regularity of contact they have had with each other (Spitze, Logan, & Robinson, 1992). However, the adult child's needs play a large part in such decision making, and the parent's co-residence often provides financial, child-rearing, and house-keeping assistance (Ward et al., 1992; Spitze & Logan, 1990; Speare & Avery, 1993).

Among married adult children, daughters or daughters-in-law are frequently the caregivers (Soldo & Agree, 1988). The greater involvement of daughters in caregiving may be partially explained by same-gender preference—that is, adult children prefer to care for the same-gender parent, and infirm elders prefer assistance from the same-gender child (Lee et al., 1993). Since the majority of elders who require assistance are mothers, this partially accounts for the predominance of daughters as caregivers (Lee, Dwyer, & Coward, 1993).

Co-Residence While spouses provide a majority of home care, the fact that the spouse co-resides with the client seems to be more important than the marital relationship itself (Tennstedt et al., 1993). The emphasis on co-residence rather than kinship relationship has implications for nontraditional family structures, such as gay and lesbian couples, single parents, and blended families. Some research on family caregiving defines "family" not according to kinship ties but in terms of a group of people who perceive that they share both an enduring commitment to and a set of mutual obligations with one another (Sankar, 1991).

Differences in Family Caregivers Client populations other than the elderly have need for caregivers. These caregivers have some problems and concerns unique to their caregiving situation. It is not the intent of this chapter to address all variations of groups or problems that exist, but a few are noted here.

Chronically Ill Children Chronically ill children are a special population presenting unique needs to their family caregivers. It is estimated that 10 to 15 percent of all children under 18 years of age have some kind of chronic physical illness (Pless & Perrin, 1985) and that 10 percent of this number have severe illness (Hobbs et al., 1985), many from the dramatic increase in survival rate due to advances in medical technology over the past decades. Not only does their survival have implications for their caregivers, but there is an ambiguity about the future that is inherent in childhood illness (Gortmaker & Sapperfield, 1984; Patterson, 1988; Cohen, 1993).

Concerns unique to family caregivers of chronically ill children include the management of parenting responsibilities of the ill child's siblings. Parents report insecurity in answering siblings' questions about the ill child and in disciplinary practices. There are increasing, and sometimes unrealistic, expectations of well siblings, expecting more than is developmentally possible. Parents report concern about their limited communication with well siblings and generally give less attention to them (Gallo, 1988). Parents need to learn to recognize cues that indicate a well sibling's need for attention, especially during transitions in the healthy child's life. Parents also need to learn how to answer questions accurately and appropriately for the child's level of understanding, and to hold more realistic expectations of siblings (Gallo, 1988).

When the child is dependent upon technology, parents experience fear and anxiety as they move into providing home care for the child. They must not only manage the equipment, such as a mechanical ventilator, but still provide a home setting that is developmentally appropriate for the child (Donar, 1988). Mobility, play, and excursions outside the home are important elements in home care for chronically ill children that must be provided by the parents.

Ethnicity The family caregiving experience is shaped by race and ethnicity, for these two factors influence one's life experiences in terms of socioeconomic status, education, marital status, health, living arrangements, and general life-style (Barresi, 1990). The number of minority older adults is increasing at a faster rate than that of the Caucasian, non-Hispanic population (U.S. Senate Special Committee on Aging, 1988). Gerontological researchers are building a body of literature on African-American, Asian-American,

Native-American, and Hispanic elders and their family caregiving experiences (Harper, 1990; Markides, 1989; Markides & Mindel, 1987). While this literature is too extensive to review here, an example of African-American family caregiving is provided to illustrate ethnic influences.

African-American caregiving is shaped by cultural precedence, historical events, and the needs of extended kin and family structure. Black elders seek assistance from the following sources in order of preference: children, other relatives, others outside the family, and, finally, formal organizations (Taylor, 1985; Taylor & Chatters, 1986). Although many forms of family structure exist, this preference for children rather than spouses as caregivers may reflect the many single-parent households in African-American families (Billingsley & McCarley, 1986; Tucker et al., 1993; Walker 1988). Consequently, African-American adults tend not to have the tangible and emotional support from the other parent to assist with caregiving.

Functional illiteracy also hampers elder African Americans in their abilities to deal with formal health care systems (Lubben & Beccera, 1988), increasing their need to use their children for assistance. The adult-child caregiver assists the parent in finding sources of formal support, in determining if the parent meets eligibility requirements for services, in completing application forms, and in corresponding or interfacing with formal providers.

Another form of caregiving among African Americans is grandparents as surrogate parents to their grandchildren for various social reasons (Burton, 1992), including the drug addiction of the children's parents. Stressors these caregivers experience include dealing with neighborhood problems (such as violence), coping with the high energy needs of their grandchildren, concern over providing long-term parenting through the child's adolescence, balancing multiple roles and multiple settings, and having little if any time for their own needs (Burton, 1992).

Roles of Caregivers   Caregiving falls primarily into the categories of care provider and care manager depending on the family's socioeconomic status (Stoller & Culter, 1993), the health status of the patient (Tennstedt et al., 1993), and the length of time caregiving is required (Sankar, 1991). Care providers perform services ranging from shopping, housework, and running errands to full-time physical care (Brody, 1985). Care managers, who tend to have competing careers, arrange for services that others will provide (USDHHS, 1990).

Of all the responsibilities of caregivers, whether as care providers or care managers, decision making is the most extensive depending on the client's own abilities and health status (Sankar, 1991). For example, clients with dementias or cognitive deficits often have difficulty making any decisions; others with aphasia may have difficulty understanding or communicating their choices. Thus, caregivers have varying degrees of responsibility for decision making regarding the countless activities in managing daily life and one's family. These include the initiation, timing, and provision and extent of services from informal and formal support systems; assessing the quality of other services the client receives; and determining who has access to the client (Sankar, 1991).

Problems and Issues of Home Caregiving

The aging of the American population, coupled with the decreased fertility of "baby boomers," and the growing number of younger individuals needing care at home has led to a predicted shortage of family caregivers, especially caretakers for the frail elderly. These trends, coupled with an increase in women in the work force, means that fewer adult daughters will be available to care for their aging parents. The cost of maintaining disabled elders in the community will shift to the public sector or to the growing fee-for-service home care industry (Soldo & Agree, 1988) (see Chapter 23, on social and health policy).

Not only is there a potential shortage of family members who can provide home care, but a shortage is predicted in paid home caretakers, especially unskilled workers who provide custodial care (Kane, 1989). Currently, "third party payers are refusing to pay for quality home care, and many elderly people . . . often cannot affort to pay enough to attract and maintain a quality work force" (Kane, 1989, p. 30). With the increased number of elderly as a percentage of the population, the increasing numbers of very old elders who often have multiple health problems, and the growing population of younger, chronically ill individuals, this situation is predicted to reach a crisis level. Increases in the number of single-parent households, childless couples, blended families, and women in the work force all influence intergenerational ties and future caregiving (Bumpass, 1990).

Impact of Chronic Illness on Families

The rewards of caregiving are challenged by disadvantages to the caregiver and family system (Haley & Pardo, 1989; Lawton et al., 1989; Stephens et al., 1988; Vitaliano et al., 1991; Zarit et al., 1980; Zarit et al., 1986). The case study of the H. family is compiled from informal interviews with this family over a five-year period. It is used to illustrate caregiver problems and issues of home care.

Caregiver Stress   When the demands of providing care for a family member are perceived as exceeding available resources, caregivers experience stress (White et al., 1992; Pruchno & Resch, 1989; Cohen & Eisdorfer, 1988; Cohen et al., 1990; Eisdorfer, 1991). Stress often leads to feelings of burden and depression. Depression is especially common for caregivers of elders with Alzheimer's dementia or individuals with AIDS or metastases with brain involvement (Cohen & Eisdorfer, 1988; Colerick & George, 1986; Vitaliano et al., 1993).

Mishel (1988a, 1990) proposes an "uncertainty in illness" theory that applies to either client or family. According to this theory, uncertainty exists when the decision maker, secondary to insufficient cues, is unable to determine the meaning of illness-related events, to assign values to objects and events, or to accurately predict outcomes.

Stress for families caring for individuals with chronic illness results from uncertainty regarding the increased need for physical care over an indefinite period (White et al., 1992; Greater New York Hospital Foundation, 1988). Such uncertainty has been found to reduce a person's sense of mastery over events, to increase a sense of danger (Mishel, 1988b), and to decrease one's sense of resourcefulness (Chilman et al., 1988).

The H. family members verbalized uncertainty about Mrs. H.'s health and ability to remain at home. With each of her hospitalizations, there was uncertainty about when the next acute episode would occur, if changed medication regimes would be more effective, and if she would be further weakened. Mr. H. voiced more and more uncertainty about his ability to continue to care for his wife at home.

Families report that they often experience extreme stress at the onset of symptoms and while awaiting diagnosis of the chronic illness. This stress increases when the client first moves in with the caregiver, resulting in loss of independence for the caregiver (Thorne, 1993).

Family caregivers also find it stressful during the ongoing caregiving experience (Greater New York Hospital Foundation, 1988) secondary to physical and intellectual changes in the client; uncertainty about aspects of the chronic disease (including possible hereditary aspects); and the loss of financial resources. Interacting with formal providers can also be a source of stress. Loss of emotional resources is another source, especially when the client was previously a source of emotional strength. Other family members contribute to emotional stressors if they do not provide sufficient, frequent assistance, or when caregiving must be balanced with responsibilities to other family members (Suitor & Pillemer, 1993).

Features of the caregiving context itself can be more detrimental to caregiver well-being than the severity or duration of the client's symptoms. Co-residence with the client was found to be associated with decreased caregiver well-being in the areas of mental health, social participation, and financial resources (George & Gwyther, 1986). However, other studies found that, whether the client co-resided with the caregiver or lived in a nursing home, family caregivers experienced depression, psychotropic drug use, and psychological distress (Cohen & Eisdorfer,

CASE STUDY

The H. Family

Mrs. H. had coronary artery disease and congestive heart failure that caused increasing fatigue, dyspnea, and angina over a five-year period. Frequent upper respiratory infections exacerbated her dyspnea. She lived at home with her husband in a small rural town, in a home they had owned since their children were small. Mr. H. was four years younger than his wife. He assumed cooking tasks in the home and was the primary caregiver for his wife, assisting her to ambulate to the bathroom for toileting and bathing, making sure her clothes were clean and accessible, and making sure she took her medicine as prescribed.

The H.s' married daughter and married son lived within a ten-minute drive of their parents' house. Both had children of their own, but assisted their parents at least once a week. The daughter did the major housecleaning for her parents, and drove them regularly to the grocery store, the frequent doctor's visits, and the pharmacy. The son assisted his father with lawn work and household repairs; he was also called upon in cases of medical emergency to be the decision maker.

Over several years, Mrs. H.'s health declined. Her upstairs bedroom became inaccessible, since stair climbing became exhausting. The living room was converted to her bedroom. She was hospitalized for a series of short-term stays for complaints of chest pain and/or difficulty breathing over this time span. Whenever she was hospitalized, the daughter and son took turns driving their father to the hospital, since he visited their mother daily.

During the next five years, these hospitalizations increased in frequency to several times yearly. She used portable oxygen at home. Initially it was only used for brief intervals during the night, and she was able to accompany her daughter for brief shopping trips or drives "to get out of the house." As

her health declined, Mrs. H. used the oxygen continuously, remaining in her room. The family got a "medi-alert" call button that Mrs. H. always wore in case she needed emergency help.

With each hospitalization, Mrs. H. returned home weaker. Mr. H. began to worry that he could no longer care for his wife at home because of her increasing weakness. He moved her commode adjacent to her wheelchair; even so, Mrs. H. had difficulty transferring from her chair to the commode. Mrs. H. was heavier than her husband; he worried about her safety, fearing that she might fall and injure herself and he would be unable to assist her. The daughter had a part-time job, but visited her parents more frequently, twice weekly. She began to express concerns about both parents' health to her brother, her friends, and her husband.

When Mrs. H. was hospitalized at the age of 78 for chest pain and difficulty breathing, the physician approached Mr. H. and his son and daughter with a request that they sign a Do Not Resuscitate (DNR) agreement. Mrs. H. had vehemently expressed, "I don't want them damn machines," so the family readily agreed to the DNR order. They were concerned for Mrs. H. since the DNR had never been brought up by the doctor before.

Mr. H. told his children that Mrs. H. would have to go to a nursing home when she was discharged from the hospital, as he could no longer care for her with her severely diminished abilities. While the family discussed this problem, they did not resolve it. After visiting Mrs. H. one evening at the hospital, in which time she was alert and talkative, the family returned to their homes. That evening Mrs. H. died. The family expressed relief that her suffering was over, that she died the way she wanted to without machines, and that the whole family did not have to struggle with the nursing home decision.

1988; Colerick & George, 1986; Dura et al., 1990).

Burdens of Caregiving   Stress can lead to a sense of burden. Caregiver burden denotes a set of negative feelings (Klein, 1989; Zarit et al., 1980) that can be defined as the subjective per-

ception of a caregiver, as related to the degree of present and potential problems being experienced in providing assistance to an individual (George, 1987). These problems often include decreased social and recreational involvement for the caregiver (see Chapter 8, on social isolation), financial difficulties, physical health problems, and depression. One study found that younger women found caregiving to be more psychologically burdensome than did older women, and that feelings of perceived burden were higher among women who had been involved in caregiving over an extended period of time (Gaynor, 1990).

Caregiver burden may change over time, as the client's chronic health problems progress. When the caregivers are elderly, they must cope with their own biological aging. Thus, there are increasing demands upon the caregiver because of aging of both caregiver and care recipient, the progression of the chronic illness, or exhaustion of resources for the family unit as a whole. When these changes occur, utilization of formal or paid help may be required to augment or substitute for the services provided by the caregiver.

Feelings of burden, especially if coupled with inadequate finances to pay for supplemental help, may lead to nursing home placement. Spouses of Alzheimer's clients who placed them in nursing homes cited the following reasons for such placement: an inability to cope with daily tasks and difficulty tolerating clients' negative behaviors. When providing home care became burdensome, caregivers then considered institutionalization as one of their care alternatives (Zarit et al., 1986).

Physical and Emotional Strain Research has demonstrated physical health changes related to caregiving. High incidences of stress-related disorders such as heart disease and hypertension were found in female caregivers (Gaynor, 1989; Gaynor, 1990; Sexton & Munro, 1985). In another study, one-third of the admissions to a hospital respite program were related directly to the caregiver's health or inability to continue providing care (Gaynor, 1989). Sleep deprivation, chronic fatigue, and depression were also found in caregivers (George & Gwyther, 1986; Zarit et al., 1980). Depression may continue even when the client dies and the family caregiver no longer has the responsibility for carrying out daily care tasks (Bodnar & Kiecolt-Glaser, 1993; Mullen, 1992).

Studies of caregivers before and after placing their family members in a nursing home have mixed results regarding the well-being of the caregiver. One study found that caregivers spent less time helping the elder and more time in desirable activities such as visiting other family members, recreation, and activities outside the home (Moss et al., 1993). Other studies found that caregivers continued to experience distress after placing the client in a nursing home (Cohen & Eisdorfer, 1988; Colerick & George, 1986; Dura et al., 1990).

Anxiety and Guilt Providing care to ill children, parents, or spouses leads to anxiety (Wade et al., 1986; Wellisch et al., 1983; Patterson, 1988). There is anxiety about the client's future health and eventual death, about the caregiver's own feelings of vulnerability and loss of control, about the effects of the illness and caregiving on other family members, and about finances (Pederson & Valanis, 1988; Patterson, 1988). Caregivers also express anxiety about their need to learn complex skills for home care, especially if they receive conflicting information from physicians and other health care providers. In fact, dealing with medical care providers can, in itself, become a source of anxiety (Pederson & Valanis, 1988; Patterson, 1988). In the case study of the H. family, the physician's introduction of the need for a DNR consent aroused anxiety, since this had never been brought up in previous hospitalizations.

Feelings of guilt, generated from the anger and frustration of the caregiving situation, can overwhelm the caregiver. For instance, anger may occur when the client lacks motivation (Thompson, Bundek, & Sobolew-Shubin, 1990) or can be secondary to the client's unpredictable, uncooperative, threatening, physically abusive, ungrateful, paranoid, or wandering behavior (Vitaliano et al., 1993). In efforts to motivate the client, the caregiver may then become highly critical. When this is unsuccessful, the caregiver becomes overprotective and does "too much" for the client (Thompson, Bundek, & Sobolew-Shubin, 1990). Thus, there seems to be a vicious cycle: The client enacts negative behaviors, the caregiver criticizes this behavior, and the negative behaviors escalate, making caregiving more difficult (Vitaliano, et al., 1993).

Criticism of the client leads to feelings of guilt when negative behaviors are disease related. Guilt may also stem from feelings that the caregiver is focusing too much on his or her own needs (Vess et al., 1988).

Parents of chronically ill children may find that physicians have little or no experience with their child's illness, because chronic illnesses in children are uncommon (Hobbs et al., 1985). Parents may experience guilt and anxiety related to the cause of the child's illness; feel that they caused the illness by defective genes or inadequate prenatal care; or blame one another (Patterson, 1988). They may worry about whether they should have more children, especially if the ill child is the firstborn (Zucman, 1982). Anxiety, guilt, and helplessness arise in parents of ill children who have pain; parents, especially fathers, wish they could take on the child's suffering and feel powerless when they cannot (Shapiro, 1983).

Feelings of anxiety and guilt are burdensome for family caregivers. They are reluctant to express their concerns to the client, since the client already has to deal with major life changes and losses (Vess et al., 1988). Many spouse caregivers are left without the emotional support from a person who was previously their closest confidant.

Caregiver Burnout A study of 510 family caregivers found that most of them seldom received assistance (George, 1987). They relied most heavily on close family members for help with client or home care and on friends for companionship (George, 1987). However, more than half of them reported needing more help from family and friends than they received (George, 1987). Caregivers are more likely to obtain help if they themselves become ill (George, 1987).

Anger Providing care to the client can be perceived as an unrewarding, unappreciated experience, especially when the care recipient "does not perceive the support as helpful; because the provider does not understand the individual's support needs; because of miscommunication by recipients and/or providers; or because of who is providing the support" (Revenson, 1990, p. 99).

Caregivers of dying patients find that the client's anger is one of the most difficult emo-tions to confront. The dying patient may verbalize anger because the caregiver will live but he or she will not. The anger may take the form of trying to control the caregiver, since controlling "is an immediate, almost tangible expression of the dying person's continued ability to have an effect on life" (Sankar, 1991, p. 132). The client can place unrealistic and unrelenting demands on the caregiver and then retaliate furiously when these demands are not met (Sankar, 1991).

Caregivers often feel unable to respond to the anger as they normally would, but instead "swallow" their feelings, creating a serious strain in some caregivers that increases their anxiety about the dying person (Sankar, 1991). As long as the caregiver feels the client is rational, the caregiver struggles with a mixture of guilt, hurt, resentment, and protective sympathy. If the client is judged to be cognitively impaired, the experience is additionally painful (Sankar, 1991), since the client cannot be held responsible for his or her anger.

Loss of Self Caregivers may experience a "loss of self," defined as "a loss of identity that comes about as a results of engulfment in the caregiver's role" (Skaff & Pearlin, 1992, p. 656). Such loss is associated with lower self-esteem, lower self-mastery, and depression (Skaff & Pearlin, 1992). When caregiving requires a great deal of vigilance and energy, little is left to invest in other roles and activities. In addition, the impaired family member may no longer be able to provide positive feedback necessary to foster positive identities in caregiving.

Spouses caring for Alzheimer's patients are more likely to experience loss of self than are adult children, possibly caused by the loss of a previously intimate marital relationship (Skaff & Pearlin, 1992). Women caregivers are also more likely to experience a loss of self than men, since retired men caregivers are more likely to view caregiving as a new job.

Younger caregivers also report more loss of self than older caregivers; they often have to give up plans for a new job, returning to school, or pursuing an intimate relationship (Skaff & Pearlin, 1992). Interestingly, the more roles caregivers had, the less they experience loss of self (Skaff & Pearlin, 1992). Being employed, married, or having children provides caregivers with roles that offer identities separate from that of caregiver.

Isolation When the client is a child, parents have problems explaining the chronic illness to the extended family and friends. Unlike adulthood, in which there are many chronic illnesses, the prevalence of any single, specific chronic illness in childhood is less than 1 per 100 children (Patterson, 1988). This fosters the family's sense of isolation, for the child and family are unlikely to know others coping with the same illness; they may feel different, isolated, and not understood (Patterson, 1988). In addition, these families can have difficulty finding the appropriate medical services for diagnosis and treatment, or they may have to travel extended distances or relocate to be near service providers, again enhancing isolation.

Other family units also undergo isolation. For example, families where there is an Alzheimer's patient or mentally ill person are often shunned or avoided by others; certain behaviors of clients alienate others, or the family may focus primarily on the disease and symptoms, which limits common grounds for socialization with others. In addition, families often isolate themselves for various reasons.

An important factor in diminishing the burden of caregiving is the need for social interaction for fun and recreation (Thompson et al., 1993). Pleasant socializing activities enhance the caregiver's sense of well-being; lack of such outside activities increases the caregiver's sense of being overburdened with the caregiver role (Thompson et al., 1993).

Elder Abuse Care recipients can be at risk for elder abuse. Causes of elder abuse perpetrated by caregivers include stress on the caregiver secondary to dealing with a dependent, difficult elderly relative; caregiver exhaustion or resentment, or frustration and anger due to caregiving demands (USDHHS, 1990).

Family systems have characteristics that contribute to elder abuse. These include lack of family support; caregiver reluctance; overcrowding; isolation; intrafamily burdens; marital conflict;

and mixed feelings among family members about institutionalizing the elder (USDHHS, 1990).

Role Changes

Caregiving roles compete with other family roles. Managing one's relations within a family can be as difficult and as stressful as the direct burdens of caregiving (Semple, 1992).

Spouse Roles Chronic illness alters marital partners' roles. The client loses the ability to carry out previous family roles, such as performance of household chores, organization of family finances, or coordination of activities, and these are assumed by the healthier caregiver (Leventhal et al., 1985). In our case study, Mr. H. took over his wife's homemaker role, including cooking and grocery shopping, when her symptoms made these tasks difficult. However, it was the adult son who took over the role of major decision maker in times of emergency.

Client and caregiver can have an ongoing struggle with dependency issues subsequent to the fatigue, pain, disability, cognitive impairments, and emotional distress that the illness imposes on the client (Burish & Bradley, 1983). While the client becomes increasingly dependent on the spouse-caregiver, the caregiver's dependence on the client-spouse decreases (Leventhal et al., 1985).

Role Reversal Adult children often find it necessary to deal with role reversal especially when the adult child cares for an impaired parent. Adult caregivers of elderly parents report conflicting values regarding caregiving versus what they desire for themselves. While they approve of extended family care for an older parent, they do not want to be dependent upon their own children, preferring nonfamily caregivers should they become ill. This value conflict is reported to be stressful (Wallahagon & Strawbridge, 1993).

Role Changes When Parents Care for Ill Children When parents are the primary caregivers of ill children, siblings report feeling that their parents are preoccupied with the ill child and not available or accessible to them (Gallo, 1988). When the ill child is cared for in the home, housing space may be reallocated for equipment needs (e.g., hospital bed, ventilator, and so forth). Siblings often feel that parents have unrealistic expectations of them, especially in terms of household responsibilities and being emotionally able to handle the upsets and crises of their sibling's illness (Gallo, 1988; Patterson, 1988).

There may be feelings of resentment regarding the parents' inattentiveness to siblings' needs and the lack of honest communication about the ill member's problems. Siblings often choose not to communicate their problems and concerns to parents, and may turn to each other for support. Family vacations, family outings, recreation, and play may be restricted because parental financial and emotional resources are channeled into care of the ill child.

Adult Sibling Roles Adult siblings also face role changes. Married daughters, who provided care to elderly parents with dementia, identified siblings and friends as sources of interpersonal support, especially friends who had also cared for an elderly relative (Suitor & Pillemer, 1993). However, siblings were overwhelmingly identified as the greatest source of interpersonal stress (Suitor & Pillemer, 1993). Even when siblings struggle jointly on decisions about their parents' care, the primary caregiver may feel singularly entitled to make decisions and resent siblings for not carrying their share of the caretaking burden. In addition, there may be unresolved feelings of rivalry from childhood, especially if siblings have not maintained close contact with each other (Suitor & Pillemer, 1993). Family caregivers report that the most painful and divisive conflicts that occur relate to decision making about the way care is provided (especially the adequacy of pain relief), the competence of professional staff, and whether treatments should be started or stopped (Sankar, 1991).

Financial Impact

Employment Over one-third of all family caregivers are employed (Soldo & Myllyluoma, 1983). Differences in caregiving often depend on the employment status of the caregiver. Adult children who work fulltime and live in separate households contribute significantly less time to caregiving than their counterparts who do not work full time (Moss et al., 1993). Caregivers, spouses or children, who either co-reside with the client or do not work full-time devote more than twice the time to caregiving than do working caregivers who do not live with the client (Moss et al., 1993). This may imply that elders who live separately from their caregivers, or who stay at home while the caregiver works, are at risk of premature institutionalization (Moss et al., 1993). While employed caregivers may experience stress from the demands of multiple roles, they seem to suffer less from a "loss of self," indicating there are benefits other than financial incentives for caregivers to maintain outside employment (Skaff & Pearlin, 1992).

Sometimes caregiving requires a wage earner to leave his or her place of employment. This is detrimental in the long run, especially for women with low or moderate earning histories, since leaving a job to care for others is associated with reduced Social Security benefits for the caregiver when she herself retires (Kingston & O'Grady-LeShane, 1993).

When the client is an ill child, it is usually the mother who terminates her employment is order to stay home and care for the child. Consequently, the father may need to work more hours to earn enough to support the family, especially with the additional financial burdens imposed by the child's illness. Parents may decline job promotions requiring relocation if needed medical services are near where they currently live (Patterson, 1988).

Public Policy The Family and Medical Leave Act of 1993 is landmark legislation addressing the needs of family caregivers. This law states that covered employees must be allowed up to twelve weeks of unpaid, job-protected leave for certain family and medical reasons including child care after a birth or adoption, care for an immediate family member or parent with a serious health condition, or a health condition of the employee that prevents performance of the job. Employees need to contact their human resources personnel to find out if their employing agency is covered by this legislation. If covered, individuals are eligible if they have worked for at least one year and for 1250 hours over the previous twelve months, and if there are less than 50 employees all living within a seventy-five mile radius (U.S. Department of Labor, 1993).

Currently there is no public financing of long-term care at home, except for hospice programs with a time-limited period during which the client is expected to die (USDHHS, 1990). Without such funding, families are often left in poverty when their financial resources are channeled into the client's health care (U.S. Senate Special Committee on Aging, 1988).

Many private insurers offer long-term care policies through employers, fraternal organizations, retirement communities, and health management organizations (*Respite Report,* 1993). Although these policies cover nursing homes, home health agencies, and day care centers, they do not cover care provided by families at home.

Federal Programs Medicare covers individuals who are 65 years of age and older, those under 65 who qualify for disability payments under Social Security, and people diagnosed with endstage renal disease (USDHHS, 1990). The Medicare program is primarily geared to institutional care of acute illness (USDHHS, 1990) with only 2 percent of the budget spent on home health services. Under the Medicare hospice benefit, clients can be admitted to the hospital for five days a 'month for caregiver respite (Sankar, 1991). However, no reimbursement is available to family members for care provided at home.

Medicaid, designed for low-income individuals or families, is administered by states under federal guidelines and focuses on meeting client needs at minimal cost. It serves as the major source of public financing for nursing home care, but requires beneficiaries to "spend down" before receiving financial assistance (USDHHS, 1990).

The majority of home care is paid for with Medicaid and Medicare money (MacAdam, 1993), making the availability and quality of home services for caregivers and clients dependent on public policies and federal programs.

Unfortunately, these programs are vulnerable to shifts in public policy, which result in changes in reimbursement rates that are critical to attracting and retaining qualified home health paraprofessionals (MacAdam, 1993). Like Medicare, Medicaid does not provide financial reimbursement to family caregivers.

Interventions

A range of strategies are used to enhance family resources needed to balance the demands and stresses of caregiving and to promote a decent quality of life for caregiver and care recipient. The literature deals primarily with resources for the elderly, since this group continues to make up the majority of those needing care in the community. However, other populations are in need of similar services.

Caregivers need various kinds of information to efficiently care for the client. Health providers are an excellent source for such information. Caregivers need to learn skills for carrying out technical tasks, including safe techniques for turning, lifting, and moving clients, and administering medications safely. For example, learning body mechanics reduces back injuries among caregivers. Caregivers also need to know where to obtain physical assistance or equipment (Chanress, 1993), legal and financial information (USDHHS, 1990), emotional support (Fink, 1993; Woods et al., 1993), adequate respite (George, 1987), and ways of avoiding burnout (USDHHS, 1990; Thompson et al., 1993; Brody, 1985).

Dealing with Growth and Development

Growth and development knowledge can be helpful for caregivers regardless of the client's age (see Chapter 2, on growth and development). Education and training programs can provide family caregivers with an understanding of normal processes through the life cycle, both physical and psychosocial. This helps caregivers understand normal versus disease-related changes they observe in the affected family member so they can more effectively deal with decision-making issues, obtain appropriate available community resources, and secure emotional support for themselves (USDHHS, 1990). Educational material is also available from specialty organizations, such as the March of Dimes, for families of recipients of different ages—for example, children and adolescents. The case study of Andrew, the ventilator-dependent child, demonstrates the importance of support and education for the parent.

Andrew's story illustrates some of the client and family needs that must be addressed. Andrew's growth, development, and social needs are addressed by his mother, their extended family, his nurses, and his therapists. As he grows older, his changing needs must be considered by individualizing the services he obtains and by treating him as normally as possible. His mother must learn about changes he will undergo and how to interface effectively with institutions such as hospitals, clinics, and schools. To achieve this, she needs various supportive services. She also needs to have her own needs met so that she can more effectively deal with Andrew's chronic condition. Andrew's restructured family, without his father, has successfully incorporated him into a coherent unit and has not allowed his illness to be a major obstacle.

Coping with Role Problems

Health professionals can assist the family in coping with role problems by emphasizing family strengths, by reflecting back stated feelings, and by asking family members open-ended questions about their expectations of each other (Payne, 1988). Realistic information about family expectations of the client and of each other can be provided. For example, fatigue is a symptom of many chronic diseases, but family members may misinterpret a client's fatigue as laziness, lack of motivation, or depression.

Families need to reintegrate their roles. They should be encouraged to verbalize and accept their feelings about caregiving responsibilities, the personal rewards of specific roles, and the lack of predictability inherent in chronic illness. When family members express anxiety or guilt about resenting their roles, they should be re-

minded to be as patient and tolerant of themselves as they feel they should be with the client (Payne, 1988).

Managing Interpersonal Interactions

Caregivers must have realistic expectations of the caregiving role (Watt & Calder, 1981). They often have many expectations that are not realistic: The chronic illness will be temporary, the client's functioning level will improve, or caregiving responsibilities will be time limited. They assume that personal reserves of energy and resources are endless and that they will never become angry, feel guilty, or become exhausted (Thorne, 1993; Sankar, 1991; Chilman et al., 1988). Such expectations often are differ from actual circumstances.

Prevention can balance unrealistic expectations. When possible, extensive planning should precede the assumption of caregiving responsibility. Circumstances such as limited health or inadequate resources need to be considered. A reasoned decision can be reached if the illness trajectory is known (see Chapter 3, on illness trajectory) and if available resources are researched. The health professional can help by assessing, teaching, counseling, and assisting the caregiver in gaining information on community agencies, health and social service departments, and finances (Watt & Calder, 1981). Such efforts ensure more realistic expectations of the caregiving role.

Attitudes of both the care receiver and the caregiver influence interpersonal interactions. Working with clients requires differentiating wants and needs (Watt & Calder, 1981). Ignoring this distinction can lead to disappointment, complaints, and distrust. Frequent irritating requests can be a means of gaining attention that could be given in other ways, thereby leading to fewer demands. The client's preferences must be respected if they are reasonable and do not consume every waking hour. If the client prefers to be alone, that wish should be respected. Clients who cannot acknowledge that they have a chronic illness present problems, since they do not try to live the most normal life possible within illness limitations. Such individuals often

CASE STUDY
Caregiving for a Ventilator-Dependent Child

Ms. L. C. is a 39-year-old white female divorced from her husband. She lives with her 2-year-old son Andrew, who has central hypoventilation syndrome (he does not breathe unassisted when asleep) and prolonged expiratory apnea (he has frequent hypoxic episodes when awake). It was Andrew's illness that led to the couple separating. After birth, Andrew was hospitalized for approximately three months with his mother remaining near the hospital rather than returning home, 70 miles away. Her absence was seen as inattentiveness and neglect by her husband. After they learned that the baby had a poor prognosis, the parents disagreed about his treatment, resulting in much conflict, domestic violence, and the eventual separation.

Home Setting. L. C. and Andrew live in a small, one-bedroom upstairs apartment on the outskirts of a small city. The living room is largely taken up with Andrew's crib and equipment: ventilator, apnea monitor, oxygen tanks, and suction equipment. Ms. C. keeps the apartment very clean to avoid respiratory irritants for her son. Toys are in every room.

Support System. Ms. C does not trust Mr. C. There is a restraining order to keep him out of the apartment, as he has stated he wishes to take Andrew off of life support. Mr. C.'s mother and sister do not acknowledge Andrew as part of the family. They visited once in the hospital after Andrew was born, but tried to take out the baby's tracheostomy tube, for in their culture only "normal" healthy babies are allowed to live.

L. C.'s mother comes to visit her daily. Her sister visits several times a week when she is off from work. Two nephews also visit once or twice weekly. Thus, there is extended family support for her from her family and much conflict from Mr. C.'s family. The consistent emotional support provided by her family keeps Ms. C. strong in her belief that her son deserves to live as normal a life as possible. She maintains a positive, almost stoic attitude about raising him at home.

Growth and Development Issues. The developmental task for this family is to incorporate the child into the family unit. The family unit itself changed after Andrew's birth given the separation of the parents due to conflicts between their values of the child's right to live. Andrew is part of his mother's extended family system. L. C. has begun to date again, which has positive implications for her meeting her own needs as well as potential long-term implications for the family unit.

Andrew is played with in developmentally appropriate ways. He is frequently held and cuddled by his mother and her extended family. He is able to get around the apartment in his walker and is taken for age-appropriate excursions outside the home with his ventilator and the nurse.

Professional Assistance for the Child. Andrew has 24-hour-a-day nursing care. Importantly, Ms. C. refers to two of the nurses as part of the family, since they have cared for him for so long. In addition, he has a special education teacher once weekly, and a physical therapist and a speech therapist who come every other week.

Assistance for the Parent Caregiver. The mother identified her need for support and counseling services. She was provided with the following information: The American Red Cross offers support groups for parents of children at home on high-tech care. The New York State Department of Health Council on Child and Adolescent Health offers a *Directory of Self-Help/Mutual Support for Children with Special Health Needs and Their Families* (1992). The National Organization of Rare Disorders is also a reference for self-help groups. The local county Mental Health Association is an additional resource for parent caregivers. L. C. is fortunate that her family allows her respite from her parenting and caregiving responsibilities. She can therefore participate in such self-help and support groups.

SOURCE: This case study is provided by Allison M. Goodell, R.N., B.S.N. staff nurse in the pediatric intensive care unit of the Children's Hospital at Albany Medical Center Hospital, Albany, New York.

need help to prevent jeopardizing their safety and health.

Learning to Take Care of Oneself

Family caregivers need to learn strategies to manage the conflicting feelings of anxiety and guilt they may experience. Open communication and a chance to vent one's feelings may reduce resentment. They need opportunities to express some of their feelings and frustration to others, found to be associated with less caregiver burden and resentment for stroke caregivers (Thompson, Bundek, & Sobolew-Shubin, 1990). Caregivers often feel that expressing such negative feelings is not in the client's best interest (Taylor & Dakof, 1988), and so they tend to avoid such discussions (Vess et al., 1988).

Taking time away from the 24-hour responsibility of caregiving is essential for those who co-reside with their clients. This requires help from others and may require a willingness to compromise some details of care or housekeeping. Caregivers may need encouragement to accept assistance from others, such as housekeeping, shopping, or sitting with the client. They should clearly specify what help they need when others make offers to assist them. The neighbor who offers to help should be allowed to help, but not to the extent that the offer will not be repeated (Chilman et al., 1988).

Caregivers also need to devote time and energy to activities other than providing care to avoid a sense of entrapment and feelings of loss of self and burnout. Attention to self helps sustain one's sense of well-being and revitalizes energy that can later be used in providing care to the client. But many caregivers feel guilty about activities that focus on themselves (Vess et al., 1988). This is unfortunate, since feeling guilty about meeting one's own needs accomplishes little. An occasional indulgence or gift can lift one's spirits immensely. Friendships and social contacts, participating in one's religious services, and attending support groups can help prevent isolation and promote well-being (Thompson et al., 1993). Caregivers need to determine their preferences and which activities they find meaningful, and then work toward creating time for them (Watt & Calder, 1981).

Caregivers need to know how to manage not only their time but their money (Watt & Calder, 1981). They need a realistic idea of the costs of living, charges for services, which services are covered under their insurance policies, and how to obtain information about their coverage. Children who are providing care need to know about their parents' finances and health insurance policies, and the extent of help the family is willing to contribute to their parents' care.

Respite

It is important for caregivers to recognize warning signs that indicate that their coping skills are overwhelmed and they need outside help. For many caregivers, the hardest step is acknowledging that one needs help; the next most difficult is extending the effort to seek help (Sankar, 1991; Chilman et al., 1988). Caregivers often feel guilty about seeking respite and delay using formal respite services until they themselves are exhausted and debilitated (Sankar, 1991). They need to see respite services as a reasonable and appropriate action, not as a sign of personal failure, if they plan to continue caregiving without being overwhelmed by the physical and social demands.

Respite is temporary relief from caregiving responsibilities. Crossman and associates (1981) define respite as "any service, whether it be day care, home care, or brief periods of institutionalization, that provides intervals of rest and relief for the caregiver." Family members may provide the primary caregiver respite by taking over some tasks; for example, daughters may assist their caregiving mothers by shopping, cleaning, and so forth. There are also formal sources of respite.

Short-Term Institutional Placement When caregiving is too physically demanding or emotionally draining, short-term institutional placement of the client may be a care alternative. Under the Medicare hospice benefit, it is possible for family caregivers to admit a client to the hospital for five days a month for caregiver respite (Sankar, 1991). Other insurance plans may have a similar benefit.

The Veterans Administration has established short-term arrangements for families of veterans so they can have brief periods of respite (Ellis & Wilson, 1983). In one particular program, the family requests to have a client admitted, and screening is done by the admission team. Medical evaluation of the client's current health status is required because the program is designed to manage only stable health conditions during the respite period. Persons whose conditions worsen during the program are transferred out of the unit. In spite of this feature, a much greater than expected number of clients were found to need maximum nursing care. Consequently, total-care patients are limited to no more than three at any given time. This program, which reinvigorates the family caregiver, is considered valuable because it delays more costly admissions, helps keep families together, and minimizes cost.

Community-Based Respite Programs Community-based respite programs provide a break for the main caregiver from some of his or her daily duties, either in the home or in an adult day care center. In the home, respite workers provide assistance for a few hours of the day, or even at night since sleep deprivation is a common problem among caregivers (Sankar, 1991).

Adult Day Care Centers Adult day care centers are one form of community-based respite program. The number of such centers in the United States has increased dramatically from 18 in 1974 to 1,700 currently (Conrad et al., 1993). Typically they are small, averaging 20 clients per day (Conrad et al., 1990).

Great variation exists in the type and amount of services that these centers provide. Using a classification system, two specialized classes of adult day care centers have been identified: Alzheimer's family care and rehabilitation (Conrad et al., 1993). Other centers offer socialization and clinical programs for disabled adults with varying degrees of independence in carrying out their activities of daily living (Conrad et al., 1993). Evaluation studies of these programs show that they have modest positive impacts on client health, satisfaction, and functional ability (Rubenstein, 1987) while providing caregivers with temporary and welcome relief from the tasks of supervising and caring for the client.

Some hospitals have initiated hospital-based day care that offers socialization and psychotherapy programs for clients with cognitive or behavioral problems while providing respite care for their families (Rubenstein, 1987).

Self-Help Groups

Self-help groups typically focus on specific client populations and related caregivers' needs. Such groups evolved because the health care system was not meeting client or family needs. Self-help groups for caregivers of the elderly have been established in many communities throughout the United States. Some are self-directed or run by volunteers; others are led by health care professionals who act as group facilitators. These groups provide information, emotional support, advocacy, or a combination of these services (USDHHS, 1990).

Support groups address such areas as skills in the care and maintenance of the disabled person and managing problems in the family; information regarding the aging process; emotional needs for recognition and support from caring people; and concrete service needs for referral and information regarding resources.

The Family Support Program of Duke University stresses that a central facility is needed for maintaining and extending support groups by providing a place where information can be disseminated, a telephone hotline can be placed, training for group facilitators can be done, and evaluating performance can be carried out (Duke University Center for the Study of Aging and Human Development, 1992). The Alzheimer's Association provides support and assistance to Alzheimer's Disease clients and their families (Alzheimer's Association, 1990) through its network of chapters, volunteers, and support groups. The National Alliance for the Mentally Ill (NAMI) focuses on families of the severely and recurrently mentally ill (NAMI, 1987).

Additional Roles for Professional Caregivers

When professionals provide services for chronically ill individuals, the family is not pushed out of the caregiving role. Provider assistance may help the caregiver to master ways of managing at home and may offer additional services to client and family based on a professional assessment.

Assessment A thorough assessment of the family's needs, problems, and personal and social resources is essential to effective intervention for the client and caregiver. Assessing psychological distress in a family caregiver as well as the caregiver's sources of support is important in assisting that person.

Because the ethnicity and culture of a family influence their values about health, family, and caregiving, and their perceptions of burden, health providers need to be sensitive to cultural dimensions of psychological distress. Assessment tools are available in the literature for use with clients and family to help identify demands of illness (Haberman et al., 1990).

Multiple methods should be used in assessing clients and caregivers: verbal self-reports, translators for clients whose primarily language is not English, forms written in the clients' language, and observation of client–family interactions (Aroian & Potsdaughter, 1989). Learning how to do culturally sensitive assessments of family caregivers may bolster the providers' confidence and skills in dealing with clients of different ethnic backgrounds. One study of community health nurses demonstrated that they lacked confidence in providing care to Black, Puerto Rican and Southeast Asian clients (Bernal & Froman, 1987).

The family's knowledge and perception of available sources of support should be explored. This includes spiritual help, formal services, how family roles and tasks are restructured, and how family priorities are changed. It also includes the quantity and quality of affective (emotional) and instrumental (tangible assistance with physical care tasks, housekeeping, and financial matters) support. During times of crisis, it is important to know what has helped the family in previous crises. Different types of support are needed at different times during the chronic illness trajectory (Woods et al., 1988).

Knowledge of services is a prerequisite to using them. Family use of different services needs to be explored and information gained about whether families have used different services in the past, and if these have been satisfactory experiences. Families may also need assistance in understanding eligibility requirements for services. Finally, families may be aware of and eligible for services such as respite, but reluctant to use them (Sankar, 1991) because of values and personal expectations of themselves as caregivers. Health professionals need to reinforce that outside services enhance family caregiving, and assist the family in providing care without exhausting their personal and family resources.

Counseling Counseling gives families support and information that they need (Woods et al., 1988). Counseling services can be combined with other programs such as day care or self-help groups. Some of the issues that caregivers need to work on during counseling include the following:

1. *The role of emotions.* Anger, frustration, and sorrow are natural emotions for family caregivers (Rolland, 1988). When they result in wishing the client would die, then guilt can ensue, further complicating matters. Caregivers may express anger at medical staff for not "fixing" the client (Doherty, 1988).
2. *Caretaker health.* Continuing to provide care requires maintaining one's own health, despite the common notion that one must be self-sacrificing. Self-care includes rest, occasional self-indulgence, and respite from responsibilities (Thompson et al., 1993; Stephens et al., 1988).
3. *Caretaker decisions.* The ultimate decision maker when conflicts arise with the client or other family members is the primary caregiver (Sankar, 1991; Thompson et al., 1993).
4. *Role changes.* Switching roles can be emotionally distressing for all concerned and can promote intrafamily conflicts (Patterson, 1988; Boss et al., 1988; Bonjean, 1988). Mutual sharing of concerns helps all to understand that such dissention is natural.
5. *Lack of improvement.* Since little that the family does results in improvement, there

is no reason to feel guilty (Rolland, 1988; Gaynor, 1990).

6. *Competing commitments.* Caregivers often feel pulled toward multiple commitments. For example, a married daughter caring for an aging patient may feel that her spouse and children are being neglected (Brody, 1985), or they may feel neglected by her (Thompson et al., 1993). Caregivers may need to change their priorities at different stages in the illness trajectory.

Formalizing and Coordinating Family Caregiving In addition to assessment and counseling, health care professionals can support family caregivers by formally recognizing their roles in caring for clients and coordinating the family caregiver role with other services (USDHHS, 1990). The health professional needs to develop a service contract with the family caregiver that identifies and delineates in writing the caregiving role. The overall service plan thus includes both the family's services and those provided by the health care agency. In this way, the family caregiver and client define their own service packages; the primary family caregiver is the case manager. The health agency fills in the "gaps" by providing services that support and enhance, not substitute for, family caregiving (USDHHS, 1990).

Many personal care tasks are shared by family caregivers and formal (paid) help, such as feeding, getting out of bed or chair, dressing, bathing, toileting, and incontinence care (Schirm, 1989). By designating the primary family caregiver as the case manager, nurses can promote a relationship in which both the family and the health care professional trust in their own competence (Schirm, 1989; Thorne & Robinson, 1989).

Summary and Conclusions

The experience of family caregiving is shaped by culture and ethnicity, which influence family size and composition, living arrangements, socioeconomic status, education, and health practices. These factors are integrated in values related to health, illness, dependency, caregiving, and family members' obligations to each other.

Family members provide most caregiving to at-home clients as long as the demands of care do not exceed the family's resources. When the definition of family extends beyond kinship bonds to people committed to each other for a long duration, the term "family caregivers" encompasses partners in such relationships as gay and lesbian couples and other co-residing individuals. A knowledge base of the caregiving practices of these client families needs to be built in order to help them enhance their caregiving skills.

Wives and daughters are most often the caregivers in families. When these women need to leave their jobs to assume caregiving tasks, especially if they have low and medium-salaried positions in the work force, they shortchange themselves in terms of decreased future Social Security benefits. Moreover, these same women may not have available caregivers should they eventually need them, since a shortage of family and paraprofessional caregivers is predicted for the future.

Health care professionals need to promote family caregivers' well-being, which is a complex, multidimensional concept that includes personal meanings (Woods et al., 1993; Birren et al., 1991; George & Gwyther, 1986). Caregivers may need assistance in clarifying their own needs and in acquiring the information, support, and services to meet those needs.

Nurses need to join with families to advocate for changes in legislation at the state and federal levels regarding caregiver needs, such as leave from employment, reimbursement for home care and respite services, research on caregiving, and training and education programs. In this way, health professionals assist family caregivers on an individual and national level.

NURSING DIAGNOSIS

Editor's Note: There are several diagnostic categories that should be considered when dealing with the problems faced by family caregivers. Prominent among them are the following.

3.2.1 Altered Role Performance

(See Chapter 4, on illness roles for definition, defining characteristics, and related factors.) The reader is directed to consider *role strain* as the most clinically applicable for the family caregiver.

3.1.2 Social Isolation

(See Chapter 8 on social isolation for definition, defining characteristics, and related factors.)

5.1.2.1.1 Ineffective Family Coping: Disabling

Definition: Behavior of significant person (family member or other primary person) that disables his or her own capacities and the client's capacities to effectively address tasks essential to either person's adaptation to the health challenge.

Defining Characteristics: Neglectful care of the client in regard to basic human needs and/or illness treatment; distortion of reality regarding the client's health problem, including extreme denial about its existence or severity; intolerance/rejection/abandonment; desertion; carrying on usual routine, disregarding client's needs, psychosomaticism; taking on illness signs of client; decisions and actions by family which are detrimental to economic or social well-being; agitation, depression, aggression, hostility; impaired restructuring of a meaningful life for self, impaired individualization, prolonged overconcern for client; neglectful relationships with other family members; client's development of helpless, inactive dependence.

Related Factors: Significant person with chronically unexpressed feelings of guilt, anxi-

ety, hostility, despair, etc; dissonant discrepancy of coping styles for dealing with adaptive tasks by the significant person and client or among significant people; highly ambivalent family relationships; arbitrary handling of family's resistance to treatment, which tends to solidify defensiveness as it fails to deal adequately with underlying anxiety.

5.1.2.1.2 Ineffective Family Coping: Compromised

Definition: A usually supportive primary person (family member or close friend) is providing insufficient, ineffective, or compromised support, comfort, assistance, or encouragement that may be needed by the client to manage or master adaptive tasks related to his or her health challenge.

Defining Characteristics:

Subjective: Client expresses or confirms a concern or complaint about significant other's response to his or her health problem; significant person describes preoccupation with personal reaction (e.g., fear, anticipatory grief, guilt, anxiety) to client's illness, disability, or to other situational or developmental crises; significant person describes or confirms an inadequate understanding or knowledge base, which interferes with effective assistive or supportive behaviors.

Objective: Significant person attempts assistive or supportive behaviors with less than satisfactory results; significant person withdraws or enters into limited or temporary personal communication with the client at the time of need; significant person displays protective behavior disproportionate (too little or too much) to the client's abilities or need for autonomy.

Related Factors: Inadequate or incorrect information or understanding by a primary person; temporary preoccupation by a significant person who is trying to manage emotional conflicts and personal suffering and is unable to perceive or act effectively in regard to client's needs; temporary family disorganization and role changes; other situational or developmental crises or situations the significant person may be facing; little support provided by client, in turn, for primary person; prolonged disease or disability progression that exhausts supportive capacity of significant people.

Editor's Note: A differential diagnosis should be made between the two ineffective family coping diagnoses. Since caregivers generally prefer keeping care recipients at home, compromised coping is more likely. However, the home situation may have deteriorated enough that the family's ability to deal with the situation may be serious. Assessment and intervention may prevent such activities as elder abuse.

STUDY QUESTIONS

1. What are the advantages for the client of being cared for at home? for the family caregiver?
2. What factors influence the cost-effectiveness of home care versus institutionalization?
3. Who are the primary providers of home care? What roles changes do they undergo?
4. How does ethnicity influence family caregiving?
5. What is the psychological impact of caregiving on the caregiver?
6. What is the financial impact of caregiving on the caregiver? How does public policy affect caregiving?
7. What kind of respite programs are available?
8. What issues need to be addressed when counseling family caregivers?
9. How can health professionals assist family caregivers?
10. How can caregivers help themselves?

References

Alzheimer's Association (1990). *The Alzheimer's Association annual report.* Chicago: Alzheimer's Association.

Aroian, K. J., & Potsdaughter, C. A. (1989). Multiple-method, cross-cultural assessment of psychological distress. *Image: The Journal of Nursing Scholarship, 21*(2), 90-93.

Barresi, C. M. (1990). Diversity in Black family caregiving: Implications for geriatric education. In M. S. Harper (Ed.), *Minority aging: Essential curricula content for selected health and allied health professions.* Health Resources and Services Administration, Department of Health and Human Services, DHHS Publication No. HRS (P-DV-90-4). Washington, D.C.: U.S. Government Printing Office.

Bernal, H., & Froman, R. (1987). The confidence of community health nurses in caring for ethnically diverse populations. *Image: The Journal of Nursing Scholarship, 19*(4), 210-204.

Billingsley, A. & McCarley, L. (1986). Afro-American families and the elderly. Paper presented at the Conference on Mental Health and the Black Elderly. Atlanta University, Atlanta.

Birren, J. E., Lubben, J. E., Rowe, J. C., & Deutchman, D. E. (Eds.) (1991). *The concept and measurement of quality of life in the frail elderly.* New York: Academic Press.

Bodnar, J. C. & Kiecolt-Glaser, J. K. (1993). Caregiver stress after bereavement: It's not over when it's over. Paper presented at the Gerontological Society of America Conference, Washington D.C.

Bonjean, M. (1988). Children and chronic illness. In C. S. Chilman, E. W. Nunally, & F. M. Cox (Ed.), *Chronic illness and disability* (pp. 141-159). Newbury Park, CA: Sage.

Boss, R., Caron, W., & Horbal, J. (1988). Alzheimer's disease and ambiguous loss. In C. S. Chilman, E. W. Nunally, & F. M. Cox (Eds.), *Chronic illness and disability.* Newbury Park, CA: Sage.

Brody, E. (1985). Parent care as normative family stress. *The Gerontologist, 25*(1), 19-29.

Bumpass, L. L. (1990). What happening to the family: Interactions between demographic and institutional change. *Demography, 27*(4), 483-498.

Burish, T. G. & Bradley, L. A. (Eds.) (1983). *Coping with chronic disease.* New York: Academic Press.

Burton, L. M. (1992). Black grandparents rearing children of drug-addicted parents: Stressors, outcomes and social service needs. *The Gerontologist, 32*(6), 744-751.

Carp, F. M. (1987). The impact of planned housing. In V. Regnier & J. Pyhoos (Eds.), *Housing the aged* (pp. 327-360). New York: Elsevier.

Chanress, N. H. (1993, April). Whither technology and aging? *Gerontology News, 2,* 10.

Chilman, C. S., Nunnally, E. W., & Cox, F. M. (1988). *Chronic illness and disability.* Newbury Park, CA: Sage.

Cohen, D., & Eisdorfer, C. (1988). Depression in family members caring for a relative with Alzheimer's disease. *Journal of the American Geriatrics Society, 38,* 227-235.

Cohen, D., Luchins, D., Eisdorfer, C., Pavenza, G., Ashdorn, J. W., Gorelick, P., Hirschman, R., Freels, S., Levy, P., Senla, T., & Shaw, H. (1990). Caring for relatives with Alzheimer's Disease: The mental health risks to spouses, adult children, and other family caregivers. *Behavior, Health, and Aging, 1*(3), 171-182.

Cohen, M. H. (1993) The unknown and the unknowable—managing sustained uncertainty. *Western Journal of Nursing Research, 15*(1), 77-96.

Colerick, F. J. & George, L. (1986). Predictors of institutionalization among caregivers and patients with Alzheimer's disease. *Journal of the American Geriatrics Society, 34,* 493-498.

Conrad, K. J., Hanrahan, P., & Hughes, S. L. (1990). Survey of adult day care in the U.S.: National and regional findings. *Research on Aging, 12,* 36-56.

Conrad, K. J., Hughes, S. L., Hanrahan, P., & Wang, S. (1993). Classification of adult day care: A cluster analysis of services and activities. *Journals of Gerontology: Social Sciences, 48*(3), S112-S122.

Coward, R., Cutler, S., & Mullens, R. (1990). Residential differences in the comparisons of the helping networks of the impaired elderly. *Family Relations, 39,* 44-50.

Crossman, L., London, C., & Barry, C. (1981). Older women caring for disabled spouses: A model for supportive services. *The Gerontologist, 21*(5), 464-470.

Doherty, W. J. (1988). Implications of chronic illness for family treatment. In C. S. Chilman, E. W. Nunnally & F. M. Cox (Eds.), *Chronic illness and disability.* Newbury Park, CA: Sage.

Donar, M. E. (1988). Community care: Pediatric home mechanical ventilation. *Holistic nursing practice, 2*(2), 68-80.

Duke University Center for the Study of Aging and Human Development (1992). *Annual report 1991-1992.* Durham, NC: Duke University.

Dura, J. R., Stukenberg, K. W. & Kiecolt-Glaser, J. K. (1990). Chronic stress and depressive disorders in older adults. *Journal of Abnormal Psychiatry, 99,* 284-290.

Eisdorfer, C. (1991). Caregiving: An emerging risk factor for emotional and physical pathology. *Bulletin of the Menninger Clinic, 55,* 238-247.

Ellis, V., & Wilson, D. (1983). Respite care in the nursing home unit of a veterans hospital. *American Journal of Nursing, 83,* 1433-1434.

Fink, S. (1993). The effects of family strengths and resources on the well-being of women providing care to an elderly parent. Paper presented to the Gerontological Society of America Conference, Washington, D.C.

Gallo, A. M. (1988). The special sibling relationship in chronic illness and disability: Parental communication with well siblings. *Holistic Nursing Practice, 2*(2), 28-37.

Gaynor, S. E. (1989). When the caregiver becomes the patient. *Geriatric Nursing, 10*(3), 120-123.

——— (1990). The long haul: The effect of home care on the caregiver. *Image: The Journal of Nursing Scholarship, 22*(4), 208-212.

George, L. (1987). Easing caregiver burden: The role of informal and formal supports. In R. A. Ward & S. S. Tobin (Eds.), *Health in aging: Sociological issues and policy directions* (pp. 133-158). New York: Spring Publishing.

George, L. K. & Gwyther, L. P. (1986). Caregiver well-being: A multidimensional examination of family caregivers of demented adults. *The Gerontologist, 26*(3), 253-259.

Gortmaker, S. & Sapperfield, J. (1984). *Care of children with chronic illness.* Philadelphia: F. D. Davis.

Greater New York Hospital Foundation (1988). *Annual report.* New York: Greater New York Hospital Foundation.

Greene, V., Lovely, M. E., & Ondrich, J. I. (1993). The cost-effectiveness of community services in a rural elderly population. *The Gerontologist, 33*(2), 177-189.

Haberman, M. R., Woods, N. F., & Packard, N. J. (1990). Demands of chronic illness: Reliability and validity assessment of a demands-of-illness inventory. *Holistic Nursing Practice, 5*(1), 25-35.

Haley, W. E., & Pardo, K. M. (1989). Relations of severity of dementia to caregiving stressors. *Psychology and Aging, 4,* 389-392.

Harper, M. S. (Ed.) (1990). *Minority aging: Essential curricula content for selected health and allied health professions.* Health Resources and Services Administration, Department of Health and Human Services, DHHS Publication No. HRS (P-DV-90-4). Washington, D.C.: U.S. Government Printing Office.

Hobbs, N., Perrin, J. M., & Ireys, H. T. (1985). *Chronically ill children and their families.* San Francisco; Jossey-Bass.

Kane, N. M. (1989). The home care crisis of the nineties. *The Gerontologist, 29*(1), 24-31.

Kingston, E. R., & O'Grady-LeShane, R. (1993). The effects of caregiving on women's Social Security benefits. *The Gerontologist, 33*(2), 230-239.

Klein, S. (1989). Caregiver burden and moral development. *Image: Journal of Nursing Scholarship, 21*(2), 94-97.

Lawton, M. P., Kleban, M. H., Moss, M., Rovine, M., & Glicksman, A. (1989). Measuring caregiving appraisal. *Journals of Gerontology: Psychological Sciences, 44,* P61-P71.

Lee, G. R., Dwyer, J. W., & Coward, R. T. (1993). Gender differences in parent care: Demographic factors and the same-gender preferences. *Journals of Gerontology: Social Sciences, 48*(1), S9-S16.

Leventhal, H., Leventhal, E. A., & Nguyen, T. V. (1985). Reactions of families to illness: Theoretical models and perspectives. In D. C. Turk & R. D. Kerns (Eds.), *Health, illness and families: A lifespan perspective.* New York: John Wiley.

Lubben, J. E., & Beccera, R. M. (1988). Social support among Blacks, Mexicans, and Chinese elderly. In D. E. Gelfand & C. M. Barresi (Eds.), *Ethnic dimensions of aging* (pp. 130-144). New York: Springer.

MacAdam, M. (1993). Home care reimbursement and effects of personnel. *The Gerontologist, 33*(1), 55-63.

Markides, K. S. (Ed.) (1989). *Aging and health: Perspectives on gender, race, ethnicity and class.* Newbury Park, CA: Sage.

Markides, K. S., & Mindel, C. H. (1987). *Aging and ethnicity.* Newbury Park, CA: Sage.

Miller, L. (1987). *Optimum service allocation in a community-based long-term care program. MMSP Evaluation.* Berkeley, CA: University of California.

Mishel, M. H. (1988a). Uncertainty in illness. *Image: The Journal of Nursing Scholarship, 20*(4), 225-232.

―――― (1988b). *Proceedings of Conference: Coping with uncertainty in illness situations: New directions in theory development and research.* Rochester, NY: Sigma Theta Tau International, University of Rochester.

―――― (1990). Reconceptualization of the uncertainty in illness theory. *Image: The Journal of Nursing Scholarship, 22*(4), 256-262.

Moss, M. S., Lawton, M. P., Kleban, M. K., & Duhamel, L. (1993). Time use of caregivers of impaired elders before and after institutionalization. *Journals of Gerontology: Social Sciences, 48*(3), S102-S111.

Mullen, J. T. (1992). The bereaved caregiver: A prospective study of changes in well-being. *The Gerontologist, 32*(5), 673-683.

National Alliance for the Mentally Ill (NAMI) (1987). *National alliance for the mentally ill.* Arlington, VA: NAMI.

New York State Department of Health (1992). *New York State directory of self-help/mutual support for children with special health needs and their families.* Albany, NY: NYS Department of Health.

O'Brien, M. E. (1989). *Anatomy of a nursing home: A new view of resident life.* Owings Mills, MD: National Health Publishing.

Pastalan, L. A. (1983). Environmental displacement: A literature reflecting old person–environment transactions. In G. D. Rowles & R. J. Ohta (Eds.), *Aging and milieu: Environmental perspectives on growing old* (pp. 189-203). New York: Academic Press.

Patterson, J. M. (1988). Chronic illness in children and the impact on families. In C. S. Chilman, E. W. Nunnally, & F. M. Cox (Eds.) *Chronic illness and disability* (pp. 69-107). Newbury Park, CA: Sage.

Payne, M. B. (1988). Utilizing role theory to assist the family with sudden disability. *Rehabilitation Nursing, 13*(4), 191-194.

Pederson, L. M., & Valanis, B. G. (1988). The effects of breast cancer on the family: A review of the literature. *Journal of Psychosocial Oncology, 6,* 95-117.

Pless, I. B., & Perrin, J. M. (1985). Issues common to a variety of illnesses. In N. Hobbs & J. M. Perrin (Eds.), *Issues in the care of children with chronic illness* (pp. 41-60). San Francisco: Jossey-Bass.

Pruchno, R. A., & Resch, N. L. (1989). Caregiving spouses: Physical and mental health in perspective. *Journal of the American Geriatrics Society, 37,* 679-705.

Respite Report (1993, Spring). Day centers can take advantage of long-term care insurance. *Respite Report,* pp. 6, 9.

Revenson, T. A. (1990). Social support among chronically ill elders: Patient and provider perspectives. In H. Giles, N. Coupland, & J. M. Wiemann (Eds.), *Communication, health and the elderly* (pp. 92–113). London: Manchester University.

Rolland, J. S. (1988). Chronic illness in children and the impact on families. In C. S. Chilman, E. W. Nunnally, & F. M. Cox, (Eds.), *Chronic illness and disability.* Newbury Park, CA: Sage.

Rubenstein, L. Z. (1987). Innovations in hospital care for elders. *Generations, XII*(1), 65-70.

Rubinstein, R. L. (1989). The home environments of older people: A description of the psychosocial processes linking person to place. *Journals of Gerontology: Social Sciences, 44*(2), S45-S53.

Sankar, A. (1991). *Dying at home: A family guide to caregiving.* Baltimore: Johns Hopkins University Press.

Schirm, V. (1989). Shared care by formal and informal caregivers for community residing elderly. *Journal of the New York State Nurses Association, 20*(1), 8-14.

Semple, S. J. (1992). Conflict in Alzheimer's caregiving families: Its dimensions and consequences. *The Gerontologist, 32*(5), 648-655.

Sexton, D., & Munro, B. (1985). Impact of a husband's chronic illness (COPD) on the spouse's life. *Research in Nursing and Health, 8,* 83-90.

Shapiro, E., & Tate, R. B. (1986). Who is really at risk of institutionalization. *The Gerontologist, 28,* 237-245.

Shapiro, J. (1983). Family reactions and coping strategies in response to the physically ill or handicapped child: A review. *Social Science in Medicine, 17*(14), 913-931.

Shumaker, S. A., & Brownell, A. (1984). Toward a theory of social support: Closing conceptual gaps. *Journal of Social Issues, 40*(1), 11-36.

Silverstein, M., & Litwak, E. (1993). A task-specific typology of intergenerational family structure in later life. *The Gerontologist, 33*(2), 258-264.

Skaff, M. M., & Pearlin, L. I. (1992). Caregiving: Role engulfment and the loss of self. *The Gerontologist, 32*(5), 656-664.

Soldo, B. J., & Agree, E. M. (1988). America's elderly. *Population Bulletin, 43*(3).

Soldo, B. J., & Myllyluoma, J. (1983). Caregivers who live with dependent elderly. *The Gerontologist, 23*(6), 605-611.

Speare, A., & Avery, R. (1993). Who helps whom in older parent-child families. *Journals of Gerontology: Social Sciences, 48*(29), S64-S73.

Spitze, G., & Logan, J. R. (1990). Sons, daughters and intergenerational support. *Journal of Marriage and the Family, 52,* 420-430.

Spitze, G., Logan, J. R., & Robinson, J. (1992). Family structure and change in living arrangements among elderly nonmarried parents. *Journals of Gerontology: Social Sciences, 47*(6), S289-S296.

Stephens, M. A. P., Norris, V. K., Kinney, J. M., Ritchie, S. W., & Grotz, R. C. (1988). Stressful situations in caregiving: Relations between caregiver coping and well-being. *Psychology and Aging, 3,* 208-209.

Stoller, E. P., & Cutler, S. J. (1993). Predictors of use of paid help among older people living in the community. *The Gerontologist, 33*(1), 31-40.

Suitor, J. J., & Pillemer, K. (1990). Transition to the status of family caregiver: A new framework for studying social support and well-being. In S. M. Stahl (Ed.), *The legacy of longevity.* Newbury Park, CA: Sage Publications.

———— (1993). Support and interpersonal stress in the social networks of married daughters caring for parents with dementia. *Journal of Gerontology: Social Sciences, 48*(1), S1-S8.

Taylor, R. J. (1985). The extended family as a source of support to elderly Blacks. *The Gerontologist, 25,* 488-495.

Taylor, R. J., & Chatters, L. M. (1986, Nov./Dec.). Patterns of informal support to elderly Black adults: Family, friends, and church members. *Social Work,* pp. 432-438.

Taylor, S. E., & Dakof, G. A. (1988). Social support and the cancer patient. In S. Spacapan & S. Oskamp (Eds.), *The social psychology of health* (pp. 95-116). Newbury Park, CA: Sage.

Tennstedt, S. L., Crawford, S., & McKinlay, J. B. (1993). Determining the pattern of community care: Is coresidence more important than caregiver relationship? *Journals of Gerontology: Social Sciences, 48*(2), S74-S83.

Thompson, S. C., Bundek, N. L., & Sobolew-Shubin, A. (1990). The caregivers of stroke patients: An investigation of factors associated with depression. *Journal of Applied Social Psychology, 20,* 115-129.

Thompson, S. C., Futterman, A. M., Gallagher-Thompson, D., Rose, J. J., & Lovett, S. B. (1993). Social support and cargiving burden in family caregivers of frail elders. *Journals of Gerontology: Social Sciences, 48*(5), S245-254.

Thorne, S. E. (1993). *Negotiating health care: The social context of chronic illness.* Newbury Park, CA: Sage.

Thorne, S. E., & Robinson, C. A. (1989). Guarded alliance: Health care relationships in chronic illness. *Image: Journal of Nursing Scholarship, 21*(3), 153-157.

Thornton, C., Dunstan, S. M., & Kemper, P. (1988). The effect of Channeling on health and long-term care costs. *Health Services Research, 23,* 129-142.

Tucker, M. B., Taylor, R. J., & Mitchell-Kernan, C. (1993). Marriage and romantic involvement among aged African Americans. *Journals of Gerontology: Social Sciences, 48*(3), S123-S132.

U.S. Department of Health and Human Services (1990). *Geriatric training curriculum for public health professionals.* Washington, D.C.: USDHHS.

U.S. Department of Labor (1993). *The family and medical leave act of 1993.* Washington, D.C.: U.S. Department of Labor, Wage and Hour Division.

U.S. Senate Special Committee on Aging (1988). *Aging America. Trends and projections.* Washington D.C.: U.S. Government Printing Office.

Vess, J. D., Moreland, J. R., Schwebel, A. I., & Kraut, E. (1988). Psychosocial needs of cancer patients: Learning from patients and their spouses. *Journal of Psychosocial Oncology, 6,* 31-51.

Vitaliano, P. P., Russo, J., Young, H. M., Becker, J., & Maiuro, R. D. (1991). The screen for caregiver burden. *The Gerontologist, 31,* 76-83.

Vitaliano, P. P., Young, H. M., Russo, J., Romano, J, & Magana-Amato, A. (1993). Does expressed emotion in spouses predict subsequent problems among care recipients with Alzheimer's disease? *Journals of Gerontology: Psychological Sciences, 48*(4), P202-P209.

Wade, D. T., Legh-Smith, J., & Hewer, R. L. (1986). Effects of living with and looking after survivors of a stroke. *British Medical Journal, 293,* 418-420.

Walker, H. A. (1988). Black-White differences in marriage and family patterns. In S. M. Dornbush & M. J. Strober (Eds.), *Feminism, children, and the new families.* New York: Guilford Press.

Wallahagen, M., & Strawbridge, W. (1993). My parent-my self: Contrasting themes in family care. Paper presented at the Gerontological Society of America Conference, Washington, D.C.

Ward, R., Logan, J. R., & Spitze, G. (1992). The influence of parent and child needs on coresidence in middle and later life. *Journal of Marriage and the Family, 54,* 209-221.

Watt, J., & Calder, A. (1981). *I love you but you drive me crazy.* Vancouver, BC: Forbes Publications.

Weissert, W., & Cready, C. M. (1989). Toward a model for improved targeting of aged at risk of institutionalization. *Health Services Research, 24,* 483-508.

Weissert, W., Gooch, K., & Cready, C. M. (1989). A prospective budgeting model for home- and community-based long-term care. *Inquiry, 26,* 116-129.

Wellisch, D. K., Fawzy, F. I., Landsvere, J., Pasnau, R. O., & Wolcott, D. L. (1983). Evaluation of psychosocial problems of homebound cancer patients: The relationships of disease and the sociodemographic variables of patients to family problems. *Journal of Psychosocial Oncology, 1,* 1-5.

White, N. E., Richter, J. M., & Fry, C. (1992). Coping, social support, and adaptation to chronic illness. *Western Journal of Nursing Research, 14*(2), 211-224.

Woods, N. F., Haberman, M. R., & Packard, N. J. (1993). Demands of illness and individual, dyadic, and family adaptation in chronic illness. *Western Journal of Nursing Research, 15*(1), 10-30.

Woods, N. F., Yates, B. C., & Primomo, J. (1988). Supporting families during chronic illness. *Image: Journal of Nursing Scholarship, 21*(1), 46-50.

Zarit, S. H. Reever, K. E., & Bach-Peterson, J. (1980). Relatives of the impaired elderly: Correlates of feelings of burden. *The Gerontologist, 20,* 649-655.

Zarit, S. H., Todd, P. A., & Zarit, J. M. (1986). Subjective burden of husbands and wives on caregivers: A longitudinal study. *The Gerontologist, 26*(3), 260-266.

Zucman, E. (1982). *Childhood disability in the family.* New York: International Exchange of Information on Rehabilitation. World Rehabilitation Fund, Inc.

Bibliography

Anderson, K. L., & Allen, W. R. (1984). Correlatives of extended household structure. *Phylon, 45,* 144-157.

Barresi, C. M., & Menon, G. (1989). Diversity in Black family caregiving. In Z. Harel, E. McKinney, & M. Williams (Eds.), *Black aged: Understanding diversity and service needs.* Washington, D.C.: National Council on Aging.

Cherlin, J. J., & Furstenberg, F. F. (1986). *The new American grandparent: A place in the family, a life apart.* New York: Basic Books.

Corbin, J. M., & Strauss, A. L. (1988). *Unending work and care: Managing chronic illness at home.* San Francisco: Jossey-Bass.

Duvall, E. (1977). *Marriage and family development* (5th ed.). Philadelphia: J. B. Lippincott.

Fife, B. (1985). A model for predicting the adaptation of families in a medical crisis: An analysis of role integration. *Image: The Journal of Nursing Scholarship, 17*(4), 108-112.

Hendrick, S., Johnson, J. R., Inui, T. S., & Diehr, P. (1991). Factors associated with participation in a randomized trial of adult day health care. *The Gerontologist, 31*(5), 607-610.

House Older Americans Caucus Subs for Defunct Aging Committee (1993, July/Aug). *Gerontology News,* p. 4.

Knafl, K. A., & Deatrick, J. A. (1986). How families manage chronic conditions: An analysis of the concept of normalization. *Research in Nursing and Health, 9,* 215-222.

Kosberg, J. J. (1988). Preventing elder abuse: Identification of high risk factors prior to placement decisions. *The Gerontologist, 27*(1), 37-53.

Moon, A., & Williams, O. (1993). Perceptions of elder abuse and help-seeking patterns among African-American, Caucasian American, and Korean-American elderly women. *The Gerontologist, 33*(3), 386-395.

National Organization for Victim Assistance (1985). The elderly crime victim. *NOVA Network Information Bulletin, 2,* 1-8.

Silverstein, M. & Waite, L. J. (1993). Are Blacks more likely than whites to receive and provide social support in middle and old age? Yes, no, and maybe so. *Journals of Gerontology: Social Sciences,* *48*(4), S212–S222.

Strauss, A. L., Fagerhaugh, S., Suczek, B., & Weiner, C. (1984). *Chronic illness and the quality of life* (2nd ed.). St. Louis: Mosby.

Thompson, S. C., & Pitts, J. S. (1992). In sickness and in health: Chronic illness, marriage, and spousal caregiving. In S. Spacapan and S. Oskamp (Eds.), *Helping and being helped: Naturalistic studies* (pp. 115–151). Newbury Park, CA: Sage.

Turner, R. (1970). *Family interaction.* New York: John Wiley.

U.S. Bureau of the Census (1989). Projections of the population of the United States, by age, sex, and race: 1988 to 2080. Current *Population Reports,* Series P-25, No. 1018. Washington, D.C.: Superintendent of Documents, U.S. Government Printing Office.

Ward, R. A., Sherman, S. R., & LaGory, M. (1984). Informal networks and knowledge of services for older persons. *Journal of Gerontology, 39*(2), 216–223.

Watzlawick, P., Beavin, J., & Jackson, D. (1967). *Pragmatics of human communication: A study of interactional patterns, pathologies and paradoxes.* New York: W. W. Norton.

Weissert, W. G. (1977). Adult day care programs in the United States. Current research projects and a survey of 10 centers. *Public Health Reports, 92,* 49–56.

CHAPTER 13

Body Image

Karna Bramble

CASE STUDY

Changes in Body Image

F. B., now 70 years of age, was just a teenager when she suffered a severe sunburn on her shoulders after a day at the beach. While initially painful, she soon recovered and continued to enjoy her summer activities. By the time school started in the fall, however, some lesions appeared on her shoulder where the original sunburn had been. F. B. paid little attention to these lesions; she was excited about returning to school, and, anyway, they were covered by her clothing. The lesions, however, did not go away but began to spread up her neck. She became sensitive about her appearance and changed the way she dressed in an attempt to hide the lesions from her classmates.

Because F. B. came from a Christian Science background, no attempt was made to seek medical intervention, and therefore the lesions remained. Over the years there were periods of remission

and exacerbations, but as she grew older the lesions became worse and spread to other parts of her body, mainly to areas that were more likely to be moist. Because the lesions were causing her physical discomfort, F. B. finally sought medical attention for her condition and was diagnosed as having Darier's disease.

While extremely careful with body hygiene, the lesions often left an unpleasant odor and intermittently areas became infected. Knowing that the lesions got worse with exposure to sun, heat, makeup, and synthetic materials, F. B. stayed at home more and more. Besides, she was embarrassed by the odor created by the lesions and medications and also by the change in her appearance. While many difficulties have confronted this client, one problem created by this chronic illness has been a lifelong change in her body image.

Introduction

Body image serves as a standard or frame of reference that individuals use when relating to themselves and their physical and social environment. Body image influences others' reactions and also affects emotions, perceptions, attitudes, and personality. It determines the limits we place

on ourselves and those others impose. Body image is a dynamic process that influences how the individual functions.

Historical Background

Body image is important for those in the health professions to understand. Although the concept has been discussed in the literature since the 1880s, not until Schilder first presented his work in 1935 did a new understanding of this concept arise. In his book, *The Image and Appearance of the Human Body,* Schilder (1950) explores the dimensions of body image and states: "The image of the human body means the picture of our own body which we form in our mind, that is to say the way in which the body appears to ourselves" (p.11). Schilder believes that the perception of one's body is based on a tridimensional image that is influenced by physiologic, psychologic, and social experiences.

Definitions

Definitions of body image, though varied, share similarities. Common to many of the definitions is the belief that body image develops in response to multiple sensory inputs (visual, tactile, proprioceptive, and kinesthetic) but also to the actions and attitudes of others. Fallon (1990) states: "Of all the ways people think of themselves, none is so essentially immediate and central as the image of their own bodies: The body is experienced as a reflection of the self. Body image is the way people perceive themselves and, equally important, the way they think others see them."

Although the concept of body image encompasses one's views of the physical structure of his or her body, it includes more than a perception of one's physical appearance. Perceptions of function, sensation, and mobility, as well as feelings and thought, also become incorporated into the body image one holds. "How one thinks and feels about one's body will influence one's social relations and one's other psychological characteristics" (Lerner & Jovanovic, 1990). Furthermore, "how we feel and think about our body influences the way that we perceive the world" (Pruzinsky & Cash, 1990).

In developing a model for understanding body image, Price (1990) presents a schematic drawing of an equilateral triangle with the three points on the triangle representing body reality, body presentation, and body ideal. *Body ideal* is similar to Schilder's original definition of body image as a picture we carry in our heads of our body's appearance and performance.

The terms *body image* and *self-concept* are frequently used interchangeably. Body image is the mental image one holds of the physical self, including attitudes and perceptions of ones's physical appearance, state of health, skills, and sexuality. "It is an integral component of self-concept, which is the total perception an individual holds of self—who one believes one is, how one believes one looks, and how one feels about one's self" (Mock, 1993).

Another similarity among the definitions of body image is the notion of *reality* and *ideality.* The view presented here is that the ideal image of oneself and the real image must coincide or be compatible. If a discrepancy exists between what is idealized and what is real, a conflict in body image that can affect personality and health may develop. If, for instance, F. B.'s idealized view of herself includes tanned, intact skin rather than the real picture of skin lesions that become worse with sun exposure, a conflict can arise.

Development of Body Image

Body image is not static, but changes and develops through the stages of the life cycle. The development of body image begins in infancy. Newborn infants have no concrete concept of body image, responding to life on the sensory or feeling level. The initial foundation for the formation of body image begins when, during the later part of infancy, infants begin to separate themselves from their caretakers.

Body image is further influenced by the interactive process the infant has with caretakers. The child's body shape influences how others will perceive and respond, which in turn determines the child's internal sense of body shape. Crucial to the development of body image throughout infancy is stimulation, the initial sense of self based on experiencing tactile and kinesthetic sensations (Pruzinsky & Cash, 1990).

Childhood is a period of dramatic changes, both in terms of size and strength. Awareness of body image expands during this time, becoming dependent on the reactions of many rather than a few. School children compare themselves with their peers in the classroom, on the playground, and at other youth-oriented activities. Early on, body shape becomes one basis for children receiving positive or negative recognition. For instance, thin children tend to be chosen as leaders; overweight children are more often left out of games and are often teased (Fontaine, 1991). Teasing, in fact, may lead to the development of body image disturbances. In addition, the reactions of adults—teachers, youth group leaders, or parents—become important.

During this period body image evolves as the child begins to develop and refine physical, motor, learning, language, and social skills. Also at this time children become more aware of sexual differences, moving from play with children of either sex to play involving only children of the same sex.

Adolescence is a time of exquisite body image sensitivity. Numerous and rapid body changes occur at this time, causing the adolescent to become preoccupied with self and body characteristics. Although such physical changes are important, the meaning that the adolescent gives to them and the way the adolescent uses his or her body may be more important. In addition, peer group recognition, acceptance, and comparison has great significance. Consequently, body image is in a constant state of revision as adolescents attempt to achieve perfect balance with their perceived view of the acceptable.

Onset of menarche may also influence body image. Girls who mature late or experience menarche after the age of 14 have a more positive body image than those who have their first menstrual period earlier, especially if it occurs before the age of 11 (Thompson, 1990). Regardless of gender, once the identity tasks are completed in adolescence, body image becomes more stable.

With adulthood, this increased stability is incorporated into the adult's sense of self. The adult is more likely to maintain this body image, regardless of whether it is positive or negative, because it affects his or her participation in daily life. This is not to say that adults cannot change their body images; rather, changing becomes more difficult because "the person perceives others' comments and behavior in relation to his already established image in order to avoid conflict and anxiety within himself" (Murray & Zentner, 1979). An adult who has a well-integrated body image is more likely to react positively to life's events.

Revising one's concept of body image accompanies the aging process. Confronted by changes that gradually develop as one ages, the adult once again has to redefine body image as visible, and not so visible. Wrinkling of skin, graying and thinning of hair, and changes in body contour are among the visible changes that remind people of their aging. Frequently, aged clients find incorporating these changes into a viable body image difficult, especially when society places more value on the attributes of youth.

Impaired sensory input due to a decrease in visual and auditory acuity can interfere with the elderly adult's interactions with the environment. The aged client may prefer to limit participation in social and family activities (because of an inability to hear or understand conversations) rather than wear a hearing aid, another visible sign of deterioration. Other changes that normally accompany aging involve reproductive functions. Although sexual activity can continue, sexual response in all phases of the cycle is slowed (see Chapter 14, on sexuality). This change in sexual response may lead elderly people to believe that they no longer are capable of enjoying sexual activity. All of these changes can affect a change in body image (Murray & Zentner, 1979).

Although body image changes throughout the life-cycle, periods of stability occur. Body image functions to provide the individual throughout life with a sense of personal identity. "It acts as a standard or frame of reference which influences people's ability to perform and the ways in which they perceive themselves, measure their continuity through life, and identify their mastery of the world" (Norris, 1978).

Influences on Body Image Concept

Changes that occur during growth and development are among the factors that influence the concept of body image. Others include one's body boundary, cultural influences, and multiple internal and external phenomena. Reactions of others also influences the concept of body image.

Body Boundaries   One's body boundary is the amount of space the individual perceives the body as occupying (Fawcett & Fry, 1980). It is the individual's interrelationship with the physical environment and differs among individuals. For some, body boundaries are well defined and separate from the surrounding environment. Others, however, cannot clearly delineate the limits of their body boundaries. An obvious example of the latter is a client who has had a stroke resulting in paralysis. Here, although the body remains intact, the individual cannot recognize that the paralyzed limb belongs to him or her.

Sexual differences also influence body boundaries. Women are said to have a more definite body boundary sense than men. Such a characteristic may stem from the fact that women receive more of their identity from their body and its function because of the importance placed on such physical attributes as breasts, legs, facial features, and hair. Men, on the other hand, are more likely to achieve an identity from their accomplishments rather than from their bodily attributes. Because of this emphasis on body, the woman may more quickly arrive at a realistic concept of her body and its boundaries than does her male counterpart (Murray, 1972a).

Body boundaries can affect interpersonal relationships. It is thought that individuals with a well-integrated sense of body boundary interact differently from those who have poorly defined boundaries. Certainly individuals who are aware of their body's boundaries are better able to judge whether a given space can be entered.

Although body boundaries influence one's concept of body image, an interplay occurs between the two. Consequently, whatever affects one will probably affect the other. A chronic illness is just one of many factors that can affect both.

Cultural Influences   Cultural background must be considered when discussing the concept of body image. Included in body image are the perception of cultural standards, the perception of how that standard is matched, and the perception of the importance placed on that match by members of the cultural group and the individual (Fallon, 1990).

In Western culture the esthetic preferences for the ideal female figure have changed over time. Prior to the 20th century, the voluptuous woman was the ideal. After World War I, this idea was transformed to a more slender, though not frail, woman. During the 1920s, when the ideal shifted from slender to flat-chested and a near absence of female secondary sex characteristics, anorexia and bulimia were first reported. This preference again changed in the 1980s when women who were tall, lean, and nearly hipless with small buttocks were idealized. Today, the preferred female body is muscular and healthy in appearance (Fontaine, 1991).

Cultural attitudes toward body weight can further affect body image. In the United States, the prevailing ideal for women is one of thinness, although there appears to be a racial difference in this preference. Rosen (1990) reported that fewer black girls, compared with white girls, felt they were overweight or were trying to lose weight; more black girls were trying to gain weight. Of further interest, when Third World immigrants come to industrialized countries such as the United States, they "have a higher rate of eating disorders than people of the same nationality who remain in their own country" (Rosen, 1990).

Mass media, as the conveyor of cultural norms, rules, and ideals, can have a powerful effect on the notion of body image. Fontaine (1991) suggests that

> The visual and print media, including television, films, videos, magazines, books, and advertising, serve as primary stimuli for encouraging thinness as well as fuel for the obsession with weight control. Fashion designers and clothing retailers also play a powerful role in shaping the cultural ideal . . . The insidious message is that life is exciting for only those people who emulate the cultural stereotype. This extreme, which is unattainable by the mast majority of women, is an ever-present threat to women's body image and self-esteem" (p. 672).

Internal and External Influences   Multiple internal and external phenomena can influence one's sense of body image. The internal environment consists of body organs and systems and those sensations that develop in response to systemic physiologic occurrences within the body (Price, 1990). Internal influences have a profound effect on the developing body image of the infant and continue to exert their influence throughout the life-cycle. The internal environment is also affected by disease entities, such as rheumatoid arthritis, systemic lupus erythematosus, or diabetes mellitus. The effects of these disease states can alter clients' perception of their bodies, causing consequent changes in body image.

External influences are also important in the development and refinement of body image. Although external influences are many, a few are worth noting. One such external influence is that of the environment, which can encompass many factors and may include weather, availability of light, surrounding decor, clothing, or people currently present. Whether one is male or female may also have an external influence on one's concept of body image. Obviously, differences between male and female body image are partly related to anatomic structure and body function. While females tend to be more critical of their appearance than males, they are generally more comfortable with bodily changes (Pruzinsky & Cash, 1990).

Another external influence relates to topological experiences, including sensations such as touch, taste, pain, thermal changes, and one's reactions to them. Other such experiences concern the surface characteristics of one's body (Norris, 1978). Relating these findings to F. B., it is possible that many external influences may be affecting her concept of body image. Certainly she must be selective in the environment in which she places herself. Her topological experiences are, additionally, distorted by the long-term effects of the skin lesions and their resultant effect of changing the body's surface. Additionally, her experiences are affected by the reactions of others to these now visible skin lesions.

Interaction with Others As suggested above, the reactions of and experiences with others can also affect one's concept of body image. Initially the groups that exert the most control over one's body image include one's parents, caretakers, other family members, significant friends, and peer groups. These attitudes, either individually or collectively, often determine one's perception of self. Thus, the more positive the opinions held by others, the more likely is the individual to develop a positive body image concept (Orr, Reznikoff, & Smith, 1989).

Others who may be less significant, such as teachers, neighbors, health care providers, and society as a whole, can also influence an individual's body image. Unfortunately, these experiences are frequently based on more superficial personal qualities (bodily appearance or appropriate behavior), and yet they may have a great effect on the individual. Other people's opinions are important, and we respond to their perceptions whether they are positive or negative. Newell (1991) suggests that "It is likely . . . that body image and its related concepts are interactive, since the physically less attractive . . . will receive less in the way of reinforcement from others, with resulting decrease in self-esteem and positive self-image." The individual reacts "to the way he thinks others see him . . . at the same time projecting to others his own body image." Interpersonal experiences can influence the role to which one is assigned, as well as determine many other aspects of oneself, including body image. "It is probably because body image is such a central concept of the human experience that it is (therefore) such an excellent indicator of a person's general health" (Castledine, 1981).

Chronicity and Body Image Modern technology has contributed to a significantly expanded life expectancy. Many who earlier might have had an untimely death or shortened life are now living longer. However, with increased longevity comes the risk of chronic illness and disability. A chronic illness may necessitate prolonged medical care, lifelong medication, or a change in life-style (for example, in one's job, activities, or physical environment). Regardless of the causative factor leading to the chronic illness or whether it is manifested outwardly (for example, skin rash) or internally (for example, diabetes), the person must incorporate a new image of self. Since adapting to a changed body image may not be easy without appropriate intervention, the intent of the remaining portions of this chapter is to address the issue of body image and its relationship to chronicity.

Body Image Problems Secondary to Chronicity

Many problems or conflicts arise when an individual's body image is threatened as a result of a chronic illness. Although it is not unusual for disturbances to develop, a conflict is more likely to occur when the individual has difficulty accepting and adapting to the changes.

External Changes

One of the problems that may arise from a chronic illness is physical disfigurement. Certainly the more visible or extensive the disfigurement, the greater the perceived threat to one's body image. Then the individual must cope not only with personal feelings about the disfigurement but with the responses of others as well (see Chapter 5, on stigma).

Facial disfigurement is one example of an external alteration that can be extremely threatening to one's body image and to others in the environment. Obviously the face is the most expressive and highly visible part of the body. Murray (1972a) notes: "There is less connection with the body image when an attribute is looked upon as a tool than when it is looked upon as a personal characteristic." In actuality, however, the face is both a tool and a personal characteristic; as a tool, it serves as one of the basic verbal and nonverbal means of communication; as a personal characteristic, it identifies the individual. Thus, when F. B. discovered that skin lesions were beginning to appear on her face, she took extreme care to camouflage them because of the value her adolescent peers placed on facial features.

Other external alterations that may affect the individual depend upon the extent of involvement and the meaning the individual and society attach to these alterations (Bernstein, 1990). Skin changes can alter one's image of self. The lesions caused by psoriasis are just one example; another is wrinkling skin and the appearance of brown, or liver, spots accompanying aging. Burn patients are prototypical of the visibly injured person. "Burns have been shown to have a more negative impact on body image; girls and women with burns generally have a more negative body image than men with burns" (Orr et al., 1989). Burns further impact on body image depending upon the percent of body surface involved or the locus of the burn injury.

Visible bodily changes can also necessitate that the individual revise body image. Again, the meaning or impact of the change determines necessity for such revision. Certainly any illness that causes a woman to lose a breast interferes with the way she views herself. If a particular feature or body part is viewed as being especially attractive, such as attractive hands, and this attractiveness is changed by a chronic illness, such as rheumatoid arthritis, body image is threatened.

Joint swelling and changes associated with many rheumatic diseases may also create problems for the individual. Poor dental hygiene or the presence of a malocclusion may be extremely damaging to an individual's perception of self. A young man once noted that having his teeth straightened was the most significant event of his life because it allowed him to smile and laugh without covering his mouth. What a tremendous effect this had not only on his body image but on his entire view of himself and his worth as a person!

Functional Limitations

Body image can also be altered by the presence of a functional limitation. Limitation of function occurs when there is a loss of a body part or a change in the functional capability of the entire body or a part of it (Norris, 1978). Any number of chronic illnesses can cause such a disability; residual effects of other illnesses, such as a fracture or joint disturbance, can be contributing factors. Loss of function can lead to decreased mobility, which in turn can foster feelings of dependence and loss of control over the environment and one's self, all of which can disrupt one's image of self. Immobility, whether permanent or temporary, contributes to changes in body image and life-style (Baird, 1985).

Loss of function can also affect an individual's ability to perform. Since so much of one's identity is tied to the ability to participate in various activities, the loss of the ability to do so may be viewed as a threat to one's body image

(Baird, 1985). This can be especially true with respect to sexual functioning, where body image problems can interfere with any phase of the sexual response cycle (Pruzinsky, 1990) For example, a woman may question her femininity or sexual attractiveness if her ability to participate in sex is limited by joint immobility caused by hip involvement from rheumatoid arthritis (see Chapter 6, on mobility). The ability to move and participate in a meaningful way is essential to one's sense of well-being; consequently, any limitation of one's functional ability may alter one's concept of body image.

Body image is threatened when the individual attaches great importance to the body part changed or lost because of chronic illness or disability. Different body parts have different meanings; whereas one might view a part as having little significance, another might attach great value to it (Norris, 1978).

Although we associate more extensive involvement with a greater degree of disturbance in body image, for some individuals even a minor loss can prove devastating. The important factor is the symbolic meaning of the change to the individual (Thompson, 1990). Even when a chronic illness produces no visible physical disfigurement, the individual can feel extremely threatened if the body part or function is held in high esteem. It is well known that a hysterectomy may prove disastrous for some women, whereas others imbue the procedure with little importance. The difference obviously lies in the fact that some women see the uterus as being essential to their femininity, and its removal therefore causes a distortion in their body image.

The consequence of experiencing a myocardial infarction (MI) also illustrates the importance an organ can have in determining whether one's self-image is threatened. Although changes produced by an MI are not physically visible, the symbolic meaning of the heart is so great and varied and its purpose so strongly attached to life, that few survive an MI without some aspect of their body image being threatened.

Another variable to consider is the meaning the treatment or rehabilitation plan has for the individual (see Chapter 24, on rehabilitation). If the individual sees the positive benefits of actively participating in the treatment program, the likelihood that chronic illness or disability will cause a changed body image is reduced.

Temporal Influences

The period over which an alteration in the body occurs can influence one's body image (Pruzinsky & Cash, 1990). In the presence of a slow, progressive disease or a gradual change in body image, the individual has time to incorporate the new body image and its resultant changes. When the changes of a chronic illness develop over time, the individual is given warning of what may likely occur and an opportunity to acknowledge and integrate the change over a longer period.

Unfortunately, individuals who experience sudden, traumatic illness have no warning of the events to come and therefore relatively little time or opportunity to cope with the change. A sudden alteration may have a greater impact on the individual, thereby making resolution of the changes in body image more difficult. For example, burn patients experience a rapid trajectory of body image change. Surgical patients, even when undergoing desired cosmetic surgery, can experience a disruption in their body image (Pruzinsky & Cash, 1990). Similarly, patients who felt well before surgery, undergoing the creation of a stoma, find adjustment to their new body image harder than others undergoing the same procedure who were ill for a prolonged period beforehand. Should there be "an immediate improvement in their quality of life, the effect on body image may be positive" (Morrall, 1990).

A person who loses functional ability through the long-term effects of rheumatoid arthritis may incorporate these changes into a revised body image more easily than one who suddenly becomes a hemiplegic as a result of a stroke. It must be recognized, however, that for some individuals even knowing what is likely to occur may not help them to adapt to the changes, because of the many other variables involved.

Influences of Other Aspects of Self

Self-esteem, identity, behavior, personality, and self-concept are closely intertwined with one's concept of body image. Consequently, any or all of these factors may become distorted if the individual fails to accept and adapt to the bodily changes accompanying chronic illness. Failure to adapt may also depend on the individual's pre-illness image; those maintaining affirmative images of themselves prior to an illness are more likely to continue to view themselves positively as opposed to those who hold more negative views beforehand (Beeken, 1978).

Cultural/Social Influences

Several years of teaching experience have demonstrated to this author that the capacity for a successful revision of body image following a chronic illness depends on one's cultural and/or social background. Each cultural and social group establishes its own norms governing the acceptable, especially in terms of physical appearance and personality attributes. Thompson (1990) points out that "the sociocultural effect on an individual's tendency to compare the self to a societally sanctioned ideal is probably very strong." If, then, a chronic illness causes an individual to differ from the group, the person may be ignored or avoided (see Chapter 5, on stigma). The attitudes of others are quickly sensed; when one cannot meet group expectations because of a chronic illness or disability, the individual's body image is likely to be threatened. The cultural or social group can also covertly or overtly discourage the individual from using public places. F. B. let her hair grow long and wears it in a bun to avoid subjecting herself to the inspection and scorn of hair stylists. She also sews many of her own clothes because in the past she found that salespersons became uneasy when they discovered that she was going to try clothes on "that" body.

The Health Team Members

The success an individual has in adapting to a new body image also depends on the members of the health team. Clients and members of the health team often view chronic illness or disability differently (Leonard, 1972). If for some reason the health team, or even one individual on it, views the change with revulsion, the client's con-

cept of body image will probably incorporate that feeling. Likewise, if the client views the bodily changes as significant in some way and the health team views them as just another example of the benefits of modern medicine in saving or prolonging life, conflict arises. The client may not comply with the treatment regimen or may otherwise attempt to make others acknowledge that the changes are important. The more the health team can help the client adapt to changes, the more likely it is that there will be an acceptable outcome in the integration of a constructive body image change.

For example, individuals who need colostomies can benefit from talking about the surgery's effects on the body before and after surgery. Providing willing assistance with stoma care until the person is ready to undertake self-care, as well as positive feedback as self-care is initiated, is a way health professionals can assist these clients in developing positive body images related to their colostomies and themselves.

Impact of Poor Adjustment

Inability to adjust to a changed body image may be manifested by the client experiencing a variety of physical or psychological symptoms. Physical symptoms can include vague subjective complaints of illness that may or may not be associated with the chronic illness. Intractable pain is another common complaint. Chronic fatigue may indicate that the client is unable to accept the reality of the changed body image and therefore expends a disproportionate amount of energy denying its existence. Other physical symptoms related to psychological problems can occur.

Psychological problems may be as varied and frequent as physical complaints; therefore, one must consider these problems in relation to the individual's concept of body image. Anger or resentment may focus on the family or health care provider. The person may also appear depressed, especially if unable to complete the grieving process for the idealized body image because of the constant reminder of the changed bodily state (see Chapter 11, on coping). Anxiety may appear in clients if a discrepancy exists between what they idealized and how they appear. Denial, as mentioned previously, is another common psychological response, as are feelings of guilt. Although these are the major psychological problems that occur, others may develop in the person having a chronic illness.

Finally, individuals with poor adjustment to body image changes may withdraw from previously enjoyed social interactions; this is especially true in burn patients in whom physical changes resulting from the burn lead to a devaluation of one's body (Orr et al., 1989).

Interventions

The goal of intervention is to help the client adapt successfully to body image changes that are taking place as a result of having a chronic illness. Many factors determine the effectiveness with which the chronically ill individual adapts to changes in body image. Regardless of whether the change results from surgery, trauma, or a disease process, the client must incorporate a new self-concept. Skillful nursing is therefore one intervention that helps clients maintain a balance between hope and despair when there is an altered body image (Harris, 1986).

However, adapting to a new body image is not necessarily a static process. The chronically ill person is continually reintegrating a new image of self, especially during periods of exacerbation or remission and particularly at times when the chronic illness that caused the original change in body image is again confronted. At such times clients may need to rework their body image.

Stages in Restructuring the Body Image

The client must work through four stages to integrate physical or functional changes into a restructured body image. As originally proposed by Lee (1970), these stages include impact, retreat, acknowledgment, and reconstruction. Individuals proceed through these stages in different ways and may return to the first stage as they revise their body image. Familiarity with

the behavior that typically occurs during each of these stages will help the health care provider to evaluate the client's progress, predict the likelihood of recovery, and determine appropriate interventions.

During the impact stage, attention focuses on the body part or disease entity causing the chronic illness. While the client is unaware of a threat to body image, he or she directs energy primarily toward coping with the disease. Consequently, a client having rheumatoid arthritis who experiences an exacerbation of the disease will attend to alleviating the symptoms rather than concentrate on the disfigurements that result from the disease.

During the retreat stage, the client becomes aware of the body changes that have occurred. However, the reality of the situation, coupled with a lack of emotional energy, becomes so overwhelming that the client retreats psychologically. The retreat phase provides the client with a "rest period during which forces are reorganized and strengthened and a point of readiness is reached for the work ahead" (Lee, 1970). Denial regarding the presence of bodily changes is the behavior manifested by the client and may range from feelings of indifference to those of euphoria.

Acknowledgment is the period when the reality of the chronic illness and the losses that have occurred are faced. Mourning for the idealized body image occurs as the client acknowledges the losses. To redefine the self-image, the individual may need solitude. This is also a time, however, when the client needs to discuss events surrounding the illness, the disability, and body image changes that are occurring. The reactions of others, including the professional's verbal and nonverbal responses, during this period are crucial to the client's progress.

Once the client has successfully acknowledged the threat to body image, reconstruction can begin. During this final stage, the client begins to assimilate a new image of self and incorporate it into daily activities of living. Adaptation to the changes imposed by chronic illness may require time because the amount of energy the client can devote to a successful reintegration may be limited. For some, it may never occur. Murray (1972a) recognizes this point and comments that "adaptation is not always positive or growth-promoting. There are those individuals who will permanently avoid the reality of having undergone change in the body." But for most, the reconstruction phase is positive, bringing about an adjustment to adaptive devices or technical procedures, a reorientation in the social aspects of life, and, finally, a reintegration of the client's body image (Lee, 1970).

Factors Influencing Adaptation

Knowledge of these stages is not sufficient to help clients adapt successfully to the problems that arise from an alteration in body image. The professional must also consider the various factors that influence adaptation if intervention is to be successful.

Age   Among the factors influencing adaptation is the client's age. Young children may find it easier to adapt to body image changes because they have not fully developed the bond between their appearance and their identity. Early in life, body image is more malleable (Pruzinsky, 1990). Body image changes in an adolescent will be viewed differently from those occurring in a young child or elderly person. Adolescence is a time when attention is normally focused on the body and how it compares with those of the peer group. At this developmental stage, body image change may be devastating and seen as extremely threatening.

One can say that bodily changes can be as devastating to an adult as it is to an adolescent, even though the variables influencing the response may be different. Body image in the adult is well developed and provides a basis for identity. Therefore, an adult may find change no easier to accept than an adolescent does, because it interferes with the individual's well-established self-image.

Adaptation to changes in body image for the older individual is complicated by the necessity to cope with changes that accompany aging (Norris, 1978). An illness that creates differences during this period in one's life may be overwhelming. Elderly individuals may also be dealing with the fears that develop because they are no longer useful in a society that (1) values physically attractive, independent people and (2) has not successfully identified a place or role for the healthy aged, let alone those who have a chronic illness.

Sex   A client's sex is another variable that needs consideration, especially when the body image change is closely perceived as a "masculine" or "feminine" characteristic. Thus, a woman who has had a mastectomy may have difficulty adapting to body image changes because of the strong association between breasts and femininity. Likewise, surgery, drug therapy, or disease that interferes with a man's ability to perform sexually may disrupt his view of himself as a man, thereby slowing his adjustment to a revised body image (see Chapter 14, on sexuality).

Interestingly, it appears that women, "more critical of their appearance and less satisfied with their bodies, are much more psychologically comfortable with body changes. Males, on the other hand, are . . . more threatened by body changes" (Fisher, 1986).

Coping Mechanisms   Previous and current coping mechanisms are aspects of a client's personality that affect the manner in which adaptation occurs. In most instances, the client's coping with the present situation is either enhanced or hampered by previous coping strategies (Price, 1990). Thus, to initiate useful interventions, the health professional must assess previous and current coping mechanisms. Even when the client does not appear to have adequate coping strategies, an important first step in working with that client is to regard the client as coping.

Prior Experience   Since past experiences exert such a tremendous influence on the client's ability to adapt to current changes, knowledge of some aspects of the client's past may help the intervention process. Areas that may provide useful information include the client's past experiences with illness and hospitalization and previous alterations in body image. Becoming aware of the amount of disparity between the pre-illness and current images of self may also facilitate intervention. Successful intervention is predicated on the health professional's understanding of what the chronic illness, body image changes, and management plan mean to the client, since these factors can dramatically influence the client's compliance with a medication regimen or rehabilitation program.

Assessment

A thorough assessment is a prerequisite to appropriate intervention. This assessment is made to determine the client's perceptions of the chronic illness and its effects on body image. It entails observing the client to determine the nature of the threat and interviewing the client to understand the meaning of the threat (McCloskey, 1976).

Assessing the client's stage of recovery is of primary importance for planning interventions. If, for instance, the client is still in a state of denial, the making of realistic teaching or rehabilitation plans may be impeded. On the other hand, the threat of the illness and its effects on the client's body image may increase the client's receptivity to help. At this point, teaching and counseling can be instrumental in helping the process of adaptation, thereby promoting a more rapid return to a higher level of functioning. Once clients reach a stage of receptiveness to the health professional's assistance, a therapeutic relationship can be established. This relationship, in turn, helps the client accept changes that have occurred, thereby facilitating progression through the recovery process.

It is the purpose of assessment to compile a complete client profile. More specifically, the health professional seeks information that will facilitate intervention. Areas worth consideration include

1. Assessing the client's definition of the current situation
2. Determining the client's knowledge of the chronic illness
3. Ascertaining the significance the client assigns to the altered body part and the client's attitude toward it
4. Discovering the client's assessment of others' responses to the changes.

The greater the number of internal and external strengths and the more positive the indications of adaptation, the more likely it is that the client will be able to revise and adapt to a changed body image. For effective intervention, assessment should include finding both positive and negative indicators of adaptation to a changed body image as well as ascertaining the client's internal and external strengths, although internal strengths depend on such factors as the client's previous adaptation to body image changes. External strengths encompass many phenomena, most important the support of family and significant others. Care providers must also assess the psychosocial background (religion, cultural orientation, social groups, occupation, and so forth) and the effect of body image changes on interactions with relevant groups.

In some client situations it may be appropriate to use one of the many assessment tools, several recently developed, that are available to measure body image disturbances (Thompson, 1990). While this section will not discuss the variety of measurement tools that exist, knowledge of their presence is important. The tool with the longest history of use (developed by Secord and Jourard in 1953 as Thompson notes) is called the "body cathexis scale." This tool asks subjects to indicate the degree of positive feeling toward various body parts.

Assessment of families is accomplished by interviewing them and observing their verbal and nonverbal interactions with the client (Leonard, 1972). Valuable to successful intervention is discovering

- Meanings the family attaches to the chronic illness and body image changes
- Perceived physical, psychological, or social losses experienced by them and by the client
- Financial stresses that are present

It is important to realize that the family, like the client, may be experiencing many reactions to the chronic illness and bodily changes. Assistance for them, via support, should be incorporated into the intervention plan so that they can be understanding of the client.

Specific Interventions

The success of intervention depends on establishing a therapeutic, supportive, professional relationship. If this relationship is to be therapeutic, health providers must identify their feelings about working with clients whose chronic illnesses encompass bodily changes. In addition, if the health professional is unable or unwilling to help clients work through their feelings about a changed body image, little therapeutic success can be expected. Acceptance of the client by the health professional, like that of the family, is important in facilitating the client's acceptance of self.

The health professional also must understand the varied dimensions that result from changes in body image, since such changes involve more than altered appearance. The person having a chronic illness that results in bodily changes needs a health care provider who is willing to serve as an advocate and to provide consistent ongoing support and care. This role requires commitment, but it also increases the probability of successful intervention.

Communication   Numerous interventions assist the client and family in adapting to body image changes. Providing the client with the opportunity to talk about the changes as they relate to the chronic illness is beneficial. The climate for such discussions should be nonthreatening and conducive to sharing. Acceptance by the health professional, demonstrated by a willingness to listen, is extremely important (Marten, 1978). In addition, clients must feel encouraged to express both positive and negative emotions. They need to talk about their emotions and experiences; through such discussions they are able to integrate a new picture of self. Consistent support by the health professional over time is the most likely way to insure a positive outcome. Family members also should have an opportunity to analyze and express their feelings, either with or without the client present. Providing opportunities for such expression is beneficial to the growth of both the client and the family.

Touch   Touching that is not perfunctory is an important intervention through which the health professional can demonstrate acceptance (Ernst & Shaw, 1980). The need for touching and being touched often supersedes the need for talking. Touch therefore provides an effective

nonverbal way of demonstrating care and concern. Used therapeutically, it can alleviate the stress and anger associated with redefining body image and can help the client feel more positive about bodily changes.

Positive Emotions   Providing an atmosphere that is conducive to positive emotions is another valuable intervention. Cousins (1983), in his work, *The Healing Heart,* suggests that positive emotions supplement the healing process. Whether expressed as "laughter, hope, faith, love, will to live, cheerfulness, humor, creativity, playfulness, confidence, (or) great expectations," positive emotions have great therapeutic value.

Visual imagery techniques can facilitate positive emotions. Imagery allows people to picture themselves differently so they can experience potential control of perceptions and feelings about their bodies (Miller, 1991).

Self-Help Groups   Experience has shown that providing an opportunity to link up with community and self-help groups can be instrumental in recovery. These groups give the client an opportunity to be with others who have the same problem and to share not only their fears and frustrations but also their successes. Group involvement helps some persons regain the confidence to socialize and to be with others. Self-help groups especially designed for the adolescent are extremely beneficial to the adolescent's process of developing an acceptable image of self.

Self-Care   Assisting clients in regaining control and feelings of self-worth is fostered by helping them assume responsibility for self-care as soon as it is feasible. The sooner the client looks at, touches, or manipulates the involved part, the sooner the adjustment process can begin. Involving the client in the planning of care and in the setting of short- and long-term goals is also important. When clients can understand, determine, and participate in self-care, they gain a sense of control over the chronic illness and resultant body changes.

Grooming is another aspect of self-care that must be encouraged. Cosmetics, clothing, wigs, and hair accessories all help to enhance one's self-image.

Other aspects of self-care that can assist clients in their rehabilitation include bibliotherapy, or reading about how others with similar problems cope, writing about one's feelings, or keeping a daily written log of experiences and reactions.

Teaching Educating the client about the chronic illness is also beneficial because knowledge dispels myths that impede adjustment (see Chapter 16, on teaching). Education can provide the means by which a client can "re-own his own health care" (Price, 1990). The knowledgeable client and family can select viable alternatives that are most appropriate for the specific aspects of their disease and adaptation, including body image changes.

Summary and Conclusions

Body image is an important concept for the health professional to understand. Many definitions have been proposed, all integrating the concept that body image serves as a frame of reference that individuals use in relating themselves to their physical and social environments. Body image is not static; it changes as the individual passes through the various stages of the life cycle. One's sense of body image is also influenced by body boundaries, culture, internal and external environments, and experiences with others.

In the presence of a chronic illness one's sense of body image can be threatened, particularly when physical disfigurement occurs. However, this sense of body image also changes in the presence of a functional limitation or when the changed or lost bodily part has great importance to the individual. Other factors that influence adaptation include the reactions of the client's cultural or social group, family, and caregivers. Inability to adjust to changed body image can result in various physical and psychological problems.

Successful intervention depends on the health professional's understanding of the recovery process. Other variables that can influence intervention include the client's age and sex, perception of the future, coping mechanisms, and past experiences with illness. A thorough assessment of the client is therefore necessary for successful intervention.

Once assessment determines how the client is adapting to the changed body image, it is possible to develop a plan of care. Establishing a therapeutic relationship with the client and family and helping the client participate in self-care are two beneficial interventions. Other interventions include touch, positive emotions, self-help groups, and teaching.

Success in adapting to body image changes varies. Awareness of factors that influence such changes and knowledge of actions that are effective can help maximize adaptation.

There is still limited knowledge of the effects of chronic illness on body image, since the focus, to date, has been primarily on the influence of acute illness and body image. The need for research on the relation between chronic illness and body image becomes apparent if health professionals are to better serve clients with chronic illnesses.

NURSING DIAGNOSIS

7.1.1 Body Image Disturbance

Definition: Disruption in the way one perceives one's body image.

Defining Characteristics:

Objective: missing body part; actual change in structure and/or function; not looking at body part; not touching body part; hiding or overexposing body part (intentional or unintentional); trauma to nonfunctioning part; change in social involvement; change in ability to estimate spatial relationship of body to environment.

Subjective: verbalization of: change in lifestyle; fear of rejection or of reaction by others; focus on past strength, function, or appearance; negative feelings about body; feelings of helplessness, hopelessness, or powerlessness; preoccupation with change or loss; emphasis on remaining strengths; heightened achievement; extension of body boundary to incorporate environmental objects; personalization of part or loss by name; depersonalization of part or loss by impersonal pronouns; refusal to verify actual change.

Related Factors: Biophysical; cognitive/perceptual; psychosocial; cultural or spiritual.

Editor's Note: The first two objective defining characteristics are cues used by the nurse to suspect a body image disturbance and not manifestation of the disturbance itself.

The related factors seem too abstract or general to assist the nurse in identifying what underlies the body image disturbance.

STUDY QUESTIONS

1. Explain the relationship of body image and self-concept.
2. Briefly describe the development of body image during the various phases of the life cycle.
3. Discuss the ways that cultural background influences one's concept of body image.
4. Describe how facial disfigurement can affect a client's body image.
5. Explain how body image can be threatened by a functional limitation.
6. Discuss the effect of a sudden, traumatic illness on a client's body image.
7. What signs and symptoms might indicate an inability to adjust to a changed body image?
8. List factors that determine the client's success in adapting to a changed body image.
9. Identify and describe the four stages of the recovery process.
10. Describe different actions the helping professional can use when intervening on behalf of the client.

References

Baird, S. E. (1985). Development of a nursing assessment tool to diagnose altered body image in immobilized patients. *Orthopaedic Nursing, 4*(1), 47-51.

Beeken, J. (1978). Body image changes in plegia. *Journal of Neurosurgical Nursing, 10,* 20-23.

Bernstein, N. R. (1990). Objective bodily damage: Disfigurement and dignity. In T. F. Cash & T. Pruzinsky (Eds.), *Body images: Development, deviance, and change* (pp. 131-148). New York: The Guilford Press.

Castledine, G. (1981). In the mind's eye . . . *Nursing Mirror, 153,* 16.

Cousins, N. (1983). *The healing heart.* New York: W. W. Norton.

Ernst, P., & Shaw, J. (1980). Touching is not taboo. *Geriatric Nursing, 10,* 193-195.

Fallon, A. (1990). Culture in the mirror: Sociocultural determinants of body image. In T. F. Cash & T. Pruzinsky (Eds.), *Body images: Development, deviance, and change* (pp 80-109). New York: The Guilford Press.

Fawcett, J. & Fry, S. (1980). Exploratory study of body image dimensionality. *Nursing Research, 29*(5), 324-327.

Fisher, S. (1986). *Development and structure of the body image.* Hillsdale, NJ: Lawrence Erlbaum Associates.

Fontaine, K. L. (1991). The conspiracy of culture: Women's issues in body size. *Nursing Clinics of North America, 26,* 669-676.

Harris, M. (1986). Helping the person with an altered self-image. *Geriatric Nursing, 16,* 90-92.

Lee, J. M. (1970). Emotional reactions to trauma. *Nursing Clinics of North America, 4,* 577-587.

Leonard, B. (1972). Body image changes in chronic illness. *Nursing Clinics of North America, 7,* 687-695.

Lerner, R. M., & Jovanovic, J. (1990). The role of body image in psychosocial development across the life span: A developmental contextual perspective. In T. F. Cash & T. Pruzinsky (Eds.), *Body images: Development, deviance, and change* (pp. 110-127). New York: The Guilford Press.

Marten, L. (1978). Self-care nursing model for patients experiencing radical changes in body image. *Journal of Gerontological Nursing, 7,* 9-13.

McCloskey, J. C. (1976). How to make the most of body image theory in nursing practice. *Nursing, 76, 6,* 68-72.

Miller, K. D. (1991). Body-image therapy. *Nursing Clinics of North America, 26,* 727-736.

Mock, V. (1993). Body image in women treated for breast cancer. *Nursing Research, 42*(3), 153-157.

Morrall, S. E. (1990). The shock of the new: Altered body image after creation of a stoma. *Professional Nurse, 5,* 529-537.

Murray, R. B., & Zentner, J. P. (1979). *Nursing assessment: Health promotion through the life span.* Englewood Cliff., NJ: Prentice-Hall.

Murray, R. L. E. (1972a). Body image development in adulthood. *Nursing Clinics of North America, 7,* 617-630.

————— (1972b). Principles of nursing intervention for the adult patient with body image changes. *Nursing Clinics of North America, 7,* 697-707.

Newell, R. (1991). Body image disturbance: Cognitive behavioral formulation and intervention. *Journal of Advanced Nursing, 16,* 1400-1405.

Norris, C. M. (1978). Body image: Its relevance to professional nursing. In C. Carlson & B. Blackwell (Eds.), *Behavioral concepts and nursing intervention.* New York: J. B. Lippincott.

Orr, D. A., Reznikoff, M., & Smith, G. M. (1989). Body image, self-esteem and depression in burn-injured adolescents and young adults. *Journal of Burn Care and Rehabilitation, 10*(5), 454-461.

Price, B. (1990). A model for body-image care. *Journal of Advanced Nursing, 15*(5), 585-593.

Pruzinsky, T. (1990). Psychopathology of body experience: Expanded perspectives. In T. F. Cash & T. Pruzinsky (Eds.), *Body images: Development, deviance, and change* (pp. 170-189). New York: The Guilford Press.

Pruzinsky, T., & Cash, T. F. (1990). Integrative themes in body-image development, deviance, and change. In T. F. Cash & T. Pruzinsky (Eds.), *Body images: Development, deviance, and change* (pp. 337-347). New York: The Guilford Press.

Rosen, J. C. (1990). Body-image disturbances in eating disorders. In T. F. Cash & T. Pruzinsky (Eds.), *Body images: Development, deviance, and change* (pp. 190-214). New York: The Guilford Press.

Schilder, P. (1950). *The image and appearance of the human body.* New York: John Wiley & Sons.

Thompson, J. K. (1990). *Body image disturbances.* New York: Pergamon Press.

Bibliography

Beaman, K., & Luzzatto, P. (1988). Psychological approaches to the treatment of skin diseases. *Nursing, 3*(29), 1061-1063.

Dewis, M. E. (1989). Spinal cord injured adolescents and young adults: The meaning of body changes. *Journal of Advanced Nursing, 14*(5), 389-396.

Erdos, D. (1992). Redefining identity when appearance is altered. *Dermatology Nursing, 4*(1), 41-46.

Ewing, G. (1989). The nursing preparation of stoma patients for self-care. *Journal of Advanced Nursing, 14*(5), 411-420.

Janelli, L. M. (1986). The realities of body image. *Journal of Gerontological Nursing, 12*(10), 23-27.

Samonds, R. J., & Cammermeyer, M. (1989). Perceptions of body image in subjects with multiple sclerosis: A pilot study. *Journal of Neuroscience Nursing, 21*(3), 190-194.

Smith, S. A. (1989). Extended body image in the ventilated patient. *Intensive Care Nursing, 5*(1), 31-38.

CHAPTER 14

Sexuality

Sheila Ostrow Flodberg • *Arlene Miller Kahn*

Introduction

Sexuality is one of the most natural and fundamental aspects of our lives, an early and basic element of our identity as human beings. It is integral to self-concept and, as such, is intrinsically involved with self-esteem and body image. It encompasses the whole person and is the sum of personality traits, ignition behaviors, physical functioning, and communications.

The need for intimacy and love, for touch and body contact, begins in utero and follows us throughout life (Hogan, 1980). Calderone (1974) suggests that sexual needs are a natural and inherent aspect of human existence and that the expression of sexuality is part of the whole person, an aspect of dignity as a human being. Sexuality transcends genitality and encompasses many kinds of expression. It has biological, psychological, and sociocultural components.

Chronic illness does not destroy one's sexuality. It may change one's perceptions of oneself as a sexual being or the ways in which one functions sexually, but it does not alter the universal lifelong need to be close to others, to be touched, and to communicate one's feelings. Adaptation to illness is a developmental crisis with many ramifications, not the least of which are sexual concerns and functioning (Bullard et al., 1980;

Mitchell, 1982; Harris, Good, & Pollard, 1982; Papadopoulos et al., 1983).

For many, sexuality and sexual expression mean being alive (Lamb & Woods, 1981). Being sexual plays an important part in the adjustment to chronic illness (Berkman, Weissman, & Frielich, 1978; Cole, 1975). Sexual expressions may change with personal needs and interpersonal experiences as a result of the limitations that affect sexual behaviors. Nursing has an obligation to help clients in their adjustment to these limitations if they want such assistance. The purpose of this chapter is to provide information that will assist nurses in this important aspect of nursing care.

Definitions of Terms

Human sexuality is a complex biological, psychosocial phenomenon. Clarifying some relevant terms will provide a better understanding of the process. The word *sex,* in the biological sense, refers to the structural and functional qualities of being male or female. For purposes of this chapter, abnormal biological sex will not be addressed. *Sex* includes the following:

1. *Genetic sex:* revealed by the chromosome count of 46XX or 46XY
2. *Gonadal sex:* the presence of ovaries or testes

3. *Hormonal sex:* the androgen-to-estrogen balance

4. *Morphology* of the internal reproductive organs and the external genitalia

Sexuality is the quality of being sexual, capable of having sexual feelings and capacity (Katchadourian, 1979). The term also refers to other aspects of an individual and includes behaviors or expected behaviors. Broadly defined, this includes any activity of an individual, including subjective experiences and those that can be observed. The behavior can have an erotic component in the form of arousal, with or without physiological concomitants (Katchadourian, 1979). It includes the interpersonal, emotional, and nongenital facets of eroticism.

Gender, or sexual identity, relates to the biological sex of a person: male or female. It also includes the personality component of one's identification of one's own gender (Katchadourian, 1979). It answers the question, What sex am I? According to Money and Ehrhardt (1972) *gender identity* is the private experience of gender role, whereas *gender role* is the public expression of gender identity.

Role, according to sociologists, is the set of societal expectations related to the way an individual in a given position should behave in fulfillment of that position. *Gender* or *sex role* can be defined as "everything a person says or does to indicate to oneself or others that one is male, female, or ambivalent. It includes mannerisms, deportment, and demeanor, and may or may not include sexual arousal and responses" (Money & Ehrhardt, 1972).

In many Western countries there is an increasing appreciation for androgyny (Fontaine, 1992). Androgeny entails flexibility in gender roles and views sexual characteristics and behaviors as human qualities common to all rather than relegated to specific genders. Androgenous persons have a flexibility that allows them to adapt better to an increasingly complex world full of roles that are rapidly changing.

Linked with sex role and identity is *sex object choice.* It refers to the choice for one's sexual activity. Although this choice is fluid during early childhood development, by adolescence most people have reached a choice decision, usually heterosexual. There are many styles of final resolution of object choice, and a state of settlement is ultimately made in adulthood (Byers, 1986).

Developmental Aspects

Human sexuality is present from conception, when sex is genetically determined, through old age (see Table 14-1) as part of a continuum. Life-cycle tasks are interdependent, yet failure to complete the psychosexual tasks at one age impedes healthy adaptation and retards growth (Erikson, 1963). When ill, a person may well regress to an earlier stage. Knowing the psychosexual tasks inherent to the developmental process assists sick or disabled persons in maintaining their identity as sexual beings (Schain, 1980).

The infant receives pleasure and sexual gratification through oral satisfaction. Through infancy and the preschool years, the child's growing awareness and mastery of the physical self include awareness of anatomical differences between male and female. Genital behavior and exploration are extended to other children, often of the opposite sex (Kolodny et al., 1979). According to Kolodny and associates (1979), inherent in many cases of adult sexual problems is a history of negative parental reactions to the discovery of childhood sexual activity. Along with awareness of the physical self, most children move from a dependency on mother through seeing the opposite-sex parent as a role object to establishing gender identity with the same-sex parent (Erikson, 1963). The child's growing awareness of sex roles within the family structure (Whaley & Wong, 1991) is influenced by parental attitudes, values, responses, and behaviors. These factors influence the child's perspective of the sexual self.

The school years are a time when children focus beyond themselves and their bodies and gain satisfaction and pleasure from mastering skills and knowledge that will be used in later years. Teachers, neighbors, and others are added as role models. Parental attitudes regarding sex are reflected by their beliefs, the physical control they demonstrate, and their approach to their child's sexual behavior, all of which can

TABLE 14-1. Sexual development through the life cycle

Age Span	Sexual Development
Conception to birth	Sex is genetically determined at conception. Gonad hormonal secretion between the 7th and 12th weeks results in biological sex determination. Brain sex typing is influenced by the hypothalamus around the time of birth (Money & Ehrhardt, 1972).
Infancy	An infant's source of pleasure is primarily oral; the sexual drive is through sucking. Male infant erections are believed to be genital excitement (Woods, 1979). Parental behavior and cues influence gender role expectations. Girl infants are more likely to be rewarded for being "good" and are more aware of visual and verbal stimuli. Boy infants are more exploratory and physically active and do not touch the care provider as much as girls do (Money & Ehrhardt, 1972).
Early childhood	There is a growing sense of body awareness and self-control; the child can differentiate male and female anatomy, including genitals. The parent of opposite sex becomes the role object, and there is early awareness of sex roles; sex role modeling begins (Maccoby & Jacklin, 1974). Genital exploration extends to other children (Kolodny et al., 1979); the child realizes that he or she can be like same-sex parent (Erikson, 1963).
School age	Teachers and neighbors also become role models. Pleasure and satisfaction expand beyond one's own body into development of skills and education. Girls show higher verbal ability and attention to details, in contrast to boys' ability to analyze and score higher in arithmetic reasoning. Girls' grades tend to be higher, but boys do inch up; by high school they test higher (Maccoby & Jacklin, 1974). Parental attitudes, beliefs, and approach to the child's sexual behavior influence the child's views and can be the basis of later sexual problems (Kolodny et al., 1979).
Adolescence	Rapid and profound biological changes lead to physical maturity, with girls maturing earlier than boys (Marshall, 1975). Impulse control between sexual urges and proscribed behaviors must be mastered. Adjustment is made to physiological changes (menses for girls, ejaculation for boys). Choice of love object is usually defined (Simon & Gagnon, 1967). Role confusion usually occurs for youngsters who have not achieved proper sexual identity earlier in life (Erikson, 1963).
Early adulthood	The desire for intimacy, including sexual intimacy, which requires adjustment and adaptation to one another (Woods, 1979), is often developed in marriage. The tasks of parenthood and vocational effectiveness become important. Successful adaptation allows the individual to be committed to concrete relationships, affiliations, and partnerships rather than distancing self from others (Erikson, 1963).
Middle adulthood	In addition to learning to separate from offspring and showing a widening concern for others, many adjustments occur during this developmental phase (Erikson, 1963). These changes influence sexuality and include concerns over body image changes, menopause, changes in sexual response, and plans for retirement. One's own values, self-concept, and assets and limitations are also reviewed (Dresen, 1975).
Old age	Although sexual involvement may be limited by declining physical capacity, lack of a sexual partner, and chronic illness, the desire for sexual activity usually continues for many older individuals (Pfeiffer & Davis, 1972; Rolf & Kleemack, 1979; Christenson & Gagnon, 1965). This can range from desire for intercourse to satisfaction with a close, caring relationship.

influence their children's views even into adulthood (McNab, 1976).

During adolescence, physical maturation progresses rapidly, with girls developing earlier than boys (Kolodny, et al., 1979; Woods, 1979). Strong sexual urges are present, and attempts at self-identity are made through projection on a love object. Impulse control must be mastered, as well as adjustment to physiological changes and secondary sex characteristics. It is now that the choice of love object is usually defined, either heterosexual or homosexual (Simon & Gagnon, 1967). If well concluded, this phase results in a strong sense of self.

A desire for intimacy and a close emotional relationship with another person, including sexual intimacy, are characteristic of early adulthood (Erikson, 1963). Acceptance of one's body image greatly affects one's ability to relate to a sexual partner. This is a time of involvement in parenthood and vocational effectiveness. The middle adult years are characterized by caring and concern for others. Physiological changes that influence sexuality occur and necessitate adjustments: visable body changes, menopause, and changes in sexual responses. Old age is a time of declining physical capacity. When it is coupled with lack of a sexual partner or chronic illness, sexual involvement becomes limited. Yet people continue to desire sexual activity (Mooradian & Greiff, 1990; Rolf & Kleemack, 1979), manifested as desire for continued intercourse or physical contact with others.

Sexual Health

At the World Health Organization (WHO) meeting on sexuality and health programs, *sexual health* was defined as "the integration of the somatic, emotional, intellectual, and social aspects of sexual being, in ways that are positive, enriching and that enhance personality, communication and love" (WHO, 1975). Included in this concept are three basic elements:

1. A capacity to enjoy sexual and reproductive behavior in accordance with a personal and social ethic
2. Freedom from fear, guilt, shame, and false information that inhibit sexual response and impair a sexual relationship

3. Freedom from organic diseases and disabilities that interfere with sexual and reproductive functions (WHO, 1975)

Maddock (1975) adds these criteria to judge sexual health:

1. Congruency between one's gender identity and a sense of comfort with the range of sex role behaviors
2. Ability to carry on an effective interpersonal relationship with both sexes, including the potential for love and commitment
3. Capacity to respond to erotic stimulation so as to make sexual activity stimulating and a positive experience
4. A high correlation between sexual behavior and congruency with one's value system

Although chronic illness and disability affect sexuality and sexual functioning, these problems are by no means limited to sick persons. Masters and Johnson (1970) reviewed their work with 790 persons, both single and married, who were physically healthy adults with a variety of sexual dysfunction problems, most "psychogenic" in origin. Like Masters and Johnson, Levine (1976) found that sexual dysfunction among married couples had an emotional component often reflecting marital discord. Communication skills were found to be important, a factor noted by Masters and Johnson (1970). In their treatment program for sexual dysfunctions, they suggest that in the middle class, sex is an expression of intimacy.

Although many sexual problems are termed *psychogenic,* dysfunction can actually be an early symptom of illness. Sparks, White, and Connelly (1980) found hormonal difficulties in 107 patients who were labeled psychogenic. The controversy between psychogenic and organic is still unclear among renal patients (Sackett, 1990). It is suggested that an early symptom of multiple sclerosis is sexual dysfunction due to disruption in spinal cord tract messages (Erkickson, Lie, & Wineinger, 1989). Among diabetics, there is a high correlation of neuropathy that may or may not precede the dysfunction (Kolodny et al., 1974; Ellenberg, 1979).

Physical impairment offen affects sexual expression through lack of energy, fear, and the general debility of chronic illness (Stockdale-Woolley, 1983; Katzim, 1990; Harris, Good, & Pollard, 1982). Impairments may be due to pain and/or difficulty with mechanic function (Yoshimo & Uchida, 1981; Buckwalter, Wernimont, & Buckwalter, 1982), might be affected by metabolic dysfunction (Procci et al., 1981), by vascular problems (Bray, Frank, & Wolfe, 1981), by neurological impairment (Berkman et al., 1978; Boller & Frank, 1982; Valleroy & Kraft, 1984), neurovascular difficulties (Kolodny et al., 1974; Ellenberg, 1979), or self-esteem and body image disturbances, as often noted in cancer patients (Jusenius, 1981; Lamb & Woods, 1981). The list is long (see Table 14-2). The dysfunctions are mainly erectile difficulties in men, arousal or

TABLE 14-2.　Effects of illness on sexuality[1]

Disorder	Mechanism for Dysfunction	Effect on Sexual Function
A.　Neurologic		M:　Erection and/or ejaculation
I.　Spinal cord surgery, trauma	Interference with afferent and efferent traits in spinal cord	F:　Orgasm and/or lubrication
Disc surgery		B:　Sexual dysfunction often an early sign
Sympathectomy	Interference with spinal nerves	Libidinal changes; increase or decrease or changes in
Multiple sclerosis		sexual behavior
II.　Cerebral cortex	Affects limbic center	
Lesion in temporal or frontal lobe		
Trauma		
Epilepsy		
B.　Vascular	Interferes with blood flow to penis	M:　Erectile difficulties
Atherosclerosis of lower part of body		
Trauma		
Sickle cell		
C.　Endocrine		
Addison's disease	Impaired feedback	B:　Decreased libido
Cushing's syndrome	mechanisms between	M:　Erection
Hypothyrodism	adrenals and pituitary; affecting androgens, general debility and fatigue	F:　Lubrication
Diabetes mellitus	Neuropathy, angiopathy	M:　Impotence
		F:　Possible lubrication
D.　Liver disease	Build-up of estrogens due to inability of liver to conjugate estrogen; general debility	M:　Decreased libido; impaired erection
		F:　Often impaired libido
E.　Systemic diseases		
Renal	Metabolic, general debility	B:　Decreased libido
Pulmonary	General debility, fatigue	M:　Erection
Cardiac	General debility; may have vascular involvement; depression and medications are involved	F:　Lubrication
Arthritis	Pain, body mechanical problems, impaired body image	
Cancer (see also Surgical conditions and Local genital disease	Pain, general debility, body image, localized disfigurement or damage to sexual organs	

TABLE 14–2. *Continued*

Disorder	Mechanism for Dysfunction	Effect on Sexual Function
F. Local genital disease (female)		
I. Vulva and vagina infection	Irritation to genital organs; pain on coitus	Decreased libido
Senile vaginitis		Dyspareunia
Allergies to spermicide sprays		Possible vaginismus
Leukoplakia		
II. Pelvic		
Pelvic inflammatory disease	Damage to genital organs, general disability, fatigue, pain in abdomen, pelvic areas	Dyspareunia: can lead to decreased libido
Endometriosis		
Tumor, cysts		
Prolapsed uterus		
III. Other		
Tight clitoris	Prevent rotation of clitoris, pain on stimulation	Orgasm impaired
G. Local genital disease (male)		
I. Conditions producing pain on coitus		
Preorgasm	Damage to external genital organs	Decreased libido
Penile trauma	Pain	May have impotence problem
Balanitis		
Phimosis		
II. Conditions causing irritation during sexual response		
Urethral pathology	Damage to reflex mechanisms	Erectile problem
Prostatitis		Premature or retarded ejaculation
III. Conditions affecting testicular function		
Orchitis	Decreased androgen level	Decreased libido
Tumor		Possible impotence
Trauma		
Contraction		
H. Surgical conditions		
I. Damage to genitals and nerve supply (males)	Destruction of nerves involved with sexual function (pudendal, sacral)	Impotence
Radical prostatectomy		
Anterior-posterior resection		
Abdominal aortic procedure		Possible ejaculation and impotence
Lumbar sympathectomy, other prostate surgery		Ejaculation / Retrograde ejaculation
II. Damage to sexual organs (female)		
Vulvectomy	Mechanical problems	Decreased libido (psychogenic)
Obstetrical trauma	Fibrotic scars, body image problems	Impaired lubrication / Dyspareunia

[1]Only a partial listing; B = both; M = male; F = female.

SOURCE: Adapted from Kaplan (1974).

lubrication problems in women, and declining libido. However, problems with ejaculation, orgasm, and reproductive ability are not uncommon, especially in neurological disorders.

Our society has become more permissive about sexual expression in general and less critical of sexual behavior among physically disabled and ill persons (Schmidt, 1982). Yet attitudes have an emotional and value component and are difficult to change. If we truly are to accept the concepts of sexual health as previously stated, our challenge is to accept the sexuality of our clients and their partners as real, and to assist them in expressing their desires for sexual contact and closeness, although that expression may be different from previous methods.

The Physiology of the Sexual Response

Female sexual response has two phases: arousal, or lubrication, and orgasm (see Figure 14-1). During the arousal stage, the walls of the vagina moisten, followed by clitoral and labial swelling; the outer one-third of the vagina contracts while the inner two-thirds expand; breasts swell, and nipples become erect (Kaplan, 1974). In the ill or disabled woman, there may be alterations in the changes in the genital area. Orgasm consists of a series of reflex, involuntary contractions of the muscles surrounding the vaginal inlet and perineal floor and the pelvic muscles. Deep pressure proprioceptors

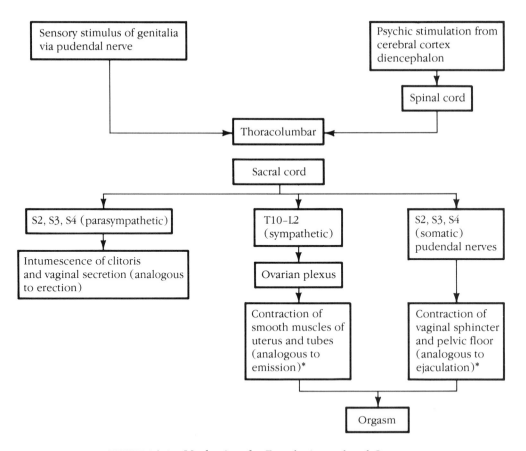

FIGURE 14-1. Mechanism for Female Arousal and Orgasm

*There is no true female counterpart of emission and ejaculation. This comparison is used because the functions are mediated by the same nerves and occur in a corresponding phase of the orgasmic cycle in both sexes.

SOURCE: Adapted from Glass (1976).

within the perineal and vaginal musculature, as well as sensory receptors, probably transmit orgastic sensations to the brain for pleasure and awareness (Kaplan, 1974).

Although it has been stated that orgasm has only one component mediated by the sympathetic nervous system, Graber and Kline-Graber (1979) suggest that it has both a sensory (afferent) component and a motor (efferent) component. They think that in an orgastic women the pubococcygeal muscles do not

effectively contract, but they are unclear as to the mechanism.

In men, the sexual response is also biphasic, with erection and ejaculatory components (see Figure 14-2). Erection involves both sensory and psychic input and occurs as a result of vasocongestion within the corpora cavernosa and the corpora spongiosium of the penis. At the same time, the skin of the scrotum tenses and the testes elevate. As in women, nipples become erect. The parasympathetic nerves are involved in

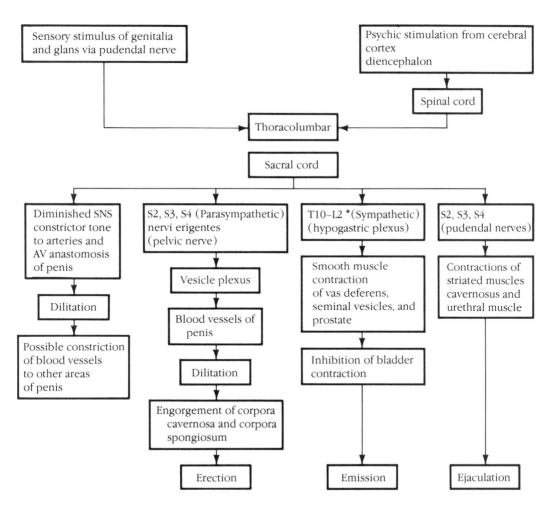

FIGURE 14-2. Mechanism of Erection and Ejaculation

*(Reflexogenic)
*T10–12 might also be involved in psychogenic erection
SOURCE: Adapted from Glass (1976).

reflexogenic erection—erection produced by direct stimulation of the genitals—whereas the sympathetic erection center mediates erection caused by mental stimuli (Boller & Frank, 1982). Weiss (1972) suggests that both centers act synergistically to produce erection. Erection requires intact neurologic and vascular reflexes. However, psychogenic erection can be found in individuals with disruptions of the spinal cord, even at the sacral nerves (Comarr, 1970).

The first part of ejaculation is called *emission.* Prior to ejaculation, semen must be expelled into the prostate urethra, a process dependent on the hypogastric sympathetic nerves. Once this occurs, it is difficult for a man to control ejaculation. This has been termed *ejaculatory inevitability* by Masters and Johnson (1970). Ejaculation is under parasympathetic control, is mediated by nervi erigentes (pelvis nerves), and involves contraction of the bulbocavernosus and ischiocavernosus muscles (Boller & Frank, 1982). With disruption to the spinal cord, this phase of sexual response is usually lacking, although spinal cord patients often report a "paraorgasm," a feeling very much like genital orgasm that occurs with sexual excitement (Glass, 1976).

Masters and Johnson have graphically depicted the human sexual response (see Figure 14-3). During the *excitement stage,* vasocongestion of the pelvic organs occur. This includes psychic and a reflexogenic stimulation that produces lubrication or an erection. During this period, heart rate, blood pressure, and breathing increases. Both sexes develop a flush of the face, neck, and trunk. The *plateau stage* is marked by increased sexual tension with heightening vasocongestion. *Orgasm* occurs by a neural reflex arc once threshold has been reached or exceeded. Following orgasm is a *resolution phase.*

With resolution, the male enters a refractory period during which further ejaculation is impossible, although erection may be maintained. There is great variability in the duration of this period between individuals. With aging, the time lengthens, as does the latency period during which the male is unable to have an erection. Females have the potential of being multiorgasmic, without dropping below the plateau stage of arousal. During resolution, the anatomic and physiological changes of the excitement and

plateau phases are reversed (Kolodny et al., 1979).

Effects of Chronic Illness on Sexual Health

Irreversible illness and disability have significant impact on many facets of life. With illness, one must deal with the direct (physiologic) and indirect (psychosocial) effects of impairment. The perceptions of illness of clients and those involved with them influence behavior, functioning, and coping. One's values, culture, and sex role patterns are also involved with adaptation. The interrelationship between these factors has a definite effect on sexuality. This section presents a broad overview of general principles related to sexual functioning and chronic illness.

Psychosocial Effects

Underlying many illnesses is depression, an emotional state in which low energy and fatigue are present. This same lack of energy is associated with extreme stress and loss. Illness, a state of loss of one's prior good health, is indeed stressful and, in fact, constitutes a deep personal insult. Sexual energy (libido) is diminished, although the mechanism through which this occurs is not clear (Kaplan, 1974). It has been suggested that the endocrine system undergoes physiological changes that accompany stress, and that depression affects brain catecholamine functioning (Kaplan, 1974). Another hypothesis is related to neuroendocrine response; during depression, plasma control levels increase. Through a feedback system, the hypothalamus-pituitary system decreases the release of gonadotropic hormone, resulting in decreased testosterone production, which depresses libido (Stockdale-Woolley, 1983; Kaplan, 1974).

Illness can sap physical as well as emotional energy. In a study of 112 women having rheumatoid arthritis, Yoshimo and Uchida (1981) found that 50 percent of the participants had decreased libido, much of it related to decreased physical energy. This same lack of energy is found among clients with chronic pulmonary disease who experience hypoxia and respiratory insufficiency (Stockdale-Woolley, 1983; Sexton &

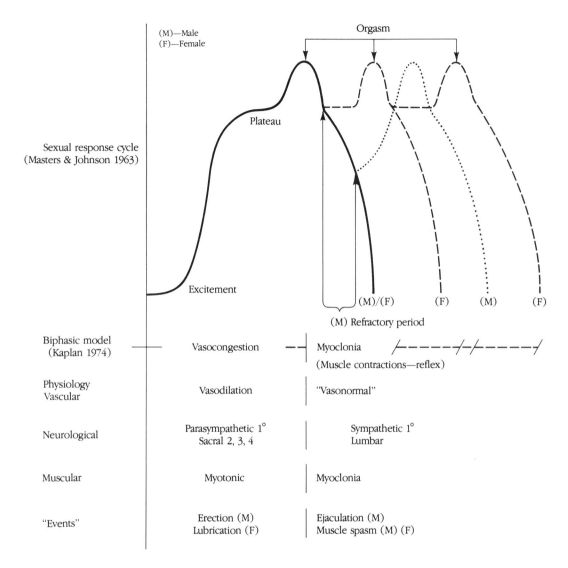

FIGURE 14-3. Sexual Response Cycle

SOURCE: Adapted from Masters, W. H., & Johnson, V. E. (1966). *Human sexual response.* Boston: Little, Brown. Used with permission.

Munro, 1988). Lack of energy and decreased libido have been reported in studies of people with multiple sclerosis (Valleroy & Kraft, 1984; Lilius, Valtonen, & Wickstrom, 1976).

Untreated renal failure produces changes in sexual functioning for both sexes. In one study, 90 percent of anemic men and 80 percent of anemic women reported decreased sexual desire and lowered physical energy levels (Levy, 1973). Abram and associates (1975) and Short and Wil-

son (1969) found that frequency of intercourse declined among individuals with chronic renal failure. These authors concluded that multiple psychogenic factors such as role reversal, dependency, economic burden of chronic illness, postdialysis lethargy, and age, as well as physiologic effects, caused the decreased energy.

In the limited research on sexuality of stroke victims, there is confusion about the finding of libidinal changes following stroke. Bray, Frank, and Wolfe (1981) and Ford and Orfiren (1976) report no change in desire after stroke, especially among individuals less than 60 years old. Goddess, Wagner, and Silverman (1979) found that libido was more diminished after strokes affecting the dominant hemisphere. In a study of hemiparesis caused by a single stroke, clients experienced important alterations in their sexual life (Boldrini et al., 1991).

Fear has a definite impact on sexual functioning. Among 66 married clients with chronic non-malignant pain, 68 percent of the women and 88 percent of the men reported a decrease in the frequency of intercourse, in part related to fear of pain acceleration (Maruta & Osborne, 1978). Persons with musculoskeletal conditions identified pain as the most significant deterent to continuing sexual activity (Blake et al., 1987). Among those who have cardiac disease, fear of pain, of another heart attack, or of sudden death deters sexual relationships (Mehta & Krop, 1979; Trelawny-Ross & Russell, 1987; Papadopoulos et al., 1983). Concerns were noted by client and partner. Sadoughi, Lesher, and Fine (1971) report a high correlation between fear of pain and decreased sexual activity in their study of a chronically ill population with disabilities that included arthritis, amputation, stroke, and emphysema.

Persons with limited mobility, either anatomical (as with amputation) or physiological (as with neurological problems in spinal cord injury or stroke), or with multiple joint involvement (as with arthritis), seem to be less sexually active. Joint stiffness in arthritis patients is a contributor to sexual difficulties (Blake et al., 1987). Hip immobility is a major mechanical impediment to sexual function for females with arthritis (Siemens & Brandzel, 1982). Wheelchairs often get in the way of sexual overtures (Glass, 1976). Persons whose limbs are paralyzed or deformed may abstain from sex because they are unable to position themselves as they formerly did (Cole, 1975). Spasticity usually does not interfere with sexual activity, according to Romano and Lassiter (1972), although they also point out that when adductor spasm is severe, intromission may be impossible for the female client (see Chapter 6, on altered mobility).

People are expected to be in control of bodily functions, especially bladder and bowel functions. When these functions are beyond one's control, and especially when the marital or sex partner has to care for the client, sexual activity has been known to decline or to cease (Glass & Padrone, 1978). Changes in attitude regarding sex can also occur among spouses of ostomate patients (Kolodny et al., 1979; Burnham, Lennard-Jones, & Brooke, 1977).

Conditions that affect sensory function can affect sexual behavior. For example, Wiig (1973) found that aphasics with relatively good receptive comprehension exhibited the fewest problems with sexual adjustment, irrespective of expressive language ability. Wiig conjectures that a client's inability to interpret body language affects sexual responses.

Few studies address sexuality in persons having congenital hearing or sight deficits (Kolodny, et al., 1979). Hearing impairment affects one's psychosocial development. Deficits in the realm of communication and social skills may predispose deaf persons to sexual adjustment problems (Fitz-Gerald & Fitz-Gerald, 1977).

Visual clues are important for sexual expression. When vision is impaired, through either congenital or acquired blindness, there may be effects on sexuality, although in this area, too, there is a paucity of research (Kolodny et al., 1979). Specially tailored sex education as well as parental and teacher attitudes may well affect outcomes related to blind persons' attitudes toward their sexuality. When blindness is acquired, attention to feelings of helplessness, depression, impaired self-esteem, and underlying disability must be addressed (Fitzgerald, 1973).

Tied into these effects is the impact of chronic illness on body image and self-esteem (see Chapter 13, on body image). Body image is the way in which one sees one's body: It is one's mental image of the self (Whaley & Wong, 1991). Body image is a fluid concept and is affected by one's perceptual apparatus of sensory experiences, along with attitudes and overtones expressed by others. Shontz (1974) identifies functions of body image that better define the concept:

1. It is a *sensory register* for integrating basic materials of cognitive and perceptual operations.

2. It is an *instrument for action,* mediating all activities.
3. It is the *source of all drives* and needs, including food, water, air, sleep, sex, and shelter.
4. It functions as a *stimulus to the self* on conscious and subconscious levels.
5. It is a *stimulus to others* and is an individual's first point of control with others.
6. It functions to *create the impression of a private world* where personal decisions are made.
7. It is an *expressive instrument* reflecting one's individuality.

When there is an insult to the perception of one's body, body image disturbance occurs. The distortion of self results as a major assault to self-esteem and body integrity. The way in which individuals see their own bodies also affects their self-concepts. A negative self-concept and diminished self-liking usually cause a person to feel unattractive or unlovable. These negative effects have been demonstrated with clients who have amputations (Reinstein, Ashley, & Miller, 1978) and among cancer patients (Lamb & Woods, 1981), ostomates (Slater, 1992), and the spinal-cord–injured (Fitting, 1978). Feeling ugly influences the sexual self-concept and in turn sexual behavior (Woods, 1979).

Whether body disruption is obvious to others (as with mastectomy or amputation), is invisible (as with a prostatectomy or hysterectomy), or results in loss of function (as with a spinal cord injury), the important factor to be assessed is the effect of the loss of that part of function on one's physical integrity, sense of wholeness, and definition as a sexual being (Derogatis, 1980).

Although many disease states and disabilities affect both the psychogenic and psychologic aspects, cancer, because of its broad effects on nearly every body system, probably best shows the direct and indirect effects (see Table 14–3).

Physiologic Effects

It is impossible to discuss all the direct sexual dysfunctions that can result from chronic illness or disability. Many of these are specific to the pathology of the disease; others result from the individual's psychosocial response. Several disease states with known sexual impact will be discussed in depth.

Diabetes Mellitus Estimates of impotency among male diabetics range from 29 to 60 percent (Manley, 1990; McCullock et al., 1980). Libido remains intact, but erectile dysfunction may gradually increase over a 6- to 24-month period (Kolodny et al., 1974; Krosnick & Poldolsky, 1981). There is no loss of the ability to ejaculate or to be aware of orgasmic sensations, nor is there a change in measures of circulatory testosterone between diabetic and nondiabetic men (Kolodny et al., 1974).

There is general agreement that the primary pathogenesis is neuropathy, involving microscopic damage to nervous fibers (Jensen, 1981; Ellenberg, 1971). Faerman and associates, (1973) found histologic changes in autonomic nerve fibers in the corpora cavernosa of impotent diabetic men at autopsy. Repeated studies have shown a high correlation between diabetic neuropathy and erectile dysfunction (Ellenberg, 1971; Jensen, 1981). Because of the microvascular angiopathy, which diabetics experience, Tyler and associates (1983) suggest that a combination of nerve and vascular damage affects potency in diabetic men. Ellenberg (1979) proposes that other vascular pathology, such as atherosclerosis or peripheral vascular disease, which limits blood supply to the penis, might affect the male diabetic's potency. Regardless of cause, if impotency appears early in the course of the disease, even with good blood glucose control, prognosis for reversal is poor, especially when neuropathy is present (Kolodny et al., 1979).

Where impotence is irreversible and definitely organic in origin, one of two types of penile prosthesis has proved beneficial (Mulcahy et al., 1990; Googe & Mook, 1983). The case study of T. R. illustrates this point.

A "new" old drug, Yohimbine, is currently used to treat impotence from organic causes (Morales et al., 1988). Yohimbine is an alpha-adrenergic blocker that stimulates norepinephrine release and thus decreases vasoconstriction of penile blood flow. In a study of men treated

TABLE 14-3.   Effect of cancer on sexuality

| Site | Dysfunction | | Reproductive Effect on Fertility | Impact on Partner |
	Organic	Psychologic[1]		
Cervix	Hysterectomy shortens vagina, usually no dysfunction, treatment of in situ with cone, resulting in no dysfunction	Sometimes	Unable to have children with hysterectomy or X-ray therapy, which will thicken vagina	May think he will contract cancer, be affected by X-ray therapy, think he caused cancer
Endometrial	Radical hysterectomy, usually no dysfunction	Sometimes	As above	As above
Ovary	In premenopausal women with bilateral oophorectomy, resulting in menopausal symptoms	Sometimes	If bilateral oophorectomy	As above
Vulva	Simple can cause introital stenosis. Radical includes clitorectomy and often has decreased range of motion and lupus erythematosus	Usually, especially altered body image	Patient usually postmenopausal	Usually
Breast	Absence of nipple arousal	Usually includes altered body image	None, unless oophorectomy and hormonal treatment were once used	Usually
Prostate	Radical resulting in impotence, retropubic and suprapubic resulting in retrograde ejaculation, hormonal manipulation and orchiectomy can alter libido	Usually altered self-image, estrogen hormone resulting in gynecomastica	Yes	Usually afraid she might develop cancer
Testicular	Retroperitoneal lymph node dissection usually resulting in retrograde ejaculation and can cause erectile dysfunction	Yes, if bilateral orchiectomy resulting in decreased libido and sexual responsiveness	Often	Usually
Bladder	Local-seldom; cystectomy in female includes anterior vagina, uterus, and urethra. Male includes prostate, bladder, urethra	Yes, altered body image with urinary incontinence	Usually yes if X-ray therapy, often patient is older male	Yes

TABLE 14-3. *Continued*

| Site | Dysfunction | | Reproductive Effect on Fertility | Impact on Partner |
	Organic	Psychologic[1]		
Colon-Rectal	If anterioposterior resection, sacral nerve involvement, results in erectile dysfunction	Yes, especially with ostomy	None, unless X-ray therapy done, sometimes with chemotherapy	Yes
Leukemia	Chemotherapy and its effects may affect erection	Sometimes, especially with fatigue	Chemotherapy affects ovulation and spermatogenesis; rebound after treatment stopped	Usually, especially if patient has decreased energy and function; may take it as rejection
Hodgkins	Libido and ability affected	Usually	As above, X-ray therapy affects testicle and ovarian function; contraception should be used because effects of chemotherapy on ovarian function and sperm maturation not understood	

[1]It is often difficult to determine the difference between psychologic and physical dysfunction since they are interrelated.
SOURCE: Adapted from Lamb & Woods (1981).

with Yohimbine, 20 percent of the subjects had complete improvement in erectile function, 23 percent experienced partial improvement, and the remaining 57 percent reported no improvement (Morales et al., 1988). The application of nitroglycerine paste to the penis has also been used effectively to produce erections in diabetic males with impotence (Owen et al., 1989).

A recent pilot study (Aloni et al., 1992) of vacuum tumescence constriction therapy shows promising results for treatment of neurologically caused impotence. Of the 30 subjects who participated in this study, 50 percent reported using the noninvasive device on a long-term basis with coital activity increases from 0.3 a week to 1.5 a week.

Until 1971, no one studied the effects of diabetes on women. In a matched sample study of 125 diabetic and 100 nondiabetic women, 35.2 percent of the diabetic women reported being anorgasmic a year prior to the study. Interestingly, they all had previously experienced or-

gasm, whereas 6 percent of the nondiabetic women had always been anorgastic. Kolodny (1971) concluded that the cause was organic rather than psychogenic. In a study of 82 insulin-dependent women and 47 controls, Tyler and coresearchers (1983) found that the diabetic women were slower to achieve vaginal lubrication. In a study of younger insulin-treated diabetic females, age 26 to 45, Jensen (1985) found no significant difference in incidence of sexual dysfunction compared to an age-matched control group.

In summary, evidence for sexual dysfunction among diabetic women is contradictory and nonconclusive. However, many previous studies may have been confounded by their failure to control for the types of diabetes. Schreiner-Engel and associates (1985) compared Type I and Type II diabetic women with healthy controls and showed that the type of diabetes was highly related to sexual responsiveness and marital satisfaction. Type I diabetes did not have a negative

CASE STUDY
The Diabetic Client

T. R. is a 63-year-old male who has had Type II diabetes for years. Until five years ago, he was using an oral hypoglycemic agent, but he is now taking 25 units NPN and 10 units regular insulin every day. His fasting blood sugar averages 180. He has had peripheral neuropathy for five years, but has no other long-term complications.

At onset of his neuropathy, T.R. began to have orgasmic dysfunction with inability to maintain erection. Over a two-year period, the problem advanced to complete inability to have an erection. His desire remained intact. This was a blow to his self-concept because he had always thought of himself as a "ladies' man" and otherwise took care of himself by maintaining his weight and physique.

On several occasions, he discussed his sexual difficulty with his nurse practitioner, who compiled a sexual history, tested hormone levels, and discussed a penile implant with him. He was referred to the urology clinic and the sexual dysfunction clinic for assessment of a penile implant, which he ultimately had. The healing process went more slowly than he had anticipated, which was discouraging to him and to his female companion. After three months the healing was complete and the prosthesis device was deemed successful. T. R. wonders why he waited "so long" to pursue coitus actively again.

---

effect on diabetic women, while Type II diabetes had a "pervasively negative impact" in a large variety of areas, including desire and relationship with sexual partner.

Diabetic women do seem more susceptible to vaginal infections, probably through a combination of increased leukocytes and elevated tissue concentrations of glucose that provide an excellent medium for bacteria. Monilia, the most common vaginal infection for diabetic women, produces decreased lubrication, pruritis, and tissue tenderness that may make intercourse painful and exudes a malodorous discharge. The reported infections may have an effect on sexual activity (Bagdade, Root, & Bulger, 1974).

Unsain and Goodwin (1982) suggest that sexual dysfunctions in female diabetics are due to an elevated stimulatory threshold before the orgasm phase. Thus, a higher level of stimulus is needed to trigger the orgasmic reflex. Kolodny and associates (1979) suggest that women experiencing orgasmic problems who were previously orgasmic might benefit from the increased stimulation of a vibrator.

Chronic Renal Disease   The degree of diminished libido, erectile dysfunction, arousal (in women), and intensity of orgasm seem to be related to the degree of disease (Abram et al., 1975; Steele, Finklestein, & Finklestein, 1976).

Procci and coresearchers (1981) reported that 50 percent of clients having uremia complained of impotence and decreased coital frequency. The researchers found no difference between clients receiving dialysis and those not receiving such therapy.

A correlation between the absence of nocturnal penile tumescence (NPT) and uremia was observed by Parker and associates (1977) and Procci and collaborators (1981). The former suggest that the absence of NPT might be related to the metabolic effects of the disease, whereas the latter suggest that age is a factor.

In a study by Berkman, Katz, and Weissman (1982) in which 50 percent of the men had severe sexual dysfunction and 22 percent had moderate dysfunction (erection and ejaculation dysfunction for both groups), there was a high correlation between declining sexual function and uremic neuropathy. Uremic men have decreased testosterone levels regardless of dialysis or control of the renal failure (Lim & Fang, 1975). After successful transplant, testosterone levels return to normal, accounting for the increased libido, but other sexual dysfunctions do not improve (Lim & Fang, 1975).

Levy (1973) reported that women who had renal transplant returned to their premorbid sexual functioning, whereas a significant percentage of the men did not. The results of a more recent study of renal transplant patients indicated that 13 of 14 subjects were able to return to work and to pre-illness activity levels and enjoyed sexual relations (Slavis et al., 1990). These subjects had received their transplants 20 years ago or longer, and all enjoyed stable renal function.

In women, chronic renal failure results in menses changes and infertility. Decreased lubrication and atrophic vaginitis may be due to an estrogen deficiency. With successful transplant, fertility improves and normal pregnancy may be possible (Feldman & Singer, 1974).

Sackett (1990) reviewed the literature on the impact of end stage renal disease on sexual functioning and concluded that while "decreased potential for orgasm, infertility, and erectile difficulties are recognized as problems, specific causal factors cannot be identified because of the many variables associated with the disease, with treatment modalities, and with the individuality of clients and their relationships with partners." In addition, she reported what while "dialysis can diminish or reverse these problems, studies do not reflect uniform improvement, probably because of the multiplicity of other factors."

Spinal Cord Injury or Lesion The level of the cord injury as well as the presence of complete or incomplete lesion determine the type of dysfunction the person experiences. In a review of the literature based on 1,296 male spinal-cord–injured individuals, 35 percent were found able to engage in intercourse, 77 percent could have erection, and in 10 percent ejaculation was preserved (Tarabulcy, 1972).

Generally speaking, clients with a lesion in the cauda equina (L2 and below) experience loss of erection but can possibly ejaculate (Boller & Frank, 1982). Among a sample of 20 males with lumbar injuries, 8 were able to have psychogenic erection, but none were able to have reflexogenic erection (Comarr, 1975). Seven had successful coitus and five achieved orgasm. For injuries above the lumbar area and complete, psychogenic erections occur infrequently, although reflexogenic and spontaneous erections are common. However, erection has a short duration, and orgasm is rarely achieved (Boller & Frank, 1982). Fertility is generally impaired, al-

though the mechanism is not clear. Usually there is impaired spermatogenesis possibly due to recurrent infections or temperature-regulation impairment in the scrotum (Comarr & Bors, 1955).

As with other areas of sexual functioning and disability, females with cord injuries have been studied less than males. In general, irrespective of the level of injury, intercourse is more possible for women than men. According to Kolodny and collaborators (1979), this funding reflects the fact that women do not require intense vasoconstrictive changes to engage in coitus. Although typical orgasm is absent in women with complete cord lesions, heightened arousal can be obtained by tactile stimulation of body parts innervated by spinal cord segments above the lesion (Griffith & Trieschmann, 1975). Within 6 to 12 months, menses returns to normal and these women have no more difficulty with conception or delivery than ablebodied women (Comarr, 1966; Goller & Paeslack, 1972). Pregnancy might be complicated by automatic dysreflexia, urinary tract infections, and premature labor (Goller & Paeslack, 1972).

Adverse Effects of Medication on Sexual Function

Table 14-4 summarizes the effects of a number of drugs (by categories) on sexual dysfunction. Much more is known about the effects of medications on men than on women, primarily because erection and ejaculation are visible and therefore more measurable than female dysfunctions, which tend to be subjectively reported (Kolodny, et al., 1979).

Soyka and Mattison (1981) reviewed the 100 most commonly prescribed drugs in 1979. Four consistent findings were changes in libido, gynecomastica, impotence, and retarded or absent ejaculation. Three drugs (amitriptyline, cyclobenzaprine, and imipramine) caused testicular swelling.

Although one tends to think of drugs as having a negative effect on sexual activity, they can also enhance function. For example, birth control pills allow women to enjoy sexual relations without fear of pregnancy. If used properly, the "pill" is considered 99 percent safe (Woods, 1979). "Once a month" and morning-after postcoital

TABLE 14–4. Some drugs that affect sexual function

Drug or Drug Category	Libidinal Change	Impotence (male) or Lubrication (female)	Gyneco-mastica or Galactorrhea	Climax Changes	Menses Change	Hormonal Change
I. Diuretics						
a. Thiazide		Impotence				
b. Spironolactone	High doses	Impotence	Gynecomastica		High doses	Antiandrogenic properties
c. Furosemide		Impotence				
II. Antihypertensives						
a. Propanolol (beta-adrenergic)	Occasional decrease	Impotence				
b. Methyldopa	Decrease	Both	Gynecomastica	F: anorgasmic M: decrease or slow ejaculation		
c. Vasodilators	Decrease with high doses					
d. Clonidine		Impotence				
e. Reserpine	Decrease		Gynecomastica	Decrease or no ejaculation		
III. Psychotropic						
a. Phenothiazines	Yes	Both	Both	Decrease or no ejaculation		
b. Thioridazine		Impotence	Galactorrhea	Decrease or no ejaculation	Yes	Increases testosterone levels
c. Trifluoperazine			Gynecomastica	Decrease or no ejaculation	Yes	
d. Haldol		Both	Both	Decrease or no ejaculation		
e. Lithium	Yes	Impotence				
f. Tricyclic antidepressants	Yes	Occasional impotence	Gynecomastica			
g. Benzodiazepines, oxazepam	Yes		Galactorrhea		Yes	Decreases testosterone levels

IV. Barbitals	Yes				
V. Aminoglycosides		Both	Gynecomastica	Yes	Increases estrogen and decreases testosterone levels
VI. Alcohol		Both			Decreases testosterone levels
VII. Cimetadine			Gynecomastica		Decreases sperm count
VIII. Anticholinergics		Some decreased lubrication, impotence			
IX. Flagyl	Yes				
X. Antiandrogens					
a. Clofibrate	Yes	Impotence	Gynecomastica		
b. Estrogens (in men)		Impotence	Gynecomastica		
XI. Steroids	Yes				
XII. Others					
a. Heroin, cocaine	Increase libido (small dose)	Impotence			
b. Marijuana		Impotence with large amounts	Gynecomastica		Decreases testosterone levels

SOURCE: Adapted from Kolodny et al. (1979), Kaplan (1974), Soyka & Mattison (1981), and Wise (1984).

drugs for men and women are being studied (Bennett, 1974; Dierassi, 1970). Chemical contraception has contributed to better understanding of sexuality in our society as well as greater enjoyment of sexual activity for both men and women.

Many drugs used for treatment of hypertension affect sexual function. Often compliance with the medication is a problem because high blood pressure is a "silent" disease. If sexual side effects occur, compliance becomes more problematic (Blackwell, 1973). Kolodny and coresearchers (1979) suggest the following guidelines when starting the client on antihypertensive therapy:

1. Obtain a good sexual history as a baseline of function.
2. Do not assume that sexual symptoms are automatically drug related. Be alert to psychological factors, other illnesses, or use of alcohol that might underlie the dysfunction.
3. Be certain to inquire about sexual problems at each visit. Such inquiries will determine dosages that can be tolerated and will be helpful in assessing sexual difficulties before the patient continues treatment.
4. Be willing to work with the patient to adjust drugs or dosages. Often blood pressure control therapy uses a combination of drugs that have different actions and therefore is less likely to be synergistic.

Whether or not to inform a client about drug-related side effects on sexual function remains a concern of health care providers. A survey of physicians revealed that 75 percent of them preferred not to tell their patients about potential side effects of prescribed medications (Ascione & Raven, 1975). However, Cyr and McLean (1978) found that 92 percent of patients want complete information about the drugs they are taking. After reviewing the literature, Meichelbaum and Turk (1987) reported that forewarning patients about possible side effects does not increase the incidence of side effects nor lead to treatment nonadherence. Based on this evidence, they conclude that "efforts at patient education should include a discussion of possible side effects in the context of a consideration of patient expectations about treatment outcomes."

Long- and short-term use of alcohol affects sexual function. Acutely, it is a central nervous system depressant, interfering with pathways of reflex transmission for sexual arousal (Farkas & Rosen, 1976). Blood alcohol levels well below intoxication levels suppress erection (Farkas & Rosen, 1976). Gordon and associates (1976) suggest that alcohol lowers circulatory testosterone levels in healthy young men.

Men who are chronic alcohol users display reduced libido, even with allowances for age. Approximately 40 percent are impotent, and 5 to 10 percent have ejaculatory difficulties (Lemere & Smith, 1973). One study of alcoholic women revealed that 30 to 40 percent had difficulty with arousal and 15 percent experienced reduction in the intensity or frequency of orgasm (Kolodny et al., 1979). Sexual problems in men are caused in part by a decreased testosterone rate as well as protein binding of testosterone. Spermatogenesis is also impaired (Van Thiel, 1976). Alcoholic women are more susceptible to cirrhosis than men, and the endocrine system probably is affected in a parallel manner (Morgan & Sherlock, 1977).

In addition to hormonal disturbances, nutritional problems found in alcoholics result in anemia (Straus, 1973) and peripheral neuropathy (Morgan & Sherlock, 1977). If the alcoholic has chronic liver disease, other physiological problems plug into the causes of sexual dysfunction.

Effects of Illness on the Sexual Partner

Prior to illness or disability, it is likely the individual was active in various social roles, contributed to the household, and was able to express sexuality in socially acceptable ways. Illness, with its many ramifications, changes former ways of functioning, often affecting interpersonal relationships, especially with those closest to the client. Sexual relationships seem to be generally impaired.

There was a decline in sexual activity among 78 percent of the chronically ill men studied by Sadoughi, Lesher, and Fine (1971). Yet 42 percent believed that their spouse wanted more sex. There was a greater decline in interest among men in this study than among women, a finding that may indicate why women clients tended to think their spouse was satisfied with the marital relationship.

Yoshimo and Uchida (1981) reported that more than 50 percent of the women in their study refused the sexual advances of their spouse. They noted a high correlation between disability and dissatisfaction with sex life for both the patient and her spouse (60 percent). Patients were anxious about their own desire as well as that of their spouse.

Harris, Good, and Pollard (1982) examined the sexual beliefs of 96 women who had gynecologic cancer and the attitudes of their partners. Sexual activity and discussions about sex declined after surgery. Partners often felt guilty and thought they caused the disease. These beliefs, along with fear of causing more pain and concern for the health of their spouse, were cited as major reasons for decreased sexual activity.

Among cardiac clients and their spouses, 51 percent expressed fear of resuming sexual activity despite the fact that 72.6 percent of these couples resumed sex at a mean of 10.8 weeks after myocardial infarction (Papadapoulos et al., 1980, 1983). Concerns included fear (previously discussed), attractiveness, safety, and the quality of sexual expression now compared to the premorbid expression.

In a study of 32 clients receiving home hemodialysis, 77 percent reported sexual dissatisfaction and genital function that resulted in less demonstrated affection and decreased sexual intercourse (Berkman et al., 1982). Abram and co-researchers (1975) reported that 45 percent of their subjects had decreased libido, potency, or both. Clients cathected and withdrew from their spouse in order to preserve their own diminished physical energy. Wives generally denied psychological effects on sexual function and tended to be defensive and protective toward their husbands.

The effects of chronic lung disease on life in general and on sexuality were examined in 128 clients (Hanson, 1982). Of these, 67 percent considered the most detrimental aspect of their illness to be the effect on the sexual aspect of their marriage. Only 40 percent thought that the emotional impact on their marriage was worsened, and many thought the disease had brought them emotionally closer to their spouse.

In instances in which illness necessitates surgery that results in physical deformity, the role of the partner is vital to the adjustment process. For example, in a study of 60 women undergoing mastectomy, the majority (70 percent) undressed in front of their partners before surgery. During the three-month period following surgery, that proportion declined to 35 percent. The follow-up study made eight years after surgery revealed that 53 percent still undressed in front of their partner. Before surgery, 76 percent were nude during sexual activity, whereas only 45 percent were eight years after surgery. However, 50 percent reported more tenderness from their partner with sex after the mastectomy than before. This study, (Frank et al., 1978) concluded that the women who adjusted better were those whose partners accepted their new body image. Similar findings were reported by Jusenius (1981), and Burnham, Lennard-Jones, and Brooke (1977). (See Chapter 13, on body image.)

Other problems for the couple include their own roles: passivity, dependence (especially if they formerly were independent), economic burdens, shame, anger, fear of abandonment and rejection, loss of friends, and fear of death. Glass (1976) proposes the question, Can a 24-hour-a-day, 7-day-a-week caregiver also be a lover? In summary, when one member of a sexual relationship is affected by illness, the partner also incurs effects.

The Social Impact on Sexuality

Every society determines which of its members may engage in sexual relations, and under what conditions such relations are approved (Siemens & Brandzel, 1982). Our society looks upon youth and beauty with favor, expecting vigor and sexual expression among this population. Many people equate illness with old age, despite the fact that illness—indeed, chronic illness—affects all age groups. Although our society has begun to look more favorably and even realistically at the sexual needs of the elderly, there still persists the erroneous belief that being old, ill, or disabled ends the need for sexual expression.

This attitude is particularly true toward persons who are institutionalized. Paradowski (1977) studied 155 residents who were chronically ill. He reports that 35 percent were involved in an active relationship, and 25 percent said that they would like to be part of a heterosexual dyad. Many of the unattached individuals reported that they masturbated. In a study of 63 residents of a nursing home, the majority believed that sexual activity was appropriate for other elderly people in nursing homes but not for themselves. Men and women had different beliefs about why the opposite sex would want sex (Wasow & Loeb, 1979). Their beliefs, no doubt, were affected by their cultural upbringing. Authors of both studies suggest that institutions should offer more privacy and opportunities for those who desire a sexual relationship.

There is a new phenomenon in our society related to the openness of homosexuality. Recent studies report that gay men and lesbian women comprise between 1 and 6 percent of the population, although some experts believe these numbers actually may be higher because of underreporting from reticent participants (Rogers, 1993). A problem confronting chronically ill, institutionalized homosexuals is insensitivity to the existence of their partners. Although space for conjugal visits is seldom provided for heterosexual couples (Paradowski, 1977), private space for homosexuals is never considered (Brossart, 1979). Brossart also suggests that homosexual partners are often denied access to intensive care units, and that often nursing homes admit only one member of a homosexual couple.

Among the various disability groups, developmental disability, formerly called mental retardation, is the largest (Chigier, 1992). In the past, people with developmental disabilities were generally deprived of relationships with the opposite sex during their reproductive years. This attitude began to change in the late 1960s and early 1970s as a result of the energetic efforts of groups like the National Association of Retarded Citizens and the Association for Persons with Severe Handicaps (Chigier, 1992). These groups directed attention both to the civil rights of the developmentally disabled and to rethinking societal definitions of "normal."

Of greater importance at that time was the effort to move institutionalized persons into community living situations (Blomberg, 1988; Kempton & Stiggall, 1989). The success of com-

munity-oriented rehabilitation resulted in a change in attitude toward the sexual behavior of the developmentally disabled (Blomberg, 1988); that is, it is now more accepted that this group of individuals have sexual needs and feelings and have the right to express them. However, it should be noted that this focus on normalization is not always accepted by parents of developmentally disabled children. A recent survey of these parents found that 53 percent of the respondents would consider sterilization for their child, and a large majority felt they alone, or in conjunction with a doctor, should be able to consent on behalf of the person with the disability. The researchers conclude that consideration needs to be given to parental anxieties about sexual and reproductive health issues that are now surfacing with the emphasis on community care.

Nurses, and other health professionals, who work with developmentally disabled individuals and their parents should be thoroughly informed about the sexual rights and sex education needs of this client population. To prepare the developmentally disabled to live as community members, an adequate sex education program must be presented to them in a timely fashion. A primary concern of such a program should be the safety needs of these individuals. Persons with developmental disabilities are four times more likely to experience sexual abuse than the nondisabled population; 99 percent of reported incidents are perpetrated by persons known to the victim (Muccigrosso, 1991).

A number of experts have suggested that the following areas be included in a sex education program for developmentally disabled children: (1) names and functions of body parts, (2) physical and emotional changes of puberty, (3) appropriate and inappropriate behavior, (4) private versus public behavior, (5) sexual intercourse and use of contraceptives, (6) possible risks and consequences of sexual activity, (7) marriage and parenthood, and (8) avoidance of sexual exploitation or abuse (Kempton & Stiggall, 1989; Muccigrosso, 1991; Blomberg, 1988).

A growing health problem facing our society is acquired immune deficiency syndrome (AIDS). The dangers of AIDS infection has, over the past ten years, changed the rules for sexual relationships across the country and the world. The incidence of AIDS is increasing steadily, but not at the exponential rate predicted at the time of discovery (*Sexual Health Promotion,* 1990). While gay men still account for the majority of AIDS cases in this country, an increasing number of cases are associated with intravenous (IV) drug use and heterosexual activity (Miller, Turner, & Moses, 1990). The number of women who are affected by the AIDS epidemic has greatly increased. Among women, although IV drug use accounts for the majority of AIDS cases, Guinan and Hardy (1987) report that the percentage of infected women who were not IV drug users increased from 12 percent in 1982 to 26 percent in 1986.

The AIDS movement has effectively transformed the relationship between society and disease because individuals with AIDS have, of necessity, been social reformers in the area of patient rights and health care (Defert, 1990). Early on in the epidemic, the medical community and society provided little help to afflicted persons and those at risk. Consequently, concerned individuals found it necessary to organize themselves into community movements to ensure food and shelter to those rendered homeless, protect the civil liberties of those threatened by discrimination, educate those at risk, and advocate for medical research and prompt access to new treatments. Individuals with AIDS are often extraordinarily informed and involved in the treatment of their disease. Because of this involvement, they serve as a force for change in the way all chronically ill individuals are perceived and treated in the medical community (Defert, 1990).

Providing Sexual Health Care

Nurses and other health providers are social beings who have a set of values and beliefs about sexual practices. How do we, or should we, treat chronically ill persons whose ways of expressing sexuality differ from our own? Regardless of our own perspective, to be effective in working with clients and their sexual concerns, it is important not to create for the couple or client a conflict with their values.

Various studies indicate that sex plays an important part in adjustment to chronic illness (Berkman, Weissman, & Frielich, 1978; Sadoughi, Lesher, & Fine, 1971; Conine, Disher, & Gilmore, 1979). It is suggested that better sexual adjustment is related to better social, physical, and psychological functioning necessary for successful rehabilitation (Berkman et al., 1978). Among spinal-cord–injured persons, the degree of sexual adjustment was found to be highly correlated with success in vocational training and employment (Conine, Disher, & Gilmore, 1979). Sick or disabled persons who view themselves as desirable and enjoy sexual behaviors that do not entirely depend on genital function have learned to value personal assets rather than to focus on disabilities (Cole, 1975).

Research further indicates that clients have sexual concerns that they want to discuss, and that they expect the health care provider to initiate the discussion (Renshaw & Karstaedt, 1988; Harris et al., 1982; Papadopoulos et al., 1980). Finally, studies indicate that they want their sexual partner included in the counseling (Hock, 1977; Hartman, Macintosh, & Englehardt, 1983). Workshops in human sexuality reflect changes in attitudes regarding sexual behavior, knowledge, and comfort in talking with clients about their sexual concerns (Frazer et al., 1982; Mims, Brown, & Lubow, 1974).

Given this information, it seems only fitting that nursing be involved in this aspect of a client's adjustment to illness. For the nursing profession, like other health professions, dealing with sexual health is a relatively new domain. There is an increasing concern among nursing educators that students receive accurate information to help them in this important role.

Based on her study of 124 nurse educators at 10 nursing schools, Fontaine (1976) made the following recommendations:

1. Hold faculty workshops on human sexuality to examine attitudes and beliefs about sex.
2. Support textbooks that examine the relationship between illness and sexual functioning.
3. Include in course content alterations in health that affect life patterns, including sexual functions.

The nurse's ability to deal with a client's sexuality depends on acceptance of her or his own sexuality, as well as acceptance of the client's (Zalar, 1975). Being comfortable with one's own sexuality allows for more sensitivity to client concerns. When the nurse conveys, verbally and nonverbally, such comfort, the client feels some leeway for the expression of feelings about the impact of illness on sexuality. The nurse who is aware of such sexual concerns also is aware of times when the client does not want to discuss sex (Payne, 1976).

The Golden and Golden study (1980) found that clients want direction and support in reestablishing sexual functioning or relationships. They make the following suggestions to health care providers:

1. Be comfortable in discussing sexual issues.
2. Know where to refer the patient and his or her partner if your knowledge is inadequate or your values based on cultural or religious beliefs differ.
3. Initiate discussion of sexual concerns at various stages of illness and treatment:
   a. When the diagnosis is being made
   b. When treatment planning occurs
   c. Early on and later along the road to recovery

The PLISSIT model is a good format to help the patient and family with sexuality. It was devised by Jack Annon, a sex therapist in Honolulu (Annon, 1976). This hierarchical model moves in accordance with the nurse's skills and the setting in which treatment is to occur. The model starts with simply giving *permission* (P) for certain behaviors such as masturbation, fantasies, or feelings. The second step is giving *limited information* (LI) related to factual information about the problem, such as telling a cardiac patient that sudden death with intercourse almost never occurs. The third step involves *specific suggestions* (SS). Here the nurse gives specific recommendations regarding a problem that has been clarified by good history taking, so that the suggestion is relevant and appropriate to the client's illness and concerns. Last comes *intensive therapy* (IT), such as sensate focus exercises (Masters & John-

son, 1970). If such therapy is beyond the nurse's capabilities, referral of the couple to a professional with more advanced training may be appropriate. The way the PLISSIT model works is illustrated by Mr. G.'s case study.

Components of a sexual history should include the nature of the problem or concerns about the marital or interpersonal relationship; previous ways of sexual expression (for example, they may not enjoy oral–genital sex); other physical health problems; medications; and use of alcohol. It is important to understand the persons' attitudes about their own bodies (Hammond & Stuart, 1980). The quality of the relationship should also be assessed. The affective tone of the relationship determines couples' perception of their sexual relationship (Frank, Anderson, & Rubenstein 1978). If premorbidity problems existed, the stress of illness will probably heighten the problems in the sexual arena or produce a deterioration or break in the relationship (Glass, 1976).

In further assessing the sexual functioning of any chronically ill person, three parameters must be considered. First is the psychological realm, involving depression, regression, self-esteem, and body image. Next are the specific aspects of physiologic functioning that can alter sexual functioning and response. Factors to consider include the disease state, which may alter sexual organs; medication; technical trappings of treatment such as a body cast; or changes in anatomy, as with radical pelvic surgery. The third area is that of organic enjoyment, in which physical functioning is intact, but the milieu is less than satisfactory. Fatigue, fear of odors or pain, decubitus, or deformities may create a less than satisfactory environment for actual pleasure (Wise, 1977).

Good communication is foremost when working with sexual problems: between client and nurse and client and partner (Kolodny et al., 1979; Mooney, Cole, & Chilgren, 1975; Lamb & Woods, 1981). Communication provides a means of discussing and defining each person's perspective of intimacy and its relation to sexual needs. Leviton (1978) defines *intimacy* as a close relationship with another, a desire to be with and enjoy that individual, perhaps a desire

CASE STUDY
Using the PLISSIT Model

Mr. G. is a 55-year-old man who has a history of angina and hypertension. Two weeks ago he had a myocardial infarction. He and his wife of 30 years have enjoyed a close relationship. Sex has been enjoyable for both of them. However, Mr. G. has been the more dominant partner, and their coital activities have been rather traditional. They both have concerns that this illness will terminate their sex life. They are afraid of sudden death or pain if they try to resume sexual activity. In addition, Mr. G. is taking a thiazide diuretic and a beta-adrenergic blocker to control his hypertension.

The nurse first initiated a discussion about sexual concerns and obtained the G.s' permission to proceed. The hospital's program for sexual activities was discussed, and the first stage was reviewed with them. Here, Mr. G. learned that masturbation is *permissible. Limited information* about cardiac activity was then given. For example, the nurse was able to tell them about the outcomes of the Hellerstein and Friedman

(1970) study on heart rate and sexual activity, as well as to inform them that with conjugal sex, Ueno (1963) found only 0.6 percent coital deaths among the 5,559 deaths he investigated.

Specific suggestions were made, including reviewing the remainder of the cardiac sexual activities program, suggesting that the G.s wait two to three hours after eating before engaging in coitus, taking a nitroglycerine tablet just prior to intercourse to prevent chest pain, and that Mrs. G. should take the superior or side-lying position so that her husband would not incur cardiac stress by the isometric effects of the male-superior position. In taking their history, the nurse learned that although Mrs. G. has enjoyed sex, she has had a difficult time with orgasm and she wonders if this situation can be changed. In this case, the nurse suggested the names of two sex therapists whom she felt might provide *more intensive therapy* to assist this couple in this more complicated realm of their sexual functioning.

---

to hold and be held, a desire to share and confide or both. In a sexual relationship, intimacy may range from being nonexistent to reaching an extreme high. Not only does intimacy vary, but so do sex acts; illness interfers with only some of them. Although illness may impose a change in actual sexual behaviors, the intimacy between the couple might be heightened if they work harder at having a good relationship. Good communications can help the client experience empathic gratification, a feeling of adequacy by pleasuring his or her partner (Cole, 1975).

In working with clients and their sexual concerns, it is important not to create in the couple or client a conflict with personal values. Remember that many people do not want to discuss sexuality (Curry, 1970), but, on the basis of the findings discussed, the nurse should open the door for discussion by using a statement such as "Many people who have experienced _____ have concerns about their sexual functioning. Do you have any problems or concerns that you would like to discuss?"

In addition to fostering communication and opening the door to discussion about sexual concerns, Lamb and Woods (1981) make these suggestions:

1. Provide anticipatory guidance. By offering information, aid the client and partner in coping more realistically with problems. This can help dispel myths.
2. Validate normalcy of sexual functioning. This helps the client to focus on alternative expressions and what might be prudent or possible, given the limitations the illness or disability imposes.
3. Educate beyond the anticipatory. This might include interventions to lessen pain, prevent pain, decrease spasms, affect timing, increase function, improve appearance or control.
4. Counsel about alternative techniques for sexual expression such as approaches, techniques, positioning, masturbation, imagery, touching, massage, and cuddling. Here the

nurse must be knowledgable about the couples' values, attitudes, and beliefs.

5. Refer to those individuals with a high level of comfort or more expertise as needed. This includes serving as a client advocate.

Many clients benefit from good counseling and accurate information (Melynk, Montgomery, & Over, 1979; McLane, Krop, & Mehta, 1980). However, we must accept the fact that we will not always be successful for a myriad of reasons, such as continued denial or lost self-esteem on the part of the client, desire to retain established beliefs or behaviors by the couple, or a partner who is negative or who sabotages efforts at sexual readjustment (Glass, 1976).

Isolation from sexuality and its paths toward intimacy can be disabling. By teaching our clients and their partners new ways to express closeness and intimacy, by helping them discover new options and erogenous zones, by working with them to accept their bodies and themselves as valuable, lovable human beings, we can help to enrich and enhance their lives (Cole, 1975).

Summary and Conclusions

Sexuality and intimacy are basic aspects of our lives. From genetic determination through old age, people find sexual gratification in many ways. Chronic illnesses can alter the opportunity and means for sexual expression. Such changes can result from interference with various physiological responses of men and women, from iatrogenic effects of treatment, or from the psychosocial effects that accompany many illnesses.

The health professional can assist the client and partner in dealing with sexual difficulties, if the client wishes such help. To be effective, professionals must be aware of their own sexuality. In addition, an adequate sexual history should be obtained as the basis of any intervention. Suggested here is the PLISSIT model, which is a useful format for helping the client and family deal with identified sexual problems. Inherent in this approach, as in most interventions, is the need for effective communication skills. The health professional can, through sensitive involvement, contribute to the clients' retaining of their sexual selves to help enhance their lives.

NURSING DIAGNOSIS

3.2.1.2.3 Sexual Dysfunction

Definition: The state in which an individual experiences a change in sexual function that is viewed as unsatisfying, unrewarding, inadequate.

Defining Characteristics: Verbalization of problem; alterations in achieving perceived sex role; actual or perceived limitation imposed by disease and/or therapy; conflicts involving values; alteration in achieving sexual satisfaction; inability to achieve desired satisfaction; seeking confirmation of desirability; alteration in relationship with significant other; change of interest in self and others.

Related Factors: Biopsychosocial alteration of sexuality; ineffectual or absent role models; phys-

ical abuse; psychosocial abuse, e.g. harmful relationships; vulnerability; values conflict; lack of privacy; lack of significant other; altered body structure or function (pregnancy, recent childbirth, drugs, surgery, anomalies, disease process, trauma, radiation); misinformation or lack of knowledge.

3.3 Altered Sexuality Patterns

Definition: The state in which an individual expresses concern regarding his/her sexuality.

Defining Characteristics: (Major characteristics) Reported difficulties, limitation, or changes in sexual behaviors or activities.

Related Factors: Knowledge/skill deficit about alternative responses to health-related transitions, altered body function or structure, illness or medical; lack of privacy; lack of significant other; ineffective or absent role models; conflicts with sexual orientation or variant preference; fear of pregnancy or of acquiring a sexually transmitted disease; impaired relationship with a significant other.

Editor's Note: The differences in definition, defining characteristics, and related factors of these two categories are inadequate to do a differential diagnosis. Their placement in the taxonomy does little to clarify matters. *Sexual dysfunction* falls under *altered role performance* (3.2.1) while *altered sexual patterns* is placed at the next level (3.3). Hopefully, there will be some study done to clarify this matter.

STUDY QUESTIONS

1. What does the word *sex* connote? What are the differences between gender identity, gender role, and sex object choice?
2. How would you explain why the steps in psychosexual development as described by Erikson are not mutually exclusive?
3. In what ways do the following affect sexual functioning: lack of energy? body image distortion? altered mobility?
4. How do the following chronic conditions affect libido or sexual functioning, including causes: diabetes mellitus? CVA? hypertension? male and female spinal cord injuries? myocardial infarction?
5. What are the various factors that affect sexual expression among alcoholics?
6. What is (are) the effect(s) of chronic illness on the sexual partner of the client? What are some of the concerns of sexual partners?

7. How does the way in which the sexual partner accepts or rejects the client's new body image affect the client's adjustment to the illness? the partner's? Explain your answer.
8. How does our society respond to the sexual needs of the chronically ill? the aged? homosexuals? Explain your answer.
9. Should the nurse or the client and partner initiate discussion about sexuality? Explain your answer.
10. Why is it important to incorporate the client's values and beliefs in sexual counseling?
11. What does the acronym PLISSIT stand for? How can the nurse use this format to counsel the client?
12. What constitutes a satisfactory sexual adjustment to chronic disease or disability? In what ways can a satisfactory sexual adjustment contribute to positive rehabilitation?

References

Abram, H. S., Lester, L. R., Sheridan, W. F., & Epstein, G. M. (1975). Sexual functioning in patients with chronic renal failure. *Journal of Nervous and Mental Disease, 160,* 220-226.

Aloni, R., Heller, L., Keren, D., Mendelson, E., Davidoff, G. (1992). Noninvasive treatment for erectile dysfunction in the neurogenically disabled population. *Journal of Sex and Marital Therapy, 18*(3), 243-249.

Annon, J. (1976). The PLISSIT model: A proposed conceptual scheme for the behavioral treatment of sexual problems. *Journal of Sex Educators and Therapists, 2,* 1-15.

Ascione, F., & Raven, R. M. (1975). Physicians' attitudes regarding patients' knowledge of prescribed medication. *Journal of American Pharmacology Association, 15,* 386-391.

Bagdade, J. D., Root, R. K., & Bulger, R. J. (1974). Impaired leukocyte function in patients with poorly controlled diabetes. *Diabetes, 23,* 9-15.

Bennett, J. P. (Ed.) (1974). Chemical contraception in the male. In *Chemical contraceptives,* New York: Columbia University Press.

Berkman, A. H., Katz, L. A., & Weissman, R. (1982). Sexuality and life-style of home dialysis patients. *Archives of Physical Medicine and Rehabilitation, 63,* 272-275.

Berkman, A. H., Weissman, R., & Frielich, M. H. (1978). Sexual adjustment of spinal cord injured veterans living in the community. *Archives of Physical Medicine and Rehabilitation, 59,* 22-23.

Blackwell, B. (1973). Patient compliance. *New England Journal of Medicine, 289,* 249-252.

Blake, D. J., Maisiak, R., Alarcon, G. S., et al. (1987). Quality of life of patients with arthritis compared to arthritis-free controls. *Journal of Rheumatology, 14,* 570-576.

Blomberg, P. S. (1988). Sex education issues for persons with developmental disabilities. *Reproductive Health Resources, 5*(4), 1-3.

Boldrini, P. Basaglia, N., & Calanca, M. C. (1991). Sexual changes in hemiparetic patients. *Archives of Physical Medicine and Rehabilitation, 72*(3), 202-207.

Boller, F., & Frank, E. (1982). *Sexual dysfunction in neurological disorders.* New York: Raven Press.

Bray, G. P., Frank, R. S., & Wolfe, T. L. (1981). Sexual functioning in stroke survivors. *Archives of Physical Medicine and Rehabilitation, 62,* 286-288.

Brossart, J. (1979). The gay patient: What should you be doing? *RN, 42*(4), 50-52.

Buckwalter, K., Wernimont, T., & Buckwalter, T. (1982). Musculoskeletal conditions and sexuality (Part II). *Sexuality and Disability, 5*(4), 195-207.

Bullard, D. G., Causey, G. G., Newman, A. B., Orloff, R., Schnaube, K., & Wallace, D. H. (1980). Sexual health care and cancer: A needs assessment. *Frontiers of Radiology Therapy and Oncology, 14,* 55-58.

Burnham, W. R., Lennard-Jones, J. E., & Brooke, B. (1977). Sexual problems among married ileostomists. *Gut, 18,* 673-677.

Byers, S. (1986). Sexuality and sexual concerns. In B. S. Johnson (Ed.), *Psychiatric-mental health nursing: Adaptation and growth* (pp. 83-98). Philadelphia: J. B. Lippincott.

Calderone, N. S. (1974). *Sexuality and human values.* New York: Association Press.

Chigier, E. (1992). Sexuality and mental retardation. *Seminars in Neurology, 12*(2), 129-134.

Christenson, C. V., & Gagnon, J. H. (1965). Sexual behavior in a group of older women. *Journal of Gerontology, 20,* 351-356.

Cole, T. E. (1975). Sexuality and physical disabilities. *Archives of Sexual Behavior, 4,* 389-403.

Comarr, A. E. (1966). Interesting observations on females with spinal cord injury. *Medical Services Journal, 22,* 651-661.

——— (1970). Sexual function among patients with spinal cord injury. *Urology International, 25,* 134-168.

——— (1975). Sexual function in spinal cord injury patients. Diagnosis and therapy. *Urology, 1,* 1-18.

Comarr, A. E., & Bors, E. (1955). Spermatocystography in patients with spinal cord injuries. *Journal of Urology, 73,* 172-178.

Conine, R., Disher, C., & Gilmore, S. (1979). Physical therapists' knowledge of sexuality of adults with spinal cord injury. *Physical Therapist, 59,* 395-398.

Curry, H. L. F. (1970). Osteoarthritis of the hip joint and sexual activity. *Annals of the Rheumatic Diseases, 29,* 288.

Cyr, J. G., & McLean, W. (1978). Patient knowledge of prescription medication. *Canadian Pharmacology Association, 17,* 361-363.

Defert, D. (1990). A new social reformer: The patient. In D. G. Ostrow (Ed.), *Behavioral aspects of AIDS.* (pp. 1-6). New York: Plenum.

Derogatis, L. R. (1980). Breast and gynecologic cancers, *Frontiers of Radiation Therapy and Oncology, 14,* 1-11.

Dierassi, C. (1970). Birth control after 1984. *Science, 169,* 941-957.

Dresen, S. E. (1975). The sexually active middle adult. *American Journal of Nursing, 75,* 1001-1011.

Ellenberg, M. (1971). Impotence in diabetes: The neurological factor. *Annals of Internal Medicine, 75,* 213-219.

——— (1977). Sexual aspects of the female diabetic. *Mt. Sinai Journal of Medicine, 44,* 495-500.

——— (1979). Sex and diabetes: A comparison between men and women. *Diabetes, 2,* 4-8.

Erikson, E. H. (1963). *Childhood and society.* New York: W. W. Norton.

Erkickson, R. P., Lie, M. R., & Wineinger, M. A. (1989). Rehabilitation in multiple sclerosis. *Mayo Clinic Proceedings, 64,* 818-828.

Faerman, K., Glaser, L., Fox, D., Jadzinsky, M. N., & Rapaport, M. (1973). Impotence and diabetes. Eighth Congress of the International Diabetes Federation, Brussels, Belgium, July 15-20, 1973.

Farkas, G. N., & Rosen, R. C. (1976). Effects of alcohol and elicited male sexual response. *Journal of Studies on Alcohol, 37,* 265-272.

Feldman, H. A., & Singer, I. (1974). Endocrinology and metabolism in uremia and dialysis: A clinical review. *Medicine, 54,* 345-376.

Fitting, M. D. (1978). Self-concept and sexuality of spinal cord injured women. *Archives of Sexual Behavior, 7,* 143-156.

Fitz-Gerald, D., & Fitz-Gerald, M. (1977). Deaf people and sexual, too! *SIECUS Report, 6*(2), 13-15.

Fitzgerald, R. G. (1973). Sexual behavior in the blind. *Medical Aspects of Human Sexuality, 7,* 60-61.

Fontaine, K. L. (1976). Human sexuality: Faculty knowledge and attitudes. *Nursing Outlook, 24,* 174-176.

——— (1992). Applying the nursing process for clients with sexual disorders. In H. S. Wilson & C. R. Kneish (Eds.) *Psychiatric nursing* (pp. 348-369). Redwood City, CA: Addison-Wesley.

Ford, A. B., & Orfiren, A. P. (1976). Sexual behavior and the chronically ill patient. *Medical Aspects of Human Behavior, 8,* 10-30.

Frank, D., Dornbush, R., Webster, S., & Kolodny, R. C. (1978). Mastectomy and sexual behavior. *Sexuality and Disability, 1,* 16-25.

Frank, E., Anderson, C., & Rubinstein, D. (1978). Frequency of sexual dysfunction in normal couples. *New England Journal of Medicine, 299,* 111-115.

Frazer, J., Albert, M., Smith, J., & Dearner, J. (1982). Impact of a human sexuality workshop in the sexual attitudes of nursing students. *Journal of Nursing Education, 21*(3), 6-13.

Glass, D. D. (1976). Sexuality and the spinal cord injured patient. In W. Oaks, G. Melchiode, & I. Ficher (Eds.), *Sex and the life cycle.* New York: Grune & Stratton.

Glass, D. D., & Padrone, F. J. (1978). Sexual adjustment in the handicapped, *Journal of Rehabilitation, 44,* 43-47.

Goddess, E. D., Wagner, N. N., & Silverman, D. R. (1979). Poststroke sexual activity of CVA patients. *Medical Aspects of Human Sexuality, 13,* 16-30.

Goldberg, S., & Lewis, M. (1972). Play behaviors in the year old infant: Early sex differences. In J. M. Bardwhich (Ed.), *Readings on the psychology of women.* New York: Harper & Row.

Golden, J. S., & Golden, M. (1980). Cancer and sex. *Frontiers of Radiation Therapy and Oncology, 14,* 59-65.

Goller, H., & Paeslack, V. (1972). Pregnancy damage and birth complications in children of paraplegic women. *Paraplegia, 10,* 213-217.

Googe, M., & Mook, T. (1983). The inflatable penile prosthesis: New developments. *American Journal of Nursing, 83*(7), 1044-1047.

Gordon, G. G., Altman, S., Southren, A., Rubin, E., & Lieber, C. (1976). Effect of ethanol administration on sex hormone metabolism in normal men. *New England Journal of Medicine, 295,* 793-797.

Graber, B., & Kline-Graber, C. (1979). Female orgasm: Role of puboccogeus muscles. *Journal of Clinical Psychiatry, 40,* 348-351.

Griffith, E. R., & Trieschmann, R. B. (1975). Sexual functioning in women with spinal cord injury. *Archives of Physical Medicine and Rehabilitation, 56,* 18-21.

Guinan, M., & Hardy, A. (1987). Epidemiology of AIDS in women in the U.S. *Journal of the American Medical Association, 257,* 2039-2042.

Hammond, D. C. & Stuart, F. M. (1980). Workshop on sexual dysfunction, University of Utah, Salt Lake City, June 11-15.

Hanson, E. I. (1982). Effects of chronic lung disease on life in general and on sexuality: Perceptions of adult patients. *Heart and Lung, 11,* 435-441.

Harris, R., Good, R. S., & Pollard, L. (1982). Sexual behavior of gynecologic cancer patients. *Archives of Sexual Behavior, 11,* 503-510.

Hartman, C., Macintosh, B., & Englehardt, B. (1983). The neglected and forgotten sexual partner of the physically handicapped. *Social Work, 28,* 370-374.

Hock, Z. (1977). Sex therapy and marital counseling for the disabled. *Archives of Physical Medicine and Rehabilitation, 85,* 413-417.

Hogan, R. (1980). *Human sexuality.* Norwalk, CT: Appleton-Century-Crofts.

Jensen, S. (1981). Diabetic sexual dysfunction: A comparative study of 160 insulin treated diabetic men and women and an age-matched control group. *Archives of Sexual Behavior, 10,* 493-504.

Jensen, S. B. (1985). Sexual dysfunction in younger insulin-treated diabetic females: A comparative study. *Diabetes Metabolism, 11*(5), 278-282.

Jusenius, K. (1981). Sexuality and gynecologic cancer. *Cancer Nursing, 4,* 479-484.

Kaplan, H. S. (1974). *The new sex therapy.* New York: New York Times Book Company.

Katchadourian, H. (1979). *Human sexuality.* Berkeley: University of California Press.

Katzin, L. (1990). Chronic illness and sexuality. *American Journal of Nursing, 90*(1), 55-59.

Kempton, W., & Stiggall, L. (1989). Sex education for persons who are mentally handicapped. *Theory into practice, 28*(3), 203-210.

Kolodny, R. C. (1971). Sexual dysfunction in diabetic females. *Diabetes,* 557-559.

Kolodny, R. C., Kahn, C. B., Goldstein, H. H., & Barnett, D. M. (1974). Sexual dysfunction in diabetic men. *Diabetes, 23,* 306-309.

Kolodny, R. C., Masters, W. H., Johnson, V. E., & Biggs, M. A. (1979). *The textbook of human sexuality for nurses.* Boston: Little, Brown.

Krosnick, F., & Poldolsky, S. (1981). Diabetes and sexual dysfunction: Restoring normal ability. *Geriatrics, 36,* 92-100.

Lamb, M. A., & Woods, N. E. (1981). Sexuality and the cancer patient. *Cancer Nursing, 4,* 137-144.

Lemere, F., & Smith, J. W. (1973). Alcohol-induced sexual impotence. *American Journal of Psychiatry, 130,* 212-213.

Levine, S. B. (1976). Marital sexual dysfunction. *Annals of Internal Medicine, 84,* 448-453.

Leviton, D. (1978). The intimacy-sexual needs of the terminally ill and the widowed. *Death Education, 2,* 261-280.

Levy, N. B. (1973). Sexual adjustment to maintenance hemodialysis and renal transplantation. *American*

Society of Artificial Internal Organs, 19, 138-143.

Lilius, H. G., Valtonen, E., & Wickstrom, J. (1976). Sexual problems in patients suffering from multiple sclerosis. *Scandinavian Journal of Social Medicine, 4,* 41-44.

Lim, V. S., & Fang, V. S. (1975). Gonadal dysfunction in uremic men: A study of hypothalamo-pituitary-testicular axis before and after renal transplantation. *American Journal of Medicine, 58,* 655-662.

Maccoby, E. E., & Jacklin, L. M. (1974). *The psychology of sex differences.* Stanford: Stanford University Press.

Maddock, J. W. (1975). Sexual health and health care. *Post-graduate Medicine, 58,* 52-58.

Manley, G. (1990). Endocrine disturbances and sexuality. In C. I. Fogel & D. Lauver (Eds.), *Sexual health promotion.* Philadelphia: W. B. Saunders.

Marshall, W. A. (1975). Growth and sexual maturation in normal puberty. *Clinics in Endocrinology and Metabolism, 4,* 3-25.

Maruta, T., & Osborne, D. (1978). Sexual activity in chronic pain. *Psychosomatics, 19,* 531-537.

Masters, W., & Johnson, V. E. (1970). *Human sexual inadequacy.* Boston: Little, Brown.

McCullock, D. K., Campbell, I. W., Wu, F. C., Prescott, R. J., & Clarke, B. F. (1980). The prevalence of diabetic impotence. *Diabetologica, 28,* 279-283.

McLane, M., Krop, H. L., & Mehta, J. (1980). Psychosexual adjustment and counseling after myocardial infarction. *Annals of Internal Medicine, 92,* 514-519.

McNab, W. L. (1976). Sexual attitude development in children and the parents' role. *Journal of School Health, 46,* 537-542.

Mehta, J., & Krop, H. (1979). The effect of myocardial infarction on sexual functioning. *Sexuality and Disability, 2,* 115-121.

Meichelbaum, D., & Turk, D. C. (1987). *Facilitating Treatment Adherence.* New York: Plenum.

Melynk, R., Montgomery, R., & Over, R. (1979). Attitude changes following a sexual counseling program for spinal cord injured persons. *Archives of Physical Medicine and Rehabilitation, 60,* 601-605.

Miller, H. G., Turner, C. F., & Moses, L. E. (Eds.) (1990). *AIDS: The second decade* (pp 1-13). Washington, D.C.: National Academy Press.

Mims, F. H., Brown, L., & Lubow, R. (1974). Human sexuality course evaluation. *Nursing Research, 25,* 187-191.

Mitchell, M. E. (1982). Sexual counseling in cardiac rehabilitation. *Journal of Rehabilitation, 48*(4), 15-18.

Money, J. (1972). Sex reassignment therapy in gender identity disorders. *International Psychiatry Clinics, 8,* 197-210.

Money, J., & Ehrhardt, A. (1972). *Man and woman: Boy and girl.* Baltimore: Johns Hopkins Press.

Mooney, T. O., Cole, T. M., & Chilgren, R. (1975). *Sexual options for paraplegics and quadraplegics,* Boston: Little Brown.

Mooradian, A. D., & Greiff, V. (1990). Sexuality in older women. *Archives of Internal Medicine, 150*(5), 1033-1038.

Morales, A., Condra, M. S., Owen, J. E., Fenemore, J., & Surridge, D. H. (1988). Oral and transcutaneous pharmacologic agents in the treatment of impotence. *Urology Clinics of North America, 15*(1), 87-93.

Morgan, M. Y., & Sherlock, S. (1977). Sex-related difference among 100 patients with alcohol liver disease. *British Medical Journal, 1,* 939-941.

Muccigrosso, L. (1991). Sexual abuse prevention strategies and programs for persons with developmental disabilities. *Sexuality and Disability, 9*(3), 261-271.

Mulcahy, J. J., Krone, R. J., Lloyd, L. K., Edson, M., & Siroky, M. B. (1990). Duraphase penile prostheses: Results of clinical trials in 63 patients. *Journal of Urology, 143*(3), 518-519.

Owen, J. A., Saunders, F., Harris, C., Fenemore, J., Reid, K., Surridge, D., Condra, M., & Morales, A. (1989). Topical nitroglycerine: A potential treatment for impotence. *Journal of Urology, 141*(3), 546-548.

Papadopoulos, G., Beaumont, C., Shelley, S., & Larrimore, P. (1983). Myocardial infarction and sexual activity of the female patient. *Archives of Internal Medicine, 14,* 1528-1530.

Papadopoulos, G., Larimore, P., Cardin, S., & Shelley, S. (1980). Sexual concerns and needs of the post coronary patient's wife. *Archives of Internal Medicine, 140,* 38-41.

Paradowski, W. (1977). Socialization patterns and sexual problems of the institutionalized chronically ill and physically disabled. *Archives of Physical Medicine and Rehabilitation, 58,* 53-59.

Parker, R. A., Bennett, W. M., Harris, R. L., Barry, J., & Porter, G. A. (1977). Nocturnal penile tumescence: Objective method for evaluation of impotence in chronic renal failure. *Clinical Dialysis Transplant Forum, 7,* 34-38.

Payne, T. (1976). Sexuality of nurses: Correlations of knowledge, attitudes and behavior. *Nursing Research, 25,* 286-292.

Pfeiffer, E., & Davis, G. C. (1972). Determinants of sexual behavior in middle and old age. *Journal of the American Geriatric Society, 20,* 151-158.

Procci, W. A., Goldstein, D. A., Adelstein, J., & Massry, S. G. (1981). Sexual dysfunction in the male with uremia: A reappraisal. *Kidney International, 19,* 317-328.

Reinstein, L., Ashley, J., & Miller, K. (1978). Sexual adjustment after lower extremity amputation. *Archives of Physical Medicine and Rehabilitation, 59,* 501-503.

Renshaw, D. C., & Karstaedt, A. (1988). Is there (sex) life after coronary bypass? *Comprehensive Therapy, 14*(4), 61-66.

Rogers, P. (1993, February 15). How many gays are there? *Newsweek,* p. 46.

Rolf, L. L., & Kleemack, D. L. (1979). Sexual activity among older persons. *Research on Aging, 1,* 389-399.

Romano, M. D., & Lassiter, R. E. (1972). Sexual counseling with the spinal cord injured. *Archives of Physical Medicine and Rehabilitation, 53,* 568-575.

Sackett, C. (1990). Genitourinary conditions and sexuality. In C. I. Fogel & D. Lauver (Eds.), *Sexual health promotion* (pp. 407-436). Philadelphia: W. B. Saunders.

Sadoughi, W., Lesher, M., & Fine, H. L. (1971). Sexual adjustment in chronically ill and disabled population: A pilot study. *Archives of Physical Medicine and Rehabilitation, 52,* 311-317.

Schmidt, G. (1982). Sex and society in the eighties. *Archives of Sexual Behavior, 11,* 91-97.

Schreiner-Engel, P., Schiavi, R. C., Vietorisz, D. De Simone-Eichel, J., & Smith, H. (1985). Diabetes and female sexuality: A comparative study of women in relationships. *Journal of Sex and Marital Therapy, 11*(3), 165-175.

Sexton, D. L., & Munro, B. J. (1988). Living with a chronic illness: The experiences of women with chronic obstructive pulmonary disease. *Western Journal of Nursing Research, 10,* 26-44.

Shontz, F. C. (1974). Body image and its disorders. *International Journal of Medicine, 5,* 461-472.

Short, N. J., & Wilson, N. P. (1969). Roles of denial in chronic hemodialysis. *Archives of General Psychiatry, 20,* 433-437.

Siemens, S., & Brandzel, R. C. (1982). *Sexuality: Nursing assessment and intervention.* Philadelphia: J. B. Lippincott.

Simon, W., & Gagnon, J. H. (1967). Homosexuality: The formulation of a sociological perspective. *Journal of Health and Human Behavior, 8,* 177-185.

Slater, M. J. (1992). What are the differences in body image between patients with a conventional stoma compared with those who have had a conventional stoma followed by a continent pouch? *Advances in Nursing, 17*(7), 841-848.

Slavis, S. A., Novick, A. C., Steinmuller, D. R., Streem, S. B., Braun W. E., Straffon, R. A., Mastroianni, B., & Graneto, D. (1990). Outcome of renal transplantation in patients with a functioning graft for 20 years or more. *Journal of Urology, 144*(1), 20-22.

Smith, L. S., Lauver, D., & Gray, P. A. (1990). Sexually transmitted diseases. In C. I. Fogel & D. Lauver (Eds.), *Sexual health promotion* (pp. 459-484). Philadelphia: W. B. Saunders.

Soyka, L. F., & Mattison, D. R. (1981). Prescription drugs that affect male sexual function. *Drug Therapy, 11,* 46-58.

Sparks, R. F., White, R. A., & Connelly, P. B. (1980). Impotence is not always psychogenic. *Journal of the American Medical Association, 243,* 750-755.

Steele, T. E., Finklestein, S. H., & Finklestein, F. O. (1976). Hemodialysis patients and spouses: Marital discord, sexual problems and depression. *Journal of Nervous and Mental Disease, 162,* 225-237.

Stockdale-Woolley, R. (1983). Sexual dysfunction and COPD: Problems and management. *Nurse Practitioner, 8,* 16-18.

Straus, D. J. (1973). Hematologic aspects of alcoholism. *Seminars in Hematology, 10,* 183-194.

Tarabulcy, E. (1972). Sexual function in the normal and in paraplegia. *Paraplegia, 10,* 201-208.

Trelawny-Ross, C., & Russell, O. (1987). Social and psychological responses to myocardial infarction: Multiple determinants of outcome at six months. *Journal of Psychosomatic Research, 31,* 125.

Tyler, G., Steel, J. M., Ewing, D. J., Bancropft, J., Warner, P., & Clarke, B. F. (1983). Sexual responsiveness in diabetic women. *Diabetologica, 24,* 166-176.

Unsain, I. C., & Goodwin, M. H. (1982). Effects on sexual function. In D. W. Guthrie & R. A. Guthrie (Eds.), *Nursing management of diabetes mellitus* (2nd ed.). St. Louis: C. V. Mosby.

Valleroy, M. L., & Kraft, H. (1984). Sexual dysfunction in multiple sclerosis. *Archives of Physical Medicine and Rehabilitation, 65,* 125-128.

Van Thiel, D. (1976). Testicular atrophy and other endocrine changes in alcoholic men. *Medical Aspects of Human Sexuality, 10,* 153-154.

Wasow, M., & Loeb, M. (1979). Sexuality in nursing homes. *Journal of the American Geriatrics Society, 27,* 73-79.

Weiss, H. D. (1972). The physiology of human penile erection. *Annals of Internal Medicine, 76,* 792, 799.

Whaley, L. F., & Wong, D. L. (1991). *Nursing care of infants and children* (3rd ed.). St. Louis: C. V. Mosby.

Wiig, E. H. (1973). Counseling the adult aphasic for sexual readjustment. *Rehabilitation Counseling Bulletin, 17,* 110-119.

Wise, T. M. (1977). Sexuality in chronic illness. *Primary Care, 4,* 199-207.

——— (1984). How drugs can help or hinder sexual function. *Drug Therapy, 14,* 51-63.

Woods, N. F. (1979). *Human sexuality in health and illness.* St. Louis: C. V. Mosby.

World Health Organization (1975). Education and treatment in human sexuality: The training of health professionals. *WHO Technical Report Series* (No. 572). Geneva: WHO.

Yoshimo, S., & Uchida, S. (1981). Sexual problems of women with rheumatoid arthritis. *Archives of Physical Medicine and Rehabilitation, 62,* 122-123.

Zalar, M. (1975, Nov./Dec.). Human sexuality: A component of total patient care. *Nursing Digest,* pp. 40-43.

Bibliography

Block, A., Molder, J., & Horsely, J. (1975). Sexual problems after myocardial infarction. *American Heart Journal, 90,* 536-537.

Brooks, M. H. (1977). Effects of diabetes on female sexual response. *Medical Aspects of Human Sexuality, 11(2),* 63-64.

Conine, T. A., & Evans, J. H. (1982). Sexual reactivation of chronically ill and disabled adults. *Journal of Allied Health, 11,* 261-270.

Druss, R. G., O'Connor, J. F., & Stern, L. O. (1969). Psychologic response to colectomy. *Archives of General Psychiatry, 20,* 419-427.

Hellerstein, H. K., & Friedman, E. H. (1970). Sexual activity and the post coronary patient. *Archives of Internal Medicine, 125,* 987-999.

Kallomaki, J. L., Markannen, T. K., & Mustonen, V. A. (1961). Sexual behavior after cerebral vascular accident. *Fertility and Sterility, 12,* 156-158.

Kass, I. (1972). Coitus induced bronchospasm. *Medical Aspects of Human Sexuality, 7,* 48.

Kimmel, D. (1978). Adult development and aging: A gay perspective. *Journal of Social Issues, 34,* 113-130.

Kinsey, A. C., Pomeroy, W. S., & Martin, C. E. (1948). *Sexual behavior in the human male.* Philadelphia: W. B. Saunders.

Kleeman, J. A. (1971). The establishment of core gender identity in normal girls. *Archives of Sexual Behavior, 1,* 103-116.

Knorr, D., & Bildingmaier, F. (1975). Gynecomastia in male adolescents. *Clinics in Endocrinology and Metabolism, 4,* 157-171.

Meltzer, H. Y., & Fang, V. S. (1976). The effect of neuroleptics on serum prolactin in schizophrenic patients. *Archives of General Psychiatry, 33,* 279-286.

Morris, D. (1972). *Intimate behavior.* New York: Random House.

Raphael, S., & Robinson, M. (1980). The older lesbian: Love relationships and friendship patterns. *Alternative Lifestyles, 3,* 207-229.

Robinson, M. (1979). The older lesbian. Master's thesis, California State University, Dominquez Hills, Carson, California.

Scott, F. B., Bradley, W. E., & Timm, G. W. (1973). Management of erectile impotence: Use of implantible penile prosthesis. *Urology, 2,* 80-82.

Schain, W. (1980). Sexual functioning, self-esteem and cancer care. *Frontiers of Radiation Therapy and Oncology, 14,* 12-19.

Small, M. P. (1978). The Small-carrion penile prosthesis. *Urology Clinics of North America, 5,* 549-562.

Story, N. L. (1974). Sexual dysfunction resulting from drug side effects. *Journal of Sexual Research, 10,* 132-149.

Strauss, A. (1976). *Chronic illness and the quality of life.* St. Louis: C. V. Mosby.

Swinburn, W. R. (1976). Sexual counseling for the arthritis. *Clinics on Rheumatic Diseases, 62,* 122-123.

Ueno, O. (1963). The so-called coition death. *Japan Journal of Legal Medicine, 17,* 333-340.

Woods, N. E. (1975). Influences on sexual adaptation to mastectomy. *Journal of Obstetric and Gynecological Nursing, 4,* 33-37.

PART III

Impact of the Health Professional

CHAPTER 15

Change Agent

Elizabeth Dixon

Introduction

Although coping with change is part of everyday living, the process of change has been studied and applied mainly to groups and institutions. Nursing literature tends to focus on the nurse's role as *change agent,* working within the health care system to bring about planned change in work environments, health organizations, and at the community level (Brooten, Hayman, & Naylor, 1988; Leddy & Pepper, 1989; Sullivan & Decker, 1988). Change tactics relating to individuals and families have dealt primarily with various psychotherapeutic and social approaches (Kanfer & Goldstein, 1980; Lippitt, 1976). There is some nursing literature, however, describing the use of change strategies as a clinical tool, and some that propose utilizing the nursing process framework to bring about planned change when interacting with individuals (Koizer & Erb, 1988; Sullivan & Decker, 1988).

Change can be viewed as an ongoing, dynamic process that involves specific strategies, not unlike the problem-solving and nursing processes. A number of change theories, mostly from leadership and management specialists, have been developed and studied to explain the process and strategies for change (Chin & Benne, 1976; Hersey & Blanchard, 1988; Lippitt, 1973).

It is assumed that effective change strategies can be learned, allowing the professional to gain the knowledge and apply the skills to promote and sustain new perceptions, attitudes, and behaviors in clients.

The purpose of this chapter is to explore imposed or chosen change through the use of change theory as a framework for understanding and assisting chronically ill clients and their families and support networks. The issue of change in the health care system, needed to further the interests of the chronically ill client population, is addressed in other texts, some of which are cited in the references.

The Change Process

Lippitt (1973) defined change as "any planned or unplanned alteration in the status quo in an organism, situation, or process." Hersey and Blanchard (1988) discussed four levels of change in people: knowledge changes, attitudinal changes, behavior changes, and group or organizational performance changes. They proposed that knowledge changes are the easiest to make, followed by attitudinal changes. Behavior changes are more difficult and time consuming than those of either knowledge or attitudes, and group or organizational performance changes are the most difficult of all. New and Couillard

(1981) agree that permanent change requires altering the attitudes and behaviors of individuals, and they go on to say that such attempts can encounter difficulty because individuals often resist change and express resistance with counterproductive behaviors such as apathy or hostility.

Change can be categorized into two broad categories: *unplanned* and *planned.* In unplanned change the change process is undirected and results are random and unpredictable. A phenomena of unplanned change is referred to as *drift,* where change is so imperceptible it is recognized only after it occurs (Reinkemeyer, 1970). Drift consists of a series of small changes in a situation that go unnoticed but have a cumulative effect that can be great and is sometimes perceived as a sudden event. For example, the chronically ill client's personal health care or eating habits may gradually deteriorate because of a lack of energy or resources and may go unrecognized until the individual becomes grossly unkempt or malnourished.

Planned change, by contrast, involves problem-solving and decision-making skills as well as interpersonal competence (Welch, 1979). It is a deliberate and conscious process that calls for planning and a purposeful attempt to effect change. Theories of planned change have many commonalities and some differences. Five theories that can be applied to situations involving individuals and families are briefly described here. A more comprehensive understanding of these theories can be obtained by reading primary references.

Force-Field Theory Kurt Lewin (1951) described three aspects of change (unfreezing, moving, and refreezing) using a systems model framework. Schein (1969) later elaborated on Lewin's work and described the physiological mechanisms for each of these aspects. During the first, *unfreezing,* people's beliefs and perceptions are shaken about a particular situation or about themselves or others in the situation. Individuals become aware of a problem and begin to see the need for different behaviors or changes to solve the problem or to cope with the situation. Once open to new ways of viewing the

situation and amenable to change, the individual is ready for the next phase.

During the *moving* phase behavioral changes actually occur as different perceptions, views, actions, values, and standards are "tried out" as part of the process of redefining the situation. During this phase, the individual begins to integrate new ways of behaving in problematic situations.

Two mechanisms, *identification* and *internalization,* that might provide individuals with new patterns of behavior during the moving phase, were described by Kelman (1958). Identification is when individuals learn and try to emulate new behavior patterns by identifying with one or more role models. Internalization is when individuals learn new behavior patterns because they are in situations in which different behaviors are required for them to be successful.

The third phase, *refreezing,* occurs when the new behaviors are integrated into the person's personality and social structures. It is important for an individual engaged in the change process to be in an environment that continually reinforces the desired change. Refreezing may be short-lived when the environment does not reinforce the new behavior patterns or is hostile toward them (Hersey & Duldt, 1989).

In force-field theory, behavior is seen as a balance of "driving" forces and "restraining" forces in opposition to each other (see Figure 15–1). Driving forces work for change, whereas restraining forces work against it. The change agent must analyze the two opposing forces and create an imbalance in favor of change by increasing driving forces, decreasing restraining forces, or doing both.

Behaviorist View Behaviorists believe that various kinds of reinforcement can be used to change behavior. Simply put, they believe human responses can be reinforced by *positive* rewards and extinguished by either *negative* punishment or an absence of reward.

Operant conditioning is based on the assumption that behavior that is followed by favorable consequences is apt to be repeated in the future when the same conditions occur. There are two kinds of reinforcement schedules that

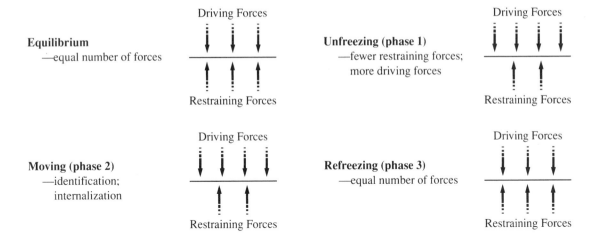

Example: Client is a 42-year-old female with multiple sclerosis. The change is whether the client will use "artificial means" for ambulation in public or continue to stay at home.

Driving forces (forces for change)

- Case manager is a home health care nurse who has change agent skills.
- Client and husband seem to have a strong relationship.
- Husband encourages client to use a walker to ambulate in the home.
- Client seems receptive to the health care system; has an appointment to meet with a physical therapist.
- Client is beginning to admit that some changes need to be made in her life-style.
- Client and husband are strongly motivated to get client out of the home and shopping again.

Restraining changes (forces against change)

- Family's lack of information about multiple sclerosis and its prognosis.
- Family's use of denial as a defense mechanism.
- Family's reluctance to use "artificial means" for ambulation.
- Client's possible low level of self-esteem.

In this example, the driving forces outweigh the restraining forces and equilibrium is disturbed. The client has entered the first phase of change—the unfreezing phase.

FIGURE 15-1. Lewin's Force-Field Model of Change

can be used with operant conditioning. With *continuous reinforcement,* individuals learn new behaviors quickly, but if the reinforcement is removed, extinction can also take place fairly soon (Hersey & Blanchard, 1988). With *intermittent reinforcement,* learning takes longer, but extinction is slower because the individual has performed the new behaviors without consistent reinforcement (Hersey & Blanchard, 1988).

Contingency contracting is an example of conditioning where rewards are contingent on the performance of desired behaviors (Steckel,

1982). A contract is developed between the client and the change agent. In the contract, behavior supporting the client's goals is reinforced; behavior opposing client goals is ignored, and whenever possible negative behavior is eliminated or changed. Important conditions of the contracting process are that power between professional and client is shared and that the client participates in identifying the means, goals, and rewards in the contract.

Aversion therapy is an example of "negative" reinforcement. It assumes that undesirable behavior can be terminated if it is accompanied or followed by sufficient noxious stimuli. Various controlled studies have used electrical shocks as aversion techniques to treat compulsive conditions, such as alcoholism, cigarette smoking, and overeating. Because of the ethical problems involved, behaviorists have expressed concern with the use of aversive techniques and have established guidelines for their appropriate use for treatment purposes (Kanfer & Goldstein, 1980).

Chin and Benne: Strategies for Change
Three general strategic categories for managing change were devised by Chin and Benne (1976). These are *power-coercive, empirical-rational,* and *normative-reeducative strategies.* The power-coercive strategy is based on the use of power or some sort of force to effect change and is useful when there is much resistance or when immediate change is critical. It frequently includes authority, political, or economic sanctions. An example of power-coercive change is legislated access to public buildings for people confined to wheelchairs, associated with a fine for noncompliance. However, results obtained with power-coercive strategies do not always last when the power to enforce the changes is removed. Guilt or shame techniques are another form of coercive strategies that health professionals have used in attempts to alter behaviors. Unfortunately, these techniques do not always produce the desired effect. The author knows one woman who stopped going to her physician because she was tired of being "insulted" about her smoking each time she saw her doctor.

The empirical-rational strategy uses knowledge as the basis for change. The change agent operates on the assumption that people are rational and make choices that promote their best interests when informed that choices are available. This strategy seems to be most effective when the client's values and beliefs do not conflict with the change. For instance, a client who values cleanliness might respond well to a comprehensive teaching plan to learn how to care effectively for her colostomy. Researchers have reported, however, that having more knowledge does not necessarily lead to changed behavior (Mazzuca, 1982).

The normative-reeducative strategy is based on the assumption that people's actions are guided by sociocultural norms and underlying values and perceptions. The psychosocial implications of the proposed change, as well as the client's level of knowledge, are attended to. Throughout the change process, clients are actively involved in defining their problems and developing solutions. An integral part of the problem-solving process is examining beliefs and assumptions that direct clients' behaviors. Skill in interpersonal relationships is an important attribute for the professional who uses this method. The change agent collaborates with the client and others involved in the change. Exploring what a disabling illness means to a client and family, and then collaborating on a plan of care that fits their personal assumptions and feelings is a normative-reeducative example. Using the previous example of the colostomy client, the nurse would first explore what having a colostomy means to the client before devising a plan with her about the best way to manage her colostomy. Contingency contracting, mentioned earlier, is another example of a normative-reeducative strategy, although the focus in contingency contracting is more on behavior and environment and less on feelings and beliefs.

Spradley's Model for Planned Change Spradley, a nurse theorist, developed a model to guide the change process (1980). She bases her model on general systems theory, which explains how a whole (system) is broken into parts and how those parts work together. Spradley advocates four principles that govern the course of change within any system: interdependence of the parts of the system, homeostasis, opposing forces, and resistance. *System interdependence* means that when one part of a system changes, all other parts of the system are affected and have to change. Thus, a chronic illness does not affect just one part of a person's life, but changes every important aspect of it. When one looks at a chronically ill person's family as a system, not only the ill person is affected; all members of the family are impacted in important ways.

Body regulatory mechanisms keep physiological and psychological functioning steady, thereby maintaining a special balance, called equilibrium or *homeostasis*. When internal or external change upsets the balance, forces within the system work to restore homeostasis (Spradley, 1980). For example, when diabetic patients are introduced to a new method of giving themselves insulin, they will be in psychological disequilibrium until homeostasis brings about a new equilibrium that incorporates the new health care practice (Spradley, 1980).

Spradley borrows the concept of driving and restraining forces from Lewin's force-field theory to describe her third principle, *opposing forces*. When driving and restraining forces are equal in strength, equilibrium exists. When opposing forces become unbalanced, if the driving forces are stronger than the restraining forces, change is brought about.

Her last principle is *resistance*. Any change, whether planned or unplanned, produces resistance. When change is being planned, strategies to deal with resistance have to be included. Thus, any major change in an ill person's life-style will produce resistance, and health professionals have to be prepared to deal with it.

Seven Steps to Planned Change   Sullivan and Decker (1988) proposed a model for managing planned change that follows the nursing process. Although this model was devised for nurse managers, it can be used as a clinical tool to assist clients. This model will be developed further in the intervention section to demonstrate its applicability to clinical practice. The seven sequential steps of the model are listed in Table 15-1.

Assessment   According to these authors, change is often planned to close a discrepancy between the desired and the actual state of affairs. A careful assessment of the discrepancy is consequently required. In this model assessment is subdivided into a three-step process. First, both opportunities and problems need to be identified and clearly defined. Second, data external and internal to the system need to be collected to recognize all driving and restraining forces. Third, analysis is done to identify resistance, potential solutions and strategies, and areas of consensus, and to help in determining which option is best.

TABLE 15-1.   Seven steps of planned change: An extension of the nursing process

Nursing Process	Change Process
Assessment	1. Identify the problem or opportunity
	2. Collect data
	3. Analyze data
Planning	4. Plan the change strategies (unfreezing)
Implementation	5. Implement the change (moving)
Evaluation	6. Evaluate effectiveness
	7. Stabilize the change (refreezing)

Added to the table by this author are the terms *unfreezing, moving,* and *refreezing*.

SOURCE: Adapted from *Effective Management in Nursing,* Third Edition, by E. Sullivan and P. Decker. Copyright © 1992 by Addison-Wesley Nursing. Used with permission.

Planning   The planning stage involves determining the who, how, and when of the needed change. Active participation of individuals involved in the change serves to decrease any resistance that can occur later. Lewin's stage of unfreezing fits here. Attitudes, habits, and ways of thinking have to soften, and boundaries must melt before changes can begin.

Implementation   When the plan is put into motion, implementation begins. This stage correlates with Lewin's moving stage. Change strategies, such as information giving, problem solving, training, collaboration, and counseling are utilized in the implementation stage. Empathy and therapeutic communication are necessary skills for the professional along with change tactics such as providing support, giving feedback, and overcoming resistance.

Evaluating and Stabilizing   The final stage of this model includes evaluating and stabilizing the change. The change agent decides if presumed benefits were achieved and determines the extent of success or failure. Once the desired change is in place, it is necessary to refreeze the situation to maintain the change. The change agent then terminates the helping relationship by delegating responsibilities for the change to members of the client's system.

Issues Relating to Change

To be effective change agents, health professionals need to be aware of the various issues and problems that can impact this role. Although there are a number of issues that relate to the process of change, only a few major ones are discussed in this section.

Resistance to Change

Resistance is perhaps one of the most important problems related to achieving change. Resistance to change can be defined as "any conduct that serves to maintain the status quo in the face of pressure to alter the status quo" (Zaltman & Duncan, 1977). People resist change because they strive to maintain consistency and predictability in their lives; the professional as change agent must be sensitive to resistance, which can be based on real or imagined consequences (Klein, 1969). Although there are many reasons individuals may resist change, New and Couillard (1981) have described five important ones. They are threatened self-interest, inaccurate perceptions, objective disagreement, psychological reactance, and low tolerance for change.

Threatened Self-Interest   When the personal costs of change outweigh personal benefits, self-interest is threatened and individuals are reluctant to change their behavior. For example, advice to change dietary habits may go unheeded if the perceived benefit of lowering cholesterol level is not as important to the client as the cost of special preparation or eliminating favorite foods. When the client's self-interests are threatened, the change agent needs to emphasize all the benefits of the change and attempt to lower or eliminate the costs.

Inaccurate Perceptions   Individuals whose perceptions are inaccurate about the nature or implications of a change may erroneously believe that the change will not make a difference or will

not be beneficial. At times, health professionals have encountered clients with incomplete or inaccurate information about their illnesses. A client who avoids certain physical activities because of the mistaken belief that such activities might intensify his or her health problem is an example of an inaccurate perception. Thus, the change agent needs to assess the client's perceptions about his illness and the pending changes, and then tactfully correct any incomplete or inaccurate information.

Objective Disagreement   A client may have accurate information that differs from the change agent's information. This difference can result in objective disagreement. When the client's judgment is based on personal experience or is more accurate than the change agent's, the client's resistance should result in reconsideration of the planned change. For instance, clients with chronic immobility problems often know alternate methods of transferring that work better for them than accepted procedures. When the change agent realizes this, the client's preferred method should be used, and no change is needed. Sometimes, however, change agents ignore objective disagreement and will not reconsider changes. All objections concerning the change should be carefully considered.

Psychological Reactance   *Psychological reactance* is a term that describes a psychological reaction to engage in behaviors that have been eliminated (Brehm, 1972). The client perceives these behaviors as now very important and desirable and tries to reestablish them. Psychological reactance explains why clients, even when they know an activity such as wearing a hearing aid will enhance their well-being, may refuse to engage in the activity although they cannot offer objective reasons for doing so. This is a difficult type of resistance to overcome, since the client does not respond well to rational explanations. Encouraging the client to engage in the change activity as often as possible may eventually wear down psychological reactance.

Low Tolerance for Change   Some individuals, because of fear of risk, low self-confidence, or little tolerance for uncertainty, may have more problems dealing with the process of change than others. Individuals with low tolerance for change may cognitively understand the need for change, but still not be able to make the emotional transition. Most professionals have met clients who thoroughly understand a technical procedure, such as giving an injection, but cannot bring themselves emotionally to actually perform it. The change agent's role becomes one of offering support and trying to improve the client's self-confidence to the point that the client can at least attempt the change behaviors. Hopefully, if the behaviors are successful, the client will continue with the change.

Alienation   Although not listed by New and Couillard, alienation (Klein, 1969) is another important reason for resistance to change. When there is a distance between the professional's theoretical knowledge and the client's experiential knowledge, the client can feel alienated from the professional. Conflicts may arise because professional and client view problems differently or because they cannot make themselves understood by one another.

Cultural and societal differences also exemplify a kind of alienation. In most health care settings, the majority of health workers are Caucasian middle- or upper-class professionals. When clients come from different socioeconomic levels or cultures, there can be very different opinions about how to manage change. What may be perceived as a very simple change by the professional may be viewed as difficult or impossible by someone who does not have the money, resources, or understanding to implement the change, or whose cultural beliefs do not fit with the proposed change. It is important that the change agent understand what the change means to the client in terms of cost and resources, and how the change fits into the client's culture and belief system. .

Ethical Implications

There are ethical implications for the professional involved in the change process, since change leads to some modification of a person's life (see Chapter 19, on nursing ethics). According to Bailey (1990), ". . . modification is

the *goal* of planned change. The professional must guard against using knowledge of the change process either to manipulate the client or to deprive the client of the right to make independent decisions."

Power   Power is a factor that must be considered during the change process. One could question whether others have the right to intervene in client choices, even when the client lacks adequate information to make valid decisions. The professional who has education and experience can broaden a client's decision-making base. Given that, it is irresponsible professional behavior to allow clients to make decisions if they are ignorant of the consequences or risks involved. The professional's responsibility goes beyond just eliminating the client's ignorance. The legitimate goal of change is a mixture of eliminating ignorance and encouraging compliance. Attempts should be made to remove all possible barriers to following sound health advice, and all tactics available to support medically recommended changes should be offered to the client. But in the end, the client has the choice to change, and this choice needs to be honored by the professional, no matter how difficult that may seem (Bailey, 1990).

Providing Information   How much information should be provided is another ethical issue, especially in today's health care setting where time spent with clients is at a premium. If too little information is given, client actions will be based on ignorance. If too much information is dispensed, a person may be overwhelmed and unable to make choices. The question arises as to the amount of information underlying the professional's decisions that should be provided. Another problem is how the professional will find the necessary time to give all available information (Bailey, 1990).

Not only is the amount of information provided important, but the individual situation must be considered. Some clients want detailed information; others cannot accept all aspects of the problem, especially in the beginning. For example, the mother of a child with newly diagnosed diabetes may be so focused on learning how to care for her child that she cannot digest information about long-term outcomes. It often requires some trial and error effort by the professional to determines the extent of information necessary to maintain the client's motivation, right to know, and sense of competency (Bailey, 1990). When time is of the essence or when the professional is not sure the client has absorbed verbal communication, written information at the level of the client's reading ability should be used to reinforce teaching and foster better client understanding (Dixon & Park, 1990).

Client Vulnerability   Some clients, especially children, the frail elderly, or debilitated adults, must depend on others to make choices. Decisions made by others, such as family members, can be based on values or beliefs that differ from those of the professional. When such differences arise, ethical conflicts can occur between the decision maker and the professional. In addition, when decisions are not in the client's best interests or do not reflect the individual's dignity, power-coercive change is in order. It may be necessary to institute legal sanctions to protect the client's status when the decision maker refuses to implement health promotion choices beneficial to the client (Bailey, 1990).

The Clinical Model of Health

Change agents need to be aware of the clinical model of health, a paradigm for health and illness. In this model, persons are perceived as physiologic systems with related functions, and the absence of disease signs and symptoms is identified as health (Koizer, Erb, & Blais, 1992). According to the clinical model, the purpose of medicine is to eradicate signs and symptoms, relieve pain and physical discomfort, and restore all body parts to "normal" physiologic functioning. Emphasis is on the diagnosis of acute disease and illness and the treatment of abnormal physiologic functioning. In contemporary medical practice, treatment is centered around technology and pharmacology; science and technological advances are seen as the answers to changing health concerns and problems.

A study done in England about disabled people's quality of life reported that doctors thought living with a disability was "terrible" (Piastro,

1993). Laypersons frequently have similar views of health and illness. Colantonio (1988) investigated the concept of health in 100 adult men and women who were asked, "What does being healthy mean to you?" More than one-third of the sample responded that being fit, that is, being able to care for oneself or to work, was being healthy. When individuals define health as both "normal" physiological functioning and an absence of any sign of illness or disease, change agents must recognize that permanent physical changes that invariably accompany chronic illness and disability will rock the belief system many clients have about health, illness, and health care services. Indeed in the clinical model paradigm, the term "chronic illness" denotes an absence of health and normalcy.

Erosion of Support Systems

Traditions and customs that govern shared pleasure and work can be the cement that holds families and loved ones together (Bailey, 1990). Well-established family traditions may be shaken by an individual's inability to manage customary activities. The couple who enjoyed bowling and skiing together has to adapt to less strenuous activities if one of them develops emphysema. Role definitions are also shaken. The husband who has always taken care of the family's finances, but now has myasthenia gravis, finds his roles as wage earner, husband, and father changed, since he can no longer work and needs increasing help with personal care. The wife's roles also change as she assumes total responsibility for managing the family's finances as well as caring for her husband. Even the children's roles change as they assume more family chores and help with their father's personal care. As the family seeks to adjust to different roles and tasks, all family members need to be included in the change process (see Chapter 4, on illness roles).

The day-to-day demands of managing chronic illness ultimately fall on the person(s) most responsible for caring for the ill individual (see Chapter 12, on family caregivers). Frequently caregiving is reported as a stress, commonly described as a burden or strain (Sayles-Cross, 1993). Identified costs to the caregiver include effects on personal/social life and physical and emotional health, financial strain, and changed perceptions about the care receiver and the value of caregiving (Sayles-Cross, 1993). Caregivers also report feelings of disgust or anger and a sense of social distance from the care receiver. When caretaking demands become overwhelming, the nurturing that the chronically ill client receives is threatened. An extreme example of this phenomenon is caretaker burnout (Bailey, 1990). It almost goes without saying that change agents have to be acutely aware of caregivers' needs, so that the change process can be used with them as much as with the chronically ill client.

Social Values

Many social institutions that once ensured care for chronically ill clients in the home have been disrupted. In the past the extended family, the wife who stayed home, the close-knit neighborhood, and church groups were all accessible for care of the chronically ill and provided encouragement as well as respite for caregivers. In today's society these supports are less available and have not been adequately replaced (Bailey, 1990). In the process of problem solving about changes affecting the chronically ill or disabled individual, there may be fewer social options than formerly available.

In general, American society reflects passive resistance to the chronically ill or disabled person through indifference rather than open hostility (Bailey, 1990). Such resistance may reflect ignorance or fear. Being in the presence of ill or disabled persons can make a well person feel vulnerable, impacting adversely on the denial about one's own susceptibility to illness (Bailey, 1990).

Reflecting societal indifference are the inadequate facilities provided the chronically ill or disabled. These range from architectural barriers through insufficient respite care centers to inadequate funding for the handicapped. Society seems to place other priorities over the needs of the chronically ill and disabled, since they represent only a small percentage of its members (Bailey, 1990). This area demands intervention by health professionals. Aligning oneself with organizations already interested in causes for the handicapped, organizing a consciousness-raising campaign, or lobbying for change on the community level can have an impact on society's indifference (see Chapter 23, on social policy).

Interventions Based on Change Theory

Nurses often have to assume the role of change agent when working with clients. The change agent has been described as a "facilitator/logician who identifies the support needed to propel a change and then provides the support" (Bailey, 1983). One can also view a change agent as "any individual or group operating to change the status quo in a system such that the individual or individuals involved must relearn how to perform their role(s)" (Zaltman & Duncan, 1977). Whenever possible, change agents work to maintain clients' sense of control and consistency while altering unacceptable or unpleasant aspects of the change (Bailey, 1990).

Seven Steps to Planned Change

A nursing model that combines various aspects of change theory is Sullivan and Decker's (1988) seven steps to planned change. These steps follow the problem-solving sequence used in the nursing process combined with aspects of Lewin's force-field theory. Strategies that can be utilized with the model are taken from behaviorist theory, Chin and Benne's strategies for change, and Spradley's systems model. In the discussion that follows, the term *client* refers to the individual and the individual's family and support system unless otherwise noted.

Assessment   "Assessment is part of each activity the nurse does for and with the patient" (Atkinson & Murray, 1986). In the acute care setting, where chronically ill clients usually stay for short periods of time and are discharged before attaining a high level of wellness, it is not always possible for health professionals to thoroughly assess and plan ahead for change, especially long-range change. For nurses who provide home health care or rehabilitation or long-term care, or who work in public health, involvement with the chronically ill is over a longer period of time. In these settings, thorough assessment and long-range planning and goal setting for change become an intregal part of nursing practice.

Clinical nurses frequently find themselves busy with very obvious problems and changes. But it should be remembered that an integral part of nursing practice is health promotion and preventive health care. Health promotion has been defined as health services and actions of health care providers to prevent health problems (Koizer, Erb, & Blais, 1992). Health professionals working with chronically ill clients must assess not only for obvious major problems but also for changes that prevent future problems and promote a healthful life-style.

Assessment is an important first step in the nursing process. Koizer, Erb, and Blais (1992) say that "assessing is a continuous process carried out during all phases of the nursing process." Even though assessment initiates the nursing process, it is important to remember that the process is cyclical, not linear, and that all steps are interrelated.

Assessment: Identify the Problem or Opportunity In the Sullivan and Decker model, assessment is divided into three phases. During early assessment, the nurse change agent is in a good position to notice slight differences in client behavior or in the client's environment that can be disturbing, before larger or more disruptive changes occur. It is important to reiterate that changes are not always negative nor do they always mean problems for the client. Many changes are positive and can offer opportunities for personal growth and development, especially if viewed as such and managed in a constructive manner.

In addition to carefully and realistically observing both client and environment, interviewing the client and others close to him or her may yield additional information that the nurse cannot observe. Joint interviews that include the family provide the opportunity to observe family interaction and gather more information. Sullivan and Decker (1988) recommend clearly ascertaining if the situation creates a problem or opportunity by asking questions of the client such as these:

• What is now happening in the client's life that is or could be a problem? What does the client see as opportunities?
• What has become different about the client's situation this last week, this last month, in the last year?
• What could the client do differently or better? What stops her or him from changing?
• Does the client feel a change is required or beneficial? If so, what kind of change and how much change?

Creative insight is another means of identifying problems or opportunities. Creative insight involves fresh ways of looking at old problems or behaviors and doing so from different perspectives. Brainstorming—coming up with all possible ideas or solutions no matter how unusual or "far out"—is one way to restructure thinking so that ideas can be combined in unique ways. Creative thinking, when used with clients, helps them look at the situation differently. There are exercises to stimulate creative thinking, and the professional might be well advised to read them and use them with clients (Covey, 1989; Hickman & Silva, 1984; von Oech, 1983).

Assessment: Collect Data The second step of the model is very important for ultimate success. Information about the problem or opportunity, clearly identified in the first step, now needs to be collected. Data can be collected in a variety of ways. Interviewing the client and asking specifically how he or she feels about the change or perceives the situation can reveal information that might not be ordinarily divulged. Careful observation of the situation, resources, or environment can reveal additional information such as assessing a wheelchair-bound client's home for wheelchair accessibility. Quantitative data, such as the number of times an event happened or the time and energy involved, should be accumulated. Other professionals more familiar with certain facets of the change may need to be consulted.

CASE STUDY
An MS Patient—The Case for Mobility

Janet Johnson is a 42-year-old woman, married with no children. She has had diagnosed multiple sclerosis (MS) for four years. Since diagnosis, she has had only two serious exacerbations. Her last exacerbation was six weeks ago and required hospitalization for three weeks. During that time, she experienced some dimness of vision, periodic shaky tremors in her hands, and muscular weakness, most pronounced in her right leg. Her walking gait became stumbling and weaving, especially when she was tired. Her primary nurse made a referral to the hospital's home health care department and wrote on the referral that she seemed to have limited understanding of the disease process, that she was hesitant to use her walker and tried to walk unaided, and that she and her husband seemed to use denial to cope with her symptoms and disability.

During her first home visit, the home health care nurse, Ms. Trevor, introduces herself and begins to establish rapport. She begins the assessment by identifying what might be the problems and potential opportunities for change. She elicits date about what recent symptoms mean to Mrs. Johnson and how her latest hospitalization has affected her and her family. She asks questions such as, "Tell me how your health has changed

in the last year and particularly the last few months?" "Do you anticipate anything different that might be needed as a result of these changes, and if so, what might it be?"

Mrs. Johnson acknowledges that her walking has gotten "worse," and she is concerned about her inability to walk very far. She admits the walker lets her ambulate around her home better, but she says she tries not to use it. She also admits it isn't helpful when she has to walk distances because she tires, even with the walker for assistance. She comments that its lucky she is "just" a housewife so she doesn't have to get out, and acknowledges that for the four months prior to hospitalization she wasn't able to leave her home to do any shopping, an activity she and her husband used to do together. He now does it alone, and neither of them likes this arrangement.

Together they identify that Mrs. Johnson's current major concern (identified problem) is her inability to leave her home and help with the shopping because she cannot ambulate any distance with or without a walker. The nurse then asks questions like, "How do you feel about making changes that are necessary to be more mobile? How did you feel when you first began using your walker?" Do you have any ideas about ways you

Data collected should answer such questions as

- How does the client feel about making a change? For example, is the client timid, fearful, anxious, excited, relieved, resigned?
- What ideas, perceptions, beliefs, and attitudes about the change does the client have? Is there any disagreement based on good information or experience?
- What are some of the benefits if this change happens? What are the costs in terms of self-esteem, time, money, or other resources?
- What are the driving forces that push or support the change and the restraining forces that hold it back or impede it?

Assessment: Analyze Data Analysis is the last part of the assessment phase. The amounts, kinds, and sources of data collected are im-

portant, but ultimately are of no value unless analyzed (Sullivan & Decker, 1988).

Concepts and themes from the collected data need to be brought together to make a logical, realistic, and convincing picture of the change necessary to solve the client's identified problem or to implement an opportunity for the client. Possible areas of resistance, motivators, and areas of agreement need to be carefully studied. All parts necessary to develop a coherent plan need to be examined, especially in relation to each other. When analyzing data, one must remember Spradley's (1980) principles for change, since a change in one part of a system affects all other parts of that system, influencing the homeostatic forces within the system that maintain or restore equilibrium.

The case study of the multiple sclerosis client demonstrates how the three steps of could get around better so you could go shopping with your husband?"

Mrs. Johnson shares how difficult it was to get used to the walker because she felt clumsy using it. She says that her husband didn't like the idea of a walker, but now encourages her to use it more to get out of the house. When asked why she doesn't like the idea of a walker, Mrs. Johnson says, "My husband doesn't want me to get too dependent on artificial things. We both know I'll be able to walk all right when my illness goes into remission again, and we want to keep my strength up so my muscles are not too weak to walk on my own."

Mrs. Johnson also tells the nurse she is going to physical therapy (PT) next week to "strengthen my muscles." Ms. Trevor obtains permission to call the doctor and physical therapist to talk about her condition. At this point, Mrs. Johnson says she isn't considering the use of a wheelchair because she would feel self-conscious and conspicuous in it, and her husband would not approve. At the end of the visit, Ms. Trevor arranges to return the following week to do some teaching about MS. As the interview ends, Mrs. Johnson acknowledges that both she and her husband thought that if doctor's orders were followed conscientiously, "the disease would go away."

In analyzing the collected data, Ms. Trevor looks for patterns so she can begin to develop a realistic plan for change with the Johnsons. She needs more data to find out what Mr. and Mrs. Johnson have been told about her disease, her future prognosis, and what might be the best mode of ambulation so she can go shopping. She plans on calling the doctor and physical therapist to gain this information. Although she agrees with the primary nurse that Mrs. Johnson needs more information about MS, she decides that Mr. Johnson has to be included in any future teaching. Ms. Trevor also agrees that husband and wife had been using denial during the long period of remission, but it is not working for them now.

Driving forces for change are (1) Mrs. Johnson's receptivity to Ms. Trevor, her doctor's advice, and using physical therapy; (2) her beginning acknowledgment that some changes need to be made in her life-style; (3) her strong relationship with her husband, who is very supportive of her independence; (4) her husband's current encouragement to use the walker to get out; and (5) her strong motivation to be as active as her disease will allow. Restraining forces against change are (1) the Johnsons' lack of information about MS; (2) their current but now ineffective use of denial as a defense mechanism; (3) their initial reluctance to use "artificial means" for ambulation; (4) and Mrs. Johnson's possible low level of self-esteem evidenced by several self-derogatory comments.

---

assessment apply. By identifying the problem and opportunity for expanding her world, collecting data on the client and factors that need consideration, and analyzing this data, a realistic picture emerges of the change necessary to solve the client's identified problem.

Plan the Change Strategy As noted, planning correlates with the unfreezing stage in Lewin's theory, since the client has acknowledged the need for change. The change agent identifies strategies that will be used to support the desired change to strengthen driving forces, decrease restraining forces, and modify resistance. The strategy or strategies that are selected should consider the client's beliefs and attitudes since beliefs and attitudes are more difficult to change than the client's knowledge level. If there are strong values, feelings, or beliefs about the change, normative-reeducative strategies are needed (Chin & Benne, 1976) to soften them before the change can be implemented.

In some cases, unfreezing may necessitate the breaking down of traditions, customs, or old ways of doing things so that the client is more ready to accept new alternatives (Hersey & Blanchard, 1988). This requires the change agent to develop an understanding of the client's traditions, as well as a trusting relationship with the client, before attempting to introduce new alternatives. Placing the client in a situation in which new behaviors are demanded may eventually change attitudes and values through the process of cognitive dissonance. Cognitive dissonance means the behavior is changed first and then, to avoid internal tension and psychological conflict, the individual modifies attitudes to correspond with the behavior (Hersey & Blanchard, 1988).

Whenever possible, the client needs to be an active participant and collaborator with the

CASE STUDY

The Overweight Client with a Cardiac Problem

Bertha Zoe is a 65-year-old individual who has been at least 50 pounds overweight much of her adult life. A month ago she had a mild heart attack, and her physician referred her to an independent nurse practitioner. After assessing the problem, gaining information about the client and her environment, and analyzing this information, the client and nurse practitioner mutually decide that a contingency contract would be an effective plan to help Mrs. Zoe lose weight. Both decide on the conditions for the contract. Mrs. Zoe agrees to visit a dietitian in the clinic and modify her diet according to the dietitian's recommendations, adhere to a daily exercise program that includes water aerobics, attend a weekly weight-control group, and use positive affirmations to increase her self-esteem. The nurse contracts to initially meet with Mrs. Zoe every two weeks for consultation and support, and both sign the contract.

The contract specifies that each time Mrs. Zoe loses 10 pounds, she is to reward herself. For the first 10 pounds she selects as a reward attending a concert, for the next 10 pounds she will purchase a new dress, and so on. Her long-term goal is to lose 50 pounds over a period of 10 months. Mrs. Zoe has never used the contract method to lose weight before, but feels it will keep her "on track" and help her reach her goals of weight loss and physical fitness.

---

change agent in formulating and deciding on the overall plan for change. If the client is too young, too frail, or incapacitated, the change agent will need to interact with the family or legal guardian. Realistic goals, as well as specific steps and actions that need to be taken by the client, should be included in the plan for change. Time limits for completion of activities and feedback mechanisms that can be used to evaluate the change process and the success of the change should also be addressed during this step.

A contingency contract can be a powerful strategy to reinforce the plan for change (Steckel, 1982). The case study of the overweight cardiac client demonstrates how a nurse can use a contingency contract to effect change.

In the case of Mrs. Zoe, dividing the weight loss into 10-pound decrements is a feedback mechanism for both client and nurse to determine whether the plan is working. Psychologically, setting the smaller weight loss goals is less threatening and more manageable for Mrs. Z. than waiting 10 months to be rewarded for losing all 50 pounds.

Implement the Change   Implementation corresponds to the moving stage of Lewin's theory; actions are undertaken that set in motion the actual change. During this step, the change agent's role is to create a supportive climate, obtain and provide feedback, act as an energizer, and overcome resistance (Sullivan & Decker, 1988). If the client lacks knowledge or skills, a teaching program utilizing an empirical-rational strategy (Chin & Benne, 1976) may be appropriate (also see Chapter 16, on teaching).

New and Couillard (1981a) outline eight techniques to deal with resistance to change: participation, coercion, manipulation, education, external agents, incentives, supportive behavior, and gradual introduction. All these techniques have advantages and disadvantages and may overcome resistance better in some situations than others. Since resistance is anticipated, the change agent needs to select those techniques most likely to be effective and incorporate them into the change process. *Participation* involves those affected by the change in the design and implementation of the change techniques. *Coercion* is the use of formal authority or power to implement and enforce the change. *Manipulation* requires utilizing information in a selective way so the change is viewed as more beneficial. *Education* employs information to help individuals see the need for and logic of the change. *External agents* are individuals not involved with those who are affected by the change and are brought in to introduce the

CASE STUDY
The Client on a Ventilator

John is on a ventilator secondary to respiratory failure. His condition has stabilized, and his family wants to take him home because doing so meets their needs and reduces the cost of care over maintaining him in the nursing home. Before the move becomes permanent, arrangements are made to have him go home for a trial period.

All persons involved in the change, including his wife, children, and others who will help, are taught how to care for him and the machinery. Arrangements are made for therapists, nurses, and home health aides to visit regularly, including some on a daily basis, to furnish support for the family. The family is also given phone numbers to contact the various professionals they deal with. Everyone involved has a clear understanding that

John will return to the nursing home after a specified time so the situation can be evaluated. Once necessary modifications are made, John will return home permanently.

During the first few days, a night nurse assists the family and provides John with necessary care. The therapists and nurses reinforce the family's growing competence. They also teach the family what to do in case of emergencies, how to obtain help, and answer questions that arise. Prior to John's return to the nursing home, the family has learned to provide most of John's care. Evaluation after his return to the nursing home identifies the family's need to rest at night, so arrangements are made to have an experienced person there.

---

change. Such agents can be effective if, for some reason, the initial change agent is not trusted. *Incentives* are rewards that are valued and can be effective if resistance is the result of threatened self-interest. *Supportive behavior* provides helpful activities such as counseling and considerate treatment during the change process and is effective for individuals with a low tolerance for change. Finally, *gradual introduction* involves employing a series of small changes over time to gradually reduce resistance.

Short-term trials or "pilot tests" are a technique used to test whether the change is practical and workable on a small scale. A successful pilot can help overcome client resistance. If unsuccessful, modifications can be made before there is a larger investment of time or resources. The case study of the client on a ventilator demonstrates the effectiveness of a short term trial.

Motivating the Client Emulating or modeling other people's behavior can be a motivator for initiating and carrying out behavior changes (Kanfer & Goldstein, 1980). Persons who have similar disabilities or problems are particularly effective models for the chronically ill. Support groups for specific disabilities, such as stroke

or multiple sclerosis clients or cancer survivors, offer support and motivation that persons without chronic illnesses cannot always provide.

Helping the client experience success is another effective motivator. Success is a reward that increases the client's belief in the ability to change, enhances the value of the change, and strengthens the changed behavior. To confirm success, clients need ongoing support and feedback from caregivers, significant others, and members of the health care system. Sometimes, the best support is simply to actively listen to the client. Recognition of success and praise are also easy-to-use, effective support tactics.

Evaluate Effectiveness All throughout the change process there should be some mechanism to determine if the change is proceeding as planned. The change agent needs to periodically monitor for the extent of success or failure and for unintended consequences or undesirable outcomes (Sullivan & Decker, 1988).

Throughout the process, clients need to receive appropriate feedback. Feedback consists of telling another person how one sees him or her, how his or her behavior appears, and how one feels about that behavior. Feedback also allows the person to see how behaviors affect others. It has been shown that monitoring and home management deteriorate when close supervision, including feedback, by the health team is discontinued (Nathan, 1983).

Feedback that is specific and direct is most helpful (Hersey & Duldt, 1989). If psychological reactance occurs, the professional may need to feed back the negative and undesirable aspects of the situation that occurred prior to the change, since, in retrospect, the client perceives the past before the change as very desirable.

Sometimes actions do not bring the intended results, or problems occur during the change that could not have been anticipated ahead of time. When this happens, the plan has to be modified to accommodate the client's needs and better fit the client's life-style. It may be necessary to reassess by gathering additional information, reanalyze the data, and plan other alternatives. The change agent can utilize techniques such as affirmations and positive self-talk to overcome negativism and help the client see progress that has already been made.

Stabilize the Change   The last stage requires stabilizing the change and refreezing the system. When the change is in place and is as acceptable as possible for the client, stabilization should occur. The change agent's role at this time is to help anticipate and plan for future threats to the new behaviors, to conduct a final evaluation of the change's impact, and to provide closure.

Until the new behaviors are internalized in the client's personality and become well-established habits, the change can be extinguished easily. Therefore, the change agent and the client need to work together to identify things that might hinder or reverse the change, and then jointly decide on strategies that can successfully manage these threats. Family and significant others have to be included in the stabilization process, for without their support the change will be difficult to maintain.

During closure it is important to briefly review what the client has been through during the change process and to address how the change process has impacted the client's life. If the professional relationship between client and change agent is to end, community resources or support systems that can assist in maintaining the change should be identified.

Murphy's Law

It is well for change agents to remember Murphy's law: "If anything can go wrong, it will" (Block, 1980). The author has taken the liberty of altering the corollaries to Murphy's law to accommodate change.

1. Change is never as easy as it looks.
2. Change always takes longer than you think.
3. If there is a possibility of several things going wrong, the one that could interfere with the change the most will be the one to go wrong.
4. If you perceive that there are four possible restraining forces and circumvent them, a fifth restraining force will promptly develop.
5. Left to themselves (drift), things tend to go from bad to worse.
6. Whenever you set out to change something, something else must be done first.
7. Every change solution breeds new problems for change.

Hill's unrevised commentaries on Murphy's law are also insightful (Block, 1980).

1. If we lose much by having things go wrong, take all possible care.
2. If we have nothing to lose by change, relax.
3. If we have everything to gain by change, relax.
4. If it doesn't matter, it does not matter.

Summary and Conclusions

This chapter explored change as a framework for understanding and assisting chronically ill clients and their families and support systems. Unplanned change and drift, a phenomenon in which a series of small changes goes unnoticed, was discussed briefly. By contrast, planned change, which is a deliberate and purposeful process of altering the status quo in a person or situation, was discussed at greater length.

Five models for planned change that health professionals can use to interact with clients and their families were presented and summarized. These included the three phases of Lewin's force-field theory; the reinforcement methods of the behaviorist view; the power-coercive, empirical-rational, and normative-re-educative strategies of Chin and Benne; Spradley's model for planned change; and Sullivan and Decker's model for planned change. Sullivan and Decker's model was used to show how change theory can be used as a clinical tool and applied to client situations. Each of the model's steps—identifying the problem or opportunity, collecting and analyzing data, planning and implementing the change strategies, and finally evaluating and stabilizing the change—were described with examples of specific change strategies.

Also discussed were reasons that clients resist change and the importance of minimizing such resistance. The change agent's role as facilitator of change and provider of necessary support during the change process was addressed. Professional ethics, the clinical model of health, erosion of support systems, and society's values about chronic illness and disability were presented as issues that can impact the change agent's role.

To use change as a clinical tool with chronically ill clients, the professional must have appropriate knowledge and skill about the change process. It is not enough to react to unplanned change; the change agent has to know how to manage change; how to assess for opportunities as well as problems; how to plan, reduce resistance, and evaluate outcomes; and when to make necessary modifications. There are many strategies for implementing change, and while it is not feasible to implement them all, the nurse needs to be skillful at those strategies and tactics that allow the greatest probability of success. For example, the normative-reeducative strategy is highly effective when interacting with chronically ill clients.

Change is never easy. Professionals who undertake planned change with their clients need to be realistic about the complexity of change, the power of resistance to it, and the potential for unintended side effects. Yet, when effectively applied, planned change can be a powerful tool for improving chronically ill clients' quality of life.

STUDY QUESTIONS

1. There are four kinds of change. What kind is the easiest to make?
2. How does planned change differ from unplanned change?
3. Describe the three phases of Lewin's force-field theory.
4. How does the change agent impact driving and restraining forces?
5. Define resistance to change.
6. What kinds of operant conditioning are discussed in this chapter? Differentiate them.
7. Discuss how normative-reeducative strategies are particularly useful with chronically ill clients and their families. Why are they more effective than power-coercive strategies?
8. What adverse effects do psychological reactance, objective resistance, and alienation have on change?
9. List the seven steps to planned change discussed in the Sullivan and Decker model. Describe one change strategy that can be used for each step.
10. Select a model of change to manage a client's situation from the ones mentioned in this chapter. Tell why you chose the model you did.

References

Atkinson, L. D., & Murray, M. E. (1986). *Understanding the nursing process* (3rd ed.). New York: Macmillan.

Bailey, B. J. (1983). Using change theory to help the diabetic. *The Diabetes Educator, 9*(3), 37-39, 56.

———— (1990). Change agent. In I. M. Lubkin (Ed.), *Chronic illness: Impact and interventions* (2nd ed.). Boston: Jones and Bartlett.

Block, A. (1980). *Murphy's law and other reasons why things go wrong!* Los Angeles: Price/Stern/Sloan.

Brehm, J. (1972). *Responses to loss of freedom: A theory of psychological reactance.* Morristown, NJ: General Learning Press.

Brooten, D. (1984). *Managerial leadership in nursing.* Philadelphia: J. B. Lippincott.

Brooten, D., Hayman, L., & Naylor, M. (1988). *Leadership for change: An action guide for nurses.* Philadelphia: J. B. Lippincott.

Chin, R., & Benne, K. (1976). General strategies for effecting changes in human systems. In W. Bennis, K. Benne, R. Chin, & K. Corey (Eds.), *The planning of change* (3rd ed.). New York: Holt, Rinehart & Winston.

Colantonio, A. (1988). Lay concepts of health. *Health Values, 12,* 3–7.

Decker, P., & Sullivan, E. (1992). Effective management in nursing (3rd ed.) Menlo Park, CA: Addison-Wesley.

Dixon, E., & Park, R. (1990, Nov./Dec.). Do patients understand written health information? *Nursing Outlook,* 278–282.

Hersey, P., & Blanchard, K. (1988). *Management of organizational behavior.* Englewood Cliffs, NJ: Prentice-Hall.

Hersey, P., & Duldt, B. (1989). *Situational leadership in nursing.* Norwalk, CT: Appleton & Lange.

Hickman, C., & Silva, M. (1984). *Creating excellence: Managing corporate culture, strategy and change in the new age.* New York: New American Library.

Kanfer, F., & Goldstein, A. (1980). *Helping people change.* New York: Pergamon Press.

Kelman, H. C. (1958). Compliance, identification and internalization: Three processes of attitude changes. *Conflict Resolution, 11,* 51–60.

Klein, D. (1969). Some notes on the dynamics of resistance to change: The defender role. in W. Bennis, K. Benne, R. Chin, & K. Corey (Eds.), *The planning of change* (2nd ed.). New York: Holt, Rinehart & Winston.

Koizer, B., & Erb, G. (1988). *Concepts and issues in nursing practice.* Menlo Park, CA: Addison-Wesley.

Koizer, B., Erb, G., & Blais, K. (1992). *Concepts and issues in nursing practice* (2nd ed.). Menlo Park, CA: Addison-Wesley.

Leddy, S., & Pepper, J. M. (1989). *Conceptual bases of professional nursing.* Philadelphia: J. B. Lippincott.

Lewin, K. (1951). *Field theory in social science.* New York: Harper & Brothers.

Lippitt, G. L. (1973). *Visualizing change: Model building and the change process.* La Jolla, CA: University Associates.

Lippitt, R. (1976). The process of utilization of social research to improve social practice. In W. Bennis, K. Benne, R. Chin, & K. Corey (Eds.), *The planning of change* (2nd ed.). New York: Holt, Rinehart & Winston.

Mazzuca, S. (1982). Does patient education in chronic disease have therapeutic value? *Journal of Chronic Disease, 35,* 521–529.

Nathan, D. M. (1983). The importance of intensive supervision in determining the efficacy of insulin pump therapy. *Diabetes Care, 6,* 295–297.

New, J. R., & Couillard, N. A. (1981a, March). Guidelines for introducing change. *The Journal of Nursing Administration,* 17–21.

———— (1981b). Guidelines for introducing change. In E. C. Hein & M. J. Nicholson (Eds.) *Contemporary leadership behavior: Selected readings* (2nd ed.). Boston: Little, Brown.

Piastro, D. B. (1993, June 27). Attitudes of others seem worst handicap the disabled face. *The Star Tribune,* Minneapolis, p. 4E.

Reinkemeyer, A. (1970). Nursing's need: Commitment to an ideology of change. *Nursing Forum, 9*(4), 340–350.

Sayles-Cross, S. (1993). Perceptions of familial caregivers of elder adults. *Image: The Journal of Nursing Scholarship, 25*(2), 88–92.

Schein, E. (1969). The mechanisms of change. in W. Bennis, K. Benne, R. Chin, & K. Corey, (Eds.), *The planning of change* (2nd ed.). New York: Holt, Rinehart & Winston.

Steckel, S. B. (1982). *Patient contracting.* Norwalk, CT: Appleton-Century-Crofts.

Spradley, B. (1980). Managing change creatively, *Journal of Nursing Administration, 10,* 32–37.

Sullivan, E., & Decker, P. (1988). *Effective management in nursing.* Menlo Park, CA: Addison-Wesley.

von Oech, R. (1983). *A whack on the side of the head.* New York: Warner Brothers.

Welch, L. B. (1979). Planned change in nursing: The theory. *Nursing Clinics of North America, 14*(2), 307–320.

Zaltman, G., & Duncan, R. (1977). *Strategies for planned change.* New York: John Wiley & Sons.

CHAPTER 16

Teaching

Audrey Bopp • Ilene Lubkin

Introduction

Health professionals have found that teaching is an important method of increasing knowledge and achieving behavioral changes that help clients cope with chronic diseases. However, teaching does not always guarantee attainment of long-term adaptation necessary for effective management. Even when teaching initially seems successful, problems may arise indicating that the desired integration of behavior, knowledge, and skills was not accomplished. This chapter addresses many of these problems and explores possible solutions.

Review of the Teaching-Learning Process

Teaching intended to create change in a client's adaptation to chronic illness is a planned activity individualized to the learner's abilities, needs, resources, and support systems. To achieve a positive outcome, this teaching process becomes an interaction between health educator and one or more clients. It encompasses four steps: (1) assessment, (2) planning, (3) implementation, and (4) evaluation.

Information collection in a teaching-learning *assessment* helps the teacher plan and implement teaching activities. Assessment data should include information about the learner's readiness and ability to learn, the learner's previous knowledge of the subject, what the learner wants to know about the subject, any incorrect information or misconceptions held by the learner, and educational needs of both learner and family.

Planning involves developing goals; determining when, where, and how the teaching process will occur; and developing a method of evaluation. It should be noted that successful outcomes are more likely when the learner is involved in the planning phase of the teaching process. *Implementation* is the actual process of teaching and utilizes a variety of teaching methods and tools. *Evaluation* enables the teacher to ascertain whether learning has occurred; it is basically a feedback loop determined by the method of evaluation developed during planning.

Review of Teaching-Learning Principles

Individual client education plans are based on identified teaching and learning principles (Pohl,

1981). (See Table 16-1.) These principles are not reviewed here; presumably the reader has some familiarity with them. In-depth information about the teaching-learning process, the principles of learning, and the principles of teaching is available in the teaching texts listed in the references and bibliography at the end of this chapter.

Learning Styles: Pedagogical versus Androgogical

Learning is classified as either *pedagogical* or *androgogical* on the basis of various assumptions about the characteristics of the learner.

TABLE 16-1. Teaching and learning principles

1. Perception is necessary for learning.
2. Conditioning is a process of learning.
3. Learning often occurs by trial and error.
4. Learning may occur through imitation.
5. Concept development is part of the learning process.
6. Motivation is necessary for learning.
7. Physical and mental readiness is necessary for learning.
8. Active participation is necessary for effective learning.
9. New learning must be based on previous knowledge and experience.
10. Learning is affected by the individual's emotional climate.
11. Repetition and reinforcement strengthen learning.
12. Success reinforces learning.
13. Good teacher–learner rapport is important in teaching.
14. Teaching requires effective communication.
15. Learning needs of clients must be determined.
16. Objectives serve as guides in planning and evaluating teaching.
17. Planning time is required for effective teaching and learning.
18. Control of the environment is an aspect of teaching.
19. Teaching skill can be acquired through practice and observation.
20. Evaluating effectiveness is a part of teaching.

SOURCE: Summarized from Pohl (1981).

Originally, pedagogy was defined as the art and science of teaching children, and androgogy as the art and science of helping adults learn. However, pedagogy and androgogy can be seen as the two ends of a spectrum, with actual teaching-learning interactions falling somewhere in between (Knowles, 1980).

Several assumptions underlie pedagogical learning. The first is that the learner is in a dependent role; the teacher takes full responsibility for determining the content, the point at which topics are introduced, the manner in which they are presented, and the student's success in learning the material. The second assumption is that learners' experiences have limited value, whereas the experiences of the teacher or other experts are highly valuable to the student. The third assumption is that people are ready to learn when society says they ought to learn. And the final assumption is that learners see education as a process of acquiring content that will be useful at a later time in life. According to the assumptions of pedagogical learning, the teacher, without input from the learner, develops the teaching plan in terms of material to be taught and the time, place, and technique of teaching. The teacher devotes little attention to the learner's past experiences, thoughts, and feelings about the material that needs to be taught (Knowles, 1980).

Androgogical learning is based on a different set of assumptions: (1) as people mature, they move from dependency to increasing self-direction, but different people do so at different rates; (2) as people mature, they accumulate an increasing reservoir of experience that becomes a rich resource for learning; (3) people become ready to learn when learning is necessary for coping with a real-life problem or task; and (4) learners consider education a process of developing increased competence to achieve their full potential and want to apply any knowledge they gain to their present living situation. In using these assumptions, the teacher takes into consideration the learner's past experiences, the learner's need for self-direction, and the learner's desire to learn about a particular topic (Knowles, 1980).

Nurses and other health educators use assumptions from both models in client education, although pedagogy predominates. However, careful assessment will help determine which set of assumptions is most appropriate to meet the needs of the individual client.

Problems and Issues in Teaching Clients

Since management of a chronic illness is a life-long undertaking, and since the management plan is often quite complex, successful learning is important to maximize outcomes. When teaching has not achieved desired change, evaluation requires determining the cause. Problems addressed in teaching texts used by health professionals are generally taken into consideration, and teaching interventions are modified to compensate for them. However, other problems occur that are not addressed in standard texts; causes appear more elusive; and clients may be considered noncompliant—but rarely is the ineffectiveness of the teaching considered. Increased awareness of teaching's role as a contributing factor in poor learning performance could enhance the health professionals' ability to successfully evaluate long-term outcomes and seek long-term solutions.

The tendency to use the pedagogical learning model more than the androgogical model may be based on time and other constraints, such as limited awareness of the learner's autonomy and values. The learner is often assumed to be dependent and likely to benefit from teaching. Although assessment occurs, the client's prior experiences (as factors that could potentiate learning) and self-identified learning needs receive less emphasis. The teacher takes responsibility for determining content and implementing the teaching plan, assuming that the learner will use presented material later. Often this approach leads to successful outcomes.

But the pedagogic method is not always effective. Long-term problems seem to emphasize the importance of androgogical learning—that is, encouraging client self-direction and responsibility. Androgogic teaching plans take into account what the client is ready and willing to learn in order to cope with client-identified long-term needs or problems. In addition, the greater integration of prior experiences allows teaching plans to have varying rates of learning and differences in life-style and need.

Regardless of which teaching model is determined more effective for long-term success, the health professional must be sensitive to potential problems. Sensitization leads to the achievement of more positive outcomes with the client whose "lack of learning" surfaces after discharge from the acute setting.

Common Problems of the Learner

If teaching is to lead to successful change, obstacles within or related to the learner must be identified and eliminated. Common learner problems include lack of readiness, physical and emotional obstacles, language barriers, and lack of motivation. The acute or chronic nature of the disease is not a factor. However, because of the characteristics of chronic illnesses, learner problems may be more frequently present in individuals having such conditions.

Lack of Readiness *Readiness* is the learner's ability in terms of physical and mental development; readiness in both respects is necessary for effective learning (Haggard, 1989). Physical readiness depends primarily on the state of the individual's neuromuscular system and is relevant chiefly to learning physical skills. Performing procedures that require fine motor coordination is impossible for the person who lacks such coordination. Mental readiness depends on the state of the individual's intellectual development; the learner must have sufficient capacity for the learning task as well as adequate ability to perceive ideas, verbalize thoughts, and conceptualize information needed for learning. If learning is to occur when physical or mental readiness is lacking in the learner, the teaching process must be adapted to the individual's developmental stage or intellectual abilities.

Physical Obstacles Discomfort, energy limitations, and decreased physical mobility are among the physical obstacles that can hinder learning for any ill person (Nurse's Reference

Library, 1987). Pain and nausea are just two of many symptoms that produce discomfort. Such symptoms draw the client's attention toward ways of gaining comfort and therefore away from learning about such things as self-management techniques. For example, clients with advanced neoplastic disorders can have severe pain; until that pain is relieved, learning is blocked.

Clients who have severe energy limitations may focus on meeting basic physiological needs. For example, individuals having chronic obstructive pulmonary disorders often use their limited energy levels to perform basic activities of daily living, with little reserve left for attention to learning activities. However, one must be careful not to assume that no learning has occurred because obvious involvement has not been noted. Individuals may be learning what needs to be learned, but on their own terms.

Physical limitations involving decreased mobility may hamper learning. This is especially true of motor skills that require involvement of the affected extremity. A client with severe rheumatoid arthritis may have difficulty mastering a physical skill that requires use of the hands.

Eliminating physical obstacles to learning is desirable but not always possible. The nurse-educator should assess these obstacles so that the teaching will provide necessary adaptation. Premedication may relieve nausea or pain, timing for high energy levels can allow for available reserves for learning, and modification of equipment can compensate for lost physical mobility. In short, timing of teaching and planning for flexibility allow individuals to circumvent physical obstacles.

Emotional Obstacles Numerous emotional obstacles affect the readiness or ability to learn. These include denial of the condition, anger, depression and withdrawal, and anxiety. In addition, lowered self-esteem may impede learning.

Denial is a normal coping mechanism that individuals use when they face overwhelming situations that are anxiety provoking (Miller, 1991). For instance, denial occurs when a serious or irreversible illness is diagnosed. Clients often think, "This might happen to others, but not to me," or "It can't be as bad as my doctor

says it is." Teaching self-care management is ineffective during denial because affected individuals cannot accept the presence or seriousness of the illness and place little value on learning to understand and manage the condition.

Anger is often present when the client begins to accept that something is wrong and that the identified chronic illness is really present. Hostility against health care providers and family is a common reaction during this phase of coping with illness. The teacher should realize that anger is a normal reaction and should not argue with, or belittle, the feelings of the learner (Anderson, 1990). A more effective strategy would be working with the client to resolve the anger and then beginning the teaching process.

Depression is also a coping mechanism used by clients with chronic illnesses. It is a reaction to the loss of valued health and well-being. Withdrawal sometimes results from this depression. While experiencing depression, clients tend to give little attention to ongoing activities, show a decreased ability to concentrate, and spend time sleeping or sitting quietly by themselves (Miller, 1991). Although these responses are not necessarily negative, the client displays little interest in learning about the illness or about self-management during periods of depression or withdrawal.

Anxiety associated with illness can obstruct learning. Fear based on an identifiable factor, such as pain or surgery, can lead to anxiety that is more free floating. Should anxiety be unrelieved, it can become severe, which in turn limits an individual's perception of events that are occurring. Attention focuses on relieving the anxiety rather than on learning (Nurse's Reference Library, 1987; Redman, 1988). For example, a newly diagnosed diabetic may be unable to master the skills of diabetic self-care, such as urine testing and diet control, because of anxiety over self-administering insulin injections.

When lowered self-esteem is displayed by persons having chronic illness, it may become an obstacle to the teaching-learning process. Lowered self-esteem leads to doubts about abilities or to feelings of inferiority, ineffectiveness, or insignificance. Consequently, lowered self-esteem can impede the client's ability to set goals or the client's sense of competence (Miller, 1991). Individuals who have low self-esteem may not believe that they are capable of carrying out the tasks required for managing their chronic illnesses. In turn, their confidence about mastering such tasks decreases.

Dealing with emotional obstacles to learning requires identifying them during the assessment process. Initially, teaching must focus on coping with and managing the activities of today rather than on following a future self-management plan. Learning to deal with present-day activities can sometimes help clients decrease anxiety and depression and increase confidence in their ability to manage their illness.

Language Barriers Language barriers have several sources (Anderson, 1990). First, there may be a difference in primary language between learner and teacher. When teacher and learner use different languages, an interpreter who can speak the client's language should be used so that the teaching plan can be implemented. Second, the learner may have limited mastery of the language used by the health educator. Health care providers sometimes forget that clients do not know the meaning of many medical words used in health care agencies. Lack of familiarity can be overcome by using terms more familiar to the learner. Third, the extent and type of the client's education influence his or her comprehension of the teaching plan. Assessment of language limitations caused by lower educational attainment leads to identifying an appropriate language level for the learner.

The reader is cautioned to remember that lack of response to teaching does not necessarily indicate limited learning capability. Rather limited response can reflect fear of appearing "dumb" if there is acknowledgment that terms being used are unfamiliar. Feedback can assure the teacher that the client understands the terminology being used.

Lack of Motivation Motivation is essential if learning is to occur. Motivation increases when the individual develops a desire to understand the illness, to perform self-care, to avoid complications, to please others, or to enjoy a higher level of wellness (Haggard, 1989; Anderson, 1990). Behaviors that indicate an individual's motivational level may be difficult to identify without a thorough assessment.

Redman (1988) lists general principles of motivation that are applicable to teaching-learning situations:

1. Incentives motivate learning.
2. Internal motivation lasts longer and is more self-directive than external motivation.
3. Learning is most effective when the learner feels a need to know.
4. Motivation is enhanced by the organization of the material.
5. Success is a more predictable motivator than failure.
6. A mild level of anxiety is useful in motivating individuals, but severe anxiety is incapacitating.

Although these principles help in motivating the client, adequate incentive to learn may be lacking if the individual has no internal inducement based on self-need.

Developmental Level and Life-Cycle Influences

Age-related differences can influence the ability to learn. These differences are most apparent when teaching a young child or an elderly person, and they point out the need for consideration of an individual's developmental level on the teaching-learning process.

Factors That Influence Learning in the Young The teaching-learning process involving a young child has problems that are not present when working with an adult. These problems are due to the physical and intellectual developmental level of the child. To promote effective learning, one must assess the child's developmental level in terms of communication ability, level of understanding, attention span, memory, and physical ability to perform necessary tasks (Schuster & Ashburn, 1986). After a thorough assessment of the child's abilities, the teacher can make an informed decision about whether the teaching should primarily involve the child alone, the family (or person responsible for the child's well-being), or both the child and the family (or responsible person).

Ability to communicate, capacity to understand concepts, and attention span vary among children, even children in similar age groups. As a child's ability to communicate increases, the effectiveness of the teaching-learning interaction with that child increases correspondingly. Children must have sufficient vocabulary to ask questions, verbalize understanding, and clarify and verify the information being taught. The child's ability to understand concepts is closely related to communication ability. Normally, at about age 5, the child begins to talk comprehensively: asks the meaning of words, is capable of memorizing, and is able to follow three-step directions in the proper sequence (Schuster & Ashburn, 1986). These skills progress rapidly as the child grows older.

The ability to attend is considered an important factor in the learning process (Schuster & Ashburn, 1986). Since attention span increases with age, the older the child, the longer the attention span. To promote maximum learning, teaching should be planned in segments that accommodate the child's actual attention span. For example, teaching a toddler or preschooler is best done in 5- to 10-minute segments, whereas teaching a school-age child may involve 30- to 40-minute segments.

Since learning cannot occur without the retention and recall of past experiences, memory plays a major role in learning. Memory is also necessary for conceptualization (Schuster & Ashburn, 1986). Obviously, the younger the child, the more limited the memory; therefore, teaching needs to be at an appropriate level for the child, given the child's ability to remember the material.

Physical growth is another consideration in teaching the child. The very young child, who has not developed fine motor coordination, cannot master the same kinds of tasks that the older, more coordinated child can. When teaching a physical skill to a child, the nurse-educator should determine if the child's motor skills have progressed to an appropriate level for mastery. Insufficient motor development impedes learning and produces frustration and a sense of failure for both the learner and the teacher (Schuster & Ashburn, 1986).

Factors That Influence Learning in the Elderly Older people are motivated to learn and to engage in activities that they consider meaningful, but they do not perform well when learning tasks they view as irrelevant or unnecessary (Hogstel, 1994). Older people learn better when they can pace learning so as to monitor both the rate and amount of incoming stimuli. They tend to be cautious and hesitant in new learning situations and commit omission errors rather than performance errors, reflecting a need to be certain of the outcome of their activities before acting. Factors that affect ability to learn in the elderly are related to physiological and memory changes that occur with aging.

Physiological Changes That Affect Learning Although sensory changes occur throughout the life span, decreases become apparent in the middle years and progress throughout the remainder of an individual's life. For example, the sense of touch is decreased in the elderly person (Hogstel, 1994), making evaluation of externally applied heat difficult; heat applied to joints affected by rheumatoid arthritis can result in a burn.

Change in visual abilities begins in middle age and continues into the older years. These changes include decreases in acuity and sensitivity to light, increased sensitivity to glare, altered color vision, and altered depth perception (Crosbie, 1990). Nurse-educators must assess the ability of the older adult to read any written teaching materials presented, since older adults may have difficulty reading such materials. These materials should be larger in size and print, and colors used in teaching aids should be warm shades of red, orange, or yellow; blues and greens should be avoided. Reading lights should be bright but diffused and properly placed (Stewart & Walton, 1992).

Age-related hearing loss, called presbycusis, is more apparent in high tones (Storandt, 1986; Hogstel, 1994). Presbycusis also influences speech intelligibility, impeding comprehension.

When communicating with older individuals who have hearing losses, the teacher should sit or stand directly facing the learner, enunciate clearly, talk slowly, and eliminate background noises, such as radios or television. Voice volume should not be raised, since this change tends to also raise the voice tone, and higher tones are the most difficult for the older person to hear. Encourage the use of hearing aids or other adaptive hearing devices for those who find them beneficial.

Endurance and muscle strength also gradually decrease with aging (Hogstel, 1994), although most older people can continue to perform daily activities. Changes in endurance and strength affect physical skills that are involved in learning activities and exercises related to the client's particular chronic condition. Also present in some older persons is a decreased sense of balance, particularly when rising quickly or acting rapidly (Hogstel, 1994). Balance should be considered in relation to activity level of the individual, and individuals should be instructed to get up or begin activities slowly.

Cardiovascular changes that accompany aging include decreased cardiac output and stroke volume; these changes do not adversely affect daily functioning. Some older people develop atheroscleroses (Hogstel, 1994) with associated decreased blood flow to the brain that alters cognitive functioning or decreases alertness; the individual's ability to absorb and process information can, therefore, be affected. Assessing the individual's level of cognition and alertness should precede teaching; after each teaching-learning interaction, retention of the material, especially by individuals known to have cognitive impairment, should be evaluated.

Memory Changes Although older persons seem to undergo minimal impairment of their ability to recall events of the distant past, a weakening in short-term memory or in the recall of recently learned information tends to occur. The greatest memory change associated with aging seems to be related to the type of recall used to form new associations (Hogstel, 1994). Since some decrease in short-term memory apparently oc-

curs, the dissemination of information needs to be planned at a slower pace and reinforced more frequently.

Lack of Compliance

The issue of noncompliance to a prescribed therapeutic plan has been identified by health care providers as a significant problem in working with chronically ill individuals. Even when health care educators provide specific and thorough teaching to improve health and manage illness, clients often do not follow the plan presented. The complexity of factors that influence compliance has been extensively studied, but many of these studies have conflicting results. Although problems related to compliance exist, these issues will not be addressed in this chapter; the reader will find a more extensive discussion of noncompliance in Chapter 10.

Locus of Control

One theory that seems to influence compliance is *locus of control,* a construct based on the assumption that an individual's beliefs about factors that influence health may be related to that individual's health behaviors (Christensen et al., 1991; Miller, 1991). People with internal locus of control ("internals") believe that their health is largely determined by their own behaviors and actions. "Externals" believe that their health is determined by factors outside their control, such as fate, chance, or other people; consequently, they tend to feel powerless or helpless in managing their illness. It is important that the client's beliefs about control of his or her health status be ascertained before teaching begins. If the client is an internal, teaching needs to encourage client follow-through on necessary externally imposed regimens. If the client is an external, teaching interventions and strategies should be geared toward assisting the individual to become more internal in relation to health care beliefs, or toward assuring the client that the health professional will be accountable for some aspects of the regimen such as scheduling appointments, validating performance, and so forth.

Sociological Influences

The degree of self-management the client demonstrates may be influenced by sociological factors. Interestingly, the literature indicates that client noncompliance is widespread across all socioeconomic groups (Miller, 1991). However, socioeconomic factors may make compliance more difficult for some clients.

Financial Resources Chronic illness can drain the client and family financially (see Chapter 22, on financial impact). Since most families have financial limitations, economic resources necessary to maintain the treatment regimen may be inadequate in relation to other needs and expenses; clients may begin to seek ways to decrease health care costs. Consequences of this effort to balance needs and finances can result in decreasing or omitting medication dosages, not purchasing needed supplies, reduced compliance with treatment regimens, or discontinuation of the treatment plan (Miller, 1991).

Time Time, like money, is finite for most people. Many treatment plans for chronic illness, such as managing an ulcerative colitis or cystic fibrosis regimen, are very time consuming. In view of other tasks and activities, the client may decide to modify, adjust, or totally omit the plan of care designed to control symptoms or exacerbations if the time requirements of the regimen are extensive (Strauss et al., 1984).

Life-Style versus Needed Change A conflict between a client's life-style and identified need to change may cause the individual to abandon the treatment plan. Clients may determine that, even though they understand the risks and results of not managing their symptoms or illness, they would rather accept those risks than institute a change in life-style.

Health care providers should assess factors and adapt the teaching plan to accommodate sociological circumstances that place clients at high risk for noncompliance. Interventions that compensate for sociological factors include providing additional physical or emotional support or scheduling and encouraging more frequent follow-up visits for reinforcement of teaching.

Dependence/Independence Conflicts and Role Loss

Chronically ill individuals often experience dependence/independence conflicts and role losses that influence their self-esteem and can be obstacles to effective learning and to mastery of self-care management. In addition, the client and family may perceive the progress of the illness differently from the health provider so that willingness to learn is affected (see Chapter 3, on illness trajectory).

Dependence/independence conflicts arise because the nature of many illnesses requires that the individual become dependent; for example, clients are dependent on medications (such as insulin), machines (such as dialysis), equipment (such as portable oxygen), or other people (caregivers who manage the clients' activities of daily living). The need to be dependent secondary to illness may be in conflict with the life-style preference or personality of the individual. Conflicts can also arise because health care providers encourage independence on the part of the client even when the client may feel a need to maintain more dependence (Miller, 1991).

Role loss can impact self-esteem and create a feeling of helplessness. Roles can be lost within the family (a mother who can no longer take care of her child), within a career (an individual who can no longer fulfill job responsibilities), or socially (an individual who can no longer attend enjoyed social activities, such as parties or ballgames). Issues that arise from role losses are best resolved prior to implementing a teaching plan (Miller, 1991).

Family Influences on Learning

The client's family and significant others are probably the single most significant determinant of success or failure for an educational plan (Haggard, 1989). Since the family is the chronically ill individual's major support system, family members have a significant impact on the individual's ability to manage illness. Family attitudes and reactions to the illness and the treatment plan influence the client's ability to learn about it. Family influence may be positive or negative.

Denial by Family Members Just as clients use denial when they are informed of serious illnesses, families also cope in this way (Haggard, 1989). Like the client, the family needs time to overcome its initial reaction and to accept the illness. However, if a lack of acceptance continues for a long time, it creates an obstacle to learning about the necessary aspects of the treatment plan. Prolonged denial by the family may also encourage continuance of the client's denial.

Sometimes the client accepts the illness, but the family continues to deny it. This situation creates difficulty for the client in implementing the treatment plan. Without family support, the client may feel the need to conceal necessary equipment and medications, or may never purchase them. Follow-up doctor or clinic appointments may not be kept, especially if transportation by family is necessary. Individuals may refrain from discussing the illness with family members, thereby being deprived of the emotional support of those persons most important to them (Haggard, 1989).

Overprotection If families overprotect the chronically ill individual, learning may be impeded (Haggard, 1989). For example, when chronically ill children are overprotected so that there are major activity restrictions, they begin to feel different from other children. This feeling can lead to frustration, anger, loneliness, or even denial. In an attempt to be like their peers, children may avoid learning or using information or skills necessary to manage their disease (Haggard, 1989; Miller, 1991).

Decision Making Involvement in the decision-making process promotes learning of a given treatment plan. However, at times, the family or health care provider makes all decisions about management of the illness without input

from the client, most frequently with children and the elderly. Without input, the client lacks a sense of control and is less likely to be motivated to learn about the plan or to perform appropriate self-management behaviors (Haggard, 1989).

Problems of the Professional as a Teacher

Even when the learner is motivated and ready to learn, ineffective teaching may impede the integration of knowledge and skills necessary for managing the illness. The professional can contribute to inadequate learning in several ways, including incorrect management of the teaching-learning process and being unable to override inherent limitations or differences in the relationship with the learner. Several areas where the teaching professional may contribute to poor learning on the part of the client are discussed here.

Inadequate Assessment Inadequate assessment often has a number of causes: poor interview or communication skills, inadequate observational skills, time limitations, or failure to consider the learner's home or social environment. The health care provider may be unaware of when an assessment has not been thorough. Nurse-educators may assume that they know what the learner needs to know; therefore, they do not assess the learner's knowledge or identify misconceptions on the part of the learner (Redman, 1988).

Individualization of the management plan should be based on each client's personal situation. Clients do not always inform health care providers of problems or limitations that exist in the home or involve their social situation. Therefore, both of these areas should be assessed before development and implementation of the teaching plan. Unless the home environment and social situation are adequate for carrying out the plan, the client is not likely to follow any plan that is developed.

Failure to Negotiate Goals Although the health care provider may have goals for the educational process, the client's goals may differ and should be given priority. Ongoing evaluation will assist the educator in recognizing when goals need to be renegotiated. Unrealistic or unclear goals lead to noncompliance (Jackson & Johnson, 1988).

Client Overload Too much material may be presented at one time, leading to client overload. Shorter sessions may prevent this by allowing the client to synthesize and formulate questions between sessions. Yawning, fidgeting, or inability to answer questions by the client may indicate overload and the need for a break in teaching (Jackson & Johnson, 1988).

Making Assumptions Assumptions about the client can be detrimental to effective teaching. Remember the following principles:

- Never assume that a client understands the disease or prescribed treatment even if it has been diagnosed for some time.
- Never assume that a client knows why a prescription drug is taken.
- Never assume that because a client is from a different socioeconomic, ethnic, or educational background that there is no motivation or ability to learn.
- Never assume that because a client has been noncompliant in the past this behavior will continue (Jackson & Johnson, 1988).

Other Factors That Impede Teaching Developing and carrying out a teaching plan can be impeded by cost limitations, time constraints, lack of support from the agency administration or physician, environmental limitations of the teaching setting, inadequate evaluation of the teaching-learning process, and sociocultural differences between teacher and learner.

Cost Limitations As agencies become more and more cost conscious, budgets are cut and "nonessential" services are omitted (Redman, 1988). Education, unfortunately, sometimes falls into the category of "nonessential." Although the cost of client education is often minimal, some financial support is necessary for the purchase of teaching materials and for salaries. Inadequate or outdated teaching materials obstruct the teaching process. Health care providers must educate administrators about the importance of client teaching and show them that the benefits of education are worth the costs.

Time Limitations Time limitations in the clinical setting pose a major problem for teaching. Usually, diagnostic procedures, activities of daily living, treatments, visits by the physician or various therapists, and other tasks have priority over teaching. It is often assumed that teaching occurs when the client is not busy with this myriad of other activities. As a result, teaching is sometimes neglected or is done immediately before the client's discharge from the facility, making assimilation of information difficult. Nurses working at the bedside have a special opportunity to catch clients at the time when they are most receptive to learning: when the client asks questions about a particular aspect of the treatment plan. Encouraging all nursing staff to be familiar with the educational plan for the client allows maximum use of time spent providing care to help achieve learning objectives (Haggard, 1989).

Lack of Administrative or Physician Support Efforts extended toward providing quality teaching often do not receive support from the agency administration or the physician. Unless the administration believes that teaching is as important as other tasks, it may be done in an unplanned, sporadic manner. Some physicians do not want their patients to be fully informed of their condition; others prefer to do all required teaching themselves. Although the physician may do an excellent job of teaching needed information, time limits make accurate client evaluation difficult. Without the involvement of other health care providers, the client may not receive needed reinforcement or answers to questions that arise when the physician is not present.

Soliciting physician cooperation and support for client education programs is important. Three strategies to promote physician support are easy access to patient education, physician endorsement, and high program visibility. The easier the access to a program, the more likely physicians are to use the program—for instance, establishing a system where the physician can simply write an order for teaching instead of completing separate forms or making additional phone calls. The medical staff needs to feel confident that information provided to the clients is accurate and appropriate and will not contradict the treatment plan. Showing actual improvement in a client's condition through teaching is the single most impressive thing that can be done to make client education visible. If the health educator publicizes proof that teaching activities make a difference, supporters among physicians and agency administration will multiply (Haggard, 1989).

Environmental Limitations Control of the environment, such as providing privacy, is the responsibility of the teacher in the teaching-learning situation. In a hospital, teaching often occurs in the client's room, which may be shared with only curtains separating the areas. Since all conversations may be heard by others, learners become reluctant to ask questions and clarify information, or are embarrassed that someone else is hearing about their problems. Privacy problems may also occur if teaching is performed in the waiting room of a clinic or physician's office while other individuals are within hearing. Other environmental factors the teacher should consider are the temperature of the setting, adequacy of lighting, presence of unnecessary noise, and interruptions. Problems with any of these factors could lead to less than ideal teaching-learning interactions (Haggard, 1989).

Inadequate Evaluation Another common problem that impedes the teaching–learning process is inadequate evaluation of teaching effectiveness (Nurse's Reference Library, 1987). Nurse-educators sometimes believe that transmission of information constitutes teaching and that learning has therefore occurred. A method of evaluation must be developed during the planning step of the teaching-learning process, and must follow each teaching session as well as the entire teaching program. Evaluation must include an objective means of determining teaching effectiveness. Asking the client "Do you understand what I have told you?" does not produce an adequate evaluation of learning.

Sociocultural Differences between Teacher and Learner Sociocultural differences between teacher and learner can impede the teaching-learning process. In this area, the teacher has two responsibilities: (1) being aware of the sociocultural beliefs of the client and incorporating them into the teaching plan, and (2) ensuring that personal sociocultural beliefs or biases do not interfere with teaching (Haggard, 1989).

Interventions to Improve Teaching

It is assumed that nurse-educators are already familiar with basic teaching methods and tools (see Table 16–2). For those who are not, many excellent teaching texts for health professionals are available that provide detailed discussion and guidance. Yet detailed and accurate teaching during early phases of illness does not always lead to demonstrable application of self-management skills. Lack of change on the part of the learner can be frustrating and disheartening to health professionals who genuinely believe they have provided effective teaching (Redman, 1988; Haggard, 1989).

The literature provides some assistance to health educators and clients in overcoming persistent learning problems. Included are suggestions for better assessment and evaluation plus some specific teaching strategies that have proven effective in achieving change in people with long-term illnesses. A few of these are discussed briefly here.

Improving Assessment and Evaluation

Several strategies suggested in the literature can improve assessment and evaluation, which are essential for effective client education. These strategies address total education programs as well as individual assessment methods and

TABLE 16-2.   Frequently used teaching methods and tools

Methods	Rationale
Demonstration and practice	For teaching skills.
Group discussion	To share information about coping and adapting; for discussing effective management strategies.
Role playing	To present a particular attitude or point of view to the learner through performance of behavior. Role play can be effective in collecting information difficult to obtain otherwise. Often used with children, it can be used in teaching adults.
One-to-one discussion	To facilitate individualization.
Lecture	To give information to a group of people. Mainly a one-way communication from the teacher to the learner. Used as a method of providing a great deal of information in a short period of time; but its effectiveness is sometimes questioned because of the lack of active participation by the learner.
Games	To review material and work through simulated situations in an interesting and exciting format. Few commercial games for clients are available, so health educators may create their own.

Commonly Used Tools[1]	Examples
Written material	Books, pamphlets, charts, self-instructional manuals, teacher-developed instruction sheets, or any written information given to the client for the purpose of teaching.
Displays	Posters, models, mounted illustrations, and other static methods of teaching—can be permanently displayed or portable to be carried to client locations.
Audiovisual materials	Audiotapes, videotapes, films, slides, overhead transparencies, flipcharts, television, computer-assisted instruction.

[1]Usually used in conjunction with verbal instruction.

SOURCE: Based on Haggard (1989) and Redmond (1988).

skills. Accurate assessment identifies important problems and issues that will influence the teaching-learning process. Evaluation provides the feedback mechanism necessary for determining weaknesses in the process. Evaluation should encompass the effectiveness of each teaching-learning interaction and the effectiveness of the total client education program.

Assessment The accuracy of the collected assessment data depends on the interviewing and observation skills of the individual making the assessment. Therefore, nurse-educators should

do periodic self-evaluation of their assessment skills so they can maintain or improve data collecting needed for the teaching-learning process. Development of a systematic assessment process will improve the quality and accuracy of the teaching plan.

Ford (1987) suggests assessment of several areas prior to preparing the teaching plan: the client's belief system, knowledge base, ability to learn, readiness to learn, and past history of compliance. In addition, assessing the following factors will help the nurse complete the database needed for developing a comprehensive teaching plan: the client's outlook on life, past history with health-related material, cultural response to illness, educational background, and fear about illness or necessary life-style changes.

Evaluation   Haggard (1989) reports several methods that can be used to evaluate the results of teaching. One simple and efficient strategy is follow-up phone calls to discharged clients; these calls can be made at set intervals to check on compliance, to review and reinforce learning, and to answer questions. Other evaluation methods include self-appraisal, in which the client and family answer questions on the use of learned behaviors, and inspection of medical records from follow-up visits for evidence of successful implementation of instruction. Physical evidence such as lab values, vital signs, changes in physical abilities, or medication compliance provides yet another way of evaluating the results of teaching.

Haggard (1989) also defines three elements that need to be evaluated to determine progam usefulness: instructor competence, cost/benefit ratios, and changes needed to enhance program effectiveness. Evaluation of these three areas identifies which parts of the program are working and which prevent the educator from capitalizing on strengths and minimizing or eliminating weaknesses.

Redman (1988) notes that program evaluation needs to focus on a series of questions based on the following six points:

1. Does the program meet stated objectives for client learning?
2. Does the program have an impact on changes in risk-factor behaviors after discharge?
3. As a result of their participation in the program, do clients believe that they can manage their own care after discharge?
4. Which teaching techniques are viewed as most helpful by clients?
5. Are physicians satisfied with the program, and do they notice differences after discharge in clients who have participated in it?
6. Are teaching staff members satisfied with the program, and do they implement it consistently?

Behavioral Strategies

Educational programs for the chronically ill tend to focus on teaching about the disease process and then on presenting a management plan, without incorporating a component for changing client behaviors. This limitation is unfortunate, since behavioral strategies have been found effective in teaching chronically ill individuals. Combining dissemination of information with behavioral strategies helps the individual gain self-management skills (Miller, 1991).

Behavioral strategies (sometimes referred to as behavioral therapy or behavior modification) use a systematic approach to analyzing assessed data to find the causes and consequences of existing behavior in order to propose effective behavioral changes. After the behavior that needs changing is identified, a technique to alter cause, reinforcer, or both, is then determined. For clients who possess self-management knowledge but are unable to change their behavior, this strategy is quite effective.

A Model for Behavioral Intervention   Mager and Pipe (1984) outline a behavioral intervention program that can serve as a model for effective change (see Figure 16–1). This model requires that ineffective behaviors be identified through assessment and then defined in behavioral terms. Factors that promote the occurrence of this behavior need to be analyzed so that possible alternatives or solutions can be explored.

Identifying the Problem   Behavioral diagnosis is a sequential process. After one expresses the ineffective behavior in behavioral terms, one needs to determine the cause of the behavior. If it is due to a knowledge deficit, then teaching can be modified or strengthened to eliminate the difficulty. One should ask if the client knows the appropriate self-management behavior.

If the client demonstrates adequate knowledge, one must next determine whether the behavior is lost or has deteriorated. This includes finding out whether the behavior is frequent or infrequent. If it is used frequently but is performed incorrectly despite regular use, periodic feedback may lead to improvement. For exam-

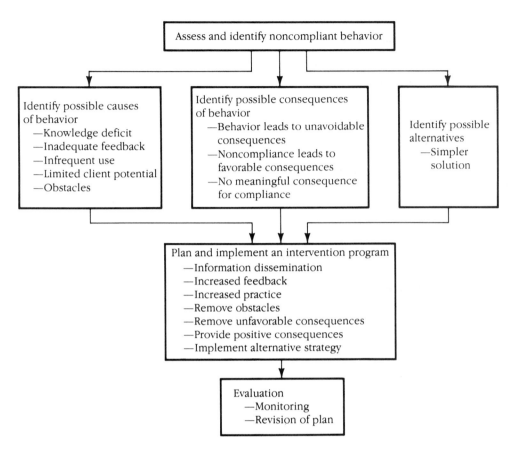

FIGURE 16-1. A Model for Behavioral Intervention

ple, a diabetic who self-injects insulin every day may be using an incorrect technique. If the behavior is used infrequently, a regular schedule of practice becomes important. For example, a family member who monitors a client's blood pressure occasionally may need to practice the technique during clinic visits.

When skill performance of the behavior is ensured, the individual's potential for carrying out the desired performance needs to be assessed as a possible cause of the unwanted behavior. Possible developmental or intellectual deficits or decreased interest that might hamper the individual's performance of desired behavior must be determined. The presence of deficits requires modification of the teaching plan so that

the client can successfully perform necessary actions. The lack of intellectual interest can be countered by stimulating the client's curiosity in such ways as identifying resources in the literature that the client can pursue and discuss.

The last major performance cause of unwanted behavior is obstacles to the performance of desired behavior. Removing these obstacles allows correction of the difficulty. For example, a diabetic who can and wants to carry out insulin injections and glucometer testing may be prevented from doing so by limited finances. Obstacles, rather than obstinacy, may be the cause.

Up to this point, the model considers only poor performance. Once performance causes are ruled out or corrected, then consequences, or lack of consequences, may underlie continued unwanted behavior. Analysis of consequences is also sequential, with the more likely being considered and corrected first.

Direct, unfavorable consequences, such as unwanted side effects, can underlie poor compliance and must be removed before satisfactory performance can be achieved. For example, clients who become nauseated every time they use a prescribed medication may be reluctant to use the medication. Solutions in this case include finding a way to control the nausea or selecting another effective medication that does not cause nausea.

If there are no unfavorable consequences, determination needs to be made as to whether nonperformance leads to more favorable consequences than the desired behavior does. Arrangements for positive reinforcement for appropriate behavior will correct the basis of such problems. For example, the child who receives more parental attention for refusing medication than for taking it may consider refusal to have a more favorable result. Correcting the behavior requires providing positive reinforcement for taking the medication.

If unwanted behavior continues, the next step is to determine whether the consequence is meaningful. If it is not, arrange a favorable result. For example, the client might receive an extra privilege for performing the desired behavior.

A final factor to consider, should neither cause nor consequence appear to influence behavior, is the possibility of alternatives such as a simpler solution to the problem. For example, would another behavior net the same outcome in terms of management of the treatment plan?

Planning and Implementing a Behavioral Program Once the underlying basis of poor performance is identified, a solution can be determined and implemented, with the selected strategy depending on the source of difficulty. The most practical, economical, and easy solution should be determined. Achieving the greatest results for the least effort is likely to increase self-management.

Several teaching strategies are applicable to the causes that underlie poor performance. For lack of knowledge, information dissemination is appropriate. When skill is inadequate, increased feedback helps, just as increased practice strengthens deteriorating skills.

Should consequences be the basis for poor learning performance, then unfavorable consequences should be removed, positive consequences or reinforcers should be provided, or obstacles to performance should be eliminated.

Finally, if neither cause nor consequence seems to underlie poor learning, one must attempt to identify and implement an alternate behavior that will net the same outcome.

Evaluation The final step in using behavioral strategies is to evaluate the entire process. Change in the specific behaviors identified during assessment should be identified, or performance of new behaviors should be clearly demonstrated. Evaluation includes continuous monitoring of client progress and identification and implementation of necessary revisions.

Contract Learning

The use of a contract is also effective in assisting clients with chronic illnesses to manage their care. With contract learning, identifying the underlying basis of poor outcomes is not emphasized; rather, the focus is on reaching agreement about preferred actions. Often called a *contingency contract,* this tool is a written plan for systematic reinforcement of specified desirable behaviors. The contract may be negotiated between the health care provider and client, or it may be a "self-contract" in which the client administers his or her own reinforcers, with another person available for support and advice if needed. A number of elements have been identified as desirable in a contingency contract (Janz, Becker, & Hartman, 1984; Knowles, 1986; Hiromoto & Dungan, 1991); most of them pertain to clarity of statement and intent (see Table 16-3).

Contingency contracting seems to be effective for chronically ill individuals for several reasons. The client becomes involved in the decision-making process regarding the treatment regimen and makes a commitment to behavior change. Everyone has the opportunity to discuss potential problems and solutions. Accountability

TABLE 16-3.   Elements desirable for
contract learning

1. Clearly stated goals must be specifically described and agreed on by all.
2. Responsibilities (behaviors) of each person must be stated in detail, including time and frequency requirements for performance of the behaviors.
3. The required behaviors should be easily observable and measured to facilitate reinforcement activities.
4. The methods of recording the behavior and the reinforcement should be identified.
5. Positive reinforcers must be clearly specified. This should also include timing and conditions for delivery of the reinforcements.
6. A detailed description of events that will occur if any person fails to fulfill the responsibilities of the contract must be provided.
7. A "bonus clause" may be included in order to provide additional reinforcers if the client exceeds the outlined responsibilities.
8. Specific dates for contract initiation and termination or renewal should be included.
9. The contract should be signed by all persons involved.

SOURCE: Based on Janz, Becker, and Hartman (1984) and Steckel (1982).

is fostered through written specification of each person's responsibilities for the client's health care; the contract elicits a formal commitment from all involved persons. The written document provides an instrument of communication for others involved in the client's care and facilities evaluation of progress by permitting comparison of activities and outcomes with the precise terms of the contract. Finally, the contingency component provides an additional incentive for achieving goals through reinforcement of the desired behaviors (Hiromoto & Dungan, 1991; Tuazon, 1992). Chapters 10 and 15, on compliance and change agent, respectively, also discuss contracting.

Other Strategies

Groups   Numerous authors have addressed the effects of group teaching and group process on the self-management of chronic illness, but suc-

cess of these groups has been limited except in terms of information dissemination. Groups, however, have succeeded in helping the chronically ill for a variety of reasons, such as providing emotional support, presenting alternatives, and sharing. Disadvantages to group sessions include the inability of the health educator to meet the special needs of individuals because group education must be tailored to meet the goals of the group (Galuk, 1990).

A study by Gonzales-Fernandez et al. (1990) of a hospital education program for hypertensives analyzed the usefulness of group education for patients with high blood pressure. The findings indicated that the group educational approach was an effective method for improving compliance and blood pressure control in the short term. Long-term compliance and control was not addressed and needs further study.

Swayze (1991) instituted a self-help group for individuals with sarcoidosis, a noncontagious multisystem chronic disorder characterized by granulomas in many organs. Although compliance was not evaluated, the self-help group sessions assisted individuals in adapting to the psychological, physiological, and medical aspects of their illness. Participants identified that the group process was instrumental in helping them to cope with problems and concerns related to the disease and with feelings of isolation and helplessness. Since feelings of isolation and helplessness are obstacles to both learning and compliance, attitude changes brought about by this self-help group process might result in improved home management of the disease.

Combination Group and Individual Teaching Sessions   A combination of group and individual teaching sessions can be used to accomplish the goals of both. Group sessions are cost effective and allow more efficient use of audiovisual aids, literature, and handouts; group interaction benefit members by enhancing motivation and providing support. Individual teaching sessions are tailored to meet individual learning needs, allow maximum interaction between educator and learner, pace sessions to optimize learning, promote simultaneous feedback, and correct misconceptions or confusion immediately.

In a study of health education methods to increase medication adherence among adults with asthma, Windsor et al. (1990) described a program that used a combination of group sessions, one-on-one sessions, and follow-up telephone calls. Each asthma client received a 30-minute one-to-one session with instruction on peak flow meter use, inhaler use, and how to use a self-help guide. In addition, all clients attended a 60-minute asthma support group session and received two telephone reinforcement calls within one month of the group session. The clients who participated in this program exhibited a significantly higher level of improvement in adherence than clients who did not.

Compliance Packaging of Medications A compliance package can be defined as a prepackaged unit that provides one treatment cycle of medication in a ready-to-use package. Compliance packaging has two primary purposes: to serve as a client education tool for health professionals, and to make it easier for clients to remember to take their medications correctly at home. The dosage units and days are usually indicated on the dosage card to remind the client when and how much medication to take. Compliance packaging is an education tool that must be combined with other components of client education such as good counseling techniques, reinforcement, and quality written medication instructions (Smith, 1989).

Discharge Planning Discharge planning can incorporate teaching to gain effective outcomes. One discharge planning program, identified as a way of decreasing hospitalizations for chronically ill individuals, used a six-step plan (Huey et al., 1981), called the METHOD discharge plan. Each letter in the word METHOD stands for one step that needs to be considered. Note that some of these steps actually involve teaching:

M—*Medication:* The client will know his or her medications's name, purpose, effect, dosage, schedule, precautions to take, and side effects that should be reported.

E—*Environment:* The client is informed that adequate homemaking and transportation services and emotional and economic support will be ensured. Physical hazards in the home will be corrected.

T—*Treatments:* The client or family member will know the purpose of treatments and will be able to demonstrate the correct technique and to report any problems that develop.

H—*Health Teaching:* The client will be able to describe the way the disease affects his or her body, to list the keys to health maintenance, and to name signs and symptoms that require medical attention.

O—*Outpatient Referral:* The client will know when and where to keep appointments and whom to call for medical help. The client and referral agencies will have copies of the discharge instruction plan.

D—*Diet:* The client will be able to describe the appropriate diet and its purpose, to name restricted foods, and to describe some typical menus.

Although this teaching strategy does not involve mechanisms to assist clients in modifying their behavior, it does present a structured plan for giving necessary self-management knowledge to client and family. This plan allows the health care educator to provide the client with needed physical, emotional, and economic support services and at the same time to furnish a copy of the management instructions to appropriate referral agencies, thereby producing a mechanism for monitoring client behaviors that can be used by persons providing the support services and by those in the referral agencies.

Summary

Teaching clients with chronic illnesses about their disease and how to manage their care can be challenging. The nurse-educator must be familiar with the general concepts of teaching and learning, as well as issues specific to the chronically ill individual. Because of the long-term nature of chronic illnesses and the complexity of their management, clients often have difficulty mastering and carrying out their treatment plans.

A number of problems make teaching less effective with the chronically ill, including problems inherent in the client, the family, the sociocultural environment, and the teacher. Only if these problems are considered can corrective teaching interventions be identified.

Although knowledge about the illness and its regimen increases the likelihood of the client successfully managing his or her care, knowledge alone does not ensure such behavior. Any number of teaching methods and tools are useful, depending on the nature of the subject being taught and on an assessment of the client's learning needs and style. Appropriateness of pedagogic or androgogic techniques also must be considered.

Effective assessment and evaluation by the health educator are prerequisites of effective teaching. Behavioral strategies based on identified specific causes or consequences of behavior can be developed to assist the client in adhering to a plan. Combining information dissemination with behavioral strategies has proved to be an effective process of the teaching-learning interaction.

Contract learning also has been proven effective for use with the chronically ill. Contracting does not require identifying the basis of poor outcomes; rather, it focuses on agreement about future behaviors by means of a written document that includes all factors of behavior, reinforcer, and responsibility for plan components.

Also mentioned is the value of groups in providing support (although they do not enhance learning) and the packaging of medications as adjuncts to improved learning for the chronically ill client. Discharge planning can incorporate aspects of a teaching plan to assist the client.

NURSING DIAGNOSIS

8.1.1 Knowledge Deficit (specify):

Definition: None provided.

Defining Characteristics: Verbalization of the problem; inaccurate follow-through of instruction; inaccurate performance of test: inappropriate or exaggerated behaviors, e.g., hysterical, hostile, agitated, apathetic.

Related Factors: Lack of exposure; lack of recall; information misinterpretation; cognitive limitation; lack of interest in learning; unfamiliarity with information resources.

Editor's Note: At the onset of an illness, clients generally lack knowledge about such things as the pathology, symptoms, effects and side effects of treatment, long-term complications, and so forth.

Teaching is a vital part of helping a client or family gain or integrate information about a disease and its management. Most of the related factors mentioned above are appropriate to this phase of the client's illness. Jenny (1987) points out that knowledge deficit is more an etiological factor than a human response, and Carpenito (1993) says that knowledge deficit is an etiological factor for other diagnoses, such as anxiety (prior to a procedure).

There are times when teaching has been done, but the client still does not demonstrate, verbally or behaviorally, that learning has occurred. Under these circumstances, knowledge deficit would be a diagnostic category and the underlying factor(s) impeding learning needs to be identified. There are a number of these factors noted in this chapter. It is suggested that NANDA rethink this diagnostic category.

STUDY QUESTIONS

1. What are the four steps of the teaching-learning process? Briefly define each.
2. In what ways are pedagogic learning and androgogic learning different? the same?
3. What are the six common obstacles to learning on the part of the learner?
4. What factors influence learning in a child? in the elderly?
5. What client factors might lead to noncompliance with the treatment regimen?
6. What factors on the part of the teacher can create problems in the teaching-learning process?
7. In what ways can assessment and evaluation be improved? Discuss them.
8. How can behavioral strategies help teach the chronically ill person? Explain the process.
9. What are the desirable elements of a contingency contract? How does contingency contracting differ from behavioral strategies?
10. What value for teaching can be found in groups? in compliance packaging of medications? How can discharge planning be used to enhance compliance?

References

Anderson, C. (1990). *Patient teaching and communicating in an information age*. Albany, NY: Delmar.

Barnes, L. P. (1992). Patient education resources. *MCN, 17,* 43.

Carpenito, L. J. (1993). *Nursing diagnosis: Application to clinical practice* (5th ed.). Philadelphia: J. B. Lippincott.

Christensen, A. J., Turner, C. W., Smith, T. W., Holman, J. M., & Gregory, M. C. (1991). Health locus of control and depression in end-stage renal disease. *Journal of Consulting and Clinical Psychology, 59*(3), 419-424.

Crosbie, J. M. (1990). Helping older learners learn. *Home Healthcare Nurse, 8*(3), 42-45.

Ford, R. D. (1987). *Patient teaching: Manual I*. Springhouse, PA: Springhouse.

Galuck, D. L. (1990). Adult education for the patient with diabetes mellitus. *Advancing Clinical Care, 5,* 33-35.

Gonzales-Fernandez, R. A., Rivera, M., Torres, D., Quiles, J., & Jackson, A. (1990). Usefulness of a systemic hypertension in-hospital educational program. *The American Journal of Cardiology, 65,* 1384-1386.

Haggard, A. (1989). *Handbook of patient education*. Rockville, MD: Aspen.

Hiromoto, B. M. & Dungan, J. (1991). Contract learning for self-care activities. *Cancer Nursing, 14*(3), 148-154.

Hogstel, M. O. (1994). *Nursing care of the older adults* (3rd ed.). New York: Delmar.

Huey, R., Loomis, J., Rosson, T., Owen, D., Kiernan, L., Madonna, M., & Quaife, M. (1981). Discharge planning: Good planning means fewer hospitalizations for the chronically ill. *Nursing 81, 11*(5), 70-75.

Jackson, J. E., & Johnson, E. A. (1988). *Patient education in home care: A practical guide to effective teaching and documentation*. Rockville, MD: Aspen.

Janz, N. K., Becker, M. H., & Hartman, P. E. (1984). Contingency contracting to enhance patient compliance: A review. *Patient Education and Counseling, 5,* 165-178.

Jenny, J. (1987). Knowledge deficit: Not a nursing diagnosis. *Image: The Journal of Nursing Scholarship, 19*(4), 184-185.

Knowles, M. S. (1980). *The modern practice of adult education: From pedagogy to androgogy*. Chicago: Association.

——— (1986). *Using learning contracts*. San Francisco: Jossey-Bass.

Mager, R. F., & Pipe, P. (1984). *Analyzing performance problems* (2nd ed.). Belmont, CA: Fearon.

Miller, J. F. (1991). *Coping with chronic illness: Overcoming powerlessness*. Philadelphia: F. A. Davis.

Nurse's Reference Library (1987). Patient teaching, *Nursing 87 Books*. Springhouse, PA: Springhouse.

Pohl, M. L. (1981). *The teaching function of the nursing practitioner* (4th ed.). Dubuque, IA: Brown.

Redman, B. K. (1988). *The process of patient teaching in nursing* (6th ed.). St. Louis: C. V. Mosby.

Schuster, C. S., & Ashburn, S. S. (1986). *The process of human development: A holistic approach* (2nd ed.). Boston: Little, Brown.

Smith, D. L. (1989). Compliance packaging: A patient education tool. *American Pharmacy, 29*(2), 42-45, 49-53.

Steckel, S. B. (1982). *Patient contracting.* Norwalk, CT: Appleton-Century-Crofts.

Stewart, K. B., & Walton, R. L. (1992). Teaching the elderly. *Nursing 92, 10,* 66-68.

Storandt, M. (1986). Psychological aspects of aging. In I. Rossman (Ed.), *Clinical geriatrics* (3rd ed.). Philadelphia: J. B. Lippincott

Strauss, A. L., Corbin, J., Fagerhaugh, S., Glaser, B., Maines, D., Suczek, B., & Wiener, C. (1984). *Chronic illness and the quality of life* (2nd ed.). St. Louis: C. V. Mosby.

Swayze, S. (1991). Helping them cope: Developing self-help groups for clients with chronic illness. *Journal of Psychosocial Nursing, 29*(5), 35-39.

Tuazon, N. C. (1992). Discharge teaching: Use this MODEL. *RN, 4,* 19-22.

Windsor, R. A., Bailey, W. C., Richards, J. M., Manzella, B., Soong, S., Brooks, M. (1990). Evaluation of the efficacy and cost effectiveness of health education methods to increase medication adherence among adults with asthma. *AJPH, 80*(12), 1519-1521.

Bibliography

Annand, F. (1993). A challenge for the 1990s: Patient education. *Today's O. R. Nurse, 15*(1), 31-35.

Barnes, L. P. (1991). Commitment to patient education. *MCN, 16,* 17.

———— (1992). The illiterate client: Strategies in patient teaching. *MCN, 17,* 127.

Bartholomew, K., Nix, M. L. (1991). An educational challenge: Focus on Behavior. *Journal of Pediatric Nursing, 6*(4), 288-289.

Bartholomew, K., & Schwartz, P. (1991). Teaching and supporting self-management of chronic illness: An example of translating theory into a family education program. *Journal of Pediatric Nursing, 6*(3), 214-215.

Bartholomew, L. K., Parcel, G. S., Seilheimer, D. K., Czyzewski, D., Spinelli, S. H., & Congdon, B. (1991). Development of a health education program to promote the self-management of cystic fibrosis. *Health Education Quarterly, 18*(4), 429-443.

Davidhizar, R. (1992). Understanding powerlessness in family member caregivers of the chronically ill. *Geriatric Nursing, 3,* 66-69.

Deatrick, J. A., & Knafl, K. A. (1990). Understanding family response to childhood chronic conditions. *Journal of Pediatric Nursing, 5*(1), 2-3.

DiMatteo, M. R., & DiNicola, D. D. (1982). *Achieving patient compliance.* New York: Pergamon.

Dixon, E., & Park, R. (1990). Do patients understand written health information? *Nursing Outlook, 38*(6), 278-281.

Donohue-Porter, P. (1989). Patient education makes all the difference. *RN, 11,* 56-60.

Dunn, S. M., Beeney, L. J., Hoskins, P. L., & Turtle, J. R. (1990). Knowledge and attitude change as predictors of metabolic improvement in diabetes education. *Social Science and Medicine, 31*(10), 1135-1141.

Eliopoulos, C. (1993). *Gerontological nursing* (3rd ed.). Philadelphia: J. B. Lippincott.

Fulton, M. L., & Coulter, S. J. (1989). Alternative means of patient education. *Nursing Management, 20*(11), 58-60.

Funnell, M. M., & Merritt, J. H. (1993). The challenges of diabetes and older adults. *Nursing Clinics of North America, 28*(1), 45-60.

Good-Reis, D. V., & Pieper, B. A. (1990). Structured vs. unstructured Teaching. *AORN Journal, 51*(5), 1334-1335, 1337-1339.

Heyduk, L. J. (1991). Medication education: Increasing patient compliance. *Journal of Psychosocial Nursing, 29*(12), 32-35.

Kazdin, A. E. (1989). *Behavior modification in applied settings* (4th ed.). Belmont, CA: Brooks-Cole.

Marshall, C. E., & Richards J. (1989). Developing culturally based patient education materials for non-reading, elderly Hispanics. *Techtrends, 34*(1), 27-30.

McCabe, B. J., Tysinger, J. W., Kreger, M., & Currwin, A. C. (1989). Strategy for designing effective patient education materials. *Journal of American Dietetic Association, 89*(9), 1290-1295.

Puntil, C. (1991). Integrating three approaches to counter resistance in a noncompliant elderly client. *Journal of Psychosocial Nursing, 29*(2), 26-32.

Rakel, B. A. (1992). Interventions related to patient teaching. *Nursing Clinics of North America, 27*(2), 397-423.

Rankin, S. H., Stallings, K. D. (1990). *Patient education: Issues, principles, practices* (2nd ed.). Philadelphia J. B. Lippincott.

Ross, F. M. (1991). Patient compliance—Whose responsibility? *Social Science and Medicine, 32*(1), 89-94.

Schofer, K. K., & Ward, C. J. (1990). Computerization of the patient education process. *Computers in Nursing, 8*(3), 116-122.

Simons, M. R. (1992). Interventions related to compliance. *Nursing Clinics of North America, 27*(2), 477-494.

Smith, C. E. (1987). *Patient education: Nurses in partnership with other health professionals.* Philadelphia: W. B. Saunders.

Squyres, W. (1985). *Patient education and health promotion in medical care.* Mountain View, CA: Mayfield.

Thorne, S. E. (1990). Constructive noncompliance in chronic illness. *Holistic Nursing Practice, 5*(1), 62-69.

Tucker, C. M. (1989). Effects of behavioral intervention with patients, nurses, and family members on dietary noncompliance in chronic hemodialysis patients. *Transplantation Proceedings, 21*(6), 3985-3988.

Williams B. (1991). Medication education. *Nursing Times, 87*(29), 50-52.

Wolfe, S. C., Schirm, V. (1992). Medication counseling for the elderly: Effects on knowledge and compliance after hospital discharge. *Geriatric Nursing, 5,* 134-138.

CHAPTER 17

Research

Karen Thornbury Labuhn

Introduction

Chronic illness presents a major challenge to nurses and other health professionals. Other chapters in this text discuss many of the problems imposed by chronic illness. These chapters offer suggestions as to how nurses and other health care professionals can assist individuals and families not only in coping with these problems but in maintaining optimal functioning and quality of life. Many of the suggested treatment approaches are based on knowledge generated by research. However, there are still many unanswered questions regarding chronicity. Ongoing research is needed to strengthen the scientific knowledge base for practice in the prevention of chronic illness and the care of the chronically ill.

This chapter presents a historical overview of health and nursing research and examines various types of research studies that contribute to the scientific knowledge base for chronic care nursing practice. Major methodologies used to address research questions about chronicity are described with examples of clinically relevant nursing research studies. Some of the advantages and challenges of research are highlighted, and suggestions are offered as to how practicing nurses can overcome barriers to participation in research and strengthen their commitment to research-based practice.

Research-Based Nursing Practice

All nurses practicing in the United States are expected to participate in research activities related to their practice. Recent American Nurses' Association (ANA) Standards of Clinical Nursing Practice clearly specify nurses' participation in research and research utilization as requirements for professional performance (ANA, 1992) (see Table 17-1). The ANA has published guidelines for appropriate research activities of nurses at different levels of education preparation (ANA, 1985, 1989; Fawcett, 1986).

Although the preponderance of nursing research studies are directed by individuals with doctoral degrees or advanced preparation in research, all nurses can actively participate in research by identifying researchable problems in their practice, collaborating with investigators on research studies relevant to their practice, and accessing and using research findings to improve patient care (Burns & Grove, 1987; Cronenwett, 1987; Fawcett, 1984; Horsley, 1985; Kirchhoff, 1983; Lindeman, 1988; Morse & Conrad, 1983; Whitney, 1986).

TABLE 17-1. ANA guidelines for research activities of nurses

Associate degree	Appreciates and values research Helps identify clinical problems for investigation Assists in data collection, using established protocols Collaborates in utilizing research in clinical practice
Baccalaureate degree	Critically evaluates research reports Understands ethical principles in research Assists investigators in identifying and accessing study subjects Provides input on data collection methods Utilizes existing research findings in practice Understands clinical research protocols of other disciplines
Master's degree	Collaborates with investigators in developing research proposals Serves as a clinical expert on the research process Evaluates clinical relevance of research findings Ensures appropriate integration of research in practice Creates a clinical practice environment to support research
Doctoral degree	Functions as an independent investigator Designs and conducts research to develop nursing theory Collaborates with clinicians and other investigators Obtains external funding for research studies Disseminates research findings to the profession and the public
Postdoctoral training	Carries out research activities of doctorally prepared nurse. Conducts programs of research in a focused practice area

SOURCE: Adapted from American Nurses' Association (1989). *Education for participation in research.* Kansas City, MO: American Nurses' Association.

Nurses who work with chronically ill individuals may be dissatisfied with the limited impact of their interventions, yet be unaware of research findings that offer possible solutions to treatment impasses or that explain why a particular treatment approach is ineffective. Even when research does not offer an immediate solution to a practice problem, it may suggest a new way of looking at the problem and thus improve clinical decision making. Research also can provide important information about the costs of new innovations or care approaches. This has important implications for chronically ill individuals and their families, health care providers, and taxpayers who carry much of the economic burden for health care. The nursing profession also benefits from documenting its cost-effectiveness because the scope of nursing practice is strongly influenced by economic considerations (Ventura et al., 1985).

Historical Perspectives: Health Research

Health research in the United States has undergone considerable growth and change since the early 1900s. In the early part of the century, research studies consisted primarily of privately funded medical investigations to find cures for infectious diseases. With the improvement in public health and the discovery of antibiotics, X rays, and other diagnostic techniques during World War II, infectious diseases were brought under better control, and attention was directed toward chronic conditions—for example, heart disease, strokes, and malignancies—which were becoming major health problems (Department of Health, Education, & Welfare [DHEW], 1979). Interest in mental disorders also increased during the post–World War II years because of the large numbers of veterans with combat-related mental problems and the discovery of tranquilizer drugs that offered hope for improved treatment.

From the 1940s to the mid-1960s, biomedical research on chronic diseases flourished in medical centers, with investigators attempting to discover the causes of specific disease conditions and on finding effective medical treatments and cures. During this time federal funding for medical research increased substantially, and the National Institutes of Health (NIH) were established to provide leadership for research endeavors. The National Cancer Institute was the first NIH institute established to investigate a specific disease. It was followed by institutes for heart and lung diseases, allergy and infectious diseases, and mental disorders in the 1940s, and by institutes for arthritis and metabolic disorders, neurologic problems, eye diseases, and environmental health problems in the 1950s and 1960s (Larson, 1984).

The growing interest in environmental, psychosocial, and behavioral risk factors in health and illness led to increasing numbers of psychologists, sociologists, nurses, and public health professionals initiating research studies and collaborating on large multidisciplinary research projects. The National Institute on Child Health and Human Development, established in 1969, and the National Institute of Aging, established in 1974, supported the development of research with a biobehavioral perspective. In 1979, the U.S. surgeon general published a national report on health promotion and disease prevention (DHEW, 1979), which stimulated federal funding agencies to sponsor a series of demonstration projects to test the effectiveness of community-based prevention programs for chronic conditions, including detection and early treatment of hypertension and promotion of healthy life-styles to prevent heart disease. Studies to determine the effectiveness of community screening programs for cancer detection and prevention also were funded (National Center for Health Statistics [NCHS], 1983).

During the 1980s and early 1990s, funding for biomedical studies continued at a high level, with emphasis on cancer and AIDS research. Research on other chronic conditions also was supported by the NIH institutes as well as by a growing number of private foundations and professional associations. Studies on the cost and quality of care emerged during this period. In 1989, The Agency for Health Care Policy and Research (AHCPR) was created to administer the Medical Treatment Effectiveness Program (MEDTEP), a federal program directed toward developing standardized measures for patient outcomes, evaluating the efficacy of medical treatments, and disseminating clinical practice guidelines. In addition to typical measures of mortality and morbidity data, quality-of-life indicators, such as functional status and emotional status, are now included in the databases (Rettig, 1991; Salive, Mayfield, & Weissman, 1990).

Since initiation of the MEDTEP program, several multidisciplinary patient outcomes research teams (PORTS) have received grants to conduct studies of medical treatment for selected problems, including several chronic conditions such as cardiovascular disease, strokes, and chronic pain (Salive et al., 1990). The current mandate of the PORTS is to identify medical practice patterns and to test methods for reducing inappropriate variations in practice (Rettig, 1991).

Development of Nursing Research

During the formative years of the NIH research programs, nursing studies focused primarily on manpower and activities of the profession rather than on health problems of individuals, families, or communities. However, there has been progressive development of nursing research focusing on care issues over the past three decades. Table 17–2 shows the major historical highlights of this trend.

Nursing graduate programs with a clinical research focus began in the 1950s with start-up funding from the federal government. During the 1960s and 1970s, small grants programs were established to support faculty research and develop research programs in graduate schools of nursing. Several surveys identified the need for a stronger research database for nursing practice. In the early 1980s, nursing research began to be recognized nationally. Increasing numbers of nurse scientists served on scientific review

TABLE 17-2.   Historical highlights

Dates	Legislation/Agency	Nursing Research Activities
1920–1940		A few case studies and patient-centered care plans appear in nursing literature.
1940–1950		Surveys on nursing needs and resources: Goldmark Report, Committee for the Grading of Nursing Schools Study, Brown's *Nursing for the Future* publication.
		World War II prompts collection of data on nursing resources and stimulates interest in documenting nursing practices. Systematic evaluation of nursing techniques are recommended.
	Division of Nursing Resources, U.S. Public Health Service (1948)	Agency is mandated to investigate nursing supply and distribution, quality and costs of nursing education, job satisfaction and turnover, patient and personnel satisfaction with care. Studies lead to published guidelines for nursing activity studies.
1950–1960		ANA conducts study of nursing activities and publishes document on functions, standards, and qualifications for nursing practice.
	Nursing Research Grants and Fellowship Program, U.S. Public Health Service (1955). Administered under NIH.	Grants provide funding for development of clinical graduate programs in nursing. A few fellowships are awarded for doctoral studies in nursing-related disciplines.
1960–1970	Institutional Training Grant Program, U.S. Public Health Service (1962). Administered under NIH until 1963, then transferred to Division of Nursing Faculty Research and Development Grants Program.	Grants increase funding for training of nurse scientists in disciplines related to nursing. Studies are conducted on nursing education and patient care issues.
		Grants provide funds for research development in 19 nursing schools and 3 other agencies. Clinical studies are initiated in interpersonal aspects of care, death and dying, and other topics.
1970–1980	Research Development Grants Program, Division of Nursing	Funds are provided to 20 nursing schools for research development. Emphasis is on generating knowledge for practice.
		WICHE Delphi study of clinical nursing research priorities identifies need for greater utilization of research in practice, development of valid and reliable research instruments, and studies on the impact of nursing interventions.
		National Academy of Science surveys doctoral programs in nursing (1977–1978) and recommends strengthening of faculty research productivity and existing doctoral programs.
	Division of Nursing Research Grants Program (component of biomedical and behavioral research grants program authorized under U.S. Public Health Service)	Grants are made available for individual nurse investigators, research conferences, and institutional research projects.
		More nurses conduct clinical studies and obtain funding from federal and private sources.

TABLE 17–2. *Continued*

Dates	Legislation/Agency	Nursing Research Activities
1980–1990	Nursing Research Grants Program, Division of Nursing	Nursing research grants are expanded to include program grants for collaborative studies, new investigator awards, research utilization studies, and small business grants.
		ANA (1981) identifies five priorities for clinical nursing research:
		1. Promoting well-being and self-care
		2. Preventing health problems
		3. Decreasing the impact of illness on coping abilities, productivity, and life satisfaction
		4. Ensuring care needs of vulnerable populations
		5. Developing cost-effective care delivery systems
		Academy of Sciences Institute of Medicine Report on Nursing and Nursing Education (1983) recommends better integration of nursing research into the scientific community and advocates a federal center for nursing research. Nursing groups lobby for an NIH institute for nursing research.
		ANA Cabinet on Nursing Research (1985) publishes *Directions for Nursing Research: Toward the 21st Century,* outlining a national research agenda for nursing.
		By 1984, more than 4,000 nurses have doctoral degrees. Doctorally prepared nurses are employed in many clinical settings as well as in universities. Nurses become more active in the political arena and are appointed to national health advisory councils.
	National Center for Nursing Research (1986)	NCNR established at NIH in 1986. Work is begun on a national nursing research agenda. Seven priority areas for research identified:
		1. Low birthweight
		2. HIV prevention and care
		3. Long-term care for elders
		4. Symptom management: pain
		5. Nursing information systems
		6. Health promotion for older children and adolescents
		7. Technology dependency across the life span
		NCNR issues program announcements and requests for applications (RFAs) for research in priority areas. Investigator-initiated proposals also are funded.
	International Center for Nursing Scholarship (1989)	Sigma Theta Tau International (SSTI) establishes Center for Nursing Scholarship in Indianapolis, IN.
1990–	Virginia Henderson International Nursing Library	Work on online library at Center for Nursing Scholarship in progress. By 1993, several on-line databases are available to users, including the *Directory of Nurse Researchers* and the *Online Journal of Knowledge Synthesis for Nursing.*
		SSTI sponsors small grants program to facilitate pilot research projects and research utilization studies. Information for research applications is disseminated to practitioners through regional conferences, professional journals, and videotapes.
		In 1993, SSTI and Mosby Company begin co-sponsoring monthly TV series, "Nursing Approach" to educate the public about current issues in professional nursing.
	National Institute for Nursing Research (1993)	NCNR becomes the National Institute for Nursing Research.

panels and were appointed to health policy committees and national advisory panels. In 1983, the National Science Foundation Institute of Medicine issued a report on nursing that recommended increased funding for nursing research and the establishment of a federal center for this purpose. Three years later the National Center for Nursing Research (NCNR) was established within the NIH. The NCNR became the National Institute for Nursing Research in 1993, establishing nursing as an integral part of the health science community (NCNR, 1993).

One of the initial tasks of the NCNR was to set priorities and guide resource allocation. Fifty nurse-scientists with research expertise in various practice areas met in a two-day invitational conference to delineate immediate research priorities. Following this conference, priority expert panels ("PEPs"), composed of multidisciplinary groups of health scientists, reviewed the scientific literature for each priority area, identified gaps in the knowledge base, and developed recommendations for research program announcements and calls for proposals. The seven priority areas established in 1988 were (1) low birthweight, (2) HIV infection, (3) long-term care for elders, (4) pain management, (5) nursing informatics, (6) health promotion for older children and adolescents, and (7) technology dependency (NCNR, 1993).

The second national conference on nursing research priorities was held in 1992, and five priority areas were targeted for 1995 through 1999: (1) nursing models for community-based care, (2) nursing interventions for HIV/AIDS, (3) cognitive impairment, (4) living with chronic illness, and (5) biobehavioral factors related to immunocompetence (NCNR, 1992). Additional program announcements were issued for 1993 research initiatives on psychosocial interventions in cancer, quality of life assessments, clinical care in nursing homes, home health care, aging and long-term care, and nursing and biological interface studies (National Institute for Nursing Research [NINR], 1993).

The NINR collaborates with the AHCPR in developmental work on patient outcomes research for nursing. The first national conference on applications of patient outcomes research for nursing was held in 1991 (NCNR, 1991). Another conference was scheduled for late 1994. Ongoing work on a Nursing Minimum Data Set (Devine & Werley, 1988; Werley et al., 1991) supports the work on patient outcomes research. The Nursing Minimum Data Set contains information that practicing nurses use across treatment settings, such as patient demographics, nursing diagnoses and interventions, treatment outcomes (resolution of nursing diagnoses or patient problems), and utilization patterns. This data set also is a prototype for development of clinical information systems (CIS) in practice settings. CIS systems will make it easier for nurses to monitor individual patients' responses to interventions and make more timely decisions about nursing practice.

Major Areas of Chronicity Research

Several broad areas of research contribute to the knowledge base needed for chronic care nursing practice. Studies to determine how environmental, psychosocial, and behavioral factors influence the development and progression of specific chronic illnesses are frequently reported in health research journals. A recent study by Polivka, Nickel, and Wilkins (1993) used epidemiological methods to compare the health histories of a sample of children with cerebral palsy and a sample of healthy children to identify exposure variables that could be risk factors for the disease. Birth weight/gestational age, APGAR scores, medication to prevent miscarriage, and urinary tract infection were found to be significantly different in the two groups of children. This study provided useful data for developing hypotheses about possible causes of cerebral palsy; it alerted nurses of the need to assess potential risk factors.

There has been extensive research on psychosocial factors influencing the course of chronic illness. Studies include patients' health beliefs and regimen adherence (Redeker, 1988; Roberson, 1992), social supports (Primomo, Yates, & Woods, 1990), and coping variables (Dodd, Dibble, & Thomas, 1993; O'Brein, 1993; Piazza et al., 1991; Raleigh, 1992). Studies of patients' health behaviors that affect disease outcomes also are frequently published. An example of health behavior research was reported by Labuhn, Lewis, and Koon (1993) on rural and urban COPD patients' smoking cessation experiences. Findings from this study showed similar smoking cessation rates for rural and urban patients. However, there were rural/urban differences in smoking cessation methods and support systems. Spouse smoking had a major impact on cessation outcomes for rural patients but not for urban patients, suggesting that smoking intervention programs for COPD patients living in rural areas need to incorporate strategies to help spouses quit smoking.

Another important area of research on chronic illness is the impact of the illness on patients and families. Studies on the trajectory of chronic illness (Corbin & Strauss, 1984); Fagerhaugh et al., 1987; Strauss et al., 1984; Wiener & Dodd, 1993) focus on disease consequences and work done by patients and other involved persons to manage the illness (see Chapter 3, on illness trajectory). The illness trajectory model has generated rich theory for nursing practice and has led to studies of illness management and coping in many diseases, such as cancer, cardiac disease, HIV, mental illness, multiple sclerosis, diabetes, and epilepsy.[1]

There is a growing body of research literature on quality-of-life studies in chronic illness,[2] both for adults (Breitmeyer et al., 1992; Burckhardt et al., 1989; Ferrell et al., 1992; McSweeny & Labuhn, 1990; Sexton & Munro, 1988; Strauss et al., 1984) and children (Neff & Dale, 1990; Whyte, 1992). The recent increase in federal funding for quality of life studies will allow more nurse investigators and other health scientists to conduct programs of research in this area.

Findings from recent caregiving studies provide useful information about specific caregiving tasks, the burdens and satisfactions of caregiving, and the characteristics of caregiver/care receiver relationships (Archbold & Stewart, 1987; Brown & Powell-Cope, 1991; Cantor, 1983; Lindgren, 1993; Sayles-Cross, 1993; Sexton & Munro, 1985; Zerwekh, 1991). Most studies on caregiving focus on spouse or family caregivers of chronically ill individuals or elders. However, caregiving acts of patients for each other also have been studied by nurse researchers. One such study conducted exploratory interviews with nursing home residents to gain information about their caregiving acts for each other; it identified four major caregiving behavior categories: protecting, supporting, confirming, and transcending (praying) (Hutchinson & Bahr, 1991). Many of the elders interviewed noted that caregiving was an important means of maintaining personal identity and self-esteem.

Another area of research that contributes to the knowledge base for chronic care nursing practice is health services research, which focuses on issues related to the delivery of care, including the cost-effectiveness of care delivery models, ethical issues, and provider concerns including staffing patterns and job satisfaction (Ingersol, Hoffart, & Schultz, 1990). Some health services research studies evaluate care delivery models such as nursing case management (see Chapter 20, on case management) and look at patient and caregivers. These studies may evaluate the relative costs and benefits of alternative care delivery models or systems. Although several research studies have demonstrated that case management is a cost-effective approach to delivering care to chronically ill patients. However, most of these studies have a weak theory base and the intervention components are not well defined. Thus, limited information is available to determine what aspects of case management are responsible for improved patient outcomes or cost savings (Lamb, 1992). Additional research is needed to examine the process and outcomes of case management and other innovative ways of delivering care to the chronically ill.

---

[1]Major findings from some of the studies on illness trajectories are reviewed in *Chronic Illness Trajectory Frameworks* edited by Woog (1991).

[2]Two new international journals, *Quality of Life Newsletter* and *Quality of Life* are good sources of information on current studies. The text, *Quality-of-Life Assessments in Clinical Trials* (Spilker, 1990), is a useful resource, since it summarizes current studies in this area for several chronic illnesses and discusses methodological issues on quality-of-life research.

Research Approaches and Methodologies

Determining whether relationships between events or variables are causal in nature is a complicated process. Research studies that attempt to establish cause need to be based on theory and carefully designed to control for possible confounding factors. Multivariate statistics are generally used to test hypotheses about causal events.[3]

Many research approaches and methodologies are used to study chronic illnesses and related phenomena. *Descriptive studies* provide data on characteristics of patients, the course of an illness, patient coping strategies, or other factors related to nursing practice. These data can then be used to improve clinical assessments, plan services, or predict staffing needs.

Correlational research studies look at relationships between variables and provide useful information about illness processes. Findings from these studies help investigators develop hypotheses about relationships between events —for example, whether cigarette smoking is associated with disease exacerbation. Statistical tests are used to determine whether findings from a study can be generalized beyond the study sample. *Survey research*, in which data are collected by questionnaires or interviews, primarily yields descriptive data, although relationships between variables can be explored during the data analysis.

Intervention studies focus on evaluating the effectiveness of practice innovations. These studies examine patient outcomes for a new treatment approach, comparing them with outcomes of usual care or comparing the relative effectiveness of different treatment approaches. Whether these studies use rigorous (experimental) or quasi-experimental designs, the interventions being tested need to be based on sound rationale or theory. One intervention study focused on testing the effectiveness of taped relaxation messages on anxiety (as measured by skin tem-

perature, heart rate, and respiratory rate) and dyspnea in patients with chronic obstructive pulmonary disease (COPD) (Gift, Moore, & Soeken, 1992). The potential benefits of music therapy and taped relaxation messages had already been documented in the literature for several populations, including critical care patients and cancer patients. In this study, 26 patients with COPD were randomized to either a control group or a treatment group. Over the four-week course of the study, both anxiety and dyspnea decreased in the treatment group but not in the control group. In addition, patients listening to the relaxation tapes also had less airway obstruction at the end of the study.

Studies that include small numbers of patients, such as in the example above, must be *replicated* before the findings can be generalized to a wider patient population (Reynolds & Haller, 1986). Usually nursing innovations are tested in a series of studies. Initially, pilot studies are conducted to test the intervention protocols, data collection procedures, and measurement tools. Then a small randomized trial is carried out. If the intervention appears to be effective, the investigators design a controlled clinical trial with a larger study sample to confirm the hypothesized effect of the innovation on the identified patient outcomes. A power analysis is used to determine the number of patients needed to statistically test the hypothesis at a given confidence level (Munro et al., 1986).

Qualitative and Quantitative Methods Both qualitative and quantitative methods have an important role in studies of chronic illness. Table 17–3 outlines and compares some of the major features of these methods.

Qualitative Research Qualitative research usually entails in-depth interviews with limited numbers of study subjects to explore illness phenomena or describe the subjective experiences of patients, caregivers, or other family members. Narrative accounts from the interviews and/or themes identified when the investigators analyze the data provide an important perspective regarding illness that cannot be captured quantitatively (Knafl & Howard, 1984). Data from qualitative studies often are used to generate the-

---

[3]For in-depth discussion of these issues, readers are encouraged to consult research methods textbooks such as those by Burns and Grove (1987); Munro, Visintainer, and Page (1986); and Valanis (1992).

TABLE 17-3. Major features of qualitative and quantitative research methods

	Qualitative	*Quantitative*
Purposes	Gathering information about a relatively unknown phenomenon; conceptualization and theory formulation; supplementing quantitative data to increase sensitivity and understanding of clients' problems; developing research instruments.	Gathering information to describe or explain phenomena when variables can be defined clearly and operationalized; testing theory, validating research instruments; formal hypothesis testing.
Types of studies	Observational studies; anthropologic or ethnographic studies; case studies; interviews. Qualitative data can be collected and studied to assess the impact of interventions, but cannot be used to test hypotheses statistically.	Observational studies; formal surveys, questionnaires with coded response options such as rating scales. Intervention studies with experimental or quasi-experimental designs. Expected outcomes of intervention are measured or categorized, using precoded formats.
Data collection	Often by participant observation. Investigators use field notes to collect narrative information or record selected data from audiotapes or videotapes. Information also can be collected from medical records, diaries, and other documents.	Survey data collected by mailed questionnaires or by telephone or face-to-face interviewing. Data in intervention studies collected by observation, participant observation, medical record review, or other recordings. Standardized protocols for intervention and data collection are used.
Data generated	Narrative descriptions (from clients' statements or observers' recordings). Information is studied for its substantive meaning. Content analysis or grounded methods are used to identify themes and/or meanings; typologies may be developed.	Numerical data or information grouped into categories. Various descriptive or inferential statistics may be used, depending on the level of data (nominal, ordinal, interval, ratio) and purpose of the study (descriptive, explanatory, hypothesis testing).
Strengths	Qualitative data provide in-depth information concerning clients' subjective experiences or other observable phenomena, thus are useful in theory construction. Case studies are easier to conduct in practice settings than are full-scale surveys or randomized experiments. Methods have been developed to ensure validity and completeness of data.	Quantitative data may be easier to interpret and are needed for hypothesis testing, since outcomes are clearly defined and measured. Procedures for assessing validity and reliability of measurement tools are well developed. Threats to validity in quasi-experimental research studies can be assessed, and control established through study design or data analysis.
Weaknesses	Methods of data collection may be less precise and not universally accepted. Funding agencies may consider qualitative methods "weaker" than quantitative methods.	Information obtained may provide limited answers to theoretical questions or may not adequately explain phenomena. Well-controlled studies are difficult to implement in practice settings. Usually need large sample of subjects for research questions to be answered, especially if results are to be generalized to wider population.

ories or develop standardized measurement tools.

Corbin and Strauss's study of couples' management of chronic illness is a good example of qualitative methods in nursing research (Corbin & Strauss, 1984). Using unstructured interviews, these investigators collected narrative information from 60 couples on their experiences with their illnesses over a period of two years. The information was organized into a meaningful conceptual framework, and guidelines were developed to assist couples in achieving effective collaboration in illness management. Another qualitative study (LeMone, 1993) explored human sexuality among adults diagnosed with diabetes mellitus (DM). Using in-depth interviews with 11 men and 8 women, the researchers documented sexuality changes associated with DM and identified strategies that individuals use to cope with these changes. Findings from the study were used to develop assessment tools that nurses can use to determine patients' emotional responses to sexuality changes.

Quantitative Research Quantitative methods are used when a research topic has been previously investigated, variables have been clearly identified, and measurement tools have been tested for validity and reliability. Quantitative methods are used in numerous investigations of chronic illness, including descriptive studies, correlational studies, and intervention studies. In the nursing literature, quantitative methods often are used to examine relationships between biopsychosocial and behavioral factors related to coping.

In a recent study, O'Brein (1993) administered several quantitative instruments[4] to 101 individuals with multiple sclerosis and used multiple regression techniques to determine the independent and combined effects of self-esteem and social support on coping. Findings from the analysis demonstrated that patients with high self-esteem used many problem-focused coping strategies, whereas those with low self-esteem were more likely to use emotion-focused coping strategies. Interestingly, individuals with the greatest degree of dysfunction had the least amount of perceived social support. This study provided useful empirical data about the wide array of strategies that patients with multiple sclerosis use to cope with the illness. The study findings also suggest that patients need more help to mobilize social supports for coping as they become increasingly disabled.

Combining Qualitative and Quantitative Methods   A growing number of nurse investigators recommend the joint use of quantitative and qualitative methods in a given research study (Breitmeyer et al., 1993; Duffy, 1987; Goodwin & Goodwin, 1984; Hasse & Myers, 1988; Hines & Young, 1987; Hoeffer & Archbold, 1983; Knafl & Breitmeyer, 1991). The term "triangulation" describes situations in which more than one research approach or method is used in a single research study. Banik (1993) describes several types of triangulation: using multiple theories to explain nursing phenomena, gathering data from multiple sources, having multiple data collectors or analysts, and using different study methods. Triangulation can be used for verification purposes or to enrich the database. For example, qualitative information from open-ended interviews can supplement findings from a quantitative analysis, helping the researcher to better understand the substantive meaning of statistical associations (Hoeffer & Archbold, 1983). If an investigator derives similar conclusions from the qualitative and quantitative data, it also helps to cross-validate the research findings.

Barriers to Research

Despite the potential benefits of research into chronic illness, only a limited number of practicing nurses initiate research in practice settings or collaborate with investigators. In addition, chronic health problems are very complex and more resistant to intervention than are most acute health problems. Although more funding for research on chronic illness is available,

---

[4]Quantitative instruments used in this study included The Ways of Coping Checklist (Lazarus & Folkman, 1984), the Tennessee Self-Concept Scale (Fitts et al., 1991), and the Norbeck Social Support Questionnaire (Norbeck et al., 1981).

financial support tends to be directed toward prevention or cure of specific diseases. In addition, most practicing nurses are unaware of research studies in their clinical areas, and many practice settings do not encourage nurses to utilize research.

Conducting Research in Practice Settings

It can be a major challenge to initiate research in practice settings or even to collaborate with investigators on research projects. The case study discussing pet therapy illustrates some of the dilemmas nurses face when they attempt to introduce research in practice. Nursing colleagues may not appreciate or value research and may be reluctant to support research activities (Champion & Leach, 1989; Goode et al., 1987). In fact, nurses graduating from education programs that do not adequately incorporate research coursework may be intimidated by research terminology and procedures and respond defensively when asked to participate in research.

Many nurses are unaware of professional expectations for research, despite the ANA's published guidelines and standards noted in Table 17-1. In addition, health care organizations have been slow to establish policies for nursing research, and many facilities do not have formal structures to facilitate nurses' involvement in research.

Limited Research Resources   A barrier to nurses' participation in research is the limited research resources in practice settings. While university-affiliated hospitals or large health care systems such as health maintenance organizations (HMOs) usually have libraries and other resources to support research activities, chronic care settings often are physically isolated from research centers and psychologically cut off from the mainstream of research. Nurses working in these settings need to network with professional colleagues and nursing organizations to obtain assistance and support for research endeavors. Without this support, it is difficult to engage in research.

Conflict of Research Versus Service Roles
Conflict between research and clinical service roles may deter some nurses from participating in research. Internal role conflict can occur because of the differing expectations of research versus patient care (Martin, 1990). For example, when collecting data for research purposes, the nurse must attempt to maintain objectivity and not bias the client's responses, whereas the nurse who functions as a practitioner intentionally attempts to influence the client's feelings and responses in order to effect positive adaptation. Competing time demands of research and clinical service are a major concern in most health care settings (Rempusheski, 1991). Because patient care normally must be given first priority in practice settings, nurses may need to volunteer their personal time to carry out research activities. In some practice settings, funds are available for clinical release time to allow nurses to participate in research. However, to actively participate, nurses generally need considerable skill to balance priorities and obtain sufficient support from colleagues and nurse managers (Rempusheski, 1991).

Recently several research publications have been introduced that are addressed to practicing nurses (Barnsteiner, 1993).[5] However, determining when research findings should be applied in the clinical practice setting is a major challenge. The long time lag between completion of research studies and their publication can limit the relevance of findings (Funk et al., 1989). Also, many nursing studies are conducted with small groups of patients and are not replicated (Reynolds & Haller, 1986; Lelean, 1982), limiting their application. Innovations based on research findings need to be systematically evaluated in the clinical setting in order to ensure their overall benefits to clients. The desired effect of a new

---

[5]Examples of research publications for practicing nurses include the quarterly *Nursing Scan in Research: Application to Clinical Practice,* which provides brief summary reports and critiques of current research studies on specific topics or clinical areas of practice; *Annual Review of Nursing Research,* which summarizes research findings from groups of studies on specific clinical topics; and Sigma Theta Tau International's new publication, *Online: Journal of Knowledge Synthesis for Nursing,* which summarizes current research information on nursing topics with recommendations for practice.

CASE STUDY
Initiating Research

Sally W., a baccalaureate nurse recently employed in a new rehabilitation center, noticed that many clients brought to the center were withdrawn and difficult to engage in treatment. Aware of reports of successful pet therapy for the elderly, Sally introduced the idea of a research study to the staff. She explained that while previous research suggested that pets could have a positive impact on an elderly patient's orientation and mood states, additional studies needed to be conducted to see if rehabilitation patients have a similar response.

Some of the staff expressed interest in pet therapy, but saw no need for a research study.

One of the nurses commented that "research is for doctors, not nurses." Another nurse reminded Sally of the difficulty in obtaining permission for research. The nurse manager could not give Sally release time to conduct research activities at the center, but was interested in the proposed research project and agreed to promote the study with the other staff and provide start-up funds for needed supplies. Sally began work on a literature review and sought guidance from a faculty member at a local university in preparing a formal research proposal.

---

nursing practice, as well as unexpected outcomes, should be compared against those of the traditional nursing practice, using well-defined outcome measures (Reynolds & Haller, 1986).

Barriers to Research Utilization

A number of authors have attempted to identify barriers to research utilization in nursing (Bircumshaw, 1990; Funk et al., 1991; King, Barnard, & Hoehn, 1981; Hefferin, Horsley, & Ventura, 1982; Kirchhoff, 1983; Levin, 1986). In a review of the literature, Champion and Leach (1989) found three major variables associated with research utilization: attitudes of nurses, availability of research findings, and support from the practice environment. Funk et al. (1991) did a factor analysis of data from a questionnaire survey of interviews with practicing nurses that was distributed to a national sample of nurse members of the American Nurses' Association. The analysis revealed four major categories of research utilization barriers: (1) nurses' research values and skills, (2) characteristics of the research, such as its quality and applicability, (3) accessibility of research findings, and (4) organizational limitations and deterrents. These barriers closely parallel elements in Rogers's theory of innovation diffusion. According to this theory, the time that it takes for a new idea (or innovation) to be accepted depends on charac-

teristics of the innovation (e.g., if it is perceived as useful), the readiness of individuals to adopt new ideas, how the innovation is communicated to potential users, and the social system in which diffusion occurs (Rogers, 1983).

Limited Access to Resources   Nurses' limited use of research findings in practice can be partially explained as an access problem (Burns & Grove, 1987; Champion & Leach, 1989; Funk, Tornquist, & Champagne, 1989). Many clinical settings have inadequate library services, and most practicing nurses have little time to conduct independent literature searches (Kirchhoff, 1983). Fortunately, computer searches are being used increasingly in practice settings to facilitate the rapid retrieval of research reports (Kilby et al., 1989; Dahlen et al., 1987). In addition, nurses are becoming more aware of how to access research articles, such as by using information services at the National Library of Medicine (Colianni, 1987). They are also developing strategies to disseminate research reports to clinical arenas. Some of these strategies are discussed in the applications section later in this chapter.

Other Barriers to Utilizing Research   Just increasing nurses' access to research journals and other resource materials does not ensure that research findings will be appropriately utilized in practice. Some nurses do not read research reports even when they are easily accessible (Bircumshaw, 1990; Champion & Leach, 1989; Hunt, 1987), which may reflect a lack of interest in research, difficulty reading and critiquing research reports, or a lack of time for planning. However, it also can be attributed to the poor packaging and dissemination of research findings. Reports in research journals use technical language and rarely contain information about practice implications (Burns & Grove, 1987; Funk, Tornquist, & Champagne, 1989; Goode et al., 1991; Tornquist et al., 1993). Presentations at research conferences are primarily addressed to investigator audiences and often focus on methodological issues that are of little interest to practitioners (Levin, 1986). Unless nurses have access to summary reports on research that contain critiques and suggestions for practice applications, they need to be skilled in reading research reports and evaluating their quality.

Interventions

The need for research-based practice has long been recognized by the nursing profession. However, for research to have a positive impact on nursing practice, *all* nurses need to be aware of research relevant to their areas of practice and know how to safely utilize research findings to benefit patients and families (Barnard, 1986; Fawcett, 1984; Lindeman, 1988; Morse & Conrad, 1983).

The 1991 accreditation standards of the Joint Commission for Accreditation of Hospitals (JCAHO) require documented evidence of procedures to incorporate new empirical knowledge into nursing practice. However, surveys conducted in the 1980s and early 1990s suggest that many nurses are not aware of new research findings in the literature and do not actively engage in research utilization activities (Hefferin et al., 1982; Kirchhoff, 1983; Brett, 1987; Coyle & Sokop, 1990). This problem is not unique to nursing; a serious time lag between knowledge development and applications in practice exists in most professional disciplines (Bohanon & Lebeau, 1986). However, the limited utilization of research in nursing has particular significance

because of the pressing need for a stronger scientific knowledge base for professional practice.

Conducting Research in Practice

There are many advantages of participating in research studies in practice settings. Research provides opportunities for continued learning of new knowledge relevant to practice. Thus, it may enhance clinical competence and self-confidence. The strong sense of professional identity that results from participation in research also may contribute to a sense of autonomy and help buffer the day-to-day stresses of nursing practice. In addition, participation in research-related activities, such as research conferences or other educational programs, provides opportunities to develop collegial relationships with individuals who have common research interests, and can lead to collaborative work on research projects or research-related activities such as nursing care standards. Another satisfying aspect of participating in research is the awareness of one's contribution to knowledge development for nursing (Green & Houston, 1993). Research-based innovations that can be generalized to patient populations beyond one's immediate practice setting can have a strong influence on professional practice.

Fostering Research in the Clinical Setting

Practicing nurses, especially staff nurses working in clinical settings, are important members of the research team (Rudy, 1991). In addition to helping investigators identify nursing problems that need to be researched, they can contribute to the design of research studies by helping the investigators in understanding the clinical significance of problems being examined, by identifying clinical variables that need to be assessed, and by determining the feasibility of carrying out research procedures in the practice setting (Nail, 1990). During study implementation, staff nurses often carry out research protocols and procedures, such as recruiting study subjects, delivering interventions, collecting data, and performing quality assurance activities. Clinical nurses' expertise also may be sought during data analysis to help identify unmeasured variables that may be contributing to unexpected study outcomes. New hypotheses can then be generated for future testing. Finally, the staff nurse perspective is essential for interpreting the clinical significance of study findings and determining appropriate applications in practice (Nail, 1990).

Despite potential barriers, increasing numbers of practicing nurses are participating in research. In a recent survey of 515 registered nurses in eight western states (Miller, Adams, & Beck, 1993), 21 percent of the respondents had participated in research activities within the past two years and 35 percent had attended research conferences. The introduction of doctorally prepared clinical nurse researchers in practice settings has supported the development of clinical research. In the mid-1980s, Knafl et al. (1987) conducted a nationwide telephone survey of 34 nurse researchers working in clinical settings who reported that they had been actively engaged in over 200 research projects over the previous two years. One-fourth of these projects involved the active participation of staff nurses.

Master's-prepared clinical nurse specialists (CNSs) also are providing strong leadership for nursing research in practice settings and are publishing reports of practice-based research in clinical and research journals (Gaits et al. 1989; Green & Houston, 1993; Hicky, 1990; Kilpack et al., 1991; Martin, 1990; Parker, Gordon, & Brannon, 1992; Rempusheski, 1991). The clinical nurse specialist is becoming a major catalyst for nursing research activities in health care organizations or systems (Martin, 1990). Martin believes that a critical mass of CNSs is necessary to support the integration of nursing research activities in practice.

In commenting on the nurse administrators' role in fostering research, Hunt et al. (1983) states:

> Nursing administration within a service setting must articulate the value of research to clinical practice by creating a climate conducive to research. This is done by incorporating research goals into departmental philosophies, beliefs, and by-laws, by including research objectives in position descriptions,

and by raising the level of research awareness and skills through nursing research committee activities and program offerings.

Promoting Research Utilization

Organized structures need to be developed in clinical practice settings to support nurses' participation in research utilization activities and to ensure the safe introduction of research-based innovations. These organizational structures are similar to those needed to support ongoing research studies in clinical settings.

Organizational issues influencing research utilization in nursing have been addressed at length in the nursing literature (Beckett, 1990; Brett, 1989; Champion & Leach, 1989; Funk, Champagne, & Tornquist, 1991; Green & Houston, 1993; Hunt et al., 1983; Hunt, 1987; Marchette, 1985; Martin, 1993). Several groups of nurse researchers have conducted studies of the research utilization process and developed strategies to integrate research findings into practice.

Federally Funded Projects   The first federally funded research utilization project, initiated in 1971, was the Western Interstate Commission for Higher Education (WICHE) Regional Program for Nursing Research Development (Krueger, Nelson, & Wolanin, 1978). Groups of nurses from various practice settings participated in a three-day workshop to learn about research utilization and the change process. Following the workshop, dyads of nurse educators and clinicians worked together to identify patient care problems, retrieve and critique research reports, develop and implement research-based care plans, and evaluate the effects of planned changes. The dyads developed research-based innovations for perioperative teaching, grief counseling, and constipation management (Burns & Grove, 1987). This project demonstrated the effectiveness of linking researchers and clinician to facilitate research utilization. Individual nurses participating in the project continued using research in practice after the project ended. However, the project had limited impact on the organizations' overall commitment to research (Krueger, Nelson, & Wolanin, 1978).

The second federally funded research utilization project, conducted from 1975 to 1980 under the auspices of the Michigan Nurses Association, was the Conduct and Utilization of Research in Nursing (CURN) study (Horsley et al., 1983). Major goals of this project were to translate research findings into clinical protocols for nursing practice and to develop organizational mechanisms to facilitate research utilization. Each published protocol describes the clinical problem being studied, the innovation under consideration, a summary of studies supporting the innovation (called the "research base"), and procedures for systematically evaluating the innovation in the practice setting. Ten CURN protocols have been published and are currently available. Those most relevant to chronic care include catheterization procedures, distress reduction, decubiti treatment, pain reduction, and mutual goal setting (CURN, 1983). The protocols are useful resources for information on both the clinical topic and the research utilization process.[6]

Other Utilization Projects The Nursing Child Assessment Satellite Training Project (NCAST), an ongoing research utilization project conducted by faculty at the University of Washington School of Nursing (King, Barnard, & Hoehn, 1981), translates research reports on childrens' health assessments into clinically meaningful terminology and disseminates findings to individual participating nurses via satellite communication systems. In addition, various other modes of communication, such as videotapes, two-way interaction by telephone, and printed resources, are being evaluated. The project initially was directed toward nurses working in patients' homes, but has now been expanded to include hospital settings. The investigators report high rates of utilization of the health assessment techniques being disseminated by satellite systems (Barnard, 1986).

Faculty at the University of North Carolina recently carried out a three-year research utiliza-

tion project that examined innovative methods of disseminating research information to practicing nurses (Funk, Tornquist, & Champagne, 1989). Methods included topic-focused conferences, monographs of conference proceedings, and an information center that could be accessed by telephone. Each conference and monograph series addressed one broad research topic where detailed summaries of research findings were presented with descriptions of major findings and practice implications. The structure of these conference sessions provided opportunity for dialogue between the researchers and clinicians on how findings could be used in practice, including strategies for evaluating the impact of research-based innovations. The monographs of conference proceedings were disseminated to participating nurses' practice settings to reinforce the learning experience and share information with other nurses.

Currently, the Orange County Research and Utilization Project (OCRUN), is being implemented by a consortium of 19 hospitals and 6 academic institutions in Southern California (OCRUN, 1992). The objective of this project is to provide a competency-driven continuing education program in research utilization to administrators, nurse managers, and clinicians. Nurse executives and administrators are offered an 8-hour course on organizational strategies to facilitate research utilization and research program development. A 16-hour course is offered to nurse educators and research facilitators that contains information on implementing research utilization projects and on teaching research utilization. Another 16-hour course, directed toward practicing nurses, includes information on identifying practice problems, conducting literature reviews, critiquing research reports, developing innovations based on research, and identifying strategies to overcome barriers to research at the unit level.

The OCRUN project has been successful in stimulating research utilization in participating hospitals, several of which are now conducting research utilization projects. Plans are under way to develop a state-wide infrastructure to support research utilization, using the OCRUN model, which will link nursing service organizations

---

[6]An additional CURN publication, *Using Research to Improve Nursing Practice: A Guide* (CURN, 1983), outlines procedures nurses can use to implement research utilization projects in the practice setting (Horsley et al., 1983).

within geographic regions and develop a dissemination network for research-based practice innovations (OCRUN, 1992).

Practice Application

The research utilization studies described above have demonstrated how research findings can be incorporated into practice in a timely and safe manner. Recent reports in the literature suggest that nurses are implementing research utilization activities in their practice settings (Crane & Horsley 1983; Gaits et al., 1989; Martin, 1990; Parker, Gordon, & Brannon, 1992; Green & Houston, 1993; Goode et al., 1989; Kerfoot & Watson, 1985; Larson, 1983; Watson, Bulechek, & McCloskey, 1987; Yeager & Shannon, 1988). Health care organizations and systems also are developing mechanisms to integrate research findings into standards of care and to support nurses' research utilization activities (Beckett, 1990; Green & Houston, 1993; Goode et al., 1987; Martin, 1993; Ohio Nurses Association, 1990; Simms, Price, & Pfoutz, 1987). Some of the strategies that have been reported in the literature are outlined in Table 17-4.

One of the recent trends is linking quality assurance and research utilization activities, which has both advantages and disadvantages (Kerfoot & Watson, 1985; Lanza, 1990). However, using quality assurance to identify practice problems and then using the research utilization process to develop and test innovation protocols to correct these problems is promising.

Utilizing Research in a Rural Setting A group of nurses at Horn Memorial Hospital in Ida Grove, Iowa, have developed an exemplary research utilization program in a rural practice setting, following recommendations from the CURN study. A research committee, consisting of staff nurses, the education director, and the director of nursing services, was established to act as a change agent and guide the process. Activities of the committee included (1) identifying practice problems, (2) gathering information from research studies, (3) ensuring that nurses have adequate knowledge to read and

TABLE 17-4.   Research utilization activities in practice settings

NURSING UNIT/CLINICAL ARENA

Conduct focus groups to clarify research values

Subscribe to research journals relevant to practice area

Develop library of research resources (videos, textbooks, reports)

Post information about research events on bulletin boards

Initiate unit-wide or arena-wide nursing research forums

Organize journal clubs for reviewing research reports

Mentor new nurses in the research utilization process

Link quality assurance and nursing research activities

Invite nurse researchers to care conferences

Obtain consultation on the research process

ORGANIZATIONAL LEVEL

Incorporate research in mission statement, philosophy, and practice standards

Specify research expectations in job descriptions and performance appraisals

Include research information in orientation sessions

Offer courses on research methods and research utilization

Provide funding for start-up research projects

Provide clinical release time for participation in research

Develop a formal research committee

Include nursing representation on institutional review boards

Ensure a critical mass of clinical nurse specialists

Foster linkages with investigators in academia and other health disciplines

Strengthen library resources/services

Develop online databases for patient outcome studies

Develop structures to disseminate research information

Sponsor nurses at selected national research conferences

Educate the public about research-based nursing practice

Hire a doctorally prepared nurse researcher

critique the literature, (4) determining whether the research is relevant to patients in the practice setting, (5) devising ways of transferring knowledge for use in clinical practice, (6) defining expected patient outcomes, (7) providing education and training as needed, and (8) evaluating the new practice protocols.

The research utilization program resulted in changed policies and procedures for taking temperatures, conducting perioperative teaching, and teaching breastfeeding (Goode et al., 1987). A study guide on research utilization was published (Goode et al., 1991), as well as a report on the organizational change process involved in research utilization (Goode & Bulechek, 1992). The Horn Memorial Group have also produced videotapes on using research in practice (Goode, 1987), critiquing research reports (Goode, 1991), and utilizing research as an organizational change process (Goode & Cipperley, 1989).

Collaboration between Practicing Nurses and Health Care Organizations To be successful, research utilization must be a collaborative endeavor between practicing nurses and the health care organizations in which they work. Individual nurses and groups of practicing nurses need to understand the importance of research-based practice and become intelligent consumers of research. An important part of their contribution to research-based practice is the systematic evaluation of current practices in light of available research findings and development and testing of new innovations based on research. The case study on integrating research into practice demonstrates how one nurse initiated a research utilization group to seek ways of integrating research findings into practice.

Nurse executives and administrators in health care organizations can support the use of research findings in practice by incorporating statements about research in mission statements, policies, and job descriptions, and by developing structures and funding mechanisms to facilitate nurses' research activities. Professional associations and government agencies can support these activities by making resources available and by educating professional colleagues and the public about the scientific knowledge base underlying professional nursing practice.

Overcoming Individual Barriers

There are several strategies that individual nurses can use to overcome their own problems associated with research. Participating in research courses and other research education experiences will facilitate the development of skills and self-confidence in research endeavors. It is not necessary to receive an advanced college degree to obtain adequate knowledge and skills in nursing research. Much knowledge can be gained through self-directed study, by continuing education courses, and in research seminars sponsored by universities, hospitals, and professional organizations. Nurses who regularly read nursing research and clinical specialty journals will have current information on new research findings and be aware of upcoming research conferences and workshops related to their areas of practice. Active participation in state nurse association activities and clinical specialty organizations can improve access to information on research education opportunities. Nursing research interest groups in many geographic locations also welcome new members.

Information on current research is becoming more accessible to practicing nurses. Articles and columns describing ongoing or recently completed research studies now appear regularly in nursing specialty journals.[7] In addition, information on accessing the database is available from Sigma Theta Tau International headquarters in Indianapolis, Indiana.

There are increasing resources that nurses can use for self-directed study in research. Several textbooks are available on research methods and statistics,[8] as well as resource materials for

[7]Journals that provide research reports with practice implications include *Nursing Scan in Research: Applications for Clinical Practice*, published by NURSCOM, Inc.; *Annual Review of Nursing Research*, and *Online: Journal of Knowledge Synthesis for Nursing*.

[8]Textbooks on research include those by Burns and Grove (1992), Leininger (1985), and Valanis (1992); on statistics they include Munro, Visintainer, and Page (1986).

CASE STUDY

Applying Research Findings in Practice

Joel S., a 35-year-old practicing R.N., had been employed at a mental health center for several years. He had worked very diligently to develop his therapeutic skills and prided himself on being open to new treatment approaches that might help his chronically ill clients. After attending a seminar on research utilization, Joel was eager to begin applying research findings to his clinical practice. He presented a report on the research seminar in a staff meeting and suggested that staff consider ways to begin accessing and using research findings to benefit patients attending the clinic. Some of Joel's colleagues were pessimistic about the new venture, while others recognized

the need for a stronger research base for their clinical decision making.

Joel organized an ongoing luncheon forum for those nurses expressing interest in research utilization activities. Most of the staff could not attend regularly because of emergency visits of clients during the noon hour. However, a small core group of staff began identifying practice problems and conducted several computer searches to obtain research articles relevant to these problems. A nurse researcher from the affiliating hospital was invited to the clinic to provide guidance in critiquing the research reports and in developing research-based practice innovations.

reading and critiquing research reports.[9] Moreover, Sigma Theta Tau International has developed a video series, the "Cameo Series," that describes nationally recognized nurse investigators' research programs and their practice implications. Some journals also advertise research lecture series and conferences.[10]

Developing Research Education Programs

Nurses can spearhead or help develop research education programs in their practice settings such as formal research courses, research seminars and conferences, unit-based journal clubs, and arena-wide research forums. It is most helpful if research education programs are instituted on an ongoing basis. All nurses should receive orientation sessions and structured inservice programs on the conduct and utilization of research. Nurses who want to be more involved in research activities can then have more focused

work sessions with colleagues in their clinical areas to identify specific practice problems and to discuss research applications.

Research committees in practice settings can be a major support for research utilization (Vessey & Campos, 1992). These committees can carry out targeted research utilization projects, develop long-range plans for program development, and facilitate the development of organizational structures to support research activities. Large health care systems need well-developed structures to ensure adequate participation in research committee work. For example, the Northwest Region of Kaiser Permanente, which has two major hospitals and over 20 outpatient settings, has implemented a region-wide nursing research committee that includes nurse representatives from all of the nursing service arenas and practice settings. Subcommittees for long-range planning, proposal review, and research facilitation in practice settings carry out much of the committee work.

Financing Nursing Research

Financial support for research is available from a variety of sources, including many grant programs administered through agencies of the federal government. Investigators usually obtain these funds by successfully competing in the grant program of the U.S. Public Health Service.

[9]Goode (1991), Phillips (1986), and Tornquist et al. (1993) are good sources for reading and critiquing research reports.

[10]The Sigma Theta Tau International publication, *Image: The Journal of Nursing Scholarship,* advertises research lecture series and conferences. The *Western Journal of Nursing Research* also publishes schedules of research conferences.

The NIH, within the Department of Health and Human Services (DHHS), is the primary funding agency for health research, with each of the institutes determining its own priorities for research and administering its own research programs. Priorities of the National Institute for Nursing Research were discussed in some detail earlier in this chapter. The Centers for Disease Control and Prevention (CDC) in Atlanta fund studies that have public health implications and recently awarded a grant to nurse investigators in Georgia to study the effect of AIDS/HIV infection in families throughout the state. Information on federal grant programs is available from research offices in universities and hospitals.

Many nurse investigators have been successful in obtaining federal grants, including some for research utilization projects in practice settings. Prospective applicants for federal funds usually establish contact with a branch officer or consultant of the potential funding agency early in proposal development to obtain guidance about program priorities and the application process. Beginning investigators may be more successful in obtaining funding if they submit a proposal in collaboration with an established investigator (e.g., a person who has previously received federal funding). Grant reviewers carefully evaluate the capabilities of the principal investigator and the total research team to determine whether the expertise is available to successfully complete the proposed study.

Nurses may be reluctant to apply for large federal grants because of the intense competition. However, gaining experience in the federal research arena can be beneficial. Even if a proposal is rejected, the investigator can learn from the reviewers' critiques. The proposal can then be improved and resubmitted for funding.

Nongovernment Funding Sources A growing number of private foundations, corporations, and other agencies are potential funding sources for nursing research. The Kellogg Foundation and the Robert Wood Johnson Foundation have funded many health research projects, including a number of nursing demonstration studies on long-term care. The Robert Wood Johnson Foundation has committed more than $5 million for research on tuberculosis during the 1990s and

another $8 million for research projects on health care policy and care delivery.

Sigma Theta Tau International has a small grants program for nursing research, and it recently started giving a few awards for dissemination of research findings in service settings (Buckwalter, 1993). In 1993, six nursing research utilization projects received awards. Other small grants programs are administered by nursing specialty organizations, such as the Oncology Nurses Society, the Oncology Nurses Foundation, the American Society of Critical Care Nurses, and the National Association of Orthopaedic Nurses. Springer Publishing Company gives an annual award for gerontological nursing research, and Mead Johnson has a perinatal grant program.[11]

Funding for nursing research in the clinical setting, especially for small pilot studies, may be limited. However, many descriptive and exploratory studies, as well as small pilot studies of nursing intervention projects, may only require funds for literature searches, supplies used in the project, and support services such as secretarial or computer assistance. Leininger (1983) provides these suggestions for how nurses can economize to limit the costs of research:

1. Use phase-in research plans, based on funding availability.
2. Borrow or rent, rather than buy, expensive equipment.
3. Use data banks for study purposes when possible.
4. Conduct multidisciplinary studies or collaborate with other investigators to share expenses.
5. Use standardized instruments and less costly data collection methods.
6. Reduce xeroxing and the use of office supplies.
7. Re-examine policies and procedures that are expensive or outdated.

Many health care institutions have developed their own internal sources of funding for small pilot studies and research utilization proj-

---

[11]The Sigma Theta Tau International newsletter, *Reflections,* is a good source of current information on small grant programs in nursing.

ects. Whether these funds are derived from developmental grants, fund-raising drives, or charitable contributions, they can support many nursing research activities. Nurses who are interested in developing strong research programs in their practice settings are encouraged to discuss their financial needs with the development staff of their respective institutions. Aggressive pursuit of funding for research often is well rewarded.

Summary and Conclusions

Research is an important component of the professional nurse's role. It contributes to the understanding of patients' health problems, assists nurses in identifying effective intervention strategies, and documents the cost-effectiveness of nursing practice. Both the conduct of research and the utilization of research findings in practice are crucial for research-based practice. Practicing nurses benefit from participating in research activities and also make important contributions to research.

Historically, nurses have not been actively involved in research activities in practice settings. However, during the past decade, there has been a steady increase in nurses' participation in research. Several areas of research contribute to the knowledge base for chronic care nursing practice, including studies on environmental, psychosocial, and behavioral factors; the impact of chronic illnesses on patients and families; and the effectiveness of nursing interventions and care delivery models. Current priorities of The National Center for Nursing Research include studies on chronic illness and quality of life, and

funding is available on a wide range of studies related to chronic care nursing practice.

Both quantitative and qualitative methods are needed for nursing research studies. These methods often can be combined in a research study to cross-validate and enrich the research findings.

Participation in research studies in the practice setting can be both rewarding and challenging. Nurses can overcome some of their individual barriers to research by taking the initiative to obtain needed information about research and by participating in research activities in the practice setting. Participation in professional associations and clinical specialty organizations also will support these efforts.

Traditionally, nursing practice has not been well grounded in research. However, several studies of research utilization in nursing have been conducted during the last decade, and nurses are beginning to make substantial progress in developing strategies to facilitate safe and timely applications of research in practice. Health care organizations and nursing administrators have an obligation to support nurses' research activities, both by developing structures to facilitate research activities and by providing sufficient start-up funding for these activities.

Currently, nursing research has greater visibility at the national level than at any time in the history of nursing. Nurse investigators are beginning to be well integrated into the scientific and political communities. Active participation of nurses in research activities in practice settings will help the profession continue obtaining the political and financial support it needs for rapid research development.

STUDY QUESTIONS

1. According to ANA guidelines, what level of educational preparation is necessary for an R.N. to participate in nursing research?
2. List three ways staff nurses can use research findings in their practice.
3. How can nursing administrators foster a positive research climate in practice settings?
4. What are the major deterrents to utilizing nursing research findings in clinical practice?

5. What are some good sources of information on (1) nursing research methods and (2) research utilization?
6. What are some of the major features of qualitative and quantitative research methods?
7. What are the two major purposes of triangulation?

References

American Nurses' Association (1989). *Education for participation in research.* Kansas City, MO: American Nurses' Association.

———— (1992). *Standards of clinical nursing practice.* Kansas City, MO: American Nurses' Association.

American Nurses' Association, Cabinet on Nursing Research (1985). *Directions for nursing research: Toward the twenty-first century.* Kansas City, MO: American Nurses' Association.

Archbold, P., & Stewart, B. (1987). Family caregiving across the life span. Paper presented at the International Nursing Research Conferences, ANA Council of Nurse Researchers. Washington, D.C., October 14.

Banik, B. J. (1993). Applying triangulation in nursing research, *Applied Nursing Research, 6*(1), 47–52.

Barnard, K. (1986). Research utilization: The clinician's role. *MCN, 11*(3), 224.

Barnsteiner, J. H. (1993). The Online Journal of Knowledge Synthesis for Nursing. *Image: The Journal of Nursing Scholarship, 20*(2), 14.

Beckett, J. E. (1990). Nursing research utilization techniques. *Journal of Nursing Administration, 20*(1), 25–30.

Bircumshaw, D. (1990). The utilization of research findings in clinical nursing practice. *Journal of Advanced Nursing, 15,* 1272–1280.

Bohanon, R. W., & Lebeau, B. F. (1986). Clinicians' use of research findings: A review of literature with implications for physical therapists. *Physical Therapy, 6,* 44–50.

Breitmeyer, B. J., Gallo, A. M., Knafl, K. A., & Zoeller, L. H. (1992). Social competence of school-aged children with chronic illnesses. *Journal of Pediatric Nursing, 7*(3), 181–188.

Brett, J. L. (1987). Use of nursing practice research findings. *Nursing Research, 12,* 226.

———— (1989). Organizational integrative mechanisms and adoption of innovations by nurses. *Nursing Research, 38*(2), 105–110.

Brown, M., & Powell-Cope, G. (1991). AIDs family caregiving: Transitions through uncertainty. *Nursing Research, 40*(6), 338–345.

Buckwalter, K. G. (1993). Sigma Theta Tau International supports nursing research dissemination. *Reflections, 19*(3), 9.

Burckhardt, C. S., Woods, S. L., Schultz, A. A., & Ziebarth, D. M. (1989). Quality of life of adults with chronic illness: A psychometric study. *Research in Nursing and Health, 12*(6), 347–354.

Burns, N., & Grove, S. K. (Eds.). (1987). Utilization of research in nursing practice. In *The practice of research: Conduct, critique and utilization* (pp. 625–668). Philadelphia: W. B. Saunders.

Cantor, M. J. (1983). Strain among caregivers: A study of experience in the United States. *The Gerontologist, 23,* 597–604.

Champion V. L., & Leach, A. (1989). Variables related to research utilization in nursing: An empirical investigation. *Journal of Advanced Nursing, 14,* 705–710.

Colianni, L. A. (1987). Information services for the nursing profession from the national library of medicine. *Journal of Professional Nursing, 6,* 372–375.

Corbin, J. M., & Strauss, A. L. (1984). Collaboration: Couples working together to manage chronic illness. *Image: The Journal of Nursing Scholarship, 16*(4), 109–115.

Coyle, L., & Sokop, A. (1990). Innovation adoption behavior among nurses. *Nursing Research, 39*(3), 176–180.

Crane, J., & Horsley, J. (1983). Research innovations in nursing: Implications for quality assurance programs. In D. L. Roice, J. C. Kruger, & R. E. Modraw (Eds.), *Organization and change in health care quality assurance.* Rockville, MD: Aspen.

Cronenwett, L. (1987). Research reflections: Research utilization in a practice setting. *Journal of Nursing Administration, 17*(7,8), 9–10.

CURN Project (1983). *Using research to improve nursing practice.* New York: Grune & Stratton. Series of clinical protocols: Clean intermittent catheterization (1982), Closed urinary drainage systems (1981), Distress reduction through sensory preparation (1981), Intravenous cannula change (1981), Mutual goal seting in patient care (1982), Pain: Deliberative nursing interventions (1982), Preventing decubitus ulcers (1981), Reducing diarrhea in tube-fed patients (1981), Structured preoperative teaching (1981).

Dahlen, R., Brundage, C., & Roth, C. (1987). Guidelines for doing a computerized literature search. *Nurse Educator, 12*(2), 17–21.

Department of Health, Education and Welfare (DHEW). (1979). *Healthy people: The surgeon general's report on health promotion and disease prevention, 1979,* DHEW Pub. No. (PHS) 79-55071, Public Health Service. Washington, DC: U.S. Government Printing Office.

Devine E. C., & Werley, H. H. (1988). Test of the Nursing Minimum Data Set: Availability of data and reliability. *Research in Nursing and Health, 11,* 97–104.

Dodd, N. J., Dibble, S. L., & Thomas, M. L. (1993). Predictors of concerns and coping strategies of cancer chemotherapy outpatients. *Applied Nursing Research, 6*(1), 2–7.

Duffy, M. (1987). Methodological triangulation: A vehicle for merging quantitative and qualitative methods. *Image: The Journal of Nursing Scholarship, 19,* 130-133.

Fagerhaugh, S., Strauss A., Suczek B., & Wiener C. (1987). *Hazards in hospital care.* San Francisco: Jossey-Bass.

Fawcett, J. (1984). Another look at utilization of nursing research. *Image: The Journal of Nursing Scholarship, 16*(2), 59-62.

———— (1986). A typology of nursing research activities according to educational preparation. *Journal of Professional Nursing, 2,* 75-78.

Ferrell, B., Grant, M., Schmidt, G. M., Rhiner, M., Whitehead, C., Fonbuena, P., & Forman, S. J. (1992). The meaning of quality of life for bone marrow transplant survivors. Part 1: The impact of bone marrow transplant on quality of life. *Cancer Nursing, 15*(3), 153-160.

Fitts, W., Adams, J., Radford, G., Richard, W., Thomas, M., & Thompson, W. (1971). *The self concept and self-actualization.* Nashville, TN: Counselor Recording & Tests.

Funk, S. G., Champagne, M. T., Wiese, R. A., & Tornquist, E. M. (1991). Barriers to using research findings in practice: The clinician's perspective. *Applied Nursing Research, 4*(2), 90-95.

Funk, S. G., Tornquist, E. M., & Champagne, M. T. (1989). A model for improving the dissemination of nursing research. *Western Journal of Nursing Research, 11*(3), 361-367.

Gaits, V., Ford, R. N., Kaplow, R., et al. (1989). Unit-based research forums: A model for the clinical nurse specialist to promote clinical research. *Clinical Nurse Specialist, 3*(2), 60-65.

Gift, A., Moore, T., & Soeken, K. (1992). Relaxation to reduce dyspnea and anxiety in COPD patients. *Nursing Research, 41*(4), 242-246.

Goode, C. (producer) (1987). *Using research in clinical nursing practice.* Ida Grove, IA: Horn Video Productions.

———— (1991). *Reading and critiquing a research report* (Videotape No. 391). Ida Grove, IA: Horn Video Productions.

Goode, C., & Bulechek, G. M. (1992). Research utilization: An organizational process that enhances quality of care. *Journal of Nursing Care Quality: Special Report,* 27-35.

Goode, C. J., Butcher, L. A., Cipperley, J. A., Ekstrom, J., Gosch, B. A., Hayes, J. E., Lovett, M. K., & Wellendorf, S. A. (1991). *Research utilization: A study guide.* Ida Grove, IA: Horn Video Productions.

Goode, C. (producer), & Cipperley, J. (associate producer) (1989). *Research utilization: A process of organizational change* (Videotape No. 289). Ida Grove, IA: Horn Video Productions.

Goode, C. J., Lovett, M. K., Hayes, J. E., & Butcher, L. A. (1987). Use of research based knowledge in clinical practice. *Journal of Nursing Administration, 17*(12), 11-18.

Goodwin, L. D., & Goodwin, W. L. (1984). Qualitative vs. quantitative research or qualitative and quantitative research? *Nursing Research, 33*(6), 378-380.

Green, S., & Houston, S. (1993). Promoting research activities: Institutional strategies. *Applied Nursing Research, 6*(2), 97-102.

Hasse, J. E., & Myers, S. T. (1988). Reconciling paradigm assumptions of qualitative and quantitative research. *Western Journal of Nursing Research, 10,* 128-137.

Hefferin, E. A., Horsley, J., & Ventura, M. R. (1982). Promoting research-based nursing: The nurse administrator's role. *Journal of Nursing Administration, 12*(5), 34-41.

Hicky, M. (1990). The role of the Clinical Nurse Specialist in the research utilization process. *Clinical Nurse Specialist, 4*(2), 93-96.

Hines, P., & Young, K. (1987). A triangulation of methods and paradigms to study nurse-given wellness care. *Nursing Research, 36,* 195-198.

Hoeffer, B., & Archbold, P. G. (1983). Problems in doing research: Interfacing quantitative and qualitative methods. *Western Journal of Nursing Research, 5*(3), 254-257.

Horsley, J. (1985). Using research in practice: The current context. *Western Journal of Nursing Research, 7*(1), 135-139.

Horsley, J., Crane, J., Crabtree, M., & Wood, D. (1983). *Using research to improve nursing practice: A guide.* New York: Grune & Stratton.

Hunt, M. (1987). The process of translating research findings into nursing practice. *Journal of Advanced Nursing, 12,* 101-110.

Hunt, V., Stark, J. L., Fisher, K. H., Joy, C., & Woldren, K. (1983). Networking: A managerial strategy for research development in a service setting. *Journal of Nursing Administration, 13*(7), 27-32.

Hutchinson, C., & Bahr, R. (1991). Types and meanings of caring behaviors among elderly nursing home residents. *Image: The Journal of Nursing Scholarship, 23*(2), 85-88.

Ingersol, G. L., Hoffart, N., Schultz, A. W. (1990). Health services research in nursing: Current status and future directions. *Nursing Economics, 8*(4), 229-238.

Kerfoot, K., & Watson, C. (1985). Research based quality assurance: The key to excellence in nursing. In

J. McClosky & H. Grace (Eds.), *Current issues in nursing.* Boston: Blackwell.

Kilby, S., Fishel, C., & Gupta, A. (1989). Access to nursing information resources. *Image: The Journal of Nursing Scholarship, 21*(1), 26-30.

Kilpack, V., Boehm, J., Smith, N., & Mudge, B. (1991). Using research-based interventions to decrease patient falls. *Applied Nursing Research, 4*(2), 50-56.

King, D., Barnard, C. E., & Hoehn, R. (1981). Disseminating the results of nursing research. *Nursing Outlook, 29*(3), 164-169.

Kirchhoff, K. T. (1983). Using research in practice: Should staff nurses be expected to use research? *Western Journal of Nursing Research, 4*(3), 245-247.

Knafl, K. A., Bevis, M. E. & Kirchhoff, K. T. (1987). Research activities of clinical nurse researchers. *Nursing Research, 36*(4), 249-252.

Knafl, K. A., & Breitmeyer, B. (1991). Triangulation in qualitative research: Issues of conceptual clarity and purpose. In J. Morse (Ed.), *Qualitative nursing research: A contemporary dialogue* (rev. ed.) (pp. 226-239). Newbury Park, CA: Sage.

Knafl, K. A., & Howard, M. J. (1984). Interpreting and reporting qualitative research. *Research in Nursing and Health, 7,* 17-24.

Krueger, J. C., Nelson, A. H., & Wolanin, M. O. (1978). *Nursing research: Development, collaboration and utilization.* Germantown, MD: Aspen.

Labuhn, K., Lewis, C., Koon, K., & Mullooly, J. (1993). Smoking cessation experiences of chronic lung disease patients living in rural and urban areas of Virginia. *Journal of Rural Health, 9*(4), 305-313.

Lamb, G. S. (1992). Conceptual and methodological issues in nurse case management research. *Advanced Nursing Science, 15*(2), 16-24.

Lanza, M. L. (1990). Research and quality assurance: Similarities and differences. *Nursing Scan in Research, 3*(2), 1-3.

Larson, E. (1983). Combining nursing quality assurance and research programs. *Journal of Nursing Administration, 13*(11), 32-35.

———— (1984). Health policy and NIH: Implications for nursing research. *Nursing Research, 33*(6), 352-356.

Lazarus, R. S., & Folkman, S. (1984). *Stress, appraisal, and coping.* New York: Springer.

Lelean, S. R. (1982). The implementation of research findings into nursing practice. *International Journal of Nursing Studies, 19*(4), 223-230.

LeMone, P. (1993). Human sexuality in adults with insulin-dependent diabetes mellitus. *Image: The Journal of Nursing Scholarship, 25*(2), 101-104.

Leininger, M. M. (1983). Creativity and challenge for nurse researchers in the economic recession. *Journal of Nursing Administration, 13*(3), 21-22.

———— (1985). *Qualitative research methods in nursing.* New York: Grune & Stratton.

Levin, R. F. (1986). Utilizing nursing research. In G. Lobiondo-Wood, & J. Haber (Eds.), *Nursing research: Critical appraisal and utilization* (pp. 294-312). St. Louis: Mosby.

Lindeman, C. (1988). Research in practice: The role of the staff nurse. *Applied Nursing Research, 1*(1), 5-7.

Lindgren, C. L. (1993). The caregiver career. *Image: The Journal of Nursing Scholarship, 25*(3), 214-219.

Marchette, L. (1985). Developing a productive nursing research program in a clinical institution. *Journal of Nursing Administration, 15*(3), 25-29.

Martin, P. A. (1993). Clinical settings need organizational support for research. *Applied Nursing Research, 6*(2), 103-104.

Martin, J. P. (1990). Implementing the research role of the clinical nurse specialist—One institution's approach. *Clinical Nurse Specialist, 4*(3), 137-140.

McSweeny, A. J., & Labuhn, K. T. (1990). Chronic obstructive pulmonary disease. In B. Spilker (Ed.), *Quality of life assessments in clinical trials* (pp. 391-418). New York: Raven Press.

Miller, B. K., Adams, D., & Beck, L. (1993). The behavioral inventory for professionalism in nursing. *Journal of Professional Nursing, 9*(5), 290-295.

Morse, J. A., & Conrad, A. (1983). Putting research into practice. *Canadian Nurse, 79*(8), 40-43.

Munro, B. H., Visintainer, M. A., & Page, E. B. (1986). *Statistical methods for health care research.* Philadelphia: J. B. Lippincott.

Nail, L. M. (1990). Involving clinicians in nursing research. *Oncology Nursing Forum, 17*(4), 621-623.

National Center for Health Statistics (1983, December). *Health, United States and prevention profile,* DHHS Pub. No. (PHS) 84-1232, Public Health Service. Washington, D.C.: U.S. Government Printing Office.

National Center for Nursing Research (1991). *Patient outcomes research: Examining the effectiveness of nursing practice: Recommendations for Future Directions.* Conference proceedings (September 11-13, 1991). U.S. Department of Health and Human Services: NCNR.

———— (1992). *Update: Initiatives for FY 1993 from the NCNR.* Bethesda, MD: Office of Information and Legislative Affairs, NCNR, NIH.

———— (1993). *Developing knowledge for practice: Challenges and opportunities,* NIH Pub. No. 93-

2416. Bethesda, MD: U.S. Department of Health and Human Services.

National Institute for Nursing Research (1993). *National nursing research agenda: Setting nursing research priorities.* Information distributed by NINR, September 23, 1993.

Neff, E. J., & Dale, J. C. (1990). Assessment of quality of life in school-aged children: A method—Phase I. *Maternal Child Nursing Journal, 19*(4), 313-320.

Norbeck, J. S., Lindsey, F., & Carrieri, V. (1981). The development of an instrument to measure social support. *Nursing Research, 30,* 264-269.

O'Brein, M. T. (1993). Multiple sclerosis: The relationship among self-esteem, social support, and coping behavior. *Applied Nursing Research, 6*(2), 54-63.

OCRUN Oration (1992). *The newsletter of the Orange County Research Utilization in Nursing Project, 1*(2).

Ohio Nurses Association (1990). *Survey of organizational support for nursing research.* Columbus, OH: Ohio Nurses' Association Assembly of Nurse Researchers.

Parker, M. E., Gordon, S. C., & Brannon, P. T. (1992). Involving nursing staff in research: A non-traditional approach. *Journal of Nursing Administration, 22*(4), 58-63.

Phillips, L.R.F. (1986). *A clinician's guide to the critique and utilization of nursing research.* Norwalk, CT: Appleton-Century-Crofts.

Piazza, D., Holcombe, J., Foote, A., Paul, P., Love, S., & Daffin, P. (1991). Hope, social support and self-esteem of patients with spinal cord injuries. *Journal of Neuroscience Nursing, 23*(4), 224-230.

Polivka, B. J., Nickel, J. T., & Wilkins, J. R. (1993). Cerebral palsy: Evaluation of a model of risk. *Research in Nursing and Health, 16,* 113-122.

Primomo, J., Yates, B. C., & Woods, N. F. (1990). Social support for women during chronic illness: The relationship among sources and types of adjustment. *Research in Nursing and Health, 13*(3), 153-156.

Raleigh, E. D. (1992). Sources of hope in chronic illness. *Oncology Nursing Forum, 19*(3), 443-448.

Redeker, N. S. (1988). Health beliefs and adherence in chronic illness. *Image: The Journal of Nursing Scholarship, 20*(1), 31-35.

Rempusheski, V. F. (1991). Incorporating research role and practice role. *Applied Nursing Research, 4*(1), 46-48.

Rettig R. (1991). History, development, and importance to nursing of outcomes research. *Journal of Nursing Quality Assurance, 5*(2), 13-17.

Reynolds, M. A., & Haller, K. B. (1986). Using research in practice: A case for replication in nursing—Part 1. *Western Journal of Nursing Research, 81,* 113-116.

Roberson, M. (1992). The meaning of compliance: Patient perspectives. *Qualitative Health Research, 2*(1), 7-26.

Rogers, E. M. (1983). *Diffusion of innovations* (3rd ed.). New York: The Free Press.

Rudy, E. B. (1991). Facilitating clinical research: Nurse-to-nurse support. *Applied Nursing Research, 4*(2), 49.

Salive, M. E., Mayfield, J. A., & Weissman, N. W. (1990). Patient outcomes research teams and the agency for health care policy and research. *HSR: Health Services Research, 25*(5), 697-708.

Sayles-Cross, S. (1993). Perceptions of familial caregivers of elder adults. *Image: The Journal of Nursing Scholarship, 25*(2), 88-92.

Sexton, D. L., & Munro, B. (1985). Impact of a husband's chronic illness (COPD) on the spouse's life. *Research in Nursing and Health, 8,* 83-90.

——— (1988). Living with a chronic illness: The experience of women with chronic obstructive pulmonary disease (COPD). *Western Journal of Nursing Research, 10*(1), 26-44.

Simms, L. M., Price, S. A., & Pfoutz, S. K. (1987). Creating the research climate: A key responsibility for nurse executives. *Nursing Economics, 5*(4), 174-178.

Spilker, B. (Ed.). (1990). *Quality of life assessments in clinical trials.* New York: Raven Press.

Strauss, A., Corbin, J., Fagerhaugh, S., Glaser, B., Maines, D., Suczek, B., & Wiener, C. (1984). *Chronic illness and the quality of life* (2nd ed.). St. Louis: C. V. Mosby.

Tornquist, E. M., Funk, S. G., Champagne, M. T., & Wiese, R. A. (1993). Advice on reading research: Overcoming the barriers. *Applied Nursing Research, 6*(4), 177-183.

Valanis, B. G. (1992). *Epidemiology in nursing and health care* (2nd ed.). Norwalk, CT: Appleton & Lange.

Ventura, M. R., Young, D. E., Feldman, M. J., Pastores, P., Pikula, S., & Yates, M. A. (1985). Cost savings as an indicator of successful nursing intervention. *Nursing Research, 34*(1), 50-53.

Vessey, J., & Campos, R. (1992). The role of the nursing research committee. *Nursing Research, 41,* 247-249.

Watson, C. A., Bulechek, G. M., & McCloskey, J. C. (1987). QAMUR: A quality assurance model using research. *Journal of Nursing Quality Assurance, 2*(1), 21-27.

Werley, H. H., Devine, E. C., Zorn, C. R., Ryan, P., & Westra, B. L. (1991). The nursing minimum data set: Abstraction tool for standardized, comparable, essential data. *American Journal of Public Health, 81*(4), 421-426.

Whitney, F. W. (1986). Turning clinical problems into research. *Heart and Lung, 15*(1), 57-59.

Whyte, D. A. (1992). A family nursing approach to the care of a child with a chronic illness. *Journal of Advanced Nursing, 17*(3), 317-327.

Wiener C. L., & Dodd M. J. (1993). Coping amid uncertainty: An illness trajectory perspective. *Scholarly Inquiry for Nursing Practice, 7*(1), 17-31.

Woog P. (1991). *The chronic illness trajectory framework: The Corbin and Strauss nursing model.* New York: Springer.

Yeager, B. H., & Shannon, T. (1988). Developing a nursing research manual. *Journal of Nursing Administration, 18*(10), 8-28.

Zerwekh, J. V. (1991). A family caregiving model for public health nursing. *Nursing Outlook, 39,* 213-217.

Bibliography

American Nurses' Association (1988). *Standards for organized nursing services.* Kansas City, MO: American Nurses' Association.

Batra, C. (1983). Motivating nurses to do nursing research. *Nursing and Health Care, 4*(1), 18-22.

Bergstrom, N., Hansen, B., Grant, M., Hanson, R., Kubo, W., Padilla, G., & Wong, H. (1984). Collaborative nursing research: Anatomy of a successful consortium. *Nursing Research, 33*(1).

Breitmeyer, B. J., Ayres, L., & Knafl, K. A. (1993). Triangulation in qualitative research: Evaluation of completeness and confirmation purposes. *Image: The Journal of Nursing Scholarship, 25*(3), 237-244.

Funk, S. G., Tornquist, E. M., Champagne, M. T., & Wiese, R. A. (1993). *Key aspects of caring for the chronically ill: Hospital and home.* New York: Springer.

Horsley, J. A., Crane, J., & Bingle, J. D. (1978). Research utilization as an organizational process. *Journal of Nursing Administration, 8*(7), 4-6.

Institute of Medicine (1983). *Nursing and nursing education: Public policies and private actions.* Washington, D.C.: National Academic Press.

Rizzuto, C., & Mitchell, M. (1988). Research in service settings: Part 1—Consortium project outcomes. *Journal of Nursing Administration, 18*(2), 32-37.

Weis, K. A. (1992). Effectiveness and outcomes research—Data sources with potential for nursing research. *Journal of Professional Nursing, 8*(4), 201.

CHAPTER 18

Alternative Modalities

Geri Neuberger • Cynthia Thorne Woods

Introduction

Persons of all ages seek help outside traditional medicine. Parents may seek help for their infants born with congenital disorders such as cerebral palsy or Down's syndrome, or individuals may seek help for chronic problems such as AIDS, migraine headaches, multiple sclerosis, arthritis, cancer, or a myriad of other incurable conditions (Goldman, 1991). Even older adults, in relatively good health, may seek alternative modalities to prolong life or enhance their level of wellness. Such actions are not necessarily reflections of noncompliance; rather, they reflect that symptoms (such as pain) or illnesses (such as terminal cancer or AIDS) may not be responding to traditional medical treatment. Under such circumstances, alternative treatment may provide a sense of control (Montbriand & Laing, 1991) and greater choice about the direction and emphasis of treatment. When the alternative option can be used in conjunction with traditional treatment, it becomes even more desirable.

In the Western world, state licensure laws have long regulated the practice of physicians, nurses, and pharmacists, but now many other providers, such as chiropractors and acupuncturists, are being regulated through licensure. At one time, only physicians diagnosed and prescribed health care. Other health professionals now diagnose and prescribe within the areas of their expertise and qualifications.

Unfortunately, many orthodox providers, including nurses, view *all* alternatives as less valid or less acceptable than more traditional practices. Such attitudes deny clients a maximum range of choices to fill their needs. In addition, alternative practitioners are frequently classed together, as if they were a single entity, and labeled as quacks, often without any prior investigation of the effectiveness of or basis for the treatment provided.

This chapter explores reasons why individuals seek alternative treatments, looks at some of the problems related to their use, and discusses some common or popular approaches.

What Are Alternative Modalities?

An alternative treatment modality is a health intervention not "approved" by the community of orthodox medicine. Individuals may seek such treatment without orders or permission from their physicians. This does not imply that all physicians object to the use of all alternative approaches but, rather, that they tend not to be prescribed or recommended.

The use of alternative treatment is not new in this country. The survival of early American colonists was due in part to their ability to use home remedies. In 1721, the city of Boston had only one doctor, and treatment was primitive, including such practices as bloodletting. For about 200 years after the arrival of the first colonists, there were no hospitals or medical schools. Choking, broken bones, hemorrhage, poisoning, gangrene, snakebite, fever, gunshot or arrow wounds, and so on, had to be treated at once by the best means known at that time (Meyer, 1973).

Folk Tradition A great number of alternative practices stem from folk tradition. Every cultural, ethnic, and religious group has, as part of its heritage, the development of a system for treating sickness. One of the authors can remember watching her maternal grandmother make a poultice of fried onions placed between sheets of flannel cloth, to be applied to the chest for upper respiratory congestion. Such treatments are passed down via tradition from one generation to the next and are numbered among choices available to an individual when sickness occurs.

From an historical viewpoint, folk medicine has provided many useful drugs and treatments. For example, lithium is a substance found in the water of natural springs; the ancient Greeks used water containing lithium salts to treat "mania and melancholy" (Kruger, 1974). In the 1970s, lithium was rediscovered as a valuable treatment for manic depression.

Another drug has an even more interesting history. An 18th century doctor was asked to examine a man suffering from heart failure and dropsy, but could offer no effective treatment. After his return from a short trip, the doctor found the man up and about with all the swelling gone. The man said he had been cured by a local charwoman who had given him an herb—foxglove. The doctor had the herb analyzed, and medicine gained a new drug, digitalis (Kruger, 1974).

Why Individuals Seek Alternative Treatment

Individuals with chronic diseases look for health care outside the traditional realm for a number of reasons: frustration with how their health and illness problems are being handled, feelings that ordered treatment is inadequate in alleviating symptoms or in correcting disease process (Furnham & Smith, 1988), preference for cultural or ethnic practices, or a desire to enhance wellness.

Pain, especially if it is chronic or intractable, motivates people to seek relief from any source. If you have ever been in pain during a long, lonely night, you have had a glimpse into the world of someone who experiences ongoing or recurrent pain. When the pain that accompanies disorders such as arthritis and late-stage cancer no longer responds adequately to medical treatment, afflicted persons may seek anything that holds a promise of relief.

Impaired mobility, which occurs with many chronic conditions such as multiple sclerosis, amyotrophic lateral sclerosis, and arthritis, is frequently given as a reason for seeking alternative treatment. Mobility limitations can create a change in one's self-concept, ability to function, and roles (see Chapter 6, on mobility); financial security may even be threatened. The failure of traditional medical treatment to improve mobility may lead people on a search for other means to greater functioning.

Negative experiences with traditional health care can create a climate of distrust. Consequently, the individual may be more likely to reject treatment provided by orthodox practitioners. Family members or others who have lost confidence in traditional treatment may encourage the client to look elsewhere. Families who consider traditional treatment ineffective may seek alternative ways to achieve improvement, regardless of cost.

When faced with the devastation and helplessness of a terminal illness, people sometimes feel there is nothing to lose and everything to gain from looking elsewhere for health care. Often, alternative practitioners offer these people hope, which in turn improves their mental status. Belief in the efficacy of a treatment is an extremely important factor in recovery or improvement.

Clients' desire for autonomy and control over their own lives in a system that seems increasingly impersonal, fragmented, and incomprehensible has also contributed to the growth of alternative methods. In fact, over the past few decades, self-care has become a trend in our society—a trend involving individuals who increasingly feel they can make decisions about enhancing their health, preventing illness, and treating disease. In fact, many American households now have self-care reference books, and household members initially treat their own symptoms rather than see a physician.

There are also people who do not want the discomfort, inconvenience, or frequency involved in traditional medical treatment. This aversion can make a "simple" treatment or "cure" seem more attractive and acceptable. Furthermore, when unhealthy life-styles underlie illness, people who cannot confront the need to change may search for unorthodox, simplistic, magical remedies.

Problems and Issues Related to Alternative Modalities

Numerous difficulties plague the client seeking relief or cure when traditional medicine has failed to improve health status or ameliorate symptoms. Quacks abound, treatment can conflict with sociocultural values, alternative methods may conflict with accepted health practices or may have no scientific basis, insurance companies may be unwilling to cover costs, and competency of practitioners may be difficult to determine. A brief discussion of each of these issues is therefore in order.

Quackery

Both clients and health professionals are faced with the perplexing problem of differentiating quackery from effective, worthwhile alternative treatment modalities. Miracle cures are often sought by people in need—people who are willing to believe in anything that is presented as effective. It is quackery that often leads people to label all alternatives as ineffective or dangerous.

Historically, quacks have promoted their treatments for their own profit (Martin et al., 1983). The Food and Drug Administration estimates that at least $2 billion are spent each year on worthless tests and treatment (Holland, 1981). To complicate the issue, quackery can occur within, as well as outside, orthodox medicine.

The Pepper Committee of the U.S. Senate defined a quack as anyone who promotes medical schemes or remedies known to be false, or which are unproven (Jarvis, 1992). Johnson (1984) reported the following six guidelines for recognizing fraudulent treatment, presented originally in the October 1984 issue of the *Harvard Medical School Health Letter* but still valid to this day:

1. Words such as *miracle, cure,* and *breakthrough* are often used.
2. Ingredients are not identified.
3. Support of experts who are not named or fully identified is asserted.
4. Claims of effectiveness for a wide variety of conditions are made.
5. The product is declared as *all natural.*
6. There are vague allusions to "public research," sometimes with an offer to supply references.

To avoid fraudulent practices, treatment goals need to be defined as clearly and realistically as possible before any proffered treatment is accepted. Questions should be asked regarding what changes or benefits are expected from such treatment. Decisions should be made in advance about how to measure the effect of the treatment in terms of expected improvement, activity tolerance, pain intensity, weight change, or dollars and time expended. When openness and trust exist between client and health care professional, the professional may be particularly helpful in identifying goals, alternatives, and methods of evaluating results of treatment.

Substitution for Known Effective Treatments

It is not uncommon for people to move to other modalities when traditional treatment is no longer effective or when the individual rejects accepted treatment in the hope of finding some miracle cure. Unfortunately, desperate people are often willing to try anything. Fortunately, many nontraditional approaches do not have negative outcomes. If value is determined by results, there are many alternatives to medical practice that are effective and lead to improvement.

Rejection of traditional treatment can create feelings of frustration among many orthodox health care professionals, feelings that may surface as anger directed at the client. Some health care providers may demand that the client choose between traditional and nontraditional methods rather than encouraging the individual to consider both, especially when the latter does not conflict with the former.

Cultural Conflict

In spite of folklore serving as the basis of many different kinds of health care, including traditional medicine, various cultural groups often do not agree with the methods and treatment offered by orthodox medicine. Disparate groups also differ in what symptoms constitute illness and what degree of impairment is necessary before one is even considered ill (Murray & Zentner, 1979). Given these factors, it is not surprising that individuals often choose familiar, and frequently effective, treatment before turning to Western methods.

Costs

Increased technology and other factors have sent health care costs soaring dramatically (Somers & Somers, 1977), leading the government to monitor the costs as well as the quality of health care services (see Chapter 22, on financial impact). Furthermore, the diseases that plague our urbanized and aging population (for instance, vascular disease, cancer, respiratory disorders, and mental illness) are not only costly to treat but not very amenable to conventional medical treatments or cures.

Rising health care costs are one factor that leads individuals to look for more cost-effective treatment. For instance, mastering relaxation or biofeedback may prove less expensive, but effective, as a treatment for migraine headaches when compared with the ongoing cost and potential dangers of the continuous use of a prescription drug. Transcutaneous electrical nerve stimulation (TENS) to control low back pain may be less expensive then the combination of prescription drugs, a back brace, and repeated hospitalization for pelvic traction.

However, not all alternative treatment modalities are effective and less expensive than traditional treatment. Regardless of the cost factor, when traditional treatment is considered superior, the health professional should share this information with the client. This, of course, means the professional must be familiar with the alternative modalities being considered. Optimally, the choice of care should be based on the client's informed decision. Even when the health professional does not agree with the client's selection, the provider should continue to be supportive and work cooperatively with both client and alternative health care provider.

Nor are all alternatives cheaper; some are more costly than traditional medical treatments. For instance, the "Mexico Cure" for arthritis may cost $300, but, when analyzed, it consists of nothing more than a few dollars' worth of cortisone and phenylbutazone. Such treatment is effective only for limited periods of time, and prolonged use of these medications can be extremely expensive and can cause serious side effects.

Payment

In addition to actual costs, payments may be adversely affected. According to *The New England Journal of Medicine,* Americans spent $13.7 billion on alternative medicine in 1990, of which $10.3 billion were out-of-pocket payments made by patients (Rock, 1993). With increasing government regulation of Medicare and Medicaid, and growing restrictions on allowable medical expenses paid by third-party providers, clients may have to pay for more and more alternative treatments themselves.

Insurance companies justify their refusal to pay for many alternative treatments on the grounds that the modality is not accepted by the medical community. This stance often forces the client to use traditional methods even though he or she feels that an alternative would be more effective. For example, an insurance company may pay for a prescription medication to curb the appetite of an obese client, but be unwilling to pay for a class in relaxation techniques to reduce the stress that may be causing the overeating, even though the client may be faced with diabetes mellitus and hypertension, both of which are related to obesity. There are times when an insurance company will consider reimbursement, especially if a primary provider makes appropriate referrals or provides data to support the benefit of an alternative modality. However, payment usually requires that a review board (often made up of physicians) approve the treatment.

Separating Fact from Fiction

Both nonprofessionals and professionals face the problem of differentiating fact from fallacy with respect to the cause and effectiveness of treatment. Reading books, magazines, and the daily newspaper is not an useful way of differentiating proven fact from hypothesis or conjecture. Some people believe that what is printed is true, since they lack the knowledge or resources to evaluate critically what they read. In addition, when medical treatment has "failed" them, they tend to believe in anything that seems to offer promise. It is this need to find help that makes people gullible.

Titles used by individuals also influence potential clients. Many books that promote various treatments or cures are written by Dr. So-and-So, yet the kind of doctorate the author holds is not listed, nor is there information on where the person's special expertise was obtained. The title *Doctor* denotes authority, special knowledge, and prestige in American society. When a suggested treatment is potentially harmful, people can be fooled into trying it because the author uses a title. This does a disservice to all legitimate health care providers, especially those outside the mainstream, because poor outcomes raise the suspicion that all alternative treatment is quackery.

Scientific versus Empirical Treatment

The scientific community makes decisions about the effectiveness of treatments based on research. A positive and exciting step was taken in April 1992, when the National Institutes of Health (NIH) established the "Office of Alternative Medicine," headed by Dr. Joseph Jacobs. Dr. Jacobs, a physician trained in traditional medicine at Yale and Dartmouth, is an expert in American Indian healing beliefs and practices. He says his charge is to look at everything from Chinese herbal medicines to changes in exercise habits, and to find the scientific basis of how they work (Rock, 1993). The establishment of this new office by NIH is a positive step for the scientific community toward objectively studying current alternative modalities.

The experimental model is used in medicine to determine if a treatment truly makes a difference. The best experimental models use a double-blind approach, so neither client nor physician knows which subjects are receiving the treatment being evaluated; the treatment group is then compared to a control group. An excellent example of this method is the Veterans Administration Cooperative Study Group study that provided convincing evidence for a step approach to hypertension management (VACSG, 1967, 1970). Good studies also control for other variables that can affect the outcome, such as age, sex, and occupation.

The Hawthorne and placebo effects, often strong and dramatic, can influence study outcomes. The *Hawthorne effect* occurs when subjects in the experimental group perform or respond better simply because they are aware of being the "experimental" group. This effect occurs because of the attention and expectations subjects feel, and not because of the independent, or treatment, variable being tested.

The *placebo effect* occurs when a subject feels better just because he or she is being treated, not because the treatment actually has any pharmacologic or physiologic effect (Brody, 1982). Feeling better is the body's response to the client's belief in the treatment, which in turn influences intrinsic neurochemical changes that have a significant physiologic impact (Levine, Gordon, & Fields, 1978). This effect is a well-accepted fact in the clinical practice of medicine. As an example, it is acknowledged that the action of a drug can be enhanced or hindered by the social context in which it is given (Berblinger, 1963).

As mentioned, the placebo effect is enhanced by a positive attitude toward the placebo's effectiveness, a phenomenon well demonstrated by faith healers. Expectations about the effects of the treatment, the extent of fear or pain, the confidence and trust placed in the practitioner, and the choice of treatment all strongly influence the client's response to any therapy. Positive placebo responses are much more likely in chronic remittent diseases or when the central nervous system is being treated (LaPatra, 1978).

But not all traditional treatment is based on science, and not all alternatives are based on word of mouth. Much of medical treatment is empirical; that is, things are tried, found effective, and used without any experimental design at all. However, more valid scientific research is done in traditional medicine than by practitioners of alternative treatments. This is in large part the result of funding provided by the federal government for such research.

Finding Competent Practitioners

An individual may decide, with or without medical approval, to try an alternative treatment modality. Once that decision is made, where does one find someone who is competent? Although many practitioners of alternative modalities are licensed, there is no licensing or certification procedure for many others. In other words, inconsistencies and gaps in standards for licensure and certification make it difficult to decide who is competent. Acupuncture is a case in point. It is considered acceptable (and even reimbursable) when acupuncture is practiced by physicians, very few of whom have had adequate training in that modality. Yet in many states, no mechanism exists for licensing Oriental practitioners, who have extensive specialized training and legitimate credentials.

Similar quandaries exist among other health disciplines. Relaxation techniques and biofeedback are being offered by many health professionals. Some are well trained, some are not. If the treatment is ordered by a primary provider, insurance payment is generally made without investigation of qualifications. One can ask if there should be some kind of regulatory system that controls who can provide certain treatments. If so, who should establish and control this system? And how do you control for the many incompetents or frauds who go unregulated?

At present, control seems unlikely. Therefore, each individual considering an alternative modality should take responsibility for seeking information to make an informed decision. However, becoming informed on competency and qualifications is a difficult task for clients and professionals alike.

Common or Popular Treatment Modalities

The health care professional should help clients reach informed treatment decisions that will be most therapeutic or meaningful to them. This requires a climate conducive to open communication about any treatment under consideration. If the health professional is not familiar with the alternative drug or treatment, efforts should be made to find unbiased or impartial information.

Clients desire a supportive environment and a sense that the professional is their advocate, who will focus on helping them live life to the fullest despite chronic illness. For the client, a full life may entail learning to live with some pain, some immobility, or the reality of his or her mortality. It may require learning ways to monitor symptoms and make appropriate adjustments in medications, activities, and so forth, in order to avoid problems.

Or it may require that professionals give clients support and show a willingness to help them make intelligent decisions on alternative treatments. Above all, clients need to feel a sense of dignity, and such feelings come largely through having control over oneself and one's environment (Prescott & Flexer, 1982; Feldman, 1990).

The rest of this section describes some alternative modalities currently in use in this country. The list is not all inclusive, nor will these modalities be presented in depth. No judgment of their validity as treatment is intended, although pros and cons are included.

Diets and Nutrients

During the last 20 years, there has been an explosion of new knowledge and scientific study of the effects of food nutrients on human health. There is now a new dietary pyramid that has replaced the basic four food groups that have long guided recommendations for human nutrition. This new pyramid reduces the amount of protein intake obtained through animal sources and puts more emphasis on the intake of fruits, vegetables, legumes, and grains. In 1990, Congress passed the Nutritional Labeling and Education Act, which will curtail many of the abuses and false claims by industries producing food and dietary supplements (Jarvis, 1992).

Diets The use of special diets[1] as part of medical management—for example, low-sodium diets for cardiac problems or calorie-controlled diets for diabetes—is well known to health professionals. Diets are also commonly used for weight control, as preventive treatment, to control symptoms such as pain, or to reverse effects of some pathologies such as arthritis or cancer. However, since food is the primary source of nutrients, the misuse of diets can create health problems.

The content, frequency, and rituals that make up dietary intake are greatly influenced by an individual's culture. Influences against certain foods are so strong that even in famine situations recipients of food packages have starved rather than eat forbidden food. Belief in the magical power of certain foods to prolong life, increase vitality, and cure illness is also widespread (Miller, 1981).

Diets can be prescribed or self-instituted. They can focus on eliminating certain foods that are considered harmful, combining certain foods for a given effect, or avoiding additives. Each diet claims different values, emphasizes different approaches, and works for different people. Because diets are so widely used for so many different reasons, only a few are described here. It is not our intent to condone or condemn any of them.

Arthritis Diets A number of the diets used by people with arthritis are basically sound from a nutritional standpoint, but they restrict the intake of certain foods that seem to increase symptoms. Clients who find relief through these diets should not be discouraged from their use, but, rather, allowed to integrate their food preferences into their medical regimens.

One such diet is presented by C. Dong, M.D., who suffered from crippling arthritis as a young adult (Dong & Banks, 1975). Based on the concept that rheumatic diseases have a food allergy component, this diet emulates simple Chinese food intake and consists primarily of rice, all seafood and vegetables, vegetable oils (particularly safflower and corn), egg whites, honey, nuts (not processed) and seeds, tea or coffee, and herbs and spices. Restricted foods include meats (except occasional white meat of chicken), fruit, dairy products, whole eggs, alcohol, and all additives, preservatives, and chemicals. Dr. Dong has found that people who consume this diet have decreased symptoms and maintain normal lab values.

Even though the medical community as a whole does not support diet as a basis for treating arthritis, a recent position statement from the American College of Rheumatology concurs that food allergies may contribute to arthritis in a small number of patients. The position statement also notes that nutritional content may alter inflammation (immune response) and that further study is needed to determine which patients, if any, may benefit from receiving specific nutrients in their diets (Panush, 1991; Delafuente, 1991).

Pritikin Diet Developed in 1974, the Pritikin diet advocates a high intake of carbohydrates and fiber, an extremely low intake of fat (less than 10 percent of total calories), low cholesterol intake (less than 100 milligrams per day), and no sugars or processed foods (Kuske, 1983). An individual on this diet who consumes approximately 1,400 calories per day meets the requirements for essential nutrients, except for recommended iron (Taylor & Anthony, 1983). Although balanced, this diet is considered less palatable to Americans who are accustomed to the flavor of a higher fat intake. Those who ad-

[1]Information on arthritis diets and Dr. Ornish's diet is courtesy of Ilene Lubkin.

here to this diet feel it is effective in reversing atherosclerotic changes.

McDougall Diet The diet designed by John McDougall, M.D., in the late 1970s is similar to, but more strict than, the Pritikin Diet. Dr. McDougall evolved his diet because of growing frustation over the many patients who did not improve with prescribed medical treatments. He also noted the state of health and longevity of the Japanese, Filipinos, and Chinese patients under his care in Hawaii. Dr. McDougall feels this diet is an alternative treatment for a number of chronic disorders, including cancer, osteoporosis, arthritis, atherosclerosis, diabetes, and hypertension (McDougall, 1985).

The McDougall diet is based on a high intake of complex carbohydrates and is low in fats, high in fiber, and contains no cholesterol. It centers around a variety of starches (rice, potatoes, sweet potatoes, corn, breads, and pasta) and contains fresh or frozen green and yellow vegetables and fruits. Not allowed on the diet are milk or milk products, eggs, meat, poultry, fish, vegetable oils or other fats, refined flour, or sugar (McDougall, 1991).

Ornish Diet Dean Ornish, M.D., directed a landmark scientific research study that showed that even severe heart disease can be reversed by changing diet and life-style without the use of drugs or surgery. The diet, combined with exercise and stress reducing methods, is based on the *type* rather than the *amount* of food ingested.

Like the Pritikin and McDougall diets, Ornish's Life Choice diet is low in fat (10 percent), high in complex carbohydrates, and high in fiber. Foods from animals are restricted, since they are high in fat and cholesterol content and low in complex carbohydrates and fiber. All plant food is allowed except those that are high in fat such as avocados, olives, nuts, and seeds. Dairy products can be used only if they are nonfat (Ornish, 1991).

Vitamin Therapy   Although not truly a dietary modification, massive doses of vitamins are used to effect nutritional and health goals. A number of vitamins are known to be "essential nutri-

ents"—that is, they cannot be synthesized by the body, must be supplied from foods, and are essential for normal body function or growth. Clearly, many disorders are due to vitamin insufficiency; these include rickets (vitamin D), pellagra (vitamin B_{12}), beriberi (vitamin B_1), and chilosis (vitamin B_2).

Many Americans consume high doses of vitamin C, vitamin A, and vitamin E in the belief that such action enhances their health. In fact, Linus Pauling recommended regular use of large doses of ascorbic acid to help prevent common colds. One text listed 28 disorders that can be alleviated or cured by taking vitamin E (Kruger, 1974).

Care should be taken in suggesting the use of massive doses of vitamins, since excessive amounts of some vitamins can cause adverse effects in the body by acting as drugs, not as nutrients. For example, it is widely believed that large doses of ascorbic acid (Vitamin C) can lead to the formation of oxalate stones. Ascorbic acid can also destroy a high percentage of vitamin B_{12} in a given meal.

Antioxidants   A growing body of knowledge related to oxygen-free radicals and their role in producing disease is beginning to influence current dietary recommendations. Free radicals—stray atoms with an unpaired electron—are created by the normal metabolism of dietary fats, strenuous exercise, and exposure to environmental pollution or radiation. Once produced, they roam the body, reacting with other body tissues, causing damage to cells through a process called "oxidation" (Fridovich, 1987). Vitamins C and E and beta-carotene have been identified as antioxidant nutrients that may protect body cells by finding and quenching free radicals before they begins their cycle of damage. Recent research on the effects of these antioxidant nutrients has added some credibility to the claims that they have protective effects (Packer, 1993).

Drugs Not Approved by the FDA

The first Pure Food and Drug Act in the United States was passed in 1906. Since that time, the federal Food and Drug Administration (FDA) has been a watchdog to protect Americans from drugs not fully tested. For example, when the drug thalidomide was used in Europe, thousands of infants were born with missing extremities. Most Americans were spared this tragedy because of our strict drug regulations (Miller, 1981).

A number of drugs used to treat some chronic diseases are illegal in this country but available in Europe and elsewhere where regulations are not as strict. If testing of such drugs were allowed in the United States, new effective treatments might be identified for use here. For instance, a Chinese herbal preparation made from "thunder god vine" is used to treat arthritis in China and has shown potent results in laboratory animals. A small human study of thunder god vine has been approved by the Food and Drug Administration (Rock, 1993).

Alternative Systems of Medical Care

A number of health practitioners provide alternative or complementary approaches to health care management. Many of these practitioners undergo extensive training to reach a level of competency and pass rigorous national and state licensing board examinations. These fields of practice have many devoted clients. Only a few are discussed here.

Chiropractic[2]   Considered by many people to be part of orthodox health care, chiropractic is seen by others as an alternative modality. Vertebral manipulation, the basis of chiropractic, has been practiced for at least two and a half millennia to treat musculoskeletal disorders and, much less frequently, visceral disease. In fact, Hippocrates used an adjusting table to treat vertebral subluxations (Anderson, 1992). Chiropractic treatment offers clients an important option to avoid chronic pain, persistent drug use, disability, or surgery for many musculoskeletal and arthritic conditions.

Today's practice of chiropractic manipulation was introduced in the late 1800s by Daniel

D. Palmer, considered the father of modern chiropractic. Palmer's extensive knowledge of medicosurgical literature led to the premise that subluxation occurs when a vertebral segment is not frankly dislocated but out of normal anatomic relationship to adjacent segments. Subluxation results in a loss of normal functioning of the nerves and leads to nerve irritation and eventual permanent muscle spasm, pain, or weakness (Waagen & Strang, 1992). Palmer's first client, a deaf employee, had an amazing portion of his hearing restored within 24 hours after being adjusted. Another of Palmer's clients, Samuel Weed, named this manipulative process *chiropractic,* from a Greek root meaning "done by hand."

Chiropractic has proved helpful in preventing rigid scar contractures. When initially laid down, scar tissue forms a random and haphazard pattern, which can lead to adhesions and poor functional biomechanical capacity. If this scar is around joints or nerve roots, stiffness results, restricting motion and creating pain. Moving and stretching new scar tissue makes it more malleable, realigning the haphazard fibers in the direction of normal biomechanical motion. The value of vertebral manipulation followed by an exercise regimen remodels the newly laid collagen before it develops into a rigid scar contracture (Cohen, Diegelmann, & Lindblad, 1992).

Although most agree that chiropractic has a valuable role in the treatment of musculoskeletal conditions, a criticism of the field is that once manipulative therapy is started, regular therapy seems to be necessary to maintain optimum health. It should be noted that many people often have serious, chronic conditions that, at best, can only be managed to reduce symptomology and pain. These people frequently enjoy a reduction or elimination of pain, musculoskeletal symptoms, and any associated drug consumption. While treatment may not be curative, it may offer the best case management possible and can be so effective that clients can decrease their treatments to occasional visits as needed.

Today, modern chiropractors are licensed primary health care providers with a wide scope of practice effective with many disorders related to the autonomic, peripheral, somatic, and central nervous systems (Anderson, 1992). Chiropractic also focuses on preventive health care

---

[2]The authors wish to thank Hugh J. Lubkin, D.C., for content on chiropractic.

and correction of traumatic, sports, or repetative stress injury. In addition, chiropractic research is currently exploring the effects of improved nerve innervation on various disease states, including internal organ dysfunction, degenerative joint disease, and postsurgical recovery.

Homeopathy Homeopathy is a system of medicine originated in the early nineteenth century by Samuel Hahnemann. It is often successful in treating various diseases, and some nonspecific, beneficial responses to low doses of nontoxic substances have been demonstrated (Buxenbaum, Neafsey, & Fournier, 1988). A characteristic goal of homeopathy is to restore the self-healing potential of the patient. Homeopathy has been advocated in nursing literature as an alternative therapy during labor and postpartum care (Swinnerton, 1991a, 1991b) and for cancer treatment using mistletoe or iscador (Mellor, 1989). The basic principle of homeopathy is as follows:

> The remedy for any case of disease or illness is the substance that, when administered systematically to a healthy person, yields precisely the symptomatology of this case . . . Homeopathy holds that when the patient receives the one remedy whose symptomatology most perfectly matches his or her own symptoms, the whole disease is removed, root and branch (Coulter, 1978).

Once a drug is selected it is then administered in the minimum effective dose, usually much less than the ordinary allopathic medication doses. Proponents cite the advantages of small dosages: rare sensitivity or toxic reactions, minimal expense, and a holistic approach (Baker, 1978). The precise matching of client symptoms with one of thousands of homeopathic remedies demands considerable time and individual attention, perhaps also contributing to the satisfaction some clients feel.

Naturopathy Naturopathy has received more attention as an alternative therapy in Canada and Europe than in the United States. It emerged around the turn of the century, began to lose favor in the late thirties, but since the 1970s has enjoyed a resurgence of interest and evolution.

Naturopaths "regard disease as a response to bodily toxins and imbalances in a person's social, psychic, and spiritual environment," and believe that the healing power of nature can restore health and emphasize preventive health, education, and client responsibility (Baer, 1992). In the past, treatments favored water therapies, diet, fasting, and exercise, but now often include other alternative modalities and may overlap with chiropractic, homeopathy, and other holistic practices.

Modalities Involving Mind Control

Relaxation/imagery, biofeedback, yoga, and transcendental meditation are addressed under this category.

Relaxation/Imagery Hans Selye, an endocrinologist and director of the Institute on Experimental Medicine and Surgery at the University of Montreal, is well known for his work related to the stress response in humans. According to Selye, chronic stress can lead to hormonal imbalance, increased blood pressure (which can lead in turn to kidney damage), and suppression of the immune system (which can lead to cancer) (Selye, 1956; Simonton, Matthews-Simonton, & Creighton, 1978). Both relaxation and imagery use the concepts in Dr. Selye's work to help reduce stress and related problems.

Relaxation There are several muscle relaxation techniques, many developed in the 1970s. Characteristics common to all of them include rhythmic breathing, decreased muscle tension, and, occasionally, an altered state of consciousness (Dimotto, 1984). A technique for progressive systemic muscle relaxation was developed in the 1930s by Dr. Edward Jacobson, inventor of electromyography. In the 1970s, a renewed trend toward holistic medicine led to an increased interest in his technique.

Progressive muscle relaxation (PMR), was developed in 1973 to produce skeletal muscle relaxation and reduce stimulation of other bodily systems (Bernstein & Borkovec, 1973). In 1975, Benson introduced the relaxation response (RR), which focuses on breathing and meditation.

Progressive relaxation involves the purposeful tensing and then relaxing of specific muscle groups (Agrar, 1983).

Progressive relaxation affects both physiological and psychological aspects of the stress response. Relaxation techniques can decrease heart rate, blood pressure, respiration, oxygen consumption, carbon dioxide production, muscle tension, and metabolic rate, and can increase peripheral vasodilation and modify peripheral temperatures (Graves & Thompson, 1978). Of 14 studies reviewed before 1984, 13 showed some positive outcomes in diverse patient populations (Snyder, 1984).

Progressive relaxation as a nursing intervention for the elderly has been found to ameliorate tension headaches (Arena et al., 1988), postoperative pain (Ceccio, 1984), anxiety related to memory loss (Yesavage, 1984; Yesavage & Jacob, 1984), and stress related to transition living (Earl, 1987). Progressive relaxation helps institutionalized elderly to increase their perception of internal focus of control and self-esteem (Bensink et al., 1992). Braden, McGlone, and Pennington's research (1993) suggests that progressive relaxation contributes to the lessening of depression and improvement of enabling skills in systemic lupus erythematosis (SLE) patients. Progressive relaxation techniques are an integral part of many other modalities such as biofeedback, autogenics, and imagery.

Imagery Guided imagery, rooted in ancient cultures and religions and used in Freudian analysis, was developed and refined as a therapeutic approach by Assagioli, an Italian psychotherapist. Guided imagery may be defined as the deliberate use of an individual's mental images, involving all five modes of perception, to effect psychological and physical well-being (Witt, 1984). Some experts apply the term *visualization* to consciously chosen images and reserve *imagery* to describe those images spontaneously occurring from the unconscious. The mechanism of guided imagery may involve a self-regulating feedback mechanism—that is, training the brain through the process of imagination (imagery) (Green & Green, 1984; Vines, 1988).

Simonton, a physician, believes that stress increases a person's susceptibility to illness and that, when compounded by an attitude of hopelessness or helplessness, it can contribute to, not cause, cancer (Simonton et al., 1978). At their clinic, the Simontons combine relaxation and imagery as a tool in conjunction with medical treatment to communicate with the unconscious, to decrease tension and stress, and to comfort and alter feelings of hopelessness and helplessness.

Though usually initiated by a relaxation exercise, techniques for employing guided imagery vary. Simonton et al. (1978) recommend positive images of the client's body, energy, goal attainment, and activities. Some nurses have advocated assisting a client to "reclaim parts of the self that have previously been disowned" by asking the client to "allow the disease, the affected organ, or the symptom to assume the form of an image" (Rancour, 1991, p. 31). The following criteria were found to result in successful guided imagery/relaxation interventions with chronic renal failure patients: "(a) intact cognitive abilities, (b) higher than normal levels of perceived stress and anxiety, (c) patient verbalization of negative expectations, and (d) patient willingness to try a guided imagery/relaxation protocol" (Horsburgh & Robinson, 1989, p. 14).

In addition, nurses have reported the effective use of guided imagery, sometimes combined with relaxation, in treating chronic arthritic pain (Varni & Gilbert, 1982), chronic hemodialysis anxiety (Alarcon et al., 1982), cancer symptoms (Lyles et al., 1982; Dixon, 1984), cancer nurses' stress (Donovan, 1981), wound healing (Holden-Lund, 1988), post-surgical depression in older adults (Leja, 1989), grief work in families (Collison & Miller, 1987), cognitive scores of nursing home residents (Abraham, Neudorfer, & Currie, 1992), abstinence from smoking (Wynd, 1992), and student nurses' anxiety (Speck, 1990).

Weinberger (1991) suggested that teaching relaxation and guided imagery to the elderly would be most effective if techniques were modified to accommodate sensory and other impairments and were prescribed in accessible settings. Relaxation techniques may be of most value before or after, rather than during, procedures.

Research on guided imagery must be evaluated carefully because of inconsistencies in the way the intervention is conceptualized and implemented and in sampling, data collection, and analysis. Yet accumulating data continue to support the use of guided imagery as a nursing intervention for redirecting physiological processes, stress and pain management, disease prevention, and health maintenance (Hahn et al., 1993).

Biofeedback Green (1978) defined biofeedback as follows:

> The presentation to a person of on-going biological information, such as heart rate, usually by means of meters, lights, or auditory signals, so that he or she can become aware of inside-the-skin behaviors. Biofeedback training means using the information in learning how to self-regulate the biological process being displayed.

Currently, biofeedback research efforts are aimed at achieving voluntary control of the autonomic nervous system and the stress response, and relieving hypertension, cardiac dysrhythmias, migraines, asthma, epilepsy, back and other pain, muscle tension, and immunologic dysfunction (Robinson, 1990).

Sensitive instruments such as electroencephalography (EEG), electromyography (EMG), thermometers, and so on, convert minute amounts of electrical energy, reflecting somatic and autonomic processes, to audible or visible signals acting in a way opposite to the way drugs act. With training and practice, many individuals learn to emit the electronic instrumentation (external feedback). These individuals develop a conscious "feedback loop" and are trained to direct perception and reaction or adjustment to bodily responses to inside-the-skin events (Green, 1978).

However, it may not be biofeedback alone that works. For instance, Dr. R. Melzack, an authority on pain, feels that pain is relieved by distraction, suggestion, relaxation, and a sense of control, all part of the biofeedback procedure (LaPatra, 1978). Holroyd (1979) stated:

> In some instances, biofeedback training may be effective because it indirectly induces the patients to alter their interactions with the environment, not because it enables them

to directly control problematic physiological responses. It is therefore crucial that treatment procedures be developed that focus on altering cognitive and behavioral responses to stress, in addition to physiological responses.

Biofeedback is a proven and valuable adjunct to many treatments and health maintenance programs, especially when combined with other approaches. It is often included as one of several components of self-management or self-regulation training, which are nursing therapies designed to involve the client in relieving tension, anxiety, and symptoms of stress disorders (Kogan & Betrus, 1984). It is important to remember that biofeedback, as well as some other self-management measures, requires higher levels of cognitive function and may not be suitable for some who are impaired.

Yoga Yoga, developed in India out of Hindu philosophy before the second century B.C., is a complex system of beliefs and practices to integrate and achieve balance of the mind and body. Like many other religions and philosophies, yoga extols the virtues of meditation in clearing the mind of thoughts, easing tensions, releasing energy, and increasing self-awareness (Kruger, 1974). The awakening of *Kundalini,* the powerful reservoir coiled like a snake at the base of the spine, results in the sensation of tremendous heat and energy. This energy is awakened and released by ascetic practices including chanting, breathing, exercises, positions, and meditation (Grisell, 1979).

The most popular and best known system of yoga is Hatha Yoga—exercises and positions (*asanas* and *mudras*) to prevent and cure disease by strengthening muscles and nerves, keeping the spine flexible, and maintaining function of the glands. Yoga also includes breathing techniques (*pranayamas*) during which the body is purified and universal energy and knowledge are drawn in. Movement and breath work in harmony.

Another variation of yogic healing is ayurvedic medicine, involving diet, herbs, and natural and Indian folk remedies. Ayurvedic medicine, based on bringing your body type in harmony with nature, endorses a diet that avoids meat, eggs, fish, and sweets (Kruger, 1974; Chopra, 1994).

Some practitioners of yoga demonstrate the benefits of relaxation and reduction of tension as a result of meditation and exercise, and some find that the dietary recommendations offer benefits. However, individual limitations and requirements, such as avoidance of spinal hyperextension or inclusion of ample dietary iron, must not be overlooked. Beneficial effects of yoga have been described for the mentally handicapped (Fields, 1991), nursing home residents and staff (Hamilton-Word, Smith, & Jessup, 1982), and patients with pleural effusion (Prakasamma & Bhaduri, 1984).

Meditation   Meditation in general is a "stylized mental technique from Vedic or Buddhist traditions repetitively practiced for the purpose of attaining a subjective experience that is frequently described as very restful, silent, and of heightened alertness, often characterized as blissful" (Jevning, Wallace, & Beidebach, 1992, p. 415).

Reputable medical research has documented the following physiologic effects of a hypometabolic state during meditation, especially by long-term practitioners: decreased blood pressure, heart and respiratory rates, oxygen consumption, carbon dioxide elimination, and neuroendocrine activation, accompanied by a rise in electrical skin resistance and alpha brain waves (Jevning et al., 1992). Prospective longitudinal studies have reported significant reduction of systolic and diastolic blood pressure in hypertensive patients, as well as improvement in hypercholesterolemia, craniomandibular muscle function, asthma, insomnia, drug dependency, and decreased cigarette smoking (Jevning et al., 1992).

Comparison in many studies of effects of different techniques on trait anxiety revealed that most treatments, such as progressive relaxation, biofeedback, and various forms of meditation, produce similar effects, except that transcendental meditation (TM) produced a significantly larger effect whereas meditation that involved concentration produced a significantly smaller effect (Eppley, Abrams, & Shear, 1989). Another study comparing 200 regular partici-

pants in TM with 600,000 similar individuals revealed lower medication utilization rates and hospital admissions for TM participants in all categories except childbirth (Orme-Johnson, 1987). However, researchers have recommended against teaching meditation techniques to populations who display very fragile self-concepts, such as borderline, schizotypal, or dissociative personalities (Persinger, 1992).

Tai Chi Chuan   Tai Chi Chuan has been described as a moving meditation (Jin, 1992). Originally developed as a martial arts form, it has been used for centuries in China as a daily exercise. Tai Chi is a series of individual dance-like moves linked together in a continuous, smooth, flowing sequence. Research on the use of Tai Chi revealed physiological and stress reduction effects similar to moderate exercise (Jin, 1992, 1989); improved postural control in the elderly (Tse & Bailey, 1992); and increased range of motion and enjoyment without adverse effects in rheumatoid arthritis patients (Van Deusen & Harlow, 1987; Kirsteins, Dietz, & Hwang, 1991). Tai Chi has been found to be beneficial for the frail elderly (Wolf et al., 1993; Wolfson et al., 1993).

Stimulation/Manipulation of the Body

Another group of alternative modalities involves body stimulation. Traditional Chinese medicine, transcutaneous electrical nerve stimulation (TENS), massage, and therapeutic touch are discussed under this heading.

Traditional Chinese Medicine/Acupuncture
Traditional Chinese medicine has been practiced for over 2,000 years and includes acupuncture, acupressure, moxibustion, and *QiGong* (treatment based on meditation). Today, traditional Chinese medicine (including acupuncture) is practiced in conjunction with Western medicine by doctors both in rural areas and in clinics and hospitals (Kruger, 1974; Dimond, 1984; Beal, 1992a, 1992b).

Traditional Chinese medicine is based on the view that all things in humanity and nature are related, that human beings are a microcosm of the universe, and that the opposing but complementary forces of yin and yang must be in harmony. The objective of traditional Chinese medicine is to maintain or restore equilibrium, to treat the cause rather than the symptoms (Bresler, Kroening, & Volen, 1978).

Energy, or life force (*qi*, or *chi'i*), is located approximately two inches below the navel and circulates through 14 meridians (channels or pathways) that pass through the body; illness is a result of an interruption or imbalance of this energy flow. Hundreds of vital points identified along the meridians each have a specific function and action, and can be stimulated by needle insertion (acupuncture), pressure (acupressure or therapeutic Chinese massage), or heat (moxibustion, which uses slow-burning sticks of herbs).

For acupuncture, needles made of stainless steel, precious metal, porcelain, or other materials, varying in diameter and length, are inserted at these points, resulting in tonification or sedation of the related organ (Kruger, 1974). Weak electric current may be applied. Described as painless, acupuncture sometimes causes sensations ranging from a dull ache to a brief sharp pain. Commonly, the presence of warmth, itching, numbness, tingling, prickling, and other sensations are viewed as evidence that the treatment is working.

Acupressure massage is the palpitating, rubbing, and kneading of flesh along the meridian lines with the fingers and heel of the hand. The ancient practice of *QiGong* begins with the patient achieving a meditative state by means of a breathing exercise. Energy is then transferred from the doctor's fingertips to the patient, without touching, and gathered by the patient to accomplish healing (Sherwin, 1992).

How traditional Chinese medicine works is a tantalizing mystery. There may be multiple mechanisms, represented by a variety of theories, including the placebo effect, hypnosis, and Melzack and Wall's gate control theory (1965), which proposes that an area within the spinal cord acts as a gate in response to electrical input from both peripheral and central nerves. Some feel that acupuncture may effect complex mobilization of the immune and inflammatory system, and others believe that it sets off subtle psychologic responses (Kruger, 1974). It has been found that some of the pain-relieving effects of

acupuncture are due to activation of endogenous endorphins (Stux & Pomeranz, 1988). Those interested in acupuncture should seek practitioners who are licensed in their states and have graduated from educational programs approved by the National Accreditation Commission for Schools and Colleges of Acupuncture.

Transcutaneous Electrical Nerve Stimulation Electrical stimulation through the skin evolved as a clinical application of Melzack and Wall's gate control theory (Moore & Blacker, 1983). Though the mechanism of action is still unclear, the stimulation of larger peripheral nerves apparently blocks transmission of pain impulses. Another possible mechanism is the release of the body's own analgesic, endorphins, as a result of nerve stimulation (Taylor et al., 1983).

TENS has been used to reduce pain associated with surgery, childbirth, and chronic disease. Studies of its application indicate that it is more successful for some types of chronic pain, such as back pain, than for others. Research has suggested beneficial effects on pain with a system of electrical stimulation called CODETRON (Fargas-Babiak, Pomeranz, & Rooney, 1992) or with auricular stimulation (Lewis et al., 1990). Proper selection of clients and thorough instruction and preparation are essential for best results. Advantages to clients include avoidance of the hazards of analgesic medication and the ability to control their own therapy (Meyer, 1982).

In recent years, electrical stimulation has also been used to enhance bone growth, to maintain some of the size and function of paralyzed muscles, and to treat chronic headaches. TENS has been recommended for use in conjunction with other modalities as analgesia for terminally ill patients (McCaffery & Wolff, 1992).

Massage In recent years, the trend toward self-awareness and getting in touch with and healing one's own body and emotions has led to incorporating massage independently or with alternative therapies. Massage is defined as the "kneading, manipulation or application of methodical pressure or friction to the body" (Lawrence, 1986, p. 10). Touch and massage are regarded as sensory integration techniques that influence the activity of the autonomic nervous system. Integration of therapeutic massage in a calm, private environment is recommended as an effective adjunct for a variety of patients in isolated and technological health care settings (White, 1988).

Japanese massage, like Chinese massage, is based on manipulation of vital spots, called *tsubo,* on the meridians for the treatment of many diseases. There are other types of Japanese massage. One, shiatsu, thought to stimulate the parasympathetic nervous system and produce relaxation, includes prolonged finger pressure and spiritual concentration (Masunaga, 1978). Japanese specialists have combined oriental *(amma)* massage with other techniques to evolve a "distinctive Japanese massage system unlike any other in the world" (Serizawa, 1978, p. 207).

A number of modern massage methods are suggestive of acupressure, but the "points" and techniques vary. The principle behind *zone therapy* is that every organ in the body has a corresponding area in one or both feet; *reflex therapy* is similar. *Polarity therapy* employs (along with exercise, diet, and "right thinking") heavy pressure by thumbs, knuckles, and elbows to special points (Pannetier, 1978). *Rolfing* is a form of very deep, intensive massage that purports to use gravity and manipulation as tools in permanently restructuring the whole body and to improve functioning and competence (Rolf, 1978). There are Swedish, Turkish, Italian, and Austrian styles of massage.

Wilhelm Reich, a psychoanalyst, combined massage with psychotherapy on the basis of his thesis that neurotics build up "compensatory muscular armor" as a defense against their repressed anxieties. *Bioenergetics,* founded by Alexander Lowen and based on Reichian therapy, incorporates massage and its associated release of tension and anger (Kruger, 1974).

Many healing capabilities are attributed to various forms of massage, including relief of pain, stress, and fatigue; stimulation of blood and lymph circulation; speeding up of waste elimination; reduction of swelling; lowering of blood pressure; and foremost, of course, relaxation of muscles (LaPatra, 1978). In fact, a study of the effects of slow-stroke back massage on hospice

clients demonstrated significant decreases in heart rate and blood pressure and increases in skin temperature, both interpreted as measures of relaxation (Meek, 1993).

Therapeutic Touch   An underlying premise for therapeutic touch (TT) is that individuals extend beyond their skin by means of an energy field (Krieger, 1979). Some have extended the concept to include other human functions, including emotion, thought, and intuition (Macrae, 1988). The science of unitary human beings (Rogers, 1986) has been used to explain the relationship between TT and mental health nursing practice (Hill & Oliver, 1993).

Krieger described TT as an act of healing or helping in which "there appears to be a transfer of energy from the healer that helps the patient to repattern his/her energy level to a state comparable to that of the healer" (Krieger, Peper, & Ancoli, 1979, p. 660). The technique of TT involves assessing the client's energy field above the skin, detecting imbalances, and correcting them. Clients have been taught to do this for themselves by Hill and Oliver (1993). Though individual treatments vary and often are combined with guided imagery and other relaxation techniques, the essential factor is the healing relationship between caregiver and patient. The practitioner focuses energy by "centering" or meditating with the intent to heal. Treatment is often described as "relying on the healing energies of the universe" (Heidt, 1991, p. 65; Payne, 1989) and as a reciprocal, open communication process between healer and patient (Heidt, 1990).

Therapeutic touch as a nursing intervention has been investigated widely (Krieger, 1990; Quinn, 1989). TT has been associated with increasing physiological relaxation, decreasing patient anxiety, and rest (Heidt, 1991) and with multidimensional, personal growth (Samarel, 1992). Nursing literature includes a growing number of recommendations of TT for broad use as a complementary modality and specifically for chronic low back pain (Smith, Airey, & Salmond, 1990), AIDS (Newshan, 1989), cancer (Mentgen, 1989), chronic skin diseases (Schulte, 1991), and rehabilitation (Payne, 1989).

Summary and Conclusions

Once health practitioners accept the right of the chronically ill client to determine what treatment modalities are most effective and meaningful, support should be given to the client's choices. Only through a willingness to accept that there are alternatives to orthodox medical practice, and that all health care providers need to be informed about them, can health professionals provide the assistance clients seek.

In the Western world, most individuals seek orthodox medical care when ill. However, this care is not always effective in controlling symptoms or prolonging life. People in need will seek ways of resolving their difficulties, and this often means alternative approaches to health care. In addition, many people follow other health practices, either because such practices are culturally correct of because they feel that their health will be enhanced. These modalities are not frequently prescribed or often approved by the medical community, often because of difficulty in explaining responses and in documenting and charging for treatment. However, many are effective, legitimate routes to health care. Problems that make it difficult to choose among valid alternatives include quackery, costs, insurance payment for treatment, determining the best treatment for the given client or situation, separating fact from fiction, and determining competency of practitioners.

In spite of these problems, clients will and do seek alternatives. Some of these alternatives have been presented. The list is only partial and meant to stimulate health care providers to explore their clients' needs in view of the ever growing availability of beneficial and effective alternative modalities.

STUDY QUESTIONS

1. What is an alternative modality?
2. Why do clients/families seek alternative treatments?
3. What is the danger of quackery, and about how much money is spent on such treatment?
4. How do the problems of effectiveness of health care, cultural conflict, false claims, and finding competent practitioners adversely affect clients and practitioners, both traditional and alternative?
5. How do costs of treatment and insurance payments influence choice of treatment?
6. Why is it important for health care practitioners to be familiar with alternative treatment modalities?
7. What characteristics are reflected in diets used to deal with chronic illnesses? What role do vitamins and antioxidants play?
8. How do chiropractors, homeopaths, and naturopaths help clients?
9. How can the following be used to enhance health or improve chronic illnesses: relaxation/imagery, biofeedback, yoga, meditation tai chi chuan, Chinese medicine/acupuncture, TENS, massage, and therapeutic touch.
10. How would you counsel a client who is interested in an alternative modality as a treatment choice?

References

Abraham, I. L., Neudorfer, M. M., & Currie, L. J. (1992). Effects of group interventions or cognition and depression in nursing home residents. *Nursing Research, 41*(4), 196–202.

Agrar, W. S. (1983). Relaxation therapy in hypertension. *Hospital Practice, 18*(50), 129–137.

Alarcon, R., Jenkens, C., Heestand, D., Scott, L., & Contor, L. (1982). The effectiveness of progressive relaxation in chronic hemodialysis patients. *Journal of Chronic Disease, 35,* 797–802.

Anderson, R. (1992). Spinal manipulation before chiropractic. In S. Haldeman (Ed.), *Principles and practice of chiropractic.* San Mateo, CA: Appleton & Lange.

Arena, J. G., Hightower, N. E., & Chang, G. C. (1988). Relaxation therapy for tension headaches in the elderly: A prospective study. *Psychology of Aging, 3*(1), 96-98.

Baer, H. A. (1992). The potential rejuvenation of American naturopathy as a consequence of the holistic health movement. *Medical Anthropology, 13*(4), 369-383.

Baker, W. P. (1978). Homeotherapeutics. In L. J. Kasloff (Ed.), *Holistic dimensions in healing: Resource guide* (pp. 49-50). Garden City, NY: Doubleday.

Beal, M. W. (1992a). Acupuncture and related treatment modalities. Part I: Theoretical background. *Journal of Nurse Midwifery, 37*(4), 254-259.

———— (1992b). Acupuncture and related treatment modalities. Part II: Applications to antepartal and intrapartal care. *Journal of Nurse Midwifery, 37*(4), 260-268.

Bensink, G. W., Godbey, K. L., Marshall, M. J., & Yarandi, H. N. (1992). Institutionalized elderly, relaxation, locus of control, self-esteem. *Journal of Gerontology Nursing, 18*(4), 30-38.

Benson, H. (1975). *The relaxation response*. New York: Avon Press.

Berblinger, K. W. (1963). The physician, patient and pill. *Psychosomatics, 4*(9), 265-269.

Bernstein, D. A., & Borkovec, T. D. (1973). *Progressive relaxation training*. Champaign, IL: Research Press.

Braden, C. J., McGlone, K., & Pennington, F. (1993). Specific psychosocial and behavioral outcomes from systemic lupus. *Health Education, 20*(1), 29-41.

Bresler, D. E., Kroening, R. J., & Volen, M. P. (1978). Acupuncture in America. In L. J. Kasloff (Ed.), *Holistic dimensions in healing: Resource guide* (pp. 132-134). Garden City, NY: Doubleday.

Brody, J. (1982). The lie that heals: The ethics of giving placebos. *Annals of Internal Medicine, 97*, 112-118.

Buxenbaum, H., Neafsey, P. J., & Fournier, D. J. (1988). Hormesis, Gompertz functions, and risk assessment. *Drug Metabolism Review, 19*(2), 195-229.

Ceccio, C. M. (1984). Postoperative pain relief through relaxation in elderly patients with fractured hips. *Orthopedic Nursing, 3*(3), 11-18.

Chopra, D. (1994). *Perfect health*. S. Lancaster, MA: Quantum Publications.

Cohen, I. K., Diegelmann, R. F., & Lindbald, W. J. (1992). *Wound healing: Biochemical and clinical aspects*. Philadelphia: W. B. Saunders.

Collison, C., & Miller, S. (1987). Using images of the future in grief work. *Image: The Journal of Nursing Scholarship, 19*(1), 9-11.

Coulter, H. J. (1978). Homeopathy. In L. J. Kasloff (Ed.), *Holistic dimensions in healing: Resource guide* (pp. 47-48). Garden City, NY: Doubleday.

Delafuente, J. C. (1991, May). Nutrients and immune responses. *Rheumatic Disease Clinics of North America, 17*(2), 203-212.

Dimond, E. G. (1984). The breaking of a profession. *The Journal of the American Medical Association, 252*, 3160-3164.

Dimotto, J. W. (1984). Relaxation. *American Journal of Nursing, 84*(6), 745-758.

Dixon, J. (1984). Effect of nursing interventions on nutritional and performance status in cancer patients. *Nursing Research, 33*(6), 330-335.

Dong, C. H., & Banks, J. (1975). *The arthritic's cookbook*. New York: Bantam.

Donovan, M. I. (1981). Study of the impact of relaxation with guided imagery on stress among cancer nurses. *Cancer Nursing, 4*(2), 121-126.

Earl, W. (1987). Relaxation groups and the aging: Suggestions for longevity. *Nursing Homes, 6*(5), 16-19.

Eppley, K. R., Abrams, A. I, & Shear, J. (1989). Differential effects of relaxation techniques on trait anxiety: A meta-analysis. *Journal of Clinical Psychology, 45*(6), 957-974.

Fargas-Babiak, A. M., Pomeranz, B., & Rooney, P. J. (1992). Acupuncture-like stimulation with Codetron for rehabilitation of patients with chronic pain syndrome and osteoarthritis. *Acupuncture Electrotherapy Research, 17*(2), 95-105.

Feldman, M. K. (1990, June). Patients who seek unorthodox medical treatment. *Minnesota Medicine, 73*, 19-25.

Fields, N. (1991). Mental handicap nursing. Promoting health: Fit for life. *Nursing Times, 87*(21), 64-65.

Fridovich, I. (1987, April). The biology of oxygen radicals: General concepts. *Proceedings of Upjohn Symposium*, 1-39.

Furnham, A., & Smith, C. (1988). Choosing alternative medicine: A comparison of the beliefs of patients visiting a general practitioner and a homeopath. *Social Science and Medicine, 26*(7), 685-689.

Goldman, B. (1991). Chronic pain and the search for alternative treatments. *Canadian Medical Association Journal, 145*(5).

Graves, H. H., & Thompson, E. A. (1978). Anxiety: A mental health vital sign. In D. C. Long, & R. A. Williams (Eds.), *Clinical practice in psychosocial nursing: Assessment and intervention*. New York: Appleton-Century-Crofts.

Green, E. (1978). Biofeedback. In Kasloff, L. J. (Ed.), *Holistic dimensions in healing: Resource guide* (pp. 169-171). Garden City, NY: Doubleday.

Green, E., & Green, A (1984) Biofeedback and transformation. *The American Theosophist, 72*(5), 142-152.

Grisell, R. D. (1979). Kundalini yoga as healing agent. In H. A. Otto and J. W. Knight (Eds.), *Dimensions in holistic healing: New frontiers in the treatment of the whole person.* Chicago: Nelson-Hall.

Hahn, Y. B., Ro, Y. J., Song, H. H., Kim, H. C., Kim, H. S., & Yoo, Y. S. (1993). The effect of thermal biofeedback and progressive muscle relaxation training in reducing blood pressure of patients with essential hypertension. *Image: The Journal of Nursing Scholarship, 28*(3), 204-207.

Hamilton-Word, V., Smith, F. W., & Jessup, E. (1982). Physical fitness on a VA nursing home unit. *Geriatric Nursing, 3*(4), 260-262.

Heidt, P. R. (1990). Openness: A qualitative analysis of nurses' and patients' experiences of therapeutic touch. *Image: The Journal of Nursing Scholarship, 22*(3), 180-186.

——— (1991). Helping Patients to rest: Clinical studies in therapeutic touch. *Holistic Nursing Practice, 5*(4), 57-66.

Hill, L., & Oliver, N. (1993). Technique integration: Therapeutic touch and theory-based mental health. *Journal of Psychosocial Nursing, 31*(2), 19-22.

Holden-Lund, C. (1988) Effect of relaxation with guided imagery on surgical stress and wound healing. *Research in Nursing and Health, 11*(4), 235-244.

Holland, J. C. (1981). Patients who seek unproven cancer remedies: A psychological perspective. *Clinical Bulletin, 11*(3), 102-105.

Holroyd, K. (1979). Stress, coping, and the treatment of stress-related illness. In J. R. McNamara (Ed.), *Behavioral approaches to medicine: Application and analysis* (pp. 191-217). New York: Plenum.

Horsburgh, M. E., & Robinson, J. A. (1989). Relaxation therapy and guided imagery in ESRD. *American Nephrology Nurses Association-Journal, 16*(1), 11-14, 19.

Jarvis, W. T. (1992). Quackery: A national scandal. *Clinical Chemistry, 38*(8), 1574-1586.

Jevning, R., Wallace, R. K., & Beidebach, M. (1992). The physiology of meditation: A review. *Neuroscience Biobehavior Review, 16*(3), 415-424.

Jin, P. (1989). Changes in heart rate, noradrenaline, cortisol and mood during Tai Chi. *Journal of Psychosomatic Research, 33*(2), 197-206.

——— (1992). Efficacy of Tai Chi, brisk walking, meditation, and reading in reducing mental and emotional stress. *Journal of Psychosomatic Research, 36*(4), 361-370.

Johnson, G. T. (1984, November 29). Studies help spot fraud in medicine. *The Kansas City Star,* p. 3B.

Kirsteins, A. E., Dietz, F., & Hwang, S. W. (1991). Tai-Chi Chuan, for rheumatoid arthritis patients. *American Journal of Physical Medicine and Rehabilitation, 70*(3), 136-141.

Kogan, H. N., & Betrus, P. A. (1984). Self-management: A nursing mode of therapeutic influence. *Advances in Nursing Science, 6*(4), 55-73.

Krieger, D. (1979). Therapeutic touch and contemporary applications. In H. A. Otto & J. W. Knight (Eds.), *Dimensions in holistic healing: New frontiers in the treatment of the whole person* (pp. 297-303). Chicago: Nelson-Hall.

——— (1990). Therapeutic touch: Two decades of research, teaching and clinical practice. *Imprint, 37*(3), 86-88.

Krieger, D., Peper, E., & Ancoli, S. (1979). The psychological indices of therapeutic touch. *American Journal of Nursing, 79,* 660-665.

Kruger, H. (1974). *Other healers, other cures: A guide to alternative medicine.* New York: Bobbs-Merrill.

Kuske, T. (1983). Quackery and fad diets. In E. Feldman (Ed.), *Nutrition in the middle and late years.* Boston: John Wright.

LaPatra, J. (1978). *Healing.* St. Louis: McGraw-Hill.

Lawrence, D. B. (1986). *Massage techniques.* New York: Knopf.

Leja, A. M. (1989). Using guided imagery to combat postsurgical depression. *Journal of Gerontology Nursing, 15*(4), 7-11.

Levine, J. D., Gordon, N. D., & Fields, H. L. (1978). The mechanisms of placebo analgesia. *Lancet, 2,* 654-657.

Lewis, S. M., Clelland, J. A., Knowles, C. J., Jackson, J. R., & Dimick, A. R. (1990). Effects of auricular acupuncture-like transcutaneous electric nerve stimulation on pain levels following wound care inpatients with burns. *Journal of Burn Care Rehabilitation, 11*(4), 322-329.

Lyles, J. N., Burish, T.G., Krozely, M. G., & Oldham, R. K. (1982). Efficacy of relaxation training and guided imagery in reducing the aversiveness of cancer chemotherapy. *Journal of Consulting and Clinical Psychology, 50*(4), 509-524.

Macrae, J. (1988). *Therapeutic touch: A practical guide.* New York: Knopf.

Martin, D. S., Allen, C. N., Cohen, R. J., Lerner, I. J., Lewis, J. P., & Pinksy, C. M. (1983). Ineffective cancer therapy: A guide for the layperson. *Journal of Clinical Oncology, 1*(2), 154-163.

Masunaga, S. (1978). Shiatsu. In L. J. Kasloff (Ed.), *Holistic dimensions in healing: Resource guide* (pp. 212-214). Garden City, NY: Doubleday.

McCaffery, M., & Wolff, M. (1992). Pain relief using cutaneous modalities, positioning, and movement. *Hospital Journal, 8*(1-2), 121-153.

McDougall, J. A. (1985). *McDougall medicine: A challenging second opinion*. Piscataway, NJ: New Century Publishers.

———— (1991). *The McDougall program*. New York: Plume.

Meek, S. S. (1993). Effects of slow stroke back massage on relaxation in hospice clients. *Image: The Journal of Nursing Scholarship, 25*(1), 17-21.

Mellor, D. (1989). Mistletoe in homeopathic cancer treatment. *Professional Nurse, 4*(12), 605-607.

Melzack, R., & Wall, P. D. (1965). Pain mechanisms: A new theory. *Science, 150,* 971.

Mentgen, J. L. (1989). Therapeutic touch: A healing art. *Journal of the Association of Pediatric Oncology Nurses, 6*(2), 29-30.

Meyer, C. (1973). *American folk medicine*. New York: Crowell.

Meyer, T. M. (1982). TENS: Relieving pain through electricity. *Nursing 82, 12*(9), 57-59.

Miller, S. A. (1981). *Nutrition and behavior*. Philadelphia: Franklin Institute Press.

Montbriand, M. J., & Laing, G. P. (1991). Alternative health care as a control strategy. *Journal of Advanced Nursing, 16,* 325-332.

Moore, D. E., & Blacker, H. M. (1983). How effective is TENS for chronic pain? *American Journal of Nursing, 83,* 1175-1177.

Murray, R., & Zentner, J. (1979). *Nursing assessment and health promotion through the life span* (2nd ed.). Englewood Cliffs, NJ: Prentice-Hall.

Newshan, G. (1989). Therapeutic touch for symptom control in persons with AIDS. *Holistic Nursing Practice, 3*(4), 45-51.

Orme-Johnson, D. (1987). Medical care utilization and the transcendental meditation program. *Psychosomatic Medicine, 49*(5), 493-507.

Ornish, D. (1991). *Eat more, weigh less*. New York: HarperCollins.

Packer, L. (1993). Health effects of nutritional antioxidants. *Free Radical Biology and Medicine 12,* 685-686.

Pannetier, P. (1978). Polarity therapy. In L. J. Kasloff (Ed.), *Holistic dimensions in healing: Resource guide* (pp. 216-217). Garden City, NY: Doubleday.

Panush, R. S. (1991, May). American College of Rheumatology position statement: Diet and arthritis. *Rheumatic Disease Clinics of North America, 17*(2), 443-444.

Payne, M. B. (1989). The use of therapeutic touch with rehabilitation clients. *Rehabilitation Nursing, 14*(2), 69-72.

Persinger, M. A. (1992). Enhanced incidence of the sensed presence in people who have learned to meditate: Support for the right hemispheric intrusion hypotheses. *Perceptual Motor Skills, 75*(3, pt. 2), 1308-1310.

Prakasamma, M., & Bhaduri, A. (1984). A study of yoga as a nursing intervention in the care of patients with pleural effusion. *Journal of Advanced Nursing, 9*(2), 127-133.

Prescott, D. M., & Flexer, A. S. (1982). *Cancer: The misguided cell*. New York: Scribner's.

Quinn, J. F. (1989) Therapeutic touch as energy exchange: Replication and extension. *Nursing Science, 2*(2), 74-78.

Rancour, P. (1991). Guided imagery: Healing when curing is out of the question. *Perspectives in Psychiatric Care, 27*(4), 30-33.

Robinson, L. (1990). Stress and anxiety. *Nursing Clinics of North America, 25*(4), 935-943.

Rock, M. (1993, Sept./Oct.). Exploring medicine's gray area. *Arthritis Today,* pp. 36-40.

Rogers, M. (1986). Science of unitary human beings. In V. M. Malinski (Ed.), *Explorations of Martha Rogers' science of unitary human beings*. (pp. 5-12) Norwalk, CT: Appleton-Century-Crofts.

Rolf, I. P. (1978). Rolfing. In L. J. Kasloff (Ed.), *Holistic dimensions in healing: Resource guide* (pp. 225-227). Garden City, NY: Doubleday.

Samarel, N. (1992). The experience of receiving therapeutic touch. *Journal of Advanced Nursing, 17*(6), 651-657.

Schulte, M.A.B. (1991). Self-care activating support: Therapeutic touch and chronic skin disease. *Dermatology Nursing, 3*(5), 335-339.

Selye, H. (1956). *The stress of life*. New York: McGraw-Hill.

Serizawa, K. (1978). Massage. In L. J. Kasloff (Ed.), *Holistic dimensions in healing: Resource guide* (pp. 206-208). Garden City, NY: Doubleday.

Sherwin, D. C. (1992). Traditional chinese medicine in rehabilitation nursing practice. *Rehabilitation Nursing, 17*(5), 253-255.

Simonton, O. C., Matthews-Simonton, S., & Creighton, J. L. (1978). *Getting well again*. New York: J. D. Tarcher.

Smith, I. W., Airey, S., & Salmond, S. W. (1990). CE Feature. Part 2: Nontechnologic strategies for coping with chronic low back pain. *Orthopedic Nursing, 9*(4), 26-34.

Snyder, M. (1984). Progressive relaxation as a nursing intervention: An analysis. *Advances in Nursing Science, 6*(3), 47-58.

Somers, A. R., & Somers, A. M. (1977). *Health & health care*. Germantown, MD: Aspen Systems.

Speck, B. J. (1990). The effect of guided imagery upon first semester nursing students. *Journal of Nursing Education, 29*(8), 346-350.

Stux, G., & Pomeranz, B. (1988). *Basics of acupuncture*. Berlin: Springer-Verlag.

Swinnerton, T. (1991a). Alternative postnatal therapies. *Nursing Times, 87*(22), 64-65.

———— (1991b). Alternative remedies during labor. *Nursing Times, 87*(9), 64-65.

Taylor, A. G., West, B. A., Simon, B., Skelton, J., & Rowlington, J. C. (1983). How effective is TENS for acute pain? *American Journal of Nursing, 83,* 1171-1174.

Taylor, K. B., & Anthony, L. E. (1983). *Clinical nutrition.* St. Louis: McGraw-Hill.

Tse, S. K., & Bailey, D. M. (1992). T'ai Chi and postural control in the well elderly. *American Journal of Occupational Therapy, 46*(4), 295-300.

Van Deusen, J., & Harlow, D. (1987). The efficacy of the ROM dance program for adults with rheumatoid arthritis. *American Journal of Occupation Therapy, 41*(2), 90-95.

Varni, J., & Gilbert, A. (1982). Self-regulation of chronic arthritis pain and long-term analgesic dependence in a hemophiliac. *Rheumatology and Rehabilitation, 11*(1), 121-126.

Veterans Administration Cooperative Study on Antihypertensive Agents (VACSG) (1967). Effects of treatment on morbidity in hypertension: 1. Results in patients with diastolic blood pressure averaging 115 through 129 mm Hg. *Journal of the American Medical Association, 202,* 1028.

———— (1970). Effects of treatment on morbidity in hypertension: 2. Results in patients with diastolic blood pressures averaging 90 through 114 mm Hg. *Journal of the American Medical Association, 213,* 1143.

Vines, S. W. (1988). The therapeutics of guided imagery. *Holistic nursing practices, 2*(3), 34-44.

Waagen, G., & Strang, V. (1992). Origin and development of traditional chiropractic philosophy. In S. Haldeman (Ed.), *Principles and practice of chiropractic.* San Mateo, CA: Appleton & Lange.

Weinberger, R. (1991). Teaching the elderly stress reduction. *Journal of Gerontology Nursing, 17*(10), 23-27.

White, J. A. (1988). Touching with intent: Therapeutic massage. *Holistic Nursing Practice, 2*(3), 63-67.

Witt, J. (1984). Relieving chronic pain. *Nurse Practitioner, 9*(1), 36-38.

Wolf, S. L, Kutner, N. G., Green, R. C., & McNeely, E. (1993). The Atlanta FICSIT study: Two exercise interventions to reduce fragility in elders. *Journal of the American Geriatric Society, 41*(3), 329-332.

Wolfson, L., Whipple, R., Judge, J., Amerman, P., Derby, C., & King, M. (1993). Training balance and strength in the elderly to improve function. *Journal of the American Geriatric Society, 41*(3), 341-343.

Wynd, C. A. (1992). Relaxation imagery used for stress reduction in the prevention of smoking relapse. *Journal of Advanced Nursing, 17*(3), 294-302.

Yesavage, J. A. (1984). Relaxation and memory training in 39 elderly patients. *American Journal of Psychiatry, 141*(10), 778-781.

Yesavage, J. A., & Jacob, R. (1984). Effects of relaxation and mnemonics memory, attention, and anxiety in the elderly. *Experimental Aging Research, 10*(4), 211-214.

Bibliography

DeJarnette, M. B. (1978). Cranial technique. In L. J. Kasloff, (Ed.), *Holistic dimensions in healing: Resource guide* (pp. 84-85). Garden City, NY: Doubleday.

Epstein, G. (1986). The image of medicine: Notes of a clinician. *Advances, 3*(1), 22-31.

Fanslow, C. A. (1983). Therapeutic touch: A healing modality throughout life. *Topics in Clinical Nursing, 5*(2), 72-79.

Feldman, E. B. (1983). *Nutrition in the middle and later years.* Boston: John Wright.

Gottlieb, R. (1978). Development vision therapy. In L. J. Kasloff (Ed.), *Holistic dimensions in healing: Resource guide* (pp. 90-91). Garden City, NY: Doubleday.

Kroening, R. J., Volen, M. P., & Bresler, D. (1979). Acupuncture: Healing the whole person. In H. A. Otto and J. W. Knight (Eds.), *Dimensions in holistic healing: New frontiers in the treatment of the whole person* (pp. 427-438). Chicago: Nelson-Hall.

Lang, P. J., Kozak, M. J., Miller, G. A., Levin, D. N., & McLean, A. (1980). Emotional imagery: Conceptual structure and pattern of somata-visceral response, *Psychophysiology, 17*(2), 179-192.

Perry, H. T. (1978). Temporomandibular joint technique. In L. J. Kasloff (Ed.), *Holistic dimensions in healing: Resource guide* (pp. 89-89). Garden City, NY: Doubleday.

Rubenfeld, I. (1978). Alexander: The use of self. In L. J. Kasloff (Ed.), *Holistic dimensions in healing: Resource guide* (pp. 222-224). Garden City, NY: Doubleday.

Vickery, D., & Fries, J. (1981). *Take care of yourself.* Reading, MA: Addison-Wesley.

CHAPTER 19

Nursing Ethics
in Chronic Illness

Beverly J. McElmurry • Barbara Harris
Susan Misner • Linda Olson

Introduction

The number and complexity of ethical issues in health care are increasing at a faster rate than our institutional mechanisms can handle. The very nature of potential ethical issues facing health care professionals demands an environment where decisions can be made that are in the best interests of clients as stakeholders. In this chapter, the operational definition of a stakeholder is anyone who has an interest in the outcome of an ethical decision or is affected by it. Therefore, chronically ill clients, their families, and significant others, as well as health care professionals who are involved in their care, should be included in the ethical decision-making process.

This chapter focuses on three important levels to consider during the process of ethical thinking about the care of persons with chronic illnesses: individual, institutional, and societal in-fluences on nursing practice. To realize such thinking, it is important to examine the nature of caring, and its influence on the relationship of nurse to client; how institutions influence the work of nurses; and societal influences on the practice of nurses. These levels of influence are often intertwined, and sometimes these associations are not apparent when one begins to think about nursing ethics.

Content herein is grounded in reflection about practice experiences; it is not a presentation of ethics from the traditional biomedical, principled reasoning approach, nor is there a focus on a particular theory or process that nurses are urged to use. By principled reasoning we mean the use of the principles of respect for autonomy, beneficence, nonmaleficence, and justice in thinking about ethical issues (see Table 19–1). What is important is that the reader think sensitively about the points raised and the issues confronted in caring for persons with chronic illnesses.

Professionals in any field are socialized by their experience and education within multiple social environments, often in ways that are

Acknowledgment: All authors have made equal contributions to this chapter.

416

TABLE 19-1. Principles of biomedical ethics

There are four traditionally used principles that apply ethical theory to ethical decision making:

1. *Principle of Respect for Autonomy*—Implies the idea of self-governance, of being one's own person, without constraints by the actions of others. Respecting another's autonomy implies that people should determine their own course of action based on a plan chosen by themselves. For example, patients have the right to refuse treatment.
2. *Principle of Beneficence*—Implies the idea of a duty to do or promote good, to confer benefits, and to contribute to the welfare of others, including their health.
3. *Principle of Nonmaleficence*—Implies the notion of "do no harm." The duty of nonmaleficence encompasses not harming others, as well as not putting others at risk for harm.
4. *Principle of Justice*—Implies the notion of fairness or that equals ought to be treated equally and unequals may be treated unequally. Principles of justice are often cited when there is concern for appropriate allocation or distribution of health care resources.

SOURCE: Adapted from Beauchamp and Childress (1983). New York: Oxford University Press.

unrecognized. The issue of professional socialization is grippingly illustrated in Jay Lifton's exhaustive study (1986) of Nazi doctors. An important aspect of his analysis is the concept of *doubling,* that is, the process of taking a humane self and joining it with a "professional self" willing to ally itself with destructive behaviors. An alternative to such negative professional socialization is to strive for the "embodied self: a self that includes a measure of unity and awareness of body and person in regard to oneself and others" (Lifton, 1986).

Key Concepts in Nursing Ethics

Nursing ethics is an emerging area of study where there is the need to fathom the questions about and criticisms that have evolved, as well as to understand the content of this area. As nursing ethics has developed, certain concepts have begun to stand out as central contributions;

three are discussed below: caring, relationships, and everyday ethics.

Caring   The concept of caring is central to the nursing profession's efforts to delineate its own ethical base of practice. Caring is also a central focus of feminist ethics, from which nursing has drawn several insights that shape the profession's development of an ethic of care.

The study of caring became popular in nursing during the 1970s, in part because of the work of Madeline Leininger, a nurse-anthropologist whose cross-cultural studies showed the importance of caring behaviors in sustaining health and well-being (Leininger, 1981). The popularity of the concept also grew in response to nurses' recognition that the boom in technological advances characteristic of health care in the 1960s and 1970s often created situations where human, spiritual, and emotional needs of clients were overshadowed by the imperative to apply all available scientific knowledge and technology to curing diseases (Carper, 1979; Engel, 1980).

Caring has since been identified as the central base of nursing practice (Gaut, 1983; Griffin, 1983; Leininger, 1988). Further, caring has been defined in a multitude of ways, although it still lacks a concise and universal definition (Morse et al., 1991). (See Table 19-2.) The central theme running through these definitions is commitment to values, attitudes, and actions that restore or maintain a patient's dignity, humanity, and well-being. These include the following ideas:

1. Caring arises out of acknowledgment of one's humanity and inherent vulnerability; it is the basis for respecting another's humanity and responding to another's vulnerability, whether manifested as physical pain and suffering, emotional or spiritual suffering, or crisis.
2. Caring is manifested through words and actions that express concern and response to needs for relief of suffering, maintenance of dignity, and search for meaning or understanding of experience.
3. Caring results in greater patient well-being, preservation of dignity, and a greater sense of meaning or understanding of self and life experiences for both nurse and patient.

TABLE 19-2. Common definitions of caring

Author	Definition
Leininger (1980)	"those human acts and processes which provide assistance to another . . . based on an interest in or concern for that human being or to meet an expressed, obvious or anticipated need." (p. 136)
Watson (1988)	"the moral idea of nursing [which] consists of transpersonal human-to-human attempts to protect, enhance, and preserve humanity." (p. 54)
Gadow (1985)	"the highest form of commitment to patients, encompassing as many different expressions of concern for the patient's well-being as we are imaginative enough to devise" (p. 8)
Gilligan (1982)	"an activity of relationship, of seeing and responding to need, taking care of the world by sustaining a web of connection so that no one is left alone." (p. 62)
Noddings (1984)	"that relation in which [one] responds as one caring out of love, natural inclination." (p. 5) Noddings calls this "natural caring" and differentiates it from "ethical caring," which occurs in professional caring relationships. Ethical caring is defined as "meeting the other morally" (p. 5). The motivation for ethical caring arises from the professional's view of self as caring, which in turn arises from previous experiences of caring and being cared for.

A more recent trend is to view caring as a core value that gives meaning to nursing practice as a moral endeavor (Gadow, 1985; Watson, 1988). Nurse scholars also define caring as a virtue of the nurse that makes ethical practice possible (Brody, 1988; Fry, 1988).

Relationship Closely associated with caring is the notion of relationship. The nurse–patient relationship historically has been an important and valued aspect of practice within the profession. One of the most frequently cited sources on the association between caring and relationship is Carol Gilligan's (1982) work toward a feminist ethic of care. Her research into the moral reasoning of girls and women suggests that many women do not use universal ethical principles as their main guide in decision making, but use their experience of relationships as the foundation of their thinking about moral and ethical concerns (Gilligan, 1982). This does not mean that all women use relationships as their only moral foundation, nor does it mean that men exclusively use principles as theirs. Rather, her findings provide evidence that people use different ways of thinking about and resolving the moral and ethical concerns that arise in their personal and professional lives.

Gilligan also provided nursing with a framework that facilitates understanding of individual nurses' experiences of ethical practice (Cooper, 1989; Parker, 1990) by suggesting that relationship is the context within which caring can occur (Benner & Wrubel, 1989; Gadow, 1988; Knowlden, 1988). For example, through participation in such a relationship, the nurse comes to know patients' needs, desires, and concerns, as well as their values and perceptions. Participation leads to a thorough understanding of the complex and individualized nature of a patient's life and situation (Gadow, 1988). The development of a mutual, genuine, and caring relationship is seen as a primary ethical responsibility of nursing (Watson, 1988). Such understanding is critical to the nurse's ability to respect patients' humanity, nurture their dignity, and participate in their ongoing attempts to make meaning of their experiences.

The nurse–patient relationship is also seen as an ethical responsibility because of its potential to significantly impact both emotional and physical health. Watson (1988), a nurse theorist, talks about the ways a caring relationship may facilitate physical or emotional restoration when it results in a free and genuine sharing of thoughts and feelings. This supposition is based on Eastern mystical philosophies of the holistic nature of persons and allows emotional expression, as well as confirmation and validation, of the client's expression of experiential meaning and self-understanding, to free energy for healing (Watson, 1988).

Contextual Influences in Decision Making
Some nonnursing ethicists refer to the building of provider–patient relationships as a means of preventing, or at least effectively addressing, ethically problematic situations. These ethicists have shown how traditional medical ethics (Table 19-1), with its emphasis on facts and emotionally detached decision making, can bypass the very information needed to make a sensitive decision (Reich, 1991). Such information includes the patient's values and perceptions of what is important to him or her.

In addition, traditional medical ethics does not place emphasis on relationships as a context for discourse or interaction between provider, patient, and family regarding health care decisions with ethical implications. The authors of this chapter value the functions of relationships and argue that patient, family, and health care providers can together offer a more natural, effective, and inclusive forum for making health care decisions that are of paramount importance to the patient and family.

Everyday Ethics   A primary characteristic of caring and relational ethics is the emphasis on the moral nature of the experience of everyday practice. Everyday ethics contrasts with biomedical ethics, which focuses on providing guidelines to the solution of recognizable ethical problems and encourages the application of the same basic rules or principles to all ethical problems.

The notion of an everyday ethics also contrasts with professional codes such as the American Nurses' Association (ANA) Code for Nurses (ANA, 1985), which enumerate standards of nursing practice (see Table 19-3). Like traditional biomedical ethics, professional codes tend to focus on problems, or breaches, in what is considered ethical practice. The ANA Code for Nurses supplies broad guidelines for practice by prescribing actions that prevent, or are an appropriate response to, potential ethical problems

TABLE 19-3.   ANA code for nurses*

1. The nurse provides services with respect for human dignity and the uniqueness of the client, unrestricted by considerations of social or economic status, personal attributes, or the nature of health problems.
2. The nurse safeguards the client's right to privacy by judiciously protecting information of a confidential nature.
3. The nurse acts to safeguard the client and the public when health care and safety are affected by the incompetent, unethical, or illegal practice of any affected person.
4. The nurse assumes responsibility and accountability for individual nursing judgments and actions.
5. The nurse maintains competence in nursing.
6. The nurse exercises informed judgment and uses individual competence and qualifications as criteria in seeking consultation, accepting responsibilities, and delegating nursing activities to others.
7. The nurse participates in activities that contribute to the ongoing development of the profession's body of knowledge.
8. The nurse participates in the profession's efforts to implement and improve standards of nursing.
9. The nurse participates in the profession's efforts to establish and maintain conditions of employment conducive to high-quality nursing care.
10. The nurse participates in the profession's effort to protect the public from misinformation and misrepresentation and to maintain the integrity of nursing.
11. The nurse collaborates with members of the health professions and other citizens in promoting community and national efforts to meet the health needs of the public.

*See American Nurses' Association (1985) for interpretive statements.
SOURCE: From American Nurses' Association (1985). Used with permission.

such as nonadherence to standards of direct patient care or instances of potential or actual abuse of patients by providers.

By contrast, caring and relational ethics focus on understanding what it is to be moral every day and in all activities. To be moral in one's life and to practice one's profession ethically does not mean simply avoiding immoral or unethical actions through adherence to codes and guidelines. Nor does it simply mean applying ethical theory and decision-making methods to problematic situations. Instead, from the nursing ethics perspective, being moral and practicing ethically means actively working to recognize and nurture the best human potential in self and others.

Problems of Nursing Ethics and Chronic Illness

What does all of this mean for health care providers working with the chronically ill? In the past few years, there has been a slowly growing recognition that current models of health care fail to adequately meet the needs of individuals with long-term illnesses. The medical model of illness and its approach to ethical decision making are grounded in a view of the client as an autonomous individual who is suffering from an acute condition (Moros et al., 1991; Cooper, 1990; Collopy et al., 1990), which is an inadequate basis for meeting the needs of individuals with chronic illnesses (Cooper, 1990; Jennings, Callahan, & Caplan, 1988). This perspective can be summarized as follows: Patients, temporarily and voluntarily, surrender their autonomy to the health care provider so that the provider, using specialized medical knowledge, is free to implement treatments to cure or eradicate the disease condition. Patients then return to their previous autonomous life, free of disease (Collopy et al., 1990).

Unlike illnesses labeled as acute, a chronic condition often entails long-term alterations of life-style and self-identity. Common dimensions include pain; suffering; and a loss of privacy, dignity, and independence. In addition, treatments for such illnesses carry their own impact on life-style and self-perception (Thorne, 1991). In essence, persons experiencing chronic illnesses can lose the ability to actualize their humanity in accustomed or preferred ways. Traditional notions of cure and autonomy cannot always address the human needs that accompany the chronic illness experience. Ways in which the concepts of nursing ethics, as currently formulated, can facilitate ethical practice with the chronically ill are discussed here.

Ethical Responses to the Chronically Ill

Living with a chronic illness requires that the illness experience be integrated into the person's identity (Collopy et al., 1990, Moros et al., 1991; Thorne, 1991). In other words, persons with chronic illnesses need to understand how the illness affects them, how they feel about that, and how to find a meaning for this reality that allows them to feel good about themselves, their lives, and inherent possibilities. This process involves coming to terms with the realities of their lives.

Nursing ethics, with its emphasis on the moral responsibility of the provider to respond to the humanness of the patient, also requires that weight be placed on being open to the variations and individuality of such expressions. Implications for the provider working with a chronically ill person are

1. To work at building a relationship so the client feels comfortable expressing thoughts and feelings that must be processed in order to make sense of, and come to terms with, the reality of his or her life (Watson, 1988).
2. To be open to variations in how clients cope, grieve, and maintain hope (Watson, 1988).
3. To be comfortable confirming the client's existence and validating his or her insights, thoughts, and feelings as human and worthwhile (Watson, 1988; Dunlop, 1986).
4. To be comfortable with the potential for shared vulnerability; the provider does not shy away from the patient's expressions of pain, suffering, or hopelessness, but accepts his or her own potential for vulnerability and limitations in alleviating the patient's pain and suffering (Benner & Wrubel, 1989; Gadow, 1988).

These are broad guidelines that speak more to attitudes, values, or a way of being than to specific actions or formulas for addressing problems. This is the crux of nursing ethics: When ethical practice is defined as an everyday process, instead of as adherence to specific guidelines to prevent or solve problems, the actu-

CASE STUDY

The Suicidal Patient

A 45-year-old man is admitted to an adult psychiatric unit following a suicide attempt. His diagnoses are major depression and pedophilia. He was arrested two months prior to admission for the sexual abuse of a 10-year-old boy. He admitted to doing this and to having a 20-year history of similar acts. Subsequently, he lost his teaching job, his wife filed for divorce, and she left the state with their three children.

The nurse who works with him on a daily basis finds that she has difficulty being around him. She feels disgusted by what he admits to having done and feels no sympathy for him, believing that, through his actions, he has brought all of these life events upon himself. She believes that all patients have a right to the same quality of care, so she goes about making sure she does everything for him that she does for her other patients. One day, after she takes his blood pressure, the patient looks up at her and says, "You don't like me very much, do you? I can see how you stand here, just counting the minutes till you can be out of here . . . I don't blame you—I don't like myself much, either."

---

alization of such practice becomes a way of being or practicing.

Stigma and Labeling   Stigma and labeling are social phenomena that hold substantial ethical implications for health care providers. Labeling refers to the process of attaching a term, often a diagnosis, to a person. When the terms have negative social connotations that affect the way clients and others perceive them, stigma occurs (see Chapter 5, on stigma).

From an ethical perspective, providers must be aware of the diagnoses, terms, and labels that can stigmatize clients. Chronic illness diagnoses that can be stigmatizing include many of the mental illnesses, such as schizophrenia and pedophilia, or physical illnesses, such as cancer and AIDS. Although diagnostic categories are useful and often necessary to determine appropriate treatment, providers must weigh the benefits of using these labels, particularly in the case of mental illness, against the negative effects of accompanying stigma. Negative effects include the client's integration of the label into a self-denigrating identity and others' negations of the client's personhood when the label colors perceptions (Goffman, 1986).

By placing emphasis on the wholeness, complexity, and individuality of persons, nursing ethics encourages providers to look beyond labels. An ethic of care, focusing on the moral responsibility to confirm and validate an individual, encourages providers to reflect on the nature of their responses and to understand their sources (Watson, 1988).

A more difficult ethical concern for providers is the situation in which a patient has a label, or stigmatizable attribute, that the provider recognizes as such but is having difficulty responding to in any but a negative manner. Consider the case study of the suicidal patient. In this case, the ANA standards of care are not compromised; the patient receives the same direct care as all of the nurse's other patients. Yet there is a difference. The nurse has made judgments in response to the label of pedophile, thereby stigmatizing him. Although she attempts to ensure that her values and judgments do not get in the way of her caregiving, something about her demeanor, perhaps in the way she provides the care, lets him know she views him negatively. This view is congruent with his view of himself.

The task facing this nurse is to determine how to respond to this patient, not just in answer to his question, but throughout the rest of his hospital stay. An ethic of care, with value placed on respecting the infinite variations of people, encourages providers to examine how their thoughts, feelings, and values influence their ability to be open to and respect the individual differences their patients bring. Values clarification exercises, in which one answers questions and practices self-reflection to determine what one values and why, would be an appropriate intervention here. Talking to a peer about the situation may also aid in values clarification and in the task of gaining the self-understanding needed to be genuinely responsive to someone who challenges the nurse's value system (Hauerwas & Burrell, 1989; Benner, 1991). An understanding of one's values fosters decision making and the process of making choices, and it is a first step in learning to deal with the ethical dilemmas in nursing practice (Davis & Aroskar, 1991; Steele, 1983).

While an ethic of care encourages providers to find ways to accept and respond to clients who have attributes that are readily stigmatizable or distasteful or go against personal beliefs or values, it does not require providers to like them. The interpretation of an ethic of care as requiring a subjective liking of patients is a source of criticism (Curzer, 1993; Olsen, 1992). There is no getting around the fact that caring does involve affect, whether it is called concern, liking, or love (Dunlop, 1986; Mayeroff, 1971). However, it is necessary to be aware of the difference between liking and concern for another.

The nurse in the case study of the suicidal patient does not have to like the patient, or even stop feeling disgusted by his behaviors. However, an ethic of care would guide the nurse toward understanding his behaviors as tragic and unfortunate, but very real, manifestations of human existence. As when providers caring for suffering and vulnerable patients are confronted with their own potential for experiencing pain and vulnerability (Gadow, 1988), this nurse must confront her own potential both to be hurt and to hurt another when she accepts the reality of the patient's hurtful behaviors towards others and his pain at her response to him. Within this confrontation are the seeds of a capacity for concern for the patient as a human being. If the nurse can act out of concern for the human needs of the patient, and if the patient can be receptive to those acts, then a caring relationship will have taken root (Gilligan, 1982; Noddings, 1984; Watson, 1988).

Compliance The nursing diagnosis of noncompliance is related to the phenomena of labeling and stigma because its use can have the same

negative effects. Noncompliance refers to failure to adhere to a treatment, regimen, or life-style change prescribed by a health care provider (see Chapter 10, on compliance). This perception has substantial ethical implications for providers who care for chronically ill individuals, most of whom find themselves confronted with a variety of treatments or life-style changes prescribed by others over the course of their illness.

Ethical implications arise from the negative connotations assigned to the label of noncompliance by health care providers (Thorne, 1991). These include considering these individuals as irrational or in denial of their illness or its seriousness (Thorne, 1991; Whitley, 1991). The elderly and the mentally ill are populations at high risk of being labeled noncompliant (Collopy et al., 1990). This is relevant for providers because of the high incidence of chronic illness among the elderly population and because of the high level of chronicity among the mentally ill (Wilson & Kneisl, 1992).

Because the label of noncompliance has such negative effects, there is an ethical responsibility to reflect on its use. Whitley (1991) noted that over 30 % of the nurses in two studies chose not to use this diagnosis because of its negative reflection on patients that overshadowed provider-related contributions to poor adherence to treatment. Examples of provider contributions to noncompliance are inadequate explanations of the use and side effects of medication or provider inattention to patients' concerns about medication and treatment. The reasons identified by these nurses for such behavior were anxiety, lack of understanding of treatment, and lack of mutual decision making about treatment between provider and client (Whitley, 1991). Thorne's (1991) study of patients' explanations for noncompliance also identifies lack of opportunity for mutual decision making as a key factor.

The importance of a provider–patient relationship is underscored by these findings, since all of these factors are amenable to nursing intervention. From an ethical perspective, each can be addressed in a relationship context: to build a relationship that holds the potential of allaying anxiety, providing useful information, and offer-

TABLE 19-4. Advance directives

There are two types of advance directives. The Living Will is a treatment directive. The power of attorney or health proxy is an appointment directive.

A Living Will	States what medical treatment one chooses to omit or refuse in the event one is unable to make decisions for oneself and is terminally ill.
A Durable Power of Attorney for Health Care	Appoints a proxy—usually a relative or trusted friend—to make medical decisions on one's behalf if one can no longer decide for oneself. It has broader applications than a living will and can apply to any illness or injury that could result in incapacitation.
The Patient Self-Determination Act	A federal law that became effective December 1, 1991. It applies to all health care institutions receiving Medicare or Medicaid funds and requires that all individuals receiving medical care must be given written information about their rights under state law to make decisions about medical care, including the right to accept or refuse medical or surgical treatment. Individuals must also be given information about their rights to formulate advance directives.

SOURCE: From American Nurses' Association (1992). Used with permission.

ing a forum for mutual decision making that respects a person's desire for self-determination. Thus, building a relationship is a responsibility that grows from acknowledging human needs in chronic illness.

Heroic Measures in Chronic Illness As medical knowledge increases and related technologies improve, fewer chronic illnesses move steadily along a downward trajectory toward a terminal phase (see Chapter 3, on illness trajectory). However, the potential to move into a terminal phase can exist at a number of points along the illness trajectory. This lack of predictability for some chronic illnesses can lead to ethical problems that most closely approximate those classical life and death ethical dilemmas characteristic of both acute and terminal care.

The questions that arise with increasing frequency are how much treatment is appropriate, and at what point should these efforts cease (Moros et al., 1991). In a sense, this is quite similar to the dilemma faced by terminally ill patients or those with severe, irreparable brain damage. Yet, because of the slow, insidious nature of physiological deterioration in many chronic illnesses, the bigger issue is identifying the point at which these questions should be asked.

Another related issue is anticipating when death is a possibility or when a significant and irretrievable loss of health or functioning will occur. In some chronic illnesses, sudden and unanticipated crises with the potential for death can arise (Hotter & McCommon, 1992). Because this can occur, providers need to consider when to initiate discussion of advance directives: living wills and power of attorney (see Table 19-4). They must also decide how to balance the need for this discussion with the patient's need to maintain hope. Providers need to think about what happens when a patient with an existing advance directive changes his or her mind during an acute crisis, particularly when mental status is altered by the condition or medication (Corley, 1992). This last point raises a further question: Can chronically ill patients make informed end-of-life decisions well before facing the actual situation? Because this can occur, providers need to consider when to initiate discussion of advance directives.

Health care providers are beginning to routinely encourage all clients, particularly those entering hospitals, to complete forms that direct desired outcomes. Although these decisions may be more clear-cut for the terminal client, this is not always so with the chronically ill client, who may view the next crisis as yet one more in a lifelong struggle with illness.

The provider committed to an ethic of care needs to gain perspective by asking for the details and context of a person's life as well as evaluating his or her personality. Such awareness provides an appreciation of how the individual deals with life, death, and illness. One chronically ill person may cope better with the uncertainty of an illness and enjoy life more by denying the possibility of a terminal complication. Another may be less anxious and enjoy life more knowing that if a catastrophic situation arises, she or he will not be kept lingering or in pain for a purpose of little or no value.

Health Care Environment Regardless of how one defines chronic illness (see Chapter 1, on what is chronicity; Table 1–1), it can be readily ascertained that a chronically ill client will be exposed to many health care organizations and be involved in many diverse relationships with health care professionals. Relationships between clients and health care providers, as well as among health care providers themselves, are important whether they occur in an acute care setting, a rehabilitation or long-term care setting, or in the community.

The work environment can influence the quality of patient care. How the nurse perceives the work environment, in relation to how difficult patient care issues or concerns are handled, is referred to as the ethical climate of the work setting. The concept of a health care organization ethical climate is a relatively new one (Christensen, 1988; Corley, 1992; Levine-Ariff & Groh, 1990).

Several sources, in business and organizational literature, and more recently in the health care and nursing literature, have indicated that the workplace influences employee attitudes and behavior. Researchers in nursing and business ethics have asserted that the culture or environment of an organization also influences the ethical behavior and beliefs of employees (Ketefian, 1985; Ketefian & Ormond, 1988; Victor & Cullen, 1987, 1988; Swider, McElmurry, & Yarling, 1985). Based on an integrative review of nursing research that focused on nurses' moral reasoning, ethical practice, and ethical decision making, Ketefian and Ormand (1988) suggested

that the work environment influences nurses' ethical practice. For example, nurses who work in a supportive work environment can feel free to voice their opinions about patient care issues or problems without fear of reprisal. In order for nurses to feel supported by their institutions, it is important that they be aware of ethical resources or consultants within their institutions who can help them with difficult ethical issues. In addition, most institutions have risk managers who can provide consultation on issues that may also have legal implications. Nurses need the professional support that is offered through consultation and position statements of their professional associations.

When choosing a place of employment, nurses should seek out those institutions where the top nursing leaders value competent nurses who take responsibility for their actions and for decision making that includes the relevant parties in the process (ANA, 1988, 1992). Since the work setting is an important influence on employee behavior, nurses should take some time to learn about the way things are done in their organization. The norms and values inherent within an organization are often referred to as the organizational culture. An organization with strong organizational culture is one in which the norms and values are well known and communicated to employees.

Others have addressed the number of constraints on ethical practice (Biordi, 1991; Davis & Aroskar, 1991; Levine-Ariff & Groh, 1990; Cassells, Silva, & Chop, 1990; Sietsema & Spradley, 1987). External constraints can arise from institutional policies and procedures, the threat of litigation, or from the authority and directives of physicians. Constraints also arise from reimbursement systems, which often control the allocation and distribution of institutional and health care resources. Internal constraints arise from personal fears, lack of confidence, feelings of low self-esteem, or lack of knowledge or awareness of resources. In addition, individual members of the health care team have personal and professional values that influence their perspectives in setting priorities and meeting the needs of chronically ill clients (Davis & Aroskar, 1991; Purtilo & Cassel, 1981). In turn, chronically ill clients have their own personal value systems that influence their decisions as well as their reasons for living.

Thus, with the increasing complexity of health care ethical issues, as well as a health care environment characterized by constraints, how does one practice in a manner in which the patient is best served and the professional is able to feel good about the decisions and actions taken in providing care?

"Nurse in the Middle"   Nurses are frequently confronted with multiple obligations to employer, physician, and patient and family when faced with difficult patient care decisions—a situation often referred to as the "nurse in the middle" problem (Jameton, 1977). Ethical issues for nurses are unique, not merely a subset of biomedical ethics, partly because of the unique nature of the relationship of nurses with clients, other health care professionals, administrators, and the health care organization itself. Since nurses constantly interact with other people in their work, they are engaged in what has been referred to as "emotional labor," work where feelings are in some way a part of job performance (Albrecht, 1990; Kerfoot, 1992).

Nurses often have difficulty recognizing ethical issues in their clinical practice. Studies have shown that health care professionals have different levels of ethical awareness and that different groups of health care professionals often perceive ethical concerns differently, depending on their perspectives (Grundstein-Amado, 1992). Ethical issues encompass more than the life and death decisions associated with termination of life support or prolongation of life that make headlines in the media. They involve our day-to-day dealings with people, the way decisions about patients are made, and the manner in which health care professionals interact with each other and with patients and families.

Costs   Economical and social costs of care for the chronically ill are an increasing subject of ethical debate secondary to the increased numbers of chronically ill populations that have evolved from technologic change (Jennings, Callahan, & Caplan, 1988). Three current problems

impeding a moral response from the health care system for this population are (1) the focus of the "medical model" on functional restoration, (2) the disproportionate focus on individualistic self-determinism, and (3) the contractual relationship between health care professionals and patients (Jennings et al., 1988). Jennings et al. (1988) state: ". . . equitable access does not mean unlimited access, either for acute or chronic care." When policies are made that ration health care, they should not discriminate against persons with chronic illness.

Some ethical issues become dilemmas, or situations in which one must choose between equally unsatisfactory alternatives (Curtin & Flaherty, 1982; Davis & Aroskar, 1991; White, 1992). When dealing with a choice between two equally unfavorable actions, there may not be a right or wrong answer. Even though not solvable, however, an ethical dilemma can be resolved through the process of critical reflection and discussion with all the parties involved in the dilemma. Ethical dilemmas give rise to questions such as "What ought I to do?" For example, we ought to prolong life, yet at the same time we ought to relieve suffering. In balancing these two competing moral claims, one must reflect on the harms and benefits that may arise from specific decisions or actions. In caring for the chronically ill, one may have to choose to initiate therapy that may have serious side effects or cause pain, yet may offer hope for prolonging life. The concept of quality of life must be weighed as well. A frequent issue confronting nurses who care for the chronically ill is that of whether to use physical or chemical restraints with patients who are in danger of falling or harming themselves. In these situations, the concern for the patient's safety (and possibly fear of legal action) must be balanced with the concern for respecting the patient's dignity.

Social Ethics and Nursing

Nurses are members of society, members of the nursing profession, and employees of health service delivery agencies—a host of roles that can be relevant to the ethical issues of chronic illness. Multiple memberships may lead to competing interests and responsibilities and, subsequently, ethical dilemmas. For instance, in the context of social responsibility, nurses may value an appropriate allocation of resources for maximum service to those with chronic illness. Yet this may compete with a professional value of equity in regard to salary compensation for nursing services (Mills, 1989).

Nurses are members of the nursing profession. Like other professions, nursing is a part of society and therefore has social responsibilities to society. As specified in the important document, *Nursing: A Social Policy Statement* (1980), there exists a social contract between society and the professions. Each nurse's authority to practice nursing is based on this social contract. In exchange for the authority to practice, society expects that professionals will act in a responsible manner that is always mindful of the public trust (ANA, 1980).

Freedom of Conscience   Compromise does not always preserve personal integrity. As with other members of society, assurance of nurses' freedom of conscience is needed. In the United States, nurses, as citizens, have legislative protection of certain rights, such as the First Amendment of the U.S. Constitution, which guarantees the right to free speech. State legal statutes may also ensure that a nurse's individual right to a code of morals, such as religious beliefs, remains protected regardless of professional role and duties. For instance, nurses who, because of their religious beliefs, refuse to participate in an abortion, would be protected from prosecution for failure to perform a professional duty (Levine-Ariff, 1990).

Accompanying nurses' rights as members of society are responsibilities regarding the public good, including those who suffer from chronic illness. As both consumers of health care and members of families, individual nurses are stakeholders in the public debates about health care, including the "right" of access to health care (see Chapter 23, on social/health policy). In light of the above, and because of their specific professional experience and knowledge, nurses have an important role in identifying and addressing ethical concerns about health issues that affect the public welfare.

Social Justice   As major health caregivers to individuals with chronic illness, nurses have a responsibility to contribute to the public health debate over issues of social justice, such as health care rationing and equal employment opportunity. There are risks to society if the chronicity of illness becomes the basis for decisions regarding the utilization of health care resources and the rationing of health care services (Moros et al., 1991). Also, when there is employment discrimination of those with a chronic illness, such as epilepsy, the talent pool of skilled workers is artificially limited, thereby confining potential benefits for society. Clearly, if nurses believe in the value of the dignity of life for all, including those with chronic illnesses, they will give attention to social injustices such as discrimination.

Social Bias in Health Care   In promoting moral social institutions, nurses must recognize when social bias affects the quality of health care services. Steele (1983) discussed the viewpoint that for some chronic conditions of women, "despite the evidence of organic etiology, a number of medical professionals continue to treat the conditions as female psychological disorders rather than exploring any biologic causes for the discomforts." The dearth of research on postpartum onsets of psychiatric syndromes may reflect this type of underlying societal discrimination against women.

Health Care and Poverty   Because chronic illness has a potential economic impact on individuals and their families, social justice issues, such as poverty, are significant for these people. The relationship between health status and poverty was recognized in a proposal of primary health care by the World Health Organization (WHO) as a strategy for "Health for All by the Year 2000" (Green, 1991). In this primary health care model, recognition is given to the interdependence of various social institutions, including the health care system, education, and industry. By including community development as a necessary component of health care, this model incorporates the responsibility to address issues of economic equity within the roles of nurses and other health professionals (Morgan & Mutalik, 1992).

Interventions for Creating an Ethical Climate

There are several interventions that can be implemented in health care organizations to create an ethical climate. These include establishing a moral community, such as a collaborative or professional practice model, or establishing institutional mechanisms, such as ethics committees or rounds, where concerns about ethical issues can be raised in a safe and nonthreatening way. The use of a leadership style that fosters ethical awareness and reflection and empowers both employees and patients to participate in important decisions, also contributes to the creation of an ethical climate.

In chronic illness, individuals need to take responsibility for their own health and to develop the capacity for directing their own care, rather than depending on health care professionals and the health care system to control the course of their disease. Rather than just serving as advocates, nurses should empower consumers by educating them to care for their own health and how to access and use the health care system (Styles, 1993). At the core of this responsibility is an atmosphere of trust and respect for each other, with people feeling free to openly raise and discuss difficult issues and decisions.

The Concept of a Moral Community

The idea of a moral community was originally expressed in the writings of Aristotle. A moral or "caring" community is one where professionals relate to and interact with one another, patients, families, and outside organizations with mutual respect and responsiveness. The best environment for patient care and staff motivation is "where there is a sense of community; that is, where there is a sense of common interest, personal bonding, and cooperative endeavor . . ." (Styles, 1993). An institution that provides such a community has moral values expressed in both its mission and its top leadership, thereby providing a framework for ethical decision making. People in such an institution interact with one another in a way that enables the institution to better carry out its mission.

An example of an institution that creates a moral community is one in which the values of the top leadership are well known and communicated to all levels of personnel. In addition, it is one in which administrators recognize their ethical obligations toward the nursing staff as well as toward patients (Christensen, 1988; Davis & Aroskar, 1991). It is important that nurses feel supported by their peers as well. Some mechanisms and strategies that can be used by nurses and their managers to support each other in dealing with the daily ethical issues in clinical practice include ethics rounds, nursing ethics committees, institutional ethics committees, continuing education in ethics, ethics resource libraries, and professional practice models, such as shared governance.

How might nurses with an interest in the care of the chronically ill participate in the development of institutions that are morally responsible? Truly comprehensive care for the chronically ill requires health care systems that are integrated with other social services (Hollingsworth & Hollingsworth, 1992). Specific policy considerations, such as employment-linked access to nursing services through employers' insurance carriers, may limit the capacity of individuals with chronic illness to achieve a maximum level of independent life-style and social productivity through decreased likelihood of "qualification" for care from nurses and other health professionals.

A particularly poignant example of the unanticipated creation of a moral community resulted when a collaborative practice model was established within an institutional setting (Pike, 1991). The mechanism of collaborative practice embodies values of mutual trust and respect between nurses and physicians through shared decision making, responsibility, and accountability for the care of patients. At Beth Israel Hospital in Boston, a 14-bed medical-surgical unit was opened to study the concept of collaborative practice between nurses and physicians. One outcome of this practice was a decrease in moral outrage, defined as "an emotional response to the inability to carry out moral choices or decisions" (Pike, 1991). Nurses freely expressed themselves, and both nurses and physicians collaborated in planning care and making decisions about patients. Within this atmosphere of mutual respect and open dialogue, nurses felt empowered to voice their views and to confront issues directly and openly. For example, there was mutual planning between nurses and physicians about a specific decision related to the use of life-prolonging measures in a terminal cancer patient with a do-not-resuscitate order (DNR).

Pike (1991) concluded that "the moral reasoning that took place incorporated a consideration of the patient's trajectory of illness, and although a moral dilemma existed, moral outrage did not occur; rather, all care providers felt that they had been able to do the right thing for this patient." Although this example occurred in an acute care setting, collaborative practice can also be established in long-term care and community health settings.

Institutional Mechanisms for Ethical Decision Making

The Joint Commission on Accreditation of Health-Care Organizations (JCAHO) now has a standard requiring the establishment of a method for nurses to address their ethical concerns, whether it be through a formal mechanism such as an institutional ethics committee (IEC) or by informal means. Some organizations have ethicists or pastoral care counselors who serve as resources for ethical decision making; in others, clinical nurse specialists often serve as experts in ethics and can be consulted when an ethical issue or concern arises. Although IECs are primarily in acute care hospitals, they are being advocated for other health care facilities, such as home care agencies or community health agencies, to provide a forum for health care professionals, patients, and families to address ethical concerns (Abel, 1990; Burger, Erlen, & Tesone, 1992).

How does the nurse become involved in an IEC and what can be expected from such a committee? First, one must recognize that these committees do not provide solutions to ethical dilemmas. Rather, they serve to promote sensitive and open dialogue about ethical issues, to

provide emotional support to those who are troubled by ethical dilemmas, and as sources of consultation and education (Oddi & Cassidy, 1990). Most IECs suggest, rather than make, policies and procedures.

The membership of an IEC should be multidisciplinary, reflecting the diversity of the health care community. Staff nurses who have knowledge of clients' wishes bring a valuable and unique perspective to the deliberations of the committee, since they spend the most time with clients and are in an excellent position to recognize ethical dilemmas. Nurses should be included as members of the committee along with other appropriate individuals such as physicians, administrators, clergy, ethicists, and social workers (Davis & Aroskar, 1991). Since the majority of ethical dilemmas in health care settings involve nurses, some organizations have established nursing bioethics committees. In assisting nurses with ethical issues and helping them to define their responsibilities when confronting such issues, a nursing bioethics committee provides education, support, and help with decision making and consultation. The committee serves as a forum through which nurses voice their concerns and identify ethical issues inherent within patient care situations (Edwards & Haddad, 1988).

Anyone concerned with the outcome of an ethical dilemma should have direct access to the consultation offered by the IEC. Concerned nurses have the moral authority to contact the committee without having to get approval from the attending physician (see ANA code, 1985). Nurses have a vital role to play and contributions to make in solving ethical problems, a responsibility that also comes from the social contract nurses and the nursing profession have to the public, as expressed in the Social Policy Statement (ANA, 1980; Murphy, 1985).

Creating Conditions for Ethical Reflection
How an organization creates conditions for ethical reflection requires one to first consider the characteristics of its moral community. Five conditions facilitate the process of ethical reflection: (1) power, (2) trust, (3) inclusion, (4) role flexibility, and (5) inquiry (Brown, 1990). Health care

professionals need access to people who can serve as role models for facilitating the ethical decision-making process. In addition, role models can help nurses think about their values, consider alternative courses of action, and respect the views of others.

The condition of power includes the rights of participants in the organization to relevant information, to participate in ethical discussions, and to say what needs to be said. The condition of trust allows members to clarify their own values and those of others. Inclusion provides stakeholders (patients, families, nurses, physicians, other health care professionals) who are concerned about the outcome of an ethical issue to be part of the discussions and debates involved in reaching a decision. Role flexibility embraces the ability to view an ethical issue from various perspectives, that is, the ability to switch roles and view the situation from the perspective of other stakeholders in the decision. Finally, the condition of inquiry allows questions to be asked so stakeholders can arrive at a good decision (Brown, 1990).

Ethical Leadership

As advocates, nurses can better deal with the ethical issues and dilemmas of the workplace that have been cited as causative factors in stress, burnout, turnover, and the tendency to leave the profession (White, 1992). To effectively advocate for patients, the nurse needs to take an active leadership role in the decision-making process. Several resources are available as guidance for the nurse in performing this role such as the ANA Code for Nurses (1985), the ANA Social Policy Statement (1980), the International Council of Nurses (ICN) Code for Nurses (1973), and the position statements (ANA, 1988, 1992) and standards (1991) of the profession. For example, the ANA publishes standards of clinical nursing practice for each nursing specialty. These standards are available for purchase from the American Nurses' Association.

Transformational leadership is the style most often associated with ethical leadership. The transformational leader empowers others to move toward mutually desirable outcomes, to take risks, and to examine their views and values in a context that is safe (Barker, 1990; Porter-O'Grady, 1993). Consumer empowerment and staff empowerment are becoming important ways of creating a milieu where quality patient care is provided and staff can participate in decision making.

Nursing ethics has an important role to play in bringing attention to, as well as drawing conclusions regarding, ethical issues in the care of the chronically ill. Many nursing ethicists have embraced the ethic of care, which differs from the traditional biomedicine approach to ethics. The ethic of care recognizes the experiences of those with chronic illness and values the nurse–patient relationship as interdependent (Cooper, 1990).

Institutional Moral Environments

In addressing the needs of the chronically ill, social institutions must strive to create an environment conducive to the conduct of moral behavior of group members. In this sense, institutions, such as health care facilities, can be viewed as possessing their own moral character.

The moral character of an organization may affect the staff's capacity to deliver effective health care, and it affects their own health (Cox & Leiter, 1992). The "absence of support at the level of primary task completion for strongly espoused organizational values may reflect unresolved conflicts regarding policy throughout the organization" (Cox & Leiter, 1992). For example, an understood value within an institution may be to maintain maximum comfort of those suffering chronic pain. However, when a coinciding concern exists about the appropriate use of narcotics, undermedication of patients for pain may result (see Chapter 7, on chronic pain).

In addition to the ethical implications in pain management, conflicts of institutional beliefs and values can create moral distress for nursing staff (Greipp, 1992). This moral distress may be relieved by options such as the application of alternative nursing care measures to address patients' pain and the recognition of current scientific limitations in keeping patients totally pain free. Even the assessment of pain has ethical implications, as when placebos are used to determine the "validity" of the client's pain, frequently creating a situation of deceit (Elander, 1991).

Serious consequences of these ethical conflicts may result, as illustrated by the debate regarding the use of aggressive medication for intractable pain. Should a nurse inadvertently give a patient a lethal dose of pain medication resulting in the patient's death, she or he might be exposed to "civil, criminal, and administrative proceedings as a result" (Pohlman, 1990).

Creating a Morally Responsive Institution
Professionals interested in creating morally responsive institutions have a role in "maintaining a reflective space (literal and figurative) within an institution, within its culture and its daily life" (Walker, 1993). There is a need for creative design and negotiation of solutions for nurses' ethical dilemmas that recognize diversity of beliefs and values occurring within specific situations. Through the encouragement of open reflection, ethical discourse is enriched and moral traditions are examined more thoroughly (Walker, 1993).

Social Approaches

Ethical conflicts require resolution in many different social contexts. As members of both social and health-related institutions, nurses need to draw attention to the contradictions between their own values and the sanctioned values of institutional policies and procedures, thereby contributing to the moral development of the institutions within which they function. Nurses have a responsibility to promote standards of ethical practice from both the institution's effects on the nurse and the nurse's effects on the institutional setting. Such effects are characterized by reciprocal relationships.

Health Care Reform   The need for health care reform has been expressed at a national level in the United States through public outcry regarding access to and costs of health care (see Chapters 22 and 23, on financial impact and social/health policy, respectively). Simultaneously, a creative challenge exists for using political action and policy development to address the need for social change that will benefit those suffering from chronic illness. Nurses, for example, are often in a unique position to nurture and interpret the values of health, knowledge, freedom of information, and equity in the distribution of health care benefits, and to advocate for the translation of these values into humanitarian environments for long-term care (Roth & Harrison, 1991). Although individual nurses advocate for moral environments in which to provide humane care for clients with chronic illness, the collective action of nurses as a group has much potential for creating beneficial social change.

Public Accountability   As members of a profession, nurses collectively have responsibilities to a public constituency. A profession includes a foundation of ethical considerations rather than just technical expertise (Behrman, 1988). Some characteristics of a profession include: specific education and expertise, a selection process assuring qualifications of membership, dedication to social service, and self-governance and self-surveillance incorporating a high code of ethics (Behrman, 1988).

Nursing's interest in ethical autonomy has been viewed, at times, as professional self-interest. However, the tradition of ethics in the nursing profession is reflected historically in Gretter's "Florence Nightingale's Pledge" (cited in Roberts & DeWitt, 1929), calling on the need to "maintain and elevate the standard of my profession." More recently, the nursing profession has been called on to provide "a new moral perspective about the goals of chronic care and the aims of public policy" (Roth & Harrison, 1991). The authors recommend the following areas for future public policy deliberation: methods of assessment of quality of life with chronic illness, mechanisms of social support for family caregivers, and the ethics of withdrawing treatment once initiated.

Ethics and Nursing Education

As a profession, nursing has the responsibility of preparing its members not only for technical expertise in clinical areas but as professionals able to discern health-related ethical considerations in the public interest. In addition, as a profession, nursing must commit to an educational program providing knowledge and skills that influence public decisions regarding health ethics and health care services (Martin, White, & Hansen, 1989).

These efforts must be based on a defined set of professional values that will guide the nursing profession in collective political action and policy development (Davis, 1988). Values of the nursing profession relevant to care of the chronically ill include (1) individual rights to health care, (2) humanistic health care, (3) maintaining as much control over one's health as possible, (4) the provision of holistic health care, and (5) the provision of health services by qualified practitioners (Davis, 1988).

Nurses as Employees

The potential for competing interests has implications for nursing's self-governance and self-surveillance as a professional group. In situations where care is provided to chronically ill individuals, the potential conflict exists between the nurse's professional role of advocating for and supporting the client and the role of employee in a health care organization. Nurses' personal beliefs and values may come into conflict with an employer's organizational policies and decisions, such as decisions to withhold food and fluids (Winslow & Winslow, 1991; Wurzbach, 1990).

As employees, nurses are frequently placed in the category of employee-at-will. The employee can be terminated for refusing to perform the job or for being unfaithful to an employer's interest. However, an employee can not be fired for refusing to perform an illegal action requested by the employer (Davis, 1986).

Institutional constraints, including nurses' employee status, have implications for nurses' ability to adequately resolve ethical conflicts (Yarling & McElmurry, 1986). There have been cases in which nurses have sustained serious consequences, such as job relocation, suspension for insubordination, and job termination for following their ethical beliefs (Blum, 1984; Witt, 1983). One reported case is that of a psychiatric nurse who alleged ethical concerns regarding the use of an orthomolecular treatment program for psychiatric patients. Following her reports

to a state agency, she was terminated from her position at the hospital where this treatment program was in place. Over two years later, a state supreme court upheld the lower court ruling awarding her a total remedy under the law, which included all compensatory and punitive damages (Witt, 1983). However, what has not been reported in the literature is that through subsequent judicial actions, the reinstatement ruling for the nurse was overturned and the actual awarding of damages never occurred. The nurse's career was destroyed (personal communication).

It has been proposed that contractual agreements for nurses as independent contractors may create options for increased professional autonomy (Borel, 1992). Another option is that collective bargaining agreements of nurse-employee groups with employers include mechanisms for addressing nurses' ethical concerns. Some nurses believe that nurse employees must be included in policy decisions via sufficient representation on hospital ethics committees. However, ethics committees have limitations because they function through case review. These committees may need further development and explanation of their operative procedural and substantive framework (Cohen, 1989). Clearly, measures need to be taken that clarify ethical issues if we are to avoid ethical conflict. Levine-Ariff (1990) advocates a "preventive ethics" approach that identifies areas of ethical diversity and institutes policies that assist in limiting or preventing ethical conflicts.

Conclusions

The ideas presented in this chapter have challenged some traditional ways of looking at ethical concerns in nursing practice. Health providers caring for others are asked to arrive at a means of deliberative reflection and response that is informed and that includes awareness of one's personal belief systems and appreciation of the institutional and social influences on those beliefs. The outcome of such reflection leads to subsequent actions.

In an interesting study of Master's-prepared nurse clinicians, Davis (1991) found that none of the nurses knew the content of the *ANA Code for Nurses*. However, when they were questioned about how they had become sensitized to ethical issues, they were able to describe sensitizing events based on clinical experience, understanding of their personal values and beliefs, participation in clinical research, and professional socialization as a student. While the clinicians had learned to live with uncertainty, the influence of differences in quality of life, the complexity of situations as well as social structure and gender, they also acknowledged that they used desensitization as a coping strategy for dealing with practice frustrations. Both the study by Davis and the historical study by Steppe (1992) of nursing in Nazi Germany illustrate important concerns. As Steppe emphasizes, nursing takes place in socially influenced settings, which in turn require nurses to have a profound understanding or appreciation of the self and others within a given context and point in time. The concept of chronicity provides an illustration of the difficulty in sorting out influences on practice.

If the foundation for a nursing ethic is the nurse–patient relationship (Yarling & McElmurry, 1986), what then governs nurses' relationships with other persons dealing with chronicity? There are areas, such as arthritis in women, which represent common chronic conditions that traditionally receive little attention in the research, practice, or education of nurses. What explains the omission? Are we aware of the personal, social, and institutional influences on the care of women with arthritis? Once we become aware of the processes that influence who makes decisions on directions in health care, we are still left with questions on how to create the moral community of nurses' willing to take socially responsible action.

STUDY QUESTIONS

1. Discuss the influences on nursing practice that need to be considered during the process of ethical thinking in the care of the chronically ill.
2. What key concepts should be considered in nursing ethics? How are they related to one another?
3. Differentiate nursing from medical ethics. How can nurses integrate both?
4. Discuss the difference between the ANA standards of care from an ethical practice of nursing. Can they be carried out concurrently? How?
5. Discuss nursing, ethics from the perspective of compliance, heroic measures, health care environments, and costs.
6. What does "nurse in the middle" mean?
7. How do social ethics affect nursing in relation to freedom of conscience, social justice, social bias in health care, and poverty?
8. Identify a situation from your clinical practice that has ethical overtones. Using interventions discussed in this chapter, how can you create an ethical climate to deal with this situation?
9. As a nurse, how can you help establish an ethical committee at your institution? Who should serve on such a committee? Why?
10. Discuss how social approaches can be used to create an ethical environment. How can education be used for this purpose?

References

Abel, P. E. (1990). Ethics committees in home health agencies. *Public Health Nursing, 7* (4), 256–259.

Albrecht, K. (1990). *Service within: Solving the middle management leadership crisis.* Homewood, IL: Dow Jones-Irwin.

American Nurses' Association (1980). *Nursing: A social policy statement.* Kansas City, MO: American Nurses' Association.

—— (1985). *Code for nurses with interpretive statements.* Kansas City, MO: American Nurses' Association.

—— (1988). *Ethics in nursing: Position statements and guidelines.* Washington, D.C.: American Nurses' Association.

—— (1991). *Standards of clinical nursing practice.* Washington, D.C.: American Nurses' Association.

———— (1992). Position statement on nursing and the Self-Determination Act. *Compendium of position statements on the nurse's role in end-of-life decisions.* Washington, D.C.: American Nurses' Association.

Barker, A. M. (1990). *Transformational nursing leadership: A vision for the future.* Baltimore: Williams & Wilkins.

Beauchamp, T. L., & Childress, J. F. (1983). *Principles of biomedical ethics.* New York: Oxford University Press.

Behrman, J. N. (1988). *Essays on ethics in business and the professions.* Englewood Cliffs, NJ: Prentice-Hall.

Benner, P. (1991). The role of experience, narrative, and community in skilled ethical comportment. *Advances in Nursing Science 14*(2), 1-21.

Benner, P., & Wrubel, J. (1989). *The primacy of caring: Stress and coping in health and illness.* Menlo Park, CA: Addison-Wesley.

Biordi, D. (1991). Ethical leadership (unpublished). University of Illinois at Chicago.

Blum, J. D. (1984). The code of nurses and wrongful discharge. *Nursing Forum, 21,* 149-152.

Borel, H. (1992). Powerquake: The registered nurse as independent contractor. *Revolution, 2*(4), 25-26, 84-89.

Brody, J. (1988). Virtue ethics, caring and nursing. *Scholarly Inquiry for Nursing Practice, 2,* 87-101.

Brown, M. T. (1990). *Working ethics: Strategies for decision making and organizational responsibility.* San Francisco: Jossey-Bass.

Burger, A. M., Erlen, J. A., & Tesone, L. (1992). Factors influencing ethical decision making in the home setting. *Home Healthcare Nurse,* 10(2), 16-20.

Carper, B. A. (1979). The ethics of caring. *Advances in Nursing Science, 1*(3), 11-19.

Cassells, J., Silva, M., & Chop, R. (1990). Administrative strategies to support staff nurses as moral agents in clinical practice. *Nursing Connections, 3*(4), 31-37.

Christensen, P. J. (1988). An ethical framework for nursing service administration. *Advances in Nursing Science, 10*(3), 46-55.

Cohen, C. B. (1989). Who will guard the guardian? *Hastings Center Report, 19*(1), 19.

Collopy, B., Dubler, N., & Zuckerman, C. (1990). The ethics of home care: Autonomy and accommodation. *Hastings Center Report, 20*(2), 1-16 (Special Suppl.).

Cooper, M. C. (1989). Gilligan's different voice: A perspective for nursing. *Journal of Professional Nursing, 5*(1), 10-16.

———— (1990). Chronic illness and nursing's ethical challenge. *Holistic Nursing Practice, 5*(1), 10-16.

Corley, M. C. (1992). The ethical case analysis: Heroic measures for patients with chronic problems. Part II: Ethical analysis. *Dimensions of Critical Care Nursing, 11*(1), 35-40.

Corley, M. C., & Raines, D. (1993). An ethical practice environment as a caring environment. *Nursing Administration Quarterly, 17*(2), 68-74.

Cox, T., & Leiter, M. (1992). The health of health care organizations. *Work and Stress, 6*(3), 219-227.

Curtin, L., & Flaherty, M. J. (1982). *Nursing ethics: Theories and pragmatics.* Bowie, MD: Brady.

Curzer, H. (1993). Is care a virtue for health care professionals? *The Journal of Medicine and Philosophy, 18,* 51-69.

Davis, A. J. (1991). The sources of a practice code of ethics for nurses. *Journal of Advanced Nursing,* 16, 1358-1362.

Davis, A. J., & Aroskar, M. A. (1991). *Ethical dilemmas and nursing practice* (3rd ed.). Norwalk, CT: Appleton & Lange.

Davis, B. G. (1986, Fall). Defining the employment rights of medical personnel within the parameters of personal conscience. *Detroit College of Law Review.*

Davis, G. C. (1988). Nursing values and health care policy. *Nursing Outlook, 36*(6), 289-292.

Dunlop, M. (1986). Is a science of caring possible? *Journal of Advanced Nursing, 11,* 671-670.

Edwards, B. J., & Haddad, A. M. (1988). Establishing a nursing bioethics committee. *Journal of Nursing Administration, 18*(3), 30-33.

Elander, G. (1991). Ethical conflicts in placebo treatment. *Journal of Advanced Nursing, 16,* 947-951.

Engel, N. (1980). Confirmation and validation: The caring that is professional nursing. *Image: The Journal of Nursing Scholarship, 12*(3), 53-56.

Fry, S. T. (1988). The role of caring in a theory of nursing ethics. *Hypatia, 4*(2), 88-103.

Gadow, S. (1985). Nurse and patient: The caring relationship. In A. Bishop & J. Scudder (Eds.), *Caring, curing, coping: Nurse-physician-patient relationships* (pp. 31-43). Birmingham, AL: University of Alabama Press.

———— (1988, October). Covenant without cure: Letting go and holding on in chronic illness. *NLN Publication* (15-2237), 5-14.

Gaut, D. (1983). Development of a theoretically adequate description of caring. *Western Journal of Nursing Research, 5*(4), 313-324.

Gilligan, C. (1982). *In a different voice.* Cambridge, MA: Harvard University Press.

Gillon, R. (1992). Caring, men and women, nurses and doctors, and health care ethics. *Journal of Medical Ethics, 18,* 171-172.

Goffman, E. (1986). *Stigma: Notes on the management of spoiled identity.* New York: Simon & Schuster.

Green, R. H. (1991). Politics, power, and poverty: Health for all in 2000 in the third world? *Social Science and Medicine, 32*(7), 745-755.

Greipp, M. E. (1992). Undermedication for pain: An ethical model. *Advances in Nursing Science, 15*(1), 44-53.

Griffin, A. (1983). A philosophical analysis of caring in nursing. *Journal of Advanced Nursing, 8,* 289-295.

Grundstein-Amado, R. (1992). Differences in ethical decision-making processes among nurses and doctors. *Journal of Advanced Nursing, 17,* 129-137.

Hauerwas, S., & Burrell, D. (1989). From system to story: An alternative pattern for rationality in ethics. In S. Hauerwas (Ed.), *Why narrative? Readings in narrative theology* (pp. 158-90). Grand Rapids, MI: Wm. B. Eerdsman.

Hollingsworth, J. R., & Hollingsworth, E. J. (1992). Challenges in the provision of care for the chronically ill. *Journal of Health Politics, Policy and Law, 17*(4), 869-878.

Hotter, A., & McCom_mon, T. (1992). The ethical care analysis: Heroic measures for patients with chronic problems. Part I: The ethical case. *Dimensions of Critical Care Nursing, 11*(1), 35-36.

International Council of Nurses (1973). *Code for nurses: Ethical concepts applied to nursing.* Geneva: International Council of Nurses.

Jameton, A. (1977, August). The nurse: When roles and rules conflict. *Hastings Center Report, 7,* 22-25.

Jennings, B., Callahan, D., & Caplan, A. L., (1988). Ethical challenges of chronic illness. *Hastings Center Report, 18*(1), 1-16.

Kerfoot, K. (1992). Preventing moral distress: Our ethical obligation. *Aspen's Advisor for Nurse Executives, 7*(5), 1, 3-5.

Ketefian, S. (1985). Professional and bureaucratic role conceptions and moral behavior among nurses. *Nursing Research, 34*(4), 248-253.

Ketefian, S., & Ormond, I. (1988). *Moral reasoning and ethical practice in nursing: An integrative review.* New York: National League for Nursing.

Knowlden, V. (1988). Nursing caring as constructed knowledge. In *Caring and nursing explorations in the feminist perspective* (pp. 318-339). Denver: Center for Human Caring, University of Colorado Health Sciences Center.

Leininger, M. (1980). Caring. A Central focus of nursing and health care services. *Nursing and Health Care, 1*(3), 135-143.

——— (1981). The phenomenon of caring: Importance, research questions, and theoretical considerations. In M. Leininger (Ed.), *Caring: An essential human need* (pp. 3-16). Thorofare, NJ: Charles B. Slack.

——— (1988). Introduction. In M. Leininger (Ed.), *Care: the essence of nursing and health.* Detroit: Wayne State University Press.

Levine-Ariff, J. (1990). Preventive ethics: The development of policies to guide decision-making. *AACN, 1*(1), 169-177.

Levine-Ariff, J., & Groh, D. H. (1990). *Creating an ethical environment.* Baltimore: Williams & Wilkins.

Lifton, R. J. (1986). *The Nazi doctors: Medical killing and the psychology of genocide.* New York: Basic Books.

Martin, E. J., White, J. E., & Hansen, M. M. (1989). Preparing students to shape health policy. *Nursing Outlook, 37*(2), 89-93.

Mayeroff, M. (1971). *On caring.* New York: Harper & Row.

Mills, M. E. (1989). Nursing compensation: The realities of seeking equity. *Nursing Economics, 7*(5), 270-272.

Moros, D. A., Rhodes, R., Baumrin, B., & Strain, J. (1991). Chronic illness and the physician-patient relationship: A response to the Hastings Center's "Ethical challenges of chronic illness." *Journal of Medicine and Philosophy, 16,* 161-181.

Morgan, R. E., & Mutalik, G. (1992). *Bringing international health back home.* Washington, D.C.: National Council for International Health.

Morse, J. M., Bottorff, J., Neander, W., & Solberg, S. (1991). Comparative analysis of conceptualizations and theories of caring. *Image: The Journal of Nursing Scholarship, 23*(2), 119-126.

Murphy, C. (1985). Nurses' views important on ethical decision team. In A. J. Davis & M. A. Aroskar (Eds.), *Ethical dilemmas confronting nurses.* Washington, D.C.: American Nurses' Association.

Murphy, J., & Gilligan, C. (1980). Moral development in late adolescence and adulthood: A critique and reconstruction of Kohlberg's theory. *Human Development, 23,* 77-104.

Noddings, N. (1984). *Caring: A feminine approach to ethics and moral education.* Berkeley, CA: University of California Press.

Oddi, L. F., & Cassidy, V. R. (1990). Participation and perception of nurse members in the hospital ethics committee. *Western Journal of Nursing Research, 12*(3), 307-317.

Olsen, D. (1992). Controversies in nursing ethics: A historical review. *Journal of Advanced Nursing, 17,* 1020-1027.

Parker, R. S. (1990). Nurses' stories: The search for a relational ethic of care. *Advances in Nursing Science, 13*(1), 31-40.

Pike, A. (1991). Moral outrage and moral discourse in nurse-physician collaboration. *Journal of Professional Nursing, 7*(6), 351-363.

Pohlman, K. J. (1990). Pain control: Euthanasia or criminal act? *AACN, 17*(3), 260-261.

Porter-O'Grady, P. (1993). Of mythspinners and mapmakers: 21st century managers. *Nursing Management, 24*(4), 52-55.

Purtilo, R. B., & Cassel, C. K. (1981). *Ethical dimensions in the health professions.* Philadelphia: W. B. Saunders.

Reich, W. (1991). Commentary: Caring as extraordinary means. *Second Opinion, 17*(1), 41-56.

Roberts, M. M., & DeWitt, K. (Eds.) (1929, May). *American Journal of Nursing,* frontispiece.

Roth, P. A., & Harrison, J. K. (1991). Orchestrating social change: An imperative in care of the chronically ill. *Journal of Medicine and Philosophy, 16*(3), 343-359.

Sietsema, M. R., & Spradley, B. (1987). Ethics and administrative decision making. *Journal of Nursing Administration, 17*(4), 28-32.

Steele, S. (1983). *Values clarification in nursing.* Norwalk, Appleton-Century-Crofts.

Steppe, H. (1992). Nursing in Nazi Germany. *Western Journal of Nursing Research, 14*(8), 744-53.

Styles, M. M. (1993). Macrotrends in nursing practice: What's in the pipeline. *The Journal of Continuing Education in Nursing, 24*(1), 7-12.

Swider, S., McElmurry, B., & Yarling, R. (1985). Ethical decision making in a bureaucratic context by senior nursing students. *Nursing Research, 34*(2), 108-112.

Thorne, S. E. (1991). Constructive noncompliance in chronic illness. *Holistic Nursing Practice, 5*(1), 62-69.

Victor, B., & Cullen, J. (1987). A theory and measure of ethical climate in organizations. *Research in Corporate Social Performance and Policy, 9,* 51-71.

———— (1988). The organizational bases of ethical work climates. *Administrative Science Quarterly, 33,* 101-125.

Walker, M. U. (1993). Keeping moral space open: New images of ethics consulting. *Hastings Center Report, 23*(2), 33-40.

Watson, J. (1988). *Human science and human care: A theory for nursing.* New York: National League for Nursing.

White, G. B. (Ed.) (1992). *Ethical dilemmas in contemporary nursing practice.* Washington, D.C.: American Nurses' Publishing.

Whitley, G. G. (1991). Noncompliance: An update. *Issues in Mental Health Nursing, 12,* 229-238.

Wilson, H. S., & Kneisl, C. R. (1992). *Psychiatric nursing* (4th ed.). Menlo Park, CA: Addison-Wesley.

Winslow, B. J., & Winslow, G. R. (1991). Integrity and compromise in nursing ethics. *The Journal of Medicine and Philosophy, 16*(3), 307-323.

Witt, P. (1983). Notes of a whistleblower. *American Journal of Nursing, 83*(12), 1649-1651.

Wurzbach, M. E. (1990). The dilemma of withholding or withdrawing nutrition. *Image: The Journal of Nursing Scholarship, 22*(4), 226-230.

Yarling, R. R., & McElmurry, B. J. (1986). The moral foundation of nursing. *Advances in Nursing Science, 8*(2), 63-73.

CHAPTER 20

Nursing Case Management

Judith Papenhausen • *Cathy Michaels*

Introduction

A major challenge facing nursing professionals during this current reactive economic climate is the development and promotion of proactive, innovative clinical nursing intervention strategies that are cost sensitive, theoretically dependable, and outcome efficacious. Currently, the pivotal driving force in the delivery of health care is cost containment, resulting in increasingly restrictive private and federal reimbursement policies.

Present cost-effectiveness strategies, such as restraints on institutional length of stay and constrictions on the range of reimbursement for health care services, may negatively influence the quality of health care delivery. Cost-containment methods have altered the distribution of health care and negatively influence people who can least likely afford private payment (Pegels, 1988; Strumpf & Knibbe, 1990). Among those who are most affected are chronically ill persons, whose labile health care status requires frequent monitoring and periodic interventions and who may require multiple hospital admissions. These clients are often discharged from acute care facilities early in the recuperative and restorative phases of their illnesses.

Increasingly, lower-cost alternatives are being chosen, including early transfer to extended care facilities or returning home with or without the support of informal caregivers or home health care. Often, these alternatives are employed before the formulation of a comprehensive health care plan that includes a support network of multidisciplinary health professionals and services to meet health care needs (Ellis & Hartley, 1988; Graham, 1989; Olivas et al., 1989a, 1989b; Zander, 1990a).

These cost-containment trends have altered the methods used to provide holistic nursing care for the chronically ill and have fostered the development of managed care and nursing case management delivery systems. Because of the diversity of their needs and the complexity of the existing health care delivery system, chronically ill clients, particularly, require professional guidance in coordinating, executing, and evaluating their health care plans. This situation has created an opportunity for the evolution of the role of the nurse case manager and the development of nursing case management models to serve selected client populations (Bower, 1992; Ethridge & Lamb, 1989; Olivas et al., 1989a; Shipp & Jay, 1988; Zander, 1988a).

Managed Care and Nursing Case Management

Managed care and *nursing case management* have become the new "buzz" words in acute care delivery (Faherty, 1990; Knollmueller, 1989). The interchangeable usage of these terms has created confusion in the literature, as they are similar in cost-effectiveness and are both guided by client outcomes. Their operational characteristics, however, are distinctly different.

Managed Care In more general usage, *managed care* broadly refers to a health care delivery system in which a group of individuals and/or organizations contract with subscribers to deliver a full range of health care services operating under a fixed level of reimbursement from an insurer source (see Chapter 23, on social/health policy). The care is provided either directly or through a contract with an outside provider at a discounted rate. (Cline, 1990; Grinnell, 1989; Halamandaris, 1990; Hereford, 1990; Olivas et al. 1989a). From the vantage point of health care delivery in an acute care setting, Etheredge (1989) offers the following definition of managed care:

> The essence of managed care is the organization of unit-based care so that specific patient outcomes can be achieved within fiscally responsible time frames (lengths of stay) while utilizing resources appropriate (in amount and sequence) to the specific case type and the individual patient (p. 3).

In other words, managed care is a strategy that can be implemented within a variety of settings and is usually based on interdisciplinary collaboration resulting in unit-based cost-effective, quality-oriented care irrespective of individual health care providers (Cohen & Cesta, 1993; Etheredge, 1989). Within a managed care system, the common or average patterns of cost and care outcomes for a specific case type (e.g., acute myocardial infarction or coronary artery bypass) are identified across the expected length of stay. This information becomes the basis for developing interdisciplinary critical pathways that stipulate cost data and clinical parameters that can then be used to monitor patient progress.

Case Management Case management differs from managed care in that an individual health care provider consistently follows an individual or a specific patient population across health care settings, collaborates with other health care team members to determine outcome goals, and provides access to and monitors utilization of resources.

Etheredge (1989, p. 2) offers the following definition of case management:

> Case management is a system of patient care delivery that focuses on the achievement of outcomes within effective time frames and with appropriate use of resources. It encompasses an entire episode of illness, crossing all settings in which the patient receives care.

Managed care can be seen as providing continuity of the plan by linking tasks and departments, while case management provides the continuity of a care provider who links people across clinical settings (Zander, 1990b). *Service management, care coordination,* and *care management* are alternate terms for case management (ANA, 1988; Bower, 1992).

Nursing Case Management Most definitions of nursing case management include (1) the use of a nurse case manager to identify high-risk/high-cost patients; (2) health assessment; (3) health care planning to improve quality and efficacy; (4) procurement, delivery, and coordination of services; and (5) monitoring of the patient's total care to ensure optimum outcomes (ANA, 1988; Bower, 1992; Desimone, 1988; Ethridge & Lamb, 1989; Knollmueller, 1989; McKenzie et al., 1989; Olivas et al., 1989a, 1988b; Shipp & Jay, 1988; Zander, 1988a, 1988b). Nursing case management models of health care delivery have, as a central theme, the premise of service brokerage.

Nursing case management has been defined as "a system, a role, a technology, a process and a service" (Bower, 1992, p. 4). Faherty (1990) states that "case management is the nursing process expanded in scope and made operational" (p. 20), and this view is supported by Zander (1990a), who sees the formal nursing process as "directly analogous to the process of case management" (p. 201). Zander (1988b) states that "nursing case management is both a model and a technology for restructuring the clinical production process and a role that facilitate cost/quality outcomes. It builds on the concept of managed care and the accountability practiced in primary nursing" (p. 503).

In various nursing case management models, the professional nurse serves clients in acute care institutions and/or home settings and provides transitional and long-term care. Important goals of the nursing case management models are

- Optimize the client's self-care capability and increase the client's self-care abilities.
- Enhance the client's quality of life, sense of autonomy, and self-determination.
- Assist the client to adjust to and manage his or her altered health state and manage his or her symptoms.
- Enable the client and family to implement a complex health care plan through the development of an interactive relationship with a nurse case manager who serves in an educative and supportive role.
- Prevent inappropriate hospitalizations and contain health care costs.
- Provide quality health care along a continuum with decreased fragmentation of services across many settings.[1]

Achieving these outcomes has particular importance to the amelioration of the psychosocial impact of chronic illness on a client's ability to adapt to an altered state of health. Persons with chronic diseases must often adjust their life patterns to provide effective self-care and to control their inherent and frequently exacerbating symptoms.

It is generally recognized that major differences exist in the patterns, characteristics, and management goals of episodic, acute health conditions compared to those that are chronic (Lubkin, 1990). Chronic illness requires increased levels of professional monitoring and supportive care to maximize the client's functioning and promote self-care activities (Cluff, 1981). Mazzuca (1982) also acknowledges the importance of client self-care or self-help in the daily management of chronic conditions.

Our current health care delivery system emphasizes the acute illness model, which seeks cure as the ultimate outcome. In this type of health delivery, health care professionals assume the responsibility for management of the client's care and practice primarily in acute care institutions. The acute illness model is an expensive and somewhat ineffective approach for clients with chronic illness. The very nature of chronic illness requires a high level of patient responsibility for successful day-to-day management (Mazzuca, 1982).

To manage chronic illness effectively requires time-intensive coordination of multiple health care professionals and services operating under common outcome goals (ANA, 1988; Bower, 1992). Increasingly, professional nurses are performing the case manager role with selected client populations. The target populations for nursing case management intervention are persons, such as the chronically ill and disabled, who are designated as high risk for the development of complex, continuous health care problems that require high-volume and diverse health care services (ANA, 1988; Bower, 1992).

Historical Development of Case Management Models

There is lack of agreement as to the origin of the case management concept, with the disciples of both mental health and social work claiming credit for its development (Applebaum & Wilson, 1988). Grau (1984) credits case management to the field of mental health. Following World War II, the notion of continuity of care was used to describe the process of delivering community services to discharged psychiatric patients (Harris & Bergman, 1988). During the 1960s, this approach was also used to assist mentally retarded clients in gaining access to services

---

[1]This list was compiled from the following sources: ANA, (1988), Bower (1992), and Shipp and Jay (1988).

and to expedite the delivery of services (Simpson, 1982).

Kemp (1981), on the other hand, suggests that case management emerged from social work. Social workers involved in rehabilitation stressed the importance of a single agent dealing with the multiple needs of disabled persons. By the early 1950s, the role of the vocational rehabilitation counsellor had emerged as separate from that of social worker, and Kemp (1981) suggests that this is the only human service profession whose scope of practice is embedded in case management. Applebaum and Wilson (1988) maintain that case management is rooted in social work, community health, and related health services.

Federally mandated cost containment has led to the recent emergence of case management models in community and acute care settings (Simpson, 1982). In the 1980s, the implementation of the prospective Medicare reimbursement system, Diagnostic Related Groups (DRGs), imposed limitations on the length of hospitalization, and stimulated growth in the home health care market. Since DRGs, home health patients have been sicker and have had more complex nursing needs after discharge from acute care settings (Graham, 1989), so that the focus of case management has been on providing services that are economically efficient (Giuliano & Poirier, 1991).

Also in the early 1980s, the Health Care Financing Administration (HCFA) and state agencies funded demonstration projects to provide community-based case management services for the elderly (Capitman, Haskins, & Bernstein, 1986; Grau, 1984). Later in that decade, the National Long-Term Care Channeling Project Study was funded to evaluate the ability of community-based case management models to provide home services to elderly clients in a cost-effective manner and thus prevent institutionalization (Carcagano & Kemper, 1988).

During the 1980s, the funding for mental health changed to a capitation system of reimbursement, resulting in the deinstitutionalization of thousands of chronic mentally ill patients (Harris & Bergman, 1989; Lamb, 1980; Schwartz, Goldman, & Churgin, 1982). This change spawned the development of community-based programs for this patient population; case man-agement and mental health services were provided through nonresidential community-based clinics. These chronically disabled, psychiatric patients could not have survived in the community without case management support services (Deitchman, 1980). Case managers serving this population came from a variety of professional disciplines, including social work, vocational rehabilitation, psychology, and nursing (Bachrach, 1989; Bond et al., 1989; Fariello & Scheidt, 1989; Kanter, 1989; Lamb, 1980; Schwartz et al., 1982).

These early projects represent the first use of nurses in the specific role of a case manager (Grau, 1984; Shipp & Jay, 1988). However, Knollmueller (1989) and others (ANA, 1988) argue that the basic tenets of case management have been practiced by community health nurses for years.

Development of Nursing Case Management

The development and use of nursing case management models proliferated by the late 1980s, with several emerging to guide practice in a variety of settings and involving many client populations (Del Bueno & Leblanc, 1989; Knollmueller, 1989; Stillwaggon, 1989). Some are primarily community health models such as the nursing center model for the provision of long-term eldercare (ANA, 1988; Bower, 1992; Dolson & Richards, 1990; DuBois, 1990; Igou et al., 1989; Miller, 1990), the home health care model (Jones et al., 1990), and the primary care model (Lajeunese, 1990), which utilizes existing home health and visiting nurse services to provide continuity of discharge planning.

Others, such as health maintenance organizations (HMO) (Abrahams, 1990; ANA, 1988; Bower, 1992) and insurance-based models (Bower, 1992; Henderson & Collard, 1988; Henderson, Souder, & Bergman, 1987; Henderson & Wallack, 1987; Knollmueller, 1989) provide case management to high-cost clients who have catastrophic illness or injury and require permanent or transitional home care. Institutional long-term case management models are used with the elderly in nursing home settings (Putney et al., 1990) and in rehabilitation and extended care settings (Blake, 1991; Loveridge, Cummings, & O'Malley, 1988).

Some acute care models developed for specific client populations such as low-birth-weight infants (Brooten et al., 1988; Mazoway, 1987), high-risk pregnant teenagers (Combs & Rusch, 1990; Korenbrot et al., 1989), and persons with acquired immune deficiency syndrome (AIDS) (ANA, 1988; Bower, 1992; Littman & Siemsen, 1989). Other acute care models have a general application for a broader range of clients (Bower, 1992; Ethridge & Lamb, 1989; Del Togno-Armansco, Olivas, & Harter, 1989; Zander, 1988a, 1988b).

The goals of all models of nursing case management are sensitive to both cost and quality; these models hold great promise for cost containment. The facilitating and gatekeeping functions of the nurse case manager have decreased the fragmentation of services across multiple settings, improved the coordination of the treatment plans across health care professionals, and prevented inappropriate hospitalizations. (ANA 1988; Bower, 1992; Ethridge, 1991; Ethridge & Lamb, 1989; McKenzie, Torkelson, & Holt, 1989; Rogers, Riordan, & Swindle, 1991; Zander, 1988b).

Characteristics of Nurse Case Managers
The legitimacy of the role of the nursing case manager is strongly supported by the literature. The Nursing Social Policy Statement (ANA, 1980) notes that an outcome of nursing intervention is the creation of a physiological, psychological, and sociocultural environment allowing the client to gain or maintain health. Zander (1990a) notes that nurses can provide case management because they have intimate access to patients and families over extended time periods, and suggests they are ideally suited for this role because of the similarities in the process of case management and nursing. With nurses in this role, case management is provided by an expert clinician with advanced educational preparation, who is with a patient throughout the entire episode of care (Zander, 1990a).

Many authorities support the view that nurses are the logical candidates to become case managers for clients having both acute and chronic physiological health problems, since professional nurses have a generalist background with a broad knowledge of both the physiologi-

cal and psychosocial ramifications of specific health conditions. Practicing nurses have experience in assessment, diagnosis, and treatment of patient responses to disease and disability, and historically they have participated in the implementation and monitoring of medical protocols in acute care and community health settings (Bower, 1992; Cronin & Maklebust, 1989; Grau, 1984; Ethridge & Lamb, 1989; Leclair, 1991; Mundinger, 1984; Zander, 1990b). After examining similarities and differences among case managers in New York City's long-term community care programs, Grau (1984, p. 374) concluded that "only the nurse case managers made case management decisions and, at the same time, provided or coordinated both health and social services."

The qualifications and training needs of case managers have been defined by several authors. Case managers require knowledge and skill in three general areas: (1) clinical expertise relative to the client's health care needs, (2) an ability to determine client resources and to negotiate for health care services, and (3) an ability to implement the steps in the process of case management. It is generally agreed that this process includes client assessment, care planning, and monitoring (Applebaum & Wilson, 1988; Le Clair, 1991; Parker & Secord, 1988; Weil, 1985). Nurse case managers should have advanced academic preparation and previous experience in clinical practice (Ethridge & Lamb, 1989; Fondiller, 1991; Graham, 1989; Henderson & Wallack, 1987; Rogers, Riordan, & Swindle, 1991).

Graduate programs to prepare nurses as case managers are being developed. Among them is the University of Virginia, which provides a curriculum of advanced concepts in community health and medical-surgical nursing, client-family assessment, health teaching, and coordination of health care services (Graham, 1989). Other universities, such as the University of Kansas, have implemented a continuing education program focusing on community based case management of the elderly (Walstedt & Blaser, 1986).[2]

---

[2]The University of Kansas program is funded through a special projects grant from the Department of Health and Human Services.

Nursing Case Management Models

Since the late 1980s, the nursing literature has depicted the development and use of nursing case management models, including discussions of the characteristics of nurse case managers, general goals and implementation guidelines for various practice models, the process of nursing case management in a variety of settings, and broad objectives and client care outcomes. Many of these models were implemented prior to systematic research to establish their specific fiscal and client-oriented quality of care outcomes. However, in the late 1980s, research documenting outcomes of nursing case management models began to appear.

The multiple models that have emerged have generic goals in common, although their focus and the exact role of the nurse case manager varies according to the client population and the nature of the institution or organization through which services are offered.

Community-Based Case Management

Of all the case management programs, community-based models for long-term clients received the earliest and most rigorous evaluation. These models developed for a variety of high-risk populations; their major focus was to broker and monitor health care services delivered in the home environment or in long-term care settings. In general, clients who require case management services in the home are the elderly or those with chronic or terminal illnesses.

Some community-based models focus only on long-term care service for the elderly. For example, in the Social-HMO model,[3] Medicare beneficiaries over 65 voluntarily enroll and receive all services covered under Medicare, as well as an extended long-term care package including skilled nursing home and home health care services. Case managers in this type of program are either nurses or social workers and have case loads of between 60 and 80 clients, half of whom require intensive contact (Abrahams, 1990).

Other community-based models provide private case management on a fee-for-service basis (Miller, 1990; Bower, 1992).[4] Fee-for-service groups provide multidimensional assessment, client and family consultation, community resource referral and coordination, and care planning services. Nurses used as case managers are often master's prepared and have advanced preparation in gerontology (Bower, 1992). The client may be either the older client or, more commonly, the primary caregiver. Fees are charged on an hourly basis (Miller, 1990).

There are community-based models that provide case management services to other populations.[5] Target populations served include technology-dependent clients who receive supportive care in their home, retirement community residents who receive direct personal care, and informal caregivers who receive respite care (Bower, 1992).

Some community-based models work exclusively with children who have special health needs and potentially chronic conditions.[6] In such models, the case manager, a public health nurse with clinical experience in pediatrics, may carry a case load of 300 to 350 children depending on the severity of the chronic conditions (Bower, 1992).

Research on Community-Based Models Early studies, such as the landmark long-term care channeling project (Kane, 1988; Kane & Kane,

[3]The Social-HMO Nurse Case Management Model is a community-based model. It was developed from a national demonstration project and is designed to provide an integration of medical and social services for older, long-term care clients.

[4]The Independent Geriatric Case Management Model, the Visiting Nurse Service (VNS) in Seattle, and Community Care Consultants (CCC) of Southfield, Michigan, are examples of fee-for-service private case management models.

[5]The Nursing Center Model developed by Trimark Health Service Inc. of Atlanta, Georgia, serves populations that require long-term care as an alternative to extended hospitalization or admission to long-term care settings.

[6]The Public Health Model, such as the one developed by the Gloucester County Health Department, New Jersey, identifies and manages children with special health needs.

1987; Kemper, 1988; Henderson & Wallack, 1987), compared community case management models to existing service models to determine if community case management services provided to high-risk elderly clients would result in a more cost-effective use of resources and decrease or prevent long-term care institutionalization. Although significant findings related to cost savings were not found, there were some significant differences between treatment and control groups on quality-of-life outcomes (Kemper, 1988).

Later studies demonstrated the fiscal advantages of long-term case management of the elderly to be 75 percent of the average cost of local institutional care (Shipp & Jay, 1988). One study of the cost of care delivery of a neighborhood team model of case management was compared to a centralized model (Eggert et al., 1991). The neighborhood team model consisted of social workers, community health nurses, and a case aide. The centralized model utilized existing hospital discharge planning and home health care agencies for service arrangement. Results indicated that the cost of providing case management care for the clients in the neighborhood team model group was 13.6 percent less expensive than the cost for the clients in the centralized model group.

Community-based management of the chronically mentally ill has demonstrated both cost savings and improvement in rate of readmission. Through case management programs, chronically mentally ill individuals receive board and care and other necessary personal and clinical services for an annual average cost of $15,000 (Harris & Bergman, 1989). This compares favorably to a average annual cost of $45,000 for institutionalized care. Bond et al. (1989) report similar cost savings and lower (32 percent) recidivism rates.

Insurance-Based Case Management

Most major private insurance carriers in the United States have implemented some form of case management primarily as a cost control measure. The first private insurer credited with the implementation of such a program initially used a form of medical management in workers' compensation cases. As group health insurance companies reviewed claims data of their insured clients, it was determined that approximately 80 percent of the total health care costs could be attributed to 20 percent of those clients (Bower, 1992). Further analysis of data led to the identification of those chronic and catastrophic diagnoses that usually result in high-cost, long-term care. These catastrophic and chronic conditions are

1. High-risk neonatal
2. Severe head trauma
3. Spinal cord injury
4. Ventilator dependency
5. Coma
6. Multiple fractures
7. AIDS
8. Severe burns
9. Cerebral vascular accidents
10. Amputations
11. Terminal illnesses
12. Substance abuse (Bower, 1992)

In private-insurance-based case management, the coordination function of the case manager is critical to controlling cost and avoiding duplication and fragmentation of services. Case management in this model begins with case identification and referral through screening activities, often initiated by the insurance company. For clients with a high-risk profile, a case manager sets up a network of communication among health care providers, health care professionals, and the client so alternatives can be explored and a plan of care determined. The case manager then monitors the plan through regular contact with the involved parties until the goals of the plan are reached, the client dies, or insurance coverage is depleted. Most of the case managers in this model are registered nurses with five years or more of clinical experience, although some companies utilize rehabilitation counsellors or social workers for this role. The average case load is 16 to 20 clients (Bower, 1992).

Research on Private (Insurance) Case Management Models Based on weekly case load reports in the literature, each of 65 Blue Cross and Blue Shield plans that used case management in 1988 saved an average of $2 million for each plan (Smith, 1990). These were high-risk, high-utilization clients. This represented an $11 savings for each dollar spent on case management services.

In addition to direct cost savings, another fiscal advantage of insurance-based case management is to stretch out patient benefits because many health insurance policies have a $500,000 to $1 million maximum lifetime benefit payout. Efficient coordination of costs and services can greatly improve the quantity and quality of health care services per health care dollar (Smith, 1990). This benefit is particularly important for clients with catastrophic and chronic conditions that may require lifetime health care support.

Within-the-Walls (Hospital-Based) Nursing Case Management

The origins of the hospital-based nurse case management model are usually attributed to the New England Medical Center (NEMC) Hospitals following a 13-year history of primary nursing and the investigation of nursing and physician practice patterns. The model entails the collaboration of physicians and staff nurses who formulate a case management plan and develop a critical pathway that indicates time-ordered client outcomes to be achieved during the acute care hospitalization (Etheredge, 1989; Zander, 1988a, 1988b, 1990a). However, with this kind of model the relationship between the nurse case manager and the client usually ends with the client's discharge from the hospital. Consequently, this model is often classified as a within-the-walls nurse case management model (Cohen & Cesta, 1993).

Since its introduction, the model has evolved, and now the case management plans and critical pathways are linked to quality improvement practices and the development of care maps for specific client groups or case types. These care maps provide for the monitoring of resource allocation, cost reimbursement systems, variances in the delivery of care, and client care outcomes (Cohen & Cesta, 1993). Many versions of within-the-walls case manage-

ment models[7] are currently being used in several acute health care facilities to lower costs, improve effective use of resources, and maintain quality of care (Olivas et al., 1989a, 1989b; Sinnenn & Schifalacqua, 1991; Cohen & Cesta, 1993; Etheredge, 1989; Fondiller, 1991; Zander, 1988a, 1990a).

The role and qualifications of the nurse case manager varies across the specific models within this classification. In some, such as the NEMC model, nurse case managers are the clients' primary caregivers and participate in the coordinating and monitoring of services throughout the hospitalization irrespective of the client's location (Cohen & Cesta, 1993). Other within-the-walls models use a form of leveled or differentiated practice based on educational preparation or clinical ladders. In these models, direct client care is provided by staff nurses, and the nurse case manager is responsible for coordinating, monitoring, and evaluating care delivery (Cohen & Cesta, 1993). The qualifications of nurse case managers in these models is typically based on clinical competency and leadership qualities; a baccalaureate degree may be required.

Research on Within-the-Walls, Hospital-Based Nurse Case Management Models Fiscal outcomes of these case management models are usually concerned with reductions in the length of hospital stay and reduction on total hospital costs. After implementation of the NEMC model, substantial savings were reported in several client-related diagnostic groups. For example, case-managed ischemic stroke patients demonstrated a 29 percent decrease in length of stay and a 47 percent decrease in the number of required intensive care unit (ICU) days, and transfer to rehabilitation services occurred 7 to 10 days sooner than the typical patterns before case management was implemented (Etheredge, 1989; Zander, 1988a).

---

[7]Other versions of within-the-walls case management include the Collaborative Case Management Model developed at Tucson Medical Center and the Coordinated Care Model developed at Saint Michael's Hospital in Milwaukee, Wisconsin.

Using the Coordinated Care Case Management Model within identified case types, there was an average decrease in the length of stay of 22 percent and a 6 percent decrease in average hospital charges in the first year of operation of the model (Sinnenn & Schifalacqua, 1991). Other positive outcomes of the use of the within-the-walls models have been suggested, such as increased patient satisfaction (Fondiller, 1991) and increased nurse satisfaction (Stillwaggon, 1989; Zander, 1988a)

Beyond-the-Walls Professional Nursing Case Management

Community-based case management models generally serve clients in their home settings or in subacute institutional settings, and within-the-walls models serve clients in acute care settings. Since the chronically ill client often needs services in both settings, health care professionals frequently pass care coordination responsibilities back and forth depending on the client's location in the health care continuum. This leads to duplication and fragmentation of services as well as greater health care costs. In addition, such change of case manager requires the development of multiple professional/client relationships.

The Professional Nurse Case Management (PNCM) Model holds great promise in alleviating these deficits, and, in the opinion of the authors, this model is most advantageous for the chronically ill. The PNCM model, developed at Carondelet St. Mary's Hospital in Tucson, Arizona, differs from other case management models because it provides continuity of case management from the acute care setting to the home setting (Bower, 1992; Ethridge, 1991; Ethridge & Lamb, 1989; Michaels, 1992).

Philosophy of PNCM   The beyond-the-walls approach is based on a belief that if high-risk, chronically ill clients are identified early during acute hospitalization, the nurse case manager can establish a continuous nurse/client/family therapeutic relationship and coordinate the entire spectrum of care in both settings for an extended and indefinite period of time. Other goals of the model include improved cost and qual-

ity outcomes (such as reduced recidivism), more appropriate service utilization, improved chronic illness management, and increased client satisfaction.

The PNCM Model blends the elements of hospital and community models by allowing for the continuity of a single nurse case manager who designs a multidisciplinary plan of care that is initiated during the client's hospitalization. The nurse case manager then follows the client into the home setting and continues to execute and monitor the plan of care (Bower, 1992; Ethridge, 1991; Ethridge & Lamb, 1989; Michaels, 1992; Rusch, 1986). The PNCM Model was an outgrowth of a centralized home health care service implemented at Carondelet St. Mary's in 1983.

Evolution of the PNCM Model   The PNCM Model developed in an interesting fashion. Using a centralized approach, acute care nurses began the discharge planning, but found their client responsibilities and relationship terminated at discharge. They noted that when home health services were required, additional client assessments and planning had to be done by a different nurse, requiring the establishment of a new professional relationship with the client. Such additional actions created a potential gap in the continuum of care during the stressful transition period from the acute care hospital to the home setting, a gap linked to the high recidivism rates seen in some chronically ill elderly clients (Ethridge & Lamb, 1989).

To deal with this problem, baccalaureate-prepared nurses with community health experience began to participate in the discharge planning process while the client was still in the acute care setting. They identified clients who had the potential for needing home health care after discharge and followed these clients to the home setting. This process was the genesis of the role, and the practice emerged from this innovation (Reisch, 1986).

The nurse case managers in the PNCM model are members of a professional group practice who serve clients 24 hours a day through a rotating on-call system shared by all members of the practice. Their present role within the PNCM model includes

1. Identifying high-risk clients, such as those who are chronically ill and those who have limited social and financial support
2. Assessing the client and family and developing a comprehensive plan of care
3. Coordinating and brokering community and agency resources
4. Collaborating with interdisciplinary health care team members and serving as the client's advocate
5. Making home visits to provide direct nursing care interventions such as emotional support, counselling, and education, designed to increase the client's self-care and symptom management abilities
6. Monitoring and evaluating client outcomes
7. Serving as the health care liaison in the event of rehospitalization (Cohen & Cesta, 1993; Ethridge & Lamb, 1989).

As the success of this approach became evident, a nursing health maintenance organization (HMO) was formed at Carondelet St. Mary's to provide expanded services to elders through various senior plan contracts, such as health assessment, education, and consultation delivered through nurse practitioners and other health care professionals at community-based nursing community health centers. These centers have become additional referral sources for the nursing case management practice group, and selected high-risk seniors are offered nurse case management services (Cohen & Cesta, 1993; Michaels, 1992).

Other PNCM Programs The PNCM Model has been implemented at St. Joseph Medical Center in Wichita, Kansas (Rogers, Riordan & Swindle, 1991), where it was initially used to serve the elderly chronically ill. This program is now exploring the use of nurse case management services for other client populations, such as chronically ill children, neonates, high-risk pregnant women, and those with psychiatric problems (Cohen & Cesta, 1993).

Another version of the beyond-the-walls approach was developed at the Medical University of South Carolina (MUSC) Medical Center in Charleston. Here, case managers are master's-prepared nurses who are speciality or service oriented. They are based in one of four clinical divisions: medical, surgical, cardiovascular, or maternal-infant. These case managers follow their clients from admission through discharge, and after discharge they follow clients during subsequent outpatient clinic visits. Bower (1992) offers, "The key characteristic of the MUSC program is that one person—the case manager—is thoroughly familiar with a patient and all aspects of the patient's care throughout the hospital stay and on subsequent admissions" (p. 35).

Research on the Professional Nursing Case Management Model The PNCM Model has demonstrated impressive reductions in the cost of providing health care to chronically ill elderly clients. Ethridge and Lamb (1989), comparing cost data on length of stay (LOS) and hospital acuity levels between case-managed and non-case-managed clients, reported that for case-managed total hip replacement clients, the average LOS was 2.1 days lower, even though the mean acuity level for the case-managed clients was higher.

Similar decreases in LOS (3.5 days) were demonstrated for historically recidivistic case-managed clients with respiratory illnesses. Those who were case managed showed a lower mean acuity level (4.4) than the non-case-managed clients (6.0). In fact, the cost per case for clients with a chronic obstructive pulmonary disease (COPD) diagnosis in 1986, the year in which nursing case management was initiated, was $6,855, but declined to $2,040 in 1988 (Ethridge & Lamb, 1989). This difference was attributed to the nurse case managers' ability to intervene earlier in an acute exacerbation of the respiratory illness. The investigators concluded that nurse case management has had a financial impact on the cost of hospitalization, a cost savings achieved both at the end of the stay (by lowering the average LOS) and at the beginning of the stay (by earlier admission of clients at a lower acuity level) (Ethridge & Lamb, 1989).

Other Studies of Financial Advantages of PNCM Using the PNCM model at St. Joseph Medical Center in Wichita, Kansas, other researchers found similar financial advantages (Rogers et al., 1991). Frail chronically ill Medicare clients (average age of 75 years with a history of frequent readmissions, extended lengths of stay, and numerous complications and multiple morbidities) showed a decrease in the mean number of admissions per client from 2.2 to 0.79 per year with the implementation of NCM. The average LOS dropped from 10.7 days to 5.3 days. The total acute care cost for all the subjects decreased from $261,638 (an average of $6,885 per client) to $35,549 for all subjects (an average $962 per client) excluding the cost of NCM. The total cost of NCM services for all subjects was $31,536, calculated at a rate of $36./hour. Rogers et al. (1991) state, "These patients as a group cost $226,089 less to care for under NCM [including NCM costs] than they had in preceding equivalent periods" (p. 34).

This initial study was continued, and additional data was obtained from subjects who entered the NCM program in the following year (Weyant, 1991). In this later study, data revealed that the number of admissions decreased from 3.05 per client to 0.88 after NCM was instituted, or 71 percent. The average LOS dropped from 9.2 days to 6.3 days, representing a 31 percent decrease. The total health care cost, for all the subjects, in an equivalent period of time decreased from $1,232,776 (an average of $9,483 per client) to $209,884 (an average of $845 per client), excluding the cost of NCM service, which ran $1,555 per year per client. This represents a decrease of 91 percent in total cost of acute care for all clients in both studies. No measurement of quality outcomes was made in either study, but Rogers et al. (1991) offered the opinion that the decrease in admission rates was due to fewer complications and less debilitation of the patients. "The most efficient inpatient care and excellent discharge planning may be in place, but if there is no one to implement, assess, modify, and otherwise make the plan work, such high-risk patients return to the hospital over and over again." (Rogers et al., 1991, p. 31).

Ethridge (1991) reported on the cost savings of case managing the care of both healthy and medically disabled seniors who were enrolled in a per capita senior plan contract through the nursing HMO at Carondelet St. Mary's Hospital and Medical Center. Seniors who meet high-risk criteria, estimated at between 5 percent and 6 percent of the total enrollees, are admitted to the PNCM services of the HMO. Admission rates per 1,000 members, yearly hospital bed days, and length of stay data were compared against national Medicare averages and revealed that in all categories the nursing HMO demonstrated better fiscal outcomes: lower admission rates (242 versus 319), fewer yearly hospital bed days (1,311 versus 2,206, and shorter length of stay (5.8 versus 7.5). Ethridge (1991) concluded that nursing-case-managed services were responsible for these changes and stated, "each patient day saved reflects a cost savings of approximately $900.00" (p. 26).

PNCM Seen from the Patient Perspective The experience of working with nurse case managers has been explored from the client's perspective (Lamb, 1992; Lamb & Stempel, 1991, 1992). Using a grounded theory approach to explore the social process of the nurse case manager–client relationship, interviews of nursing case-managed subjects were tape-recorded and verbatim responses coded and analyzed. Three distinctive stages or phases of the process were identified by the subjects. These phases were bonding, working together, and changing.

The *bonding phase* consisted of establishing the nurse/client relationship (Lamb & Stempel, 1991, 1992). Early in the phase, the nurse case manager was viewed as an expert who could assist in the assessment and stabilization of physiological problems related to disease exacerbation, and could facilitate access to needed health care services. As the client became more physically stable, the relationship became progressively more holistic and focused on emotional and spiritual concerns. The nurse case manager moved from being an expert outsider to an "insider-expert," a notion coined by Lamb and Stempel (1991, 1992) based on clients' phrases describing their relationship with nurse case managers. Clients characterized the actions of the nurse case manager as "comforting," "supporting," "caring," and "going beyond" the expected duties of a nurse (Lamb & Stempel, 1992, p. 3).

In the *working* and *changing phases* of the process, clients' attitudes, reactions, and behaviors that contribute to exacerbation of their illnesses or prevent them from using the health care system effectively are identified (Lamb & Stempel, 1992). Specific management strategies are explored and cooperatively developed. Modification in the client's cognitive attitudes seems to arise from a "sense of consistency and emotional support," and the nurse case manager promotes the client's "competence and self worth" (Lamb & Stempel, 1992, p. 4). Clients note that the case manager makes them feel worthwhile, improves their outlook, and provides a sense of being highly supported (Lamb & Stempel, 1992). Changes in client behaviors occur in two major areas: learning improved self-care activities and mastering the ability to more appropriately access health care services.

Clients reported an improved ability to recognize the signs of exacerbation of their symptoms and responded by seeking early assistance. They also reported improved adherence to medication and other health-related regimens. At the termination of nursing case management services, "many reached a level of independence where they acted as their own insider-expert, recognizing the symptoms of exacerbation and accessing the health care system in a timely and appropriate way" (Lamb & Stempel, 1992, p. 5).

Another study explored client and informal caregiver satisfaction with nursing case management services (Lamb, 1992b). Telephone interviews were conducted with clients and family members who had worked with a nurse case manager for a minimum of two months through a senior managed-care plan. Subjects were asked if the nursing case manager had been helpful and to describe a helpful experience. Subjects described nurse case manager attributes as caring, advocative, encouraging, and giving, and noted that their activities or functions were supportive, educative, and assistive. The outcomes identified by clients were an increase in self-care skills and illness management, an increase in their sense of well-being, and an increase in their ability to access health care services.

Intervention

It is important to demonstrate how one nurse case management model works. Since these au-

thors strongly believe that the PNCM model is the most effective approach for people with chronic disease, the Carondelet health care program is presented.

The Carondelet Approach[8]

At Carondelet, PNCMs establish partnerships with people at high risk for managing their health concerns. The PNCM moves across health care settings and across time. Unlike care given in hospitals and through home health, PNCM services are not limited to a single episode of illness, but are available at any point in time to help people with chronic disease avoid or minimize acute illness.

The PNCM provides direct nursing care focused on enhancing individuals' self-care ability, and it brokers access to health care and supportive services. Each PNCM caseload averages about 40 clients needing varying levels of service that range from weekly to monthly visits. Referrals are accepted for a designated geographic area.

Payment Services are paid for in three ways. First, a portion of the dollars accrued to inpatient nursing care is earmarked for PNCM services. Second, individual PNCM services are established through individual contracts with insurers. And third, system-wide managed care contracts are established. Recently, these contracts have been based on capitated payment, allowing the PNCM to accrue a contracted amount of money each month for each managed-care enrollee. The resultant pool of money pays for PNCM services.

General Outcomes Clients who partner with PNCMs tend to use hospital services less, which enhances quality of life while reducing the cost of health care. In addition, clients speak positively about their partnership. They say they learn earlier to identify signs and symptoms of illness and learn more strategies to avoid or minimize illness. They acknowledge that the relationship is pivotal to their learning.

---

[8]The intervention section of this chapter is based on the practice of Cathy Michaels, Ph.D., PNCM.

CASE STUDY
Jane

Jane lived alone. She had been referred by a hospital staff nurse to the PNCM program when she came into the hospital emergency room by ambulance for hemorrhoid treatment. Assessment showed that she had a long history of emphysema, and she demonstrated both judgment impairment and short-term memory deficit. Unfortunately, judgment impairment can also compound the effects of short-term memory deficit. For instance, when Jane received a large bill, she wanted to pay it off, leaving herself without funds to buy food for the rest of the month. This required developing a plan to pay her bills a little at a time. However, she often forgot about the plan, so the PNCM learned to ask her about her bills via phone between home visits.

As with other seniors, Jane's emotional challenge played out in depression and anxiety. She felt anxious about being short of breath (SOB), and being SOB increased her anxiety. Both her long-standing depression and her anxiety further challenged her memory and judgment. Prior to working with the PNCM, her closest ally had been the ambulance team, which she could call day or night.

Jane needed to take additional diuretics at home two days in a row to counteract a buildup of body fluids. To ensure her taking the Lasix, the PNCM scheduled visits for two consecutive days rather than the usual weekly one. The extra visit allowed the PNCM to compensate for Jane's memory deficit and provided an opportunity to evaluate the effect of the medication. The PNCM was concerned that Jane's short-term memory deficit would not enable her to follow through with this temporary change and could, consequently, precipitate an unnecessary bout with congestive heart failure. In this way, the additional visit was preventive.

Patient Selection: High-Risk Profile Most often the people in need of PNCM service are seniors who demonstrate a high-risk profile characterized by (1) having a serious chronic disease that may be life-threatening, (2) being cognitively challenged, (3) being emotionally challenged, and (4) having inadequate caregiver support. Cognitive challenge usually plays out as short-term memory deficit and judgment impairment, while emotional challenge is often associated with depression and anxiety. Many times, this client lives alone. But whether there is no one available or the caregiver does not have the necessary knowledge, skills, and abilities, there is inadequate caregiver support.

The medical diagnoses that most frequently accompany this high risk profile are congestive heart failure (CHF), chronic obstructive pulmonary disease (COPD), terminal cancer, and diabetes. In general, there is a mismatch between the individual's health care burden and the ability to manage the disease and day-to-day activities. The health care needs of this population are greater than those of the general population as a whole.

Referrals Clients may be referred to PNCM from the community, from the hospital, or from a skilled nursing facility. It is not uncommon for other nurses, physicians, and social workers to refer clients who match the high-risk profile, but individuals may refer themselves or be referred by friends, neighbors, or family.

The case study of Jane is an example of the interplay of cognitive impairment and the need to adapt a prescribed regimen. Jane presents a classic profile of a senior who needs nurse case management.

PNCM Service

Partnership In order to develop a meaningful plan of care, a partnership needs to be established between the client and the PNCM. They must know one another. The PNCM needs to know the client's health concerns, how body changes are perceived, what knowledge exists for initiating and following up with self-care strategies (like relaxation) or those prescribed by the physician or other health care professionals. The

CASE STUDY

Eric

Eric is an 85-year-old who was hospitalized for a month with fulminating pneumonia and empyema. He was also a diabetic. While hospitalized he required insulin, but on discharge was able to return to oral hypoglycemics, specifically Diabeta. Three months later, he decided he was well enough to stop his oral hypoglycemic. He even informed his PNCM that he had seen newspaper evidence that diabetes could be cured. Moreover, he told her that his sister had written and informed him about a lady who cured her diabetes by taking cedar berries. He was convinced he too would be cured. His plan was to go to every health food store in town until he found cedar berries.

A process needed to be identified that would assist his learning about diabetes as a chronic condition while acknowledging that treatment was his choice and responsibility. It was finally

determined not to reinforce his choice for taking or not taking the Diabeta, but to encourage his learning to monitor his blood sugar levels. In that way, he would gain knowledge of whether his blood sugar was staying at a satisfactory level or if it was getting too high. Eric liked the idea and decided to learn to monitor his blood sugar. Until he mastered the monitor, he decided to continue with the Diabeta.

A glucometer was obtained at a discount, and over several weeks he learned how to check his blood sugar levels. After several months of checking his blood sugar on a daily basis, he realized that his blood sugar levels fluctuated, and he confessed he was doing so well that he did not want to "rock the boat." Although Eric continued with his oral hypoglycemics and blood sugar monitoring, he never gave up the idea that his diabetes would be cured.

PNCM needs to know how the client managed before and whether the chronic disease is accepted or ignored until it reaches a crisis. Also important is knowing if the client can focus beyond the chronic disease to other aspects of life. The client must feel respected for his or her learning.

In turn, the client needs to know about the PNCM. Is there a genuine sense of caring, or is this just a job? Is there active listening, a willingness to really help when needed, or just a wish to provide information and move on? Will the client's ability or inability to learn be accepted, or will there just be negative judgment and criticism?

It may take two or three months for all these questions to be answered and respect to develop between the client and the PNCM. When the client feels respected as a person learning to live with chronic disease, the partnership is grounded. The case study about Eric demonstrates the evolution of a trusting relationship.

Direct Nursing Service   As the partnership is being established, health status, well-being, and

self-care ability are assessed. In fact, assessment is ongoing and includes gaining knowledge of clients' health perceptions and behaviors. It is interesting to note that a client's perception of health often blends with behavior that is practiced. Evaluation of well-being offers insight into how safe and valued the client feels. Review of self-care ability provides a picture of the client's capability for carrying out activities of daily living. The case study of Carlos demonstrates how trust was evolved and assessment done.

Creating and Reaching Goals   Clients are helped to improved health, self-care ability, and well-being through PNCM services. The goal is to sufficiently bolster self-care activity so that the health care burden can be managed with the least number of resources. This begins by the client identifying what is most troublesome. Then an approach is created to resolve or minimize the issue and concern.

Many times, it is not easy to discern what is troubling the client. Clients tend to "lump" concerns together. Active listening, focusing on themes, and reframing what is said allows the

CASE STUDY
Carlos

When Carlos first became a client, he always said he was fine. Over time, it became possible to discern a difference in his voice when he was in pain. When this occurred, it became time to ask questions to discover more about his pain, if he was having chest pressure or more shortness of breath. Because Carlos has many chronic diseases, including lung cancer, COPD, CHF, and diabetes, he needs to be quickly evaluated for any significant change in health status if he is to receive preventive care. When necessary this means rapid access to his physician for symptom control to help prevent hospitalization. Or he may need to be hospitalized at a lower level of illness acuity.

Given his situation, his sense of well-being is continually reassessed. As a Native American, he has enduring faith in the Great Spirit. He believes that Spirit will decide when "it is his time to go."

In the meantime, he, his wife, and his PNCM explore ways to maximize his comfort. Recently he achieved more consistent pain control with transdermal patches, using morphine elixir for breakthrough pain. Now his sense of well-being is even stronger.

Because of his debilitating chronic diseases and the effect of his analgesics, his self-care ability needs to be regularly reassessed. He remains safe walking around the house, managing his oxygen delivery, and mobilizing help when he needs it. Because of his forgetfulness, his wife organizes his medications in a box. Since she works, she checks on him frequently by phone. Periodically, the need for support services is explored with Carlos and his wife. However, the informal support provided by his wife, other family members, and his neighbor is enough to maintain him.

---

client to feel heard. Over time, the client's full range of concerns is identified and dealt with. Only safety issues take precedence over patient concerns. The case study of Laury demonstrates how concerns are identified and resolution evolves.

Brokering Services

Clients often need to access health care and supportive services. This is done through the process of brokering or matching need to service. Brokering seems straightforward: A need is identified, a match is made to a service, and an evaluation is done on how the person benefited. But it is not that simple, because, before a service can be provided, the client's feelings about it must be explored. This means not only identifying whether the need is troublesome or not, but also agreeing on how it could be resolved or minimized. For instance, one patient agreed she did not have the energy needed to carry out meal preparation and personal hygiene, especially after her monthly chemotherapy. But she fiercely resisted having anyone help her with

personal care. She feared an aide would make all the decisions: what to eat, what to wear, what time to sleep.

Health care services commonly brokered include physician office visits, home health, routine screening (like mammography), and routine preventive services (like flu shots and securing durable medical equipment). Other services that are frequently brokered include home-delivered meals, housekeeping, personal support, and respite.

Summary and Conclusions

The growing challenge during the current economic climate involves developing cost-sensitive and outcome-efficacious interventions especially for the chronically ill individual who needs ongoing monitoring and periodic interventions, acute and long term. Lower-cost alternatives have evolved so that holistic nursing care can be provided, including the development of managed care and case management.

CASE STUDY
Laury

Laury had endstage COPD. Because she was unable to get enough oxygen into her body to carry out activities, she had many concerns about how to manage. She was concerned about her bills, grocery shopping, food preparation, personal hygiene, getting to her physician, shortness-of-breath, and dying. But talking to her made it apparent that it was the swelling in her legs and feet from CHF that was most troublesome.

From the first visit, it was apparent that Laury did not have the energy to consider more than one issue at a time. The PNCM approached complex situations like hers slowly and simply, allowing her to take the lead. Despite her endstage COPD, Laury was fiercely independent. She wanted

help, but she did not want her life taken over by someone telling her what was wrong and how to resolve it.

Laury not only had endstage COPD; 27 pertinent nursing diagnoses had been identified. It was overwhelming trying to develop a plan of care that addressed them all. Once the paperwork was put aside, it became possible to focus on what was the most troublesome issue to her each time she was visited. That issue was then translated into a nursing diagnosis and a resolution was mutually determined. Over time many of the original 27 diagnoses were addressed, including anxiety, health maintenance deficit, and self-care deficit.

Managed care encompasses the use of groups of individuals or organizations contracting with subscribers to deliver health care services under a fixed level of reimbursement. It provides continuity by linking tasks and departments. Case management, on the other hand, provides a consistent individual health care provider who works across health care settings to achieve desired outcomes for clients. In other words, case management links people across clinical settings.

Nursing case management has evolved to help the client deal with the psychosocial impact of chronic illness and to adapt to an altered state of health. Nurse case managers have both acute and chronic health care experience and knowledge in the physiological and psychosocial ramifications of specific health conditions. They have a generalist background in assessment, diagnosis, and treatment of diseases, and experience in implementing and monitoring medical protocols.

There are several nursing case management models that have developed to guide practice in various settings and to assist various patient populations. These include community health models, home health care models, health mainte-

nance organizations or other hospital-based models, and insurance-based models. All of them are sensitive to both cost and quality and hold promise for cost containment. Each provides cost savings and reduced recidivism. However, they function in either the community or in institutions, resulting in duplication and fragmentation of services.

Only the Professional Nurse Case Management (PNCM) Model, favored by these authors, deals with clients both in the community and in institutions, providing the continuity of a single health care provider for the client. In general, PNCM nursing interventions focus on enhancing the client's sense of competence and self worth. Specifically, self-care strategies and others used to monitor and manage illness symptoms are cooperatively developed by the client and the PNCM.

The PNCM Model has demonstrated impressive reductions in the cost of providing health care to chronically ill elderly clients. The explanation for these client outcomes and the accompanying cost benefits seems embedded in the professional nursing process. Central to the process is partnership.

STUDY QUESTIONS

1. Differentiate managed care and case management.
2. State four goals or objectives of nursing case management.
3. What are the reasons that nurses are able to become nurse case managers?
4. What kinds of client populations are usually served by community-based case models?
5. What kinds of high-risk populations are served by insurance-based case management models?
6. What are the major differences between within-the-walls and beyond-the-walls models

of nursing case management? What are the advantages of each?

7. Discuss the financial outcomes of each of the types of case management models (community based, insurance-based, within-the-walls, beyond-the-walls).
8. Select a client you have worked with, and identify how that individual would be helped (or hindered) through the use of at least one of the models discussed in this chapter.

References

Abrahams, R. (1990). The Social HMO: Case management in an integrated acute and long-term care system. *Caring, 9*(8), 30-39.

American Nurses' Association (1980). *Nursing: A social policy statement.* Kansas City, MO: American Nurses' Association.

——— (1988). *Nursing case management,* Publication No. NS-32. Kansas City, MO: American Nurses' Association.

Applebaum, R. A., & Wilson, N. L. (1988). Training needs for providing case management for the long-term care client: Lessons from the national channeling demonstration. *The Gerontologist, 28*(2), 172-176.

Bachrach, L. L. (1989). Case management: Toward a shared definition. *Hospital and Community Psychiatry, 40*(9), 883-884.

Blake, K. (1991). Rehabilitation nursing program management. *Nursing Management, 22*(1), 42-44.

Bond, G. R., Witheridge, T. F., Wasmer, D., McRae, S. A., Mayes, J., & Ward, R. S. (1989). A comparison of two crisis housing alternatives to psychiatric hospitalization. *Hospital and Community Psychiatry, 40*(2), 177-183.

Bower, K. A. (1988). Managed care: Controlling costs, guaranteeing outcomes. *Definition, 3*(3), 1-3.

——— (1992). *Case Management by nurses.* Kansas City, MO: American Nurses' Publishing.

Brooten, D., Brown, L., Munro, B., York, R., Cohen, S., Roncoli, M., & Hollingsworth, A. (1988). Early discharge and specialist transitional care. *Image: The Journal of Nursing Scholarship, 20*(2), 64-68.

Capitman, J. A., Haskins, B., & Bernstein, J. (1986). Case management approaches in coordinated community-oriented long-term care demonstrations. *The Gerontologist, 26*(4), 398-404.

Carcagano, G. J., & Kemper, P. (1988). An overview of the channeling demonstration and its evaluation. *Health Services Research, 23*(1), 1-22.

Cline, B. G. (1990). Case management: Organizational models and administrative methods. *Caring, 9*(7), 14-18.

Cluff, L. (1981). Chronic disease, function and the quality of care. *Journal of Chronic Disease, 34,* 299-304.

Cohen, E. L., & Cesta, T. G. (1993). *Nursing case management: From concept to evaluation.* St. Louis: Mosby.

Combs, J. A., & Rusch, S. C. (1990) Creating a healing environment. *Health Progress, 71*(4), 38-41.

Cronin, C., & Maklebust, J. (1989). Case-managed care: Capitalizing on the CNS. *Nursing Management, 20*(3), 38-47.

Deitchman, W. S. (1980). How many case managers does it take to screw in a light bulb? *Hospital and Community Psychiatry, 31*(11), 788-789.

Del Bueno, D. J., & Leblanc, D. (1989). Nurse managed care: One approach. *Journal of Nursing Administration, 19*(11), 24-25.

Del Togno-Armansco, V., Olivas, G. S., & Harter, S. (1989). Developing an integrated nursing case management model. *Nursing Management, 20*(10), 26-29.

Desimone, B. (1988). The case for case management. *Continuing Care, 3*(7), 22-23.

Dolson, R., & Richards, L. (1990). Area agencies on aging: The community care connection. *Caring, 9*(8), 18-23.

DuBois, M. M. (1990). Community-based homecare programs are not for everyone—yet. *Caring, 9*(7), 24-27.

Eggert, G. M., Zimmer, J. G., Hall, W. J., & Friedman,

B. (1991). Case Management: A randomized controlled study comparing a neighborhood team and a centralized indivdual model. *Health Services Research, 26*(4), 471-507.

Ellis, J. R., & Hartley, C. L. (1988). *Nursing in today's world, challenges, issues and trends* (3rd ed.). Philadelphia: J. B. Lippincott.

Etheredge, M. L. (1989). *Collaborative care: Nursing case management.* Chicago: American Hospital Publishing.

Ethridge, P. (1991). A nursing HMO: Carondelet St. Mary's experience. *Nursing Management, 22*(7), 22-27.

Ethridge, P., & Lamb, G. (1989). Professional nursing case management improves quality, access and costs. *Nursing Management, 20*(3), 30-35.

Faherty, B. (1990). Case management the latest buzzword: What it is, and what it isn't. *Caring, 9*(7), 20-22.

Fariello, D., & Scheidt, S. (1989). Clinical case management of the dually diagnosed patient. *Hospital and Community Psychiatry, 40*(10), 1065-1067.

Fondiller, S. H. (1991). How case management is changing the picture. *American Journal of Nursing, 91*(1), 64-80.

Giuliano, K. K., & Poirier, C. E. (1991). Nursing case management: Criitcal pathways to desirable outcomes. *Nursing Management, 22*(3), 52-55.

Graham, B. (1989). Preparing case managers. *Caring, 7*(2), 22-23.

Grau, L. (1984). Case management and the nurse. *Geriatric Nursing, 5*(6), 372-375.

Grinnell, S. K. (1989). Post conference reflections: Autonomy and independence for health professionals? *Journal of Allied Health, 18*(1), 115-121.

Halamandaris, V. J. (1990). The paradox of case management. *Caring, 9*,(8), 4-7.

Harris, M., & Bergman, H. (1989). Capitation financing for the chronic mentally ill: A case management approach. *Hospital and Community Psychiatry, 39*(1), 68-72.

Henderson, M. G., & Collard, A. (1988). Measuring quality in medical case management programs. *Quality Review Bulletin, 14*(2), 33-39.

Henderson, M. G., Souder, B. A., & Bergman, A. (1987). Measuring the efficiencies of managed care. *Business and Health, 4*(12), 43-46.

Henderson, M. G., & Wallack, S. S. (1987). Evaluating case management for catastrophic illness. *Business and Health, 4*(3), 7-11.

Hereford, R. W. (1990). Private-pay case management: Let the seller beware. *Caring, 9*(8), 8-12.

Igou, J. F., Hawkins, J. W., Johnson, E. E., & Utley, Q. E. (1989). Nurse-managed approach to care. *Geriatric Nursing, 10*(1), 32-34.

Jones, K., Kopjo, R., Goodneer-Laff, L., & Weber, C. (1990). Gaining control in a changing environment. *Caring, 9*(7), 38-42.

Kane, R. (1988). The noblest experiment of them all: Learning from the National Channeling Evaluation. *Health Services Research, 23*(1), 189-198.

Kane, R. A., & Kane, R. L. (1987). *Long-term care: Principles, programs and policies.* New York: Springer.

Kanter, J. (1989). Clinical case management: Definition, principles, components. *Hospital and Community Psychiatry, 40*(4), 361-368.

Kemp, B. J. (1981). The case management model of human services delivery. In E. L. Pan, T. E. Baker, & C. L. Vash (Eds.), *Annual review of rehabilitation, 2,* (pp. 212-236). New York: Springer.

Kemper, P. (1988). Overview of findings. *Health Services Research, 23*(1), 161-174.

Knollmueller, R. (1989). Case management: What's in a name? *Nursing Management, 20*(10), 38-42.

Korenbrot, C. C., Showstack, J., Loomis, A., & Brindis, C. (1989). Birth weight outcomes in a teenage pregnancy case management project. *Journal of Adolescent Health Care, 10*(2), 97-104.

Lajeunesse, D. A. (1990). Case management: A primary nursing approach. *Caring, 9*(8), 13-16.

Lamb, G. S. (1992). Nursing case management satisfaction survey. Unpublished raw data.

Lamb, G. S., & Stempel, J. E. (1991, October). *Nursing case management: The patient's experience.* Paper presented at the meeting of the American Nurses' Association Council of Nurse Researchers' International Nursing Research Conference, Los Angeles, CA.

———— (1992). *Working with the nurse case manager: Growing as Insider-Expert.* Unpublished manuscript.

Lamb, H. R. (1980). Therapist-case managers: More than brokers of services. *Hospital and Community Psychiatry, 31*(11), 762-764.

Leclair. C. L. (1991). Introducing and accounting for RN case management. *Nursing Management, 22*(3), 44-49.

Littman, E., & Siemsen, J. (1989). AIDS case management: A model for smaller communities. *Caring, 7*(11), 26-31.

Loveridge, C. E., Cummings, S. H., & O'Malley, J. (1988). Developing case management in a primary nursing system. *Journal of Nursing Administration, 18*(10), 36-39.

Lubkin, I. (Ed.) (1990). *Chronic Illness: Impact and interventions* (2nd ed.) Boston: Jones and Bartlett.

Mazoway, J. M. (1987). Early intervention in high cost care. *Business and Health, 4*(3), 12-16.

Mazzuca, S. (1982). Does patient education in chronic disease have a therapeutic value? *Journal of Chronic Disease, 35*(9), 521-529.

McKenzie, C. B., Torkelson, N. G., & Holt, M. A. (1989). Care and cost: Nursing case management improves both. *Nursing Management, 20*(10), 30-34.

Michaels, C. (1992). Carondelet St. Mary's experience. *Nursing Clinics of North America, 27*(1), 77-85.

Miller, K. (1990). Fee-for-service case management. *Caring, 9*(8), 46-49.

Mundinger, M. O. (1984). Community based care: Who will be the case managers. *Nursing Outlook, 32*(6), 294-295.

Olivas, G. S., Del Togno-Armanasco, V., Erickson, J. R., & Harter, S. (1989a). Case management: A bottom-line care delivery model. Part I: The concept. *Journal of Nursing Administration, 19*(11), 16-20.

——— (1989b). Case management: A bottom-line care delivery model. Part II: Adaptation of the model. *Journal of Nursing Administration, 19*(12), 2-17.

Parker, M., & Secord, L. J. (1988). Private geriatric case management: Current trends and future directions. In K. Fisher & E. Wiseman (Eds.), *Case management: Guiding patients through the health care maze* (pp. 27-32). Chicago: Joint Commission on Accreditation of Healthcare Organizations.

Pegels, C. C. (1988). *Health care and the older citizen, economic, demographic and financial aspects.* Rockville, MD.: Aspen.

Putney, K. A., Hauner, J., Hall, T., & Kobb, R. (1990). Case management in long-term care: New directions for professional nursing. *Journal of Gerontological Nursing, 16*(12), 30-33.

Reisch, S. (1986). Continuity of care: From hospital unit into home. *Nursing Management, 17*(12), 38-41.

Rogers, M., Riordan, J., & Swindle, D. (1991). Community-based nursing case management pays off. *Nursing Management, 22*(3), 30-34.

Rusch, S. (1986). Continuity of Care: From hospital unit into home. *Nursing Management, 17*(12), 38-41.

Schwartz, S. R., Goldman, H. H., & Churgin, S. (1982). Case management for the chronic mentally ill: Models and dimensions. *Hospital and Community Psychiatry, 33*(12), 1006-1009.

Shipp. M. K., & Jay, T. M. (1988). Case management and long term care. *Caring, 7*(3), 42-44.

Simpson, D. F. (1982). *Case management in long-term programs.* Washington D.C.: The Center for the Study of Social Policy.

Sinnenn, M. T., & Schifalacqua, M. M. (1991). Coordinated care in a community hospital. *Nursing Management, 22*(3), 38-42.

Smith, M. L. (1990). Blue cross blue shield: Individual case management: A win-win proposition. *Caring, 9*(8), 26-28.

Stillwaggon, C. A. (1989). The impact of nurse managed care on the cost of nurse practice and nurse satisfaction. *Journal of Nursing Administration, 19*(11), 21-27.

Strumpf, N. E., & Knibbe, K. K. (1990). Long-term care, fulfilling promises to the elderly. In J. C. McCloskey & H. K. Grace (Eds.), *Current issues in nursing* (pp. 215-225). St. Louis: C. V. Mosby.

Walstedt, P., & Blaser, W. (1986). Nurse case management for the frail elderly: A curriculum to prepare nurses for that role. *Home Healthcare Nurse, 4*(2), 30-35.

Weil, M. (1985). Professional and eduational issues in case management practice. In M. Weil, & J. Karl and Associates (Eds.), *Case management in human service practice* (pp. 357-390). San Francisco: Jossey-Bass.

Weyant, J. (1991, February). *St. Joseph Medical Center in Wichita, Community-based nurse case management department report.* Paper presented at a meeting of nurse case managers, Tuscon, AZ.

Zander, K. (1988a). Nursing case management: Strategic management of cost and quality outcomes. *Journal of Nursing Administration, 18*(5), 23-29.

——— (1988b). Nursing case management: Resolving the DRG paradox. *Nursing Clinics of North America, 23*(3), 503-520.

——— (1990a). Case management a golden opportunity for whom? In J. C. McCloskey & H. K. Grace (Eds.), *Current issues in nursing* (3rd ed.) (pp. 199-204). St. Louis: C. V. Mosby.

——— (1990b). Differentiating managed care and case management. *Definition, 5*(2), 1-2.

Bibliography

Bawden, E. L. (1990). Reaching out to the chronically mentally ill homeless. *Journal of Psychosocial Nursing and Mental Health Services, 28*(3), 6-13.

Calogero, M. A. (1990). Individual case management and the blue cross and blue shield system. *The Case Manager, 1*(1), 25-27.

Evaluation of the National Long Term Care Demonstation (1988). (Special Issue). *Health Services Review, 23*(1), 1-199.

Harris, M., & Bergman, H. C. (1988). Misconceptions about the use of case management services by the chronic mentally ill: A utilization analysis. *Hospital and Community Psychiatry, 39*(12), 1276-1280.

Lamb, G. S. (1992a). *Conceptual and methodological issues in nurse case management research.* Manuscript submitted for publication.

Ryan, N. (1982). Service coordination and monitoring. In J. Quinn, S. R. Schwartz, H. H. Goldman, & S. Churgin (1982). Case management for the chronic mentally ill: Models and dimensions. *Hospital and Community Psychiatry, 33*(12), 1006-1009.

Staebler, R. (1990a). Case management: What is it? *Caring, 9*(7), 1.

———— (1990b). Case management: Who's doing it? *Caring, 9*(8), 1.

PART IV

Impact of the System

CHAPTER 21

Agency Maze

Deborah Burton

Introduction

The complex needs of the chronically ill usually exceed the resources that can be provided by families and friends alone. Learning to negotiate community networks of health, social, and support services can be extremely confusing for the client and family. The situation is similar to that of a mouse trying to find its way out of a maze. The term *agency maze* is deliberately selected, as it very appropriately describes the complex of community resources for the chronically ill.

There are two approaches to successfully negotiating this agency maze: (1) trial and error, which can be frustrating and inefficient, and can lead to a sense of powerlessness; and (2) understanding the structure and function of the maze and planning accordingly. The latter is, of course, the preferred option.

Rapidly evolving technology and more aggressive preventive services have allowed many people to survive what were once fatal acute illnesses, leaving them to deal with chronic conditions. For example, the diagnoses of cancer

Acknowledgment: The author wishes to thank M. L. Friedemann, R.N., Ph.D., and B. Scheffer, R.N., Ph.D., for their contribution to earlier editions of this text. Special thanks are given for their model, *Dealing with the Agency Maze.*

and diabetes are no longer associated with a prognosis of imminent death. Even AIDS is being reconceptualized as a chronic illness (Fee & Fox, 1992; Smith, 1987). These changes present new challenges to today's acute care focused health care delivery system. Supporting those living with chronic illness means shifting emphasis from cure to adaptation and maintaining independence (Calahan, 1992; CDC, 1993).

The shift toward chronicity, longer lives, and an aging citizenry has dramatically influenced political trends. Equal access to health care was the political issue of the 1960s and 1970s. The health care delivery system responded by increasing services. As a result, mental health centers, neighborhood clinics, and regional programs—heart, cancer, and stroke programs—were established. The increased costs were absorbed by a healthy and growing economy (Lewis, 1983).

In the 1980s, however, this political trend was reversed. Federal health planning efforts fell short on containing costs, and inflation in the health care industry skyrocketed out of control (see Chapter 22). Medicare and Medicaid spending increased tremendously, at a time when the federal budget was plagued by an economic recession that could no longer absorb increasing costs. As a result, health care cost containment emerged as the policy dilemma for the 1990s (DHHS, 1993). Early national reform efforts emphasized both cost containment and access to a basic benefit package of health care services for every American (Clinton & Gore, 1992).

Despite reform initiatives that advocate for more community-based services and for improved integration of services among organizations and agencies, the problem of agency complexity will by no means be resolved. No basic benefit package can affordably cover *every* health, social, emotional, spiritual, and mental health support service needed by the chronically ill. Nor will agencies and services ever be so well integrated that coordination of care and services can be complete and flawless.

As the numbers and scope of agency services have expanded, the roles of health care professionals have evolved to meet emerging needs. For example, nurses serve as case managers, administrators, health planners, and evaluators. Other health care providers, such as social workers and psychologists, have expanded roles that include liaison or facilitator of community support groups. Pharmacists no longer only "count pills"; they are increasingly involved in client education, community support, and problem solving.

A number of comprehensive case management projects initiated in the 1980s have demonstrated track records not only in supporting complex, vulnerable clients in the community but in reducing costs. Two model programs are On Lok and ACCESS. On Lok is a San Francisco-based agency that draws funds from block grants and the private sector and serves as a model that may work elsewhere. Its outreach programs are locally controlled by a community board to provide consumer input. On Lok provides a service package of medical, rehabilitation, maintenance, and custodial care for clients with functional deficits. An innovative, cost-saving idea that is incorporated in the project is monetary compensation for participating caretaking family members, which reduces the need for hospitalization and provides a means by which the family can care for loved ones at home (Rucklin, Norris, & Eggert, 1982). ACCESS (Assessment for Community Care Services) is a comparable project in the state of New York that has managed to keep the daily cost for care at approximately 52 percent of the institutional rates allowed by Medicaid (Eggert, Bowlyow, & Nichole, 1980; Palmer & Vogel, 1985).

Comprehensive health care has advantages for both client and professional. Clients are spared anxiety and frustration in finding their way through the agency maze; caregivers are provided help in handling referrals more effectively. Comprehensive service packages are often more effective in meeting clients' needs than are referrals to multiple agencies. In addition, the caregiver's time is saved in locating resources. The case study on innovative resources demonstrates the way one family benefited from health care innovations.

Problems, Unresolved Issues, and Negative Effects

In spite of many exciting innovations in community health care, there is slow progress in meeting client needs, which also has a negative impact on professionals who provide services. Several issues contribute to this slow progress: fragmentation of services, lack of communication between agencies and caregivers, unaffordable costs for services, and politics. Left unresolved, these issues have a negative effect on both clients and professionals.

Although there is more health care provided now than there was 20 or 30 years ago, good health care is becoming more of a privilege of the wealthy than a right for all. It still remains to be seen just how much these pervasive problems will be addressed and resolved through reform initiatives. However, an explicit commitment to the notion that adequate health care is a basic right rather than a privilege was made by the Clinton administration (Clinton & Gore, 1992).

Client Needs

Deinstitutionalization of the chronically mentally ill from state mental hospitals began in the 1960s (Caton, 1981) under the assumption that money would be saved. However, poor planning left communities unprepared to deal with this influx of newly discharged patients. Confusion and needless suffering followed, and it is debatable whether costs were saved in the long run. The deinstitutionalization movement did survive, and community residential care of the chronically mentally ill is likely to last (Stroul, 1989).

CASE STUDY
Innovative Resources

Bobby, the only son of Eva and Robert F., suffers from severe cerebral palsy and is wheelchair bound. He cannot speak because of poor muscle control, although he has always been able to make his wants known by signs and sounds. When Bobby was very young, a visiting nurse taught Eva how to provide basic physical care and alerted the family to their right to have Bobby evaluated by the public school system for special preschool training. As a result, Bobby became part of a program staffed by special education professionals. The family was taught how to work with Bobby in improving daily living skills, bowel and bladder control, and discipline.

When Bobby reached school age, the preschool staff helped the family adjust to a new program administered by the local university. This program had not only special education faculty and students but physical therapists, speech therapists, and other allied health professionals. Team functions were designed to maximize the child's potential, work cooperatively with the parents, and provide liaison between parents and the staffs

of the neurology and orthopedic clinics that treated Bobby. The family was fortunate to have a special education student work with them for several months. She taught Eva and Robert many ways to make physical care for Bobby easier. She helped find funding for a patient lift and a specially equipped transport van.

Bobby was also provided with a small electronic communication device, and he learned to activate special meaningful sounds in order to communicate. His ability to operate the device at age 11 was a major turning point for the family. Now that he could communicate, frustration was reduced, and his potential for further development was greatly enhanced. Eva and Robert are extremely grateful for the care and concern of these health caregivers. Eva feels obliged to contribute service to other families. She has established a cerebral palsy support group and has become involved in community-wide fund raising for the university program, so that more children can have a new way of living.

SOURCE: From Friedemann and Scheffer (1990).

Developments with care of the chronically physically ill appear to have taken a similar course. Hospital cost containment efforts and the advent of Diagnostic Related Groups (DRGs) have resulted in early hospital discharges. Consequently, families and extended care facilities are now called upon to assume care for the chronically ill and the elderly in communities. Home health care agencies and services have proliferated in response to this movement (Wasik, Bryant, & Lyons, 1990).

Needs of the Chronically Ill The community-based health care delivery system is faced with the challenge of organizing and delivering available resources to help meet the needs of the dependent chronically ill—needs that can be categorized in four groups: clinical care, psychological/spiritual, rehabilitation, and optimal functioning in activities of daily living (ADLs) (see Table 21-1). Clinical care needs include assistance in obtaining proper medical diagnoses and clinical treatment and supervision. Psycho-

logical/spiritual needs include adjusting emotionally and spiritually to the situation and adapting to the ongoing illness. Rehabilitation needs require specialized assistance for restoring and maintaining body functions and life-style. ADL needs require creative problem solving so the client can achieve as much independence and autonomy as possible.

Client education is fundamental to addressing all four categories of needs (see Chapters 10 and 16, on compliance and teaching, respectively). Knowledge about their particular illness and treatment increases the likelihood of clients successfully managing their own care. In a community where complex sets of health needs are being addressed by many agencies and providers, ensuring that the client is receiving accurate, adequate, and appropriate information is critical to achieving maximal functioning and independence.

It is also important to differentiate between models of care for the chronically *physically* ill and for the chronically *mentally* ill. Although

TABLE 21-1.   Needs of the chronically ill

CLINICAL NEEDS	
Physical illness	Supervision of treatment regimen
	Maintenance of physical care
	Understanding purpose of treatment
	Skillful clinical interventions
	Obtaining necessary equipment and supplies
Mental/emotional illness	Ongoing monitoring of medication
	Monitoring of behavior changes
	Assistance with administration of medication
PSYCHOLOGICAL/SPIRITUAL NEEDS	
Physical and mental/emotional illness	Emotional support from family and friends
	Help with acceptance of limitations
	Help to feel like a productive member of the family and community
	Assistance in gaining positive self-concept and body image
	Avoidance of unduly restrictive and overprotective parenting (children)
	Maximizing independence
	Encouragement to express feelings
	Consistency and continuity of care to provide a sense of security
	Opportunity to participate in religious activities and counseling
	Help with acceptance of chronicity of illness
REHABILITATION NEEDS	
Physical illness	Rehabilitation training: exercises, vocational training
	Supervision of prescribed rehabilitation program
	Coordination, long-term follow-up, and evaluation of rehabilitation program
Mental/emotional illness	Assistance in coping with life stressors
	Identifying and locating support systems
	Learning social and job skills
NEEDS FOR OPTIMAL FUNCTIONING IN ACTIVITIES OF DAILY LIVING	
Physical and mental/emotional illness	Identification of client supports within family and social network
	Evaluation of client's total functioning level in the environment
	Help in developing strength in self-care
	Assistance with daily self-care as necessary

SOURCE: Modified from Friedemann and Scheffer (1990).

the needs of the two groups are similar, rehabilitation goals for the chronically mentally impaired can be quite different, particularly in the areas of self-sufficiency and productivity. The deinstitutionalization movement was a disappointment in terms of community-based rehabilitation and resocialization. The original goals for care were to relearn community living, to become achievement and success oriented, and to maintain employment. Unfortunately, for clients who had spent many years in an institutional environment, these goals were unrealistic because many had become very dependent. As a result, rehabilitation aims have had to be adjusted over time. Now, emphasis is placed on strengthening and supporting present functional levels by ensuring that clients can perform the physical, emotional, intellectual, and social skills needed to live in a community with the least amount of required support from professional providers (Anthony & Lieberman, 1986; Stroul, 1989).

It should also be mentioned that that physical rehabilitation is integrally connected with psychological functioning for both the physically and mentally impaired. Without motivation to restore health and increase independence, a client is unlikely to progress with meeting therapeutic objectives. Conversely, tangible progress with restoring physical functioning can lead to increased motivation with continuing treatment.

Effects on the Client The primary effects on clients and families lost in an agency maze are confusion, difficulty in perceiving their complex needs, and feelings of powerlessness. Frustration results when they find out that they do not qualify for a service, that no such service is available in the area, that they cannot obtain satisfactory services, or that they cannot afford services. Often clients get false or contradictory information about services and later discover that the agency cannot meet their needs. When assistance in locating agencies is not forthcoming, clients may give up trying to establish contact. In addition, without adequate information to make knowledgeable choices, clients are likely to become confused or discouraged by the large selection of agencies that offer similar services (Preston, 1992).

Once a client has decided to accept a service, satisfaction is not guaranteed. For example, because of a lack of adequate funds for private care, a mentally ill family member may need to be sent to a state hospital, where treatment may include heavy sedation that results in a marked reduction in activity participation. Family members consequently may become distressed because they have no power to influence care and no alternative services from which to choose.

Disadvantaged clients often find community-based services have long waiting lists for counseling, or medical clinics may be staffed with doctors and nurses who are to busy to listen to a client's problem.

In many instances, lack of communication among health professionals and agencies can leave clients with either no referral or one that is useless, such as one to an agency that no longer exists. Referrals are sometimes done hastily, without exploring what the client actually needs or wants.

Clients in need of prolonged services can find their savings depleted over time. Although medical insurance usually covers part or all of hospitalization expenses, outpatient and home care is inadequately covered under private insurance plans, Medicare, and Medicaid (Dimond, 1991; DHHS, 1993). When Medicare or Medicaid clients cannot afford coinsurance and deductibles, they may not seek health care except in an emergency. The elderly are particularly affected by this problem, and some communities have set up special clinics or have private physicians who volunteer their services to meet the medical needs of this cohort. However, many senior citizens do not have access to such care or may not know that such services exist.

Many chronically ill individuals are caught in loopholes in the system and go without care or supportive help. Some people no longer qualify for Medicaid or Medicare; others do not have private insurance coverage because they are self-employed or unemployed; and many run out of insurance benefits if they need long-term rehabilitation or support services (see Chapter 22, on financial impact). For example, many clients no longer needing skilled nursing care do not qualify for home care services meaning they must pay most of costs for support services from privately run companies.

A last problem worth mentioning is the client's frustration about repeated data collection. Clients in need of several services are forced to have a lengthy interview with each agency they contact and give the same information many times. Unfortunately, sharing data among agencies is difficult because of legal restrictions to maintain client confidentiality. Agencies are required to get a written consent from the client before treatment information can be released (Knollmueller, 1988). Some hospitals have relatively free information exchange with agencies, such as the Visiting Nurses Association in their states, and use release-of-information forms. But many agencies prefer to develop their own database for each client. Much valuable information is necessarily lost in the archives of agencies, and much time is wasted. Often, only the clients and their families know all the historical facts of the illness and treatments and sometimes report overlapping services, useless treatments, and resulting frustration and anger.

Fragmentation

Demand for specialized health services has changed rapidly. At times, responses by health planners have been rushed, erratic, and disorganized. These responses have been attempts to find solutions to local health needs by well-meaning professionals and consumers. In addition, the federal government has encouraged development of community health agencies, many of which have strong profit motives. Today's health care delivery system comprises thousands of federal, state, and local agencies offering services in competition with one another for funding. Consequently, some level of fragmentation is inevitable and can lead to unnecessary duplication and unequal distribution of services. The Clinton administration promised increased efficiency, reduction in unnecessary paperwork and forms, and access to a comprehensive set of health care services for every American. However, until and unless *all* levels of service are covered, and as long as a reform strategy includes incentives for competition, some fragmentation will persist. These problems will likely be even more pronounced in rural areas (Clinton & Gore, 1992; Gore, 1993; OTA, 1990).

Lack of Communication

Adequate communication between agencies and health professionals is difficult to achieve in a complex, changing, and fragmented delivery system. Many agencies function autonomously and within an individual budget. Caregivers may have knowledge of few other agencies that complement or augment their services. Consequently, referrals are made according to a fixed routing system to a few commonly used referral sources. These referral patterns are simple, but they overlook community services that could better meet individual clients' needs and leave little room for creativity.

Of particular importance is inadequate communication between hospitals and home health agencies. Some essential referrals are never made or they are made too late even when critical to clients, thereby preventing smooth transitions. For example, discharging a client on a Friday or over the weekend without prior arrangements can be dangerous if community support services cannot be accessed until Monday. Clients may require rehospitalization because family members are not sufficiently skilled in taking care of them or because of a lack of coordination and family education regarding caregiving, resulting in overwhelmed family members. In addition, lack of communication can lead to frustration for professionals, confusing or contradictory messages being given to families, disruption of care, insufficient education of caregivers, and a general sense on the part of the client of a lack of support (Haddad & Kapp, 1991).

Costs of Service

Fragmentation and duplication of services, technological advances, and sophisticated care delivery models have driven up the costs of care. Cuts in government funds have eroded public services for the poor and disadvantaged. For example, the limited payment by Medicaid for nursing home care is insufficient to pay costs. Private insurance companies have increased premiums and reduced or eliminated third-party coverage for nonacute care services.

The Clinton administration proposed sweeping reform with emphasis on client-centered care; coordination of services through local networks or "alliances" for care; and basic coverage to be guaranteed for everyone irrespective of health status, income, age, or amount of services used (Clinton & Gore, 1992). While these initiatives would have solved many of the fragmentation and cost barriers to achieving comprehensive community care, the cost to taxpayers likely would be prohibitive, and politics often limit the extent to which plans can be fully implemented.

Politics and Power

Competition among governments, providers, service agencies, institutions, and legislative bodies is accentuated as reform initiatives take shape. The considerable lobbying power of the medical profession and hospital industry is, in part, at the root of expensive technological developments—a system that emphasizes acute institutional and specialty care rather than community-based and primary care. It is yet to be seen whether this historical political clout can withstand growing legislative and consumer demands to control costs in health care and to provide everyone with basic affordable services (Maraldo, 1990).

As public funds have diminished, institutions have turned to private funding sources. Competition is stiff, and funding decisions are not always made on the basis of need or rationality. Because of the nature of grant funding cycles and time-limited demonstration project initiatives, the community care system is constantly in a state of flux. Agencies must survive despite shrinking public resources, legislation that may be driven by partisan politics, grant-funding criteria that may not represent community priorities, and growing competition. Just keeping abreast of available services, third-party coverage for needed services, and eligibility criteria for specific services within a community at any given time can represent an agency maze.

People who are satisfied with or benefit from comprehensive health care still remain threatened by the political and financial issues described. Chronically ill clients need consistency and a sense of security, which are hard to find in a system submerged in constant changes in rules and regulations. Agencies fighting for survival reduce the number of staff personnel or cut services. This influences the quality of care all clients receive. The ultimate threat to clients is the closing of an entire agency on which they depend. Many clients who lose their support system in this manner feel betrayed and angry, depressed and disillusioned. They may not have the energy to establish contact with other agencies, especially if they see their future there as equally uncertain.

Impact on the Professional

Hard-working, well-meaning professionals can become disheartened in their attempts to connect clients with services. Often there are no services available to address individual client needs; at other times, waiting lists are discouragingly long. In addition, selected agencies do not always perform at the level of quality promised. Over time, professionals become frustrated, dis-

illusioned, and can suffer burnout. Professional disappointment can become acute where extensive energy has been invested in preparing a client for referral. For example, a nurse or social worker may counsel a depressed client for a long time, long enough to overcome barriers to accepting help from mental health professionals. If the client walks out angrily after one or two counseling sessions because a counselor is perceived as insensitive to the client's problem, the referring caregiver may feel demoralized and may give up trying.

The intake process required by most agencies frequently involves filling out lengthy forms and collecting statements from other health professionals verifying the client's condition. This process can discourage professional caregivers from making referrals. In addition, the complex referral systems in many metropolitan areas require advanced skills or unrealistic amounts of time to accomplish.

Professionals may lack information about performance and service quality of specific agencies and the preparation and credentials of their staff. Communication about new agencies or services may be inadequate, and because a community's services can change so rapidly, professionals may be unable to keep up to date with information regarding available services. Making referrals represents only a small proportion of the workload for many professionals, which may account for the limited time and energy available to keep informed. These problems not only may cause professionals to feel frustrated, but can cause them to become as confused as their clients. However, development of specialized referral and case management agencies will help in addressing these issues.

Availability of Community Resources

Two significant trends are presently influencing availability of, and access to, community resources. The first, cost control measures and shrinking public funds, has affected nearly every state and federal health agency. Expenditures of public funds have not kept up with the increased demand for services. Medicare and Medicaid, which have provided coverage for periodic

hospitalization and limited coverage for extended care and home care, are still the basic
funding sources for care for the poor and the
elderly (Moon, 1987). Faced with severe cut-
backs and cost control measures, both systems
are struggling for their very survival. For example, state psychiatric hospitals continue to serve
as the only temporary resource for intermittent
acute phases of many mental disorders, and they
are confronted by serious administrative and financial difficulties. In many cases, psychiatric
services have been reduced to minimum standard levels. Other agencies dependent on government funding, such as public health
departments, community mental health centers,
schools, courts, and prisons, have been forced
to drastically reduce health services.

The second trend, the boom in the home
health care industry, is directly related to the
first trend. Cuts in Medicare and Medicaid,
reduced lengths of hospital stays, as well as a
growing consumerism movement have led to
increased demands for services to support the
chronically ill in their homes with the goal
of keeping them there as long as possible
(Stanhope & Lancaster, 1992; DHHS, 1993;
Wasik, Bryant, & Lyons, 1990). Despite methodological limitations and difficulty with comparing diverse services, there is a growing body
of evidence that comprehensive home-based
services for complex clients and families can
reduce costs in both the long and short run
(GAO, 1990; Palmer & Vogel, 1985).

There is a growing community-level response to the need for more out-of-hospital supports. Table 21–2 outlines examples of these
actions, many of which also reflect growing demands on the part of consumers. Most of these
responses rely on some form of voluntary effort.
In fact, their very survival and success are heavily
dependent on continued volunteer efforts as
funds diminish. This dependency on volunteers
and local support explains one distinct advantage enjoyed by wealthier urban communities
over more rural areas: Because more funds and
volunteer resources are available, more services
and agencies tend to be located in urban areas.
Overall, despite the best of intentions on the
part of all communities, the actions outlined in
Table 21–2 have served to complicate the agency
maze.

Interventions

Earlier sections of this chapter briefly introduced
a multitude of problems and unresolved issues
facing the chronically ill, their families, and
health care professionals who must deal with
agencies. Solutions to these administrative, economic, political, and communication challenges
cannot be adequately addressed within a few
pages. The reader is encouraged to read Chapter
22, on financial impact, and to seek more comprehensive publications for in-depth analyses of
these problems and suggested solutions. In the
remaining sections of this chapter, we will view
the positive effects of agencies on clients and
professionals and introduce a model that can be
used by health care providers to get into, around,
and through the agency maze.

Positive Effects on the Client
and Professional

Community-level agencies have had extremely
positive influences on the lives of clients, families, and health care professionals. Clients and
families benefit from services that emphasize humanness, health promotion, self-care, and independence, all within a familiar environment.

Expanded home health services and community-based support programs are providing professionals with sufficient resources to match
client needs with available services. These networks are also leading to the development of
new or expanded professional roles within the
community: case managers, discharge planners,
managed care specialists, home health care
nurses, and community health educators and
consultants (Preston, 1992; Stanhope & Lancaster, 1992; Werley, Drago, & Hadley, 1990).

Humane Care Increased emphasis on the
nonphysical needs of the chronically ill have positively affected the health care system as a whole.
This is evidenced by the restructuring of education for nurses and other health professionals
to focus on psychosocial aspects of client care
(Stanhope & Lancaster, 1992). Care is aimed at
assessing and intervening with identified health-
related problems in all aspects of the client's
life, including social support, coping, sexuality,

TABLE 21-2. Creative community responses to chronic illness needs

Problem	Community Responses
Scarcity of funds	• More aggressive and expanded fund-raising efforts aimed at corporate and philanthropic organizations • Expanded use of volunteer resources, such as crisis counseling, friendly visitors, Meals on Wheels • Involvement of churches in offering community services • Increased volunteerism on the part of physicians, nurses, and dentists • More emphasis by existing services on case management services to oversee and coordinate care • Growth of self-help and support groups to provide mutual support for and assistance with coping and self-care (ostomy, diabetes, smoking cessation, mastectomy groups, and so forth)
Need for more home care services	• New private business enterprises offering comprehensive community-based care services, including home care, homemaker, adult day care, and extended care • Existing voluntary and nonprofit organizations offering supportive community services such as transportation, shopping, housekeeping, and friendly visiting
Lack of resources to meet psychosocial needs	• Rise of self-help and support groups • Specialized summer camp and retreat programs for children and families that provide education and counseling, including leukemia, epilepsy, and diabetes • Increased volunteerism by counselors, therapists, and clergy

SOURCE: Adapted from Friedemann and Scheffer (1990).

spiritual issues, nutrition, and knowledge of community resources. This is in contrast to earlier nursing roles, which focused primarily on the execution of physician orders.

At the community level, nursing services often include a case management function (see Chapter 20, on case management). Nursing case management is used to implement the nursing care plan through coordination of care across services and agencies, as well as to carry out advocacy for the client and evaluation of the community care being received (American Nurses' Association, 1988).

Health Maintenance, Health Promotion, and Rehabilitation The shift toward both chronicity and the growing numbers of elderly has brought about changes in the structure of health care delivery systems. Most notable is the rapid growth of health maintenance organizations (HMOs) that charge a flat rate per subscriber for comprehensive health services, irrespective of the actual costs of care. These services include inpatient, outpatient, ambulatory, psychiatric, long-term, home health, and hospice care. Based on a community rating principle, where risk is spread throughout a group of subscribers, HMOs have built-in incentives to deliver care that is inexpensive and efficient (see Chapter 23, on social/health policy). The HMO model is increasing in popularity and holds promise for the future because it emphasizes prevention and cost controls and services are coordinated, which greatly reduces the complexity of services that must be negotiated by its members (Jacobs, 1991). The chronically ill benefit from the available assistance of social workers, therapists, dietitians, and counselors, all within the same organization and covered within the member subscription rate.

Other traditional health services are also reorganizing care to offer more comprehensive service models. Many hospitals have established home health and hospice services and have expanded ambulatory care services to include educational programs and psychosocial and other support services. Case management and care co-ordination services are offered to the chronically ill to improve efficiency and reduce the agency maze burden (ANA, 1988). Client benefits from these changes include easy access to care, links with support systems with similarly afflicted individuals, and an overall improvement in the extent to which their comprehensive health needs are being adequately addressed (Berkowitz, Halfon, & Klee, 1992).

Support Services and Increased Quality of Life   Home health agencies and services have increased in number and have expanded services to a more comprehensive approach. Home health aides, trained to provide basic care such as baths, linen changes, cooking, and simple health care procedures are now widely available. Home-making services, which include housekeeping, shopping, meal preparation, and transportation, are also available to maintain the chronically ill in their home environments. Adult day care and respite programs are available to give families and caregivers a "break" from the demands of caregiving.

Transportation, which can be essential to a client's sense of well-being, is often provided by community groups, churches, and other organizations. Transportation enhances participation in social activities, church services, and community activities. Such participation provides mental stimulation and a sense of belonging. In addition, involvement with others can reduce social isolation and increase the feeling of independence and self-worth. However, in rural areas, where social isolation is often a problem even for those who do not have chronic conditions, transportation services are not as readily available. Unfortunately, the lack of available comprehensive support services in rural areas only compounds the complexity of the agency maze, leaving gaps in the continuum of needed services for rural chronically ill residents (Office of Technology Assessment, 1990).

Dealing with the Agency Maze

This final section of the chapter is devoted to negotiating the agency maze itself. Friedemann and Scheffer's model (1990), "Dealing with the

Agency Maze" (Figure 21–1) is a framework designed to help client and professional minimize the confusion, frustration, and discouragement that comes from inadequate interaction with agencies by linking needs with resources in the community. The following diagram illustrates the need–resource linking relationship among client, caregiver, and community resources.

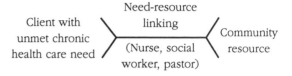

A health care professional's skill in linking needs with community resources can mean the difference between client independence or dependence and possible institutionalization. Like the mouse in the maze mentioned earlier, professional caregivers who enter this maze without experience or adequate knowledge can easily become frustrated and disillusioned, although with luck some may eventually find their way through, albeit inefficiently.

Although the diagram implies that any health professional can successfully link clients and resources, the hospital-based staff nurse usually refers clients to those most commonly involved in referrals to community resources: hospital discharge planners, social workers, nurse case managers, home care coordinators, community health nurses, and hospice nurses. However, an understanding of both the agency maze and the linking process can enable hospital staff nurses to better plan for client discharge, starting from the first day of an admission. Professional caregivers can gain an understanding of community resources and the linking process via help and support of others, and sometimes through trial-and-error learning. However, inexperienced caregivers, unfamiliar with the maze, may be faced with other urgent problems and have little time to experiment with the system.

Figure 21–1 offers a "path" through the maze of resource procurement and linking. Following this path also allows the professional to leave the maze with increased knowledge and experience. Each step is outlined in detail.

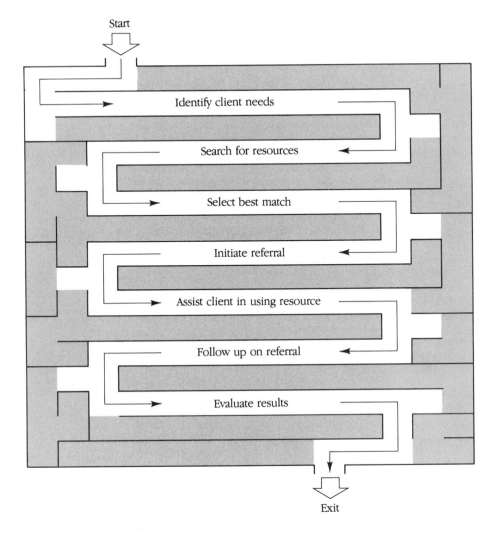

FIGURE 21-1. Dealing with the Agency Maze

SOURCE: From Friedemann and Scheffer (1990).

Identify Client Needs

The process of identifying needs corresponds directly to the first step in any problem-solving approach: the assessment of the problem. A comprehensive database should be collected from a variety of sources: clients, significant others, the physician, the hospital, medical records, service agencies, agency referral forms, other providers, and so on. Assessment comprises the accurate collection of information and determination of which information is essential. for example, a critical factor in assessment is determining the client's financial status, since ability to pay affects eligibility for services. Unfortunately, questions about income can be perceived by caregiver and client as prying into private matters. Justifying the need for asking such questions requires recognizing the value of financial data for agency selection. Practicing with a friend or colleague to find words that are comfortable to use is often helpful. The client can be prepared for such

CASE STUDY

Mrs. Kim: Assessment and Categorizing Needs

Mrs. Kim, a 45-year-old former schoolteacher, has multiple sclerosis (MS), which was diagnosed eight years ago. She is married, has two children ages 12 and 8, and lives in a suburban community with a large selection of service agencies. Mrs. Kim has to be hospitalized periodically for treat-ment but, with the support of her family and community resources, she is able to remain at home. The community health nurse collected data and determined corresponding needs (see Table 21–3).

---

questioning by explaining the purpose and need for such questions. For example,

> Mr. Green, there is one more area of informa-tion I need to ask about. It is sometimes diffi-cult for people to talk about money matters, but the information is needed in our plan-ning. It will help us to determine what agency to select: a public one, a tax-supported one without fees, or one that charges for services or has a sliding fee scale. We want the agency that can do the job best.

Once assessment is complete, the caregiver, cli-ent, and family list all identified needs in the following four categories: clinical care, psy-chological/spiritual, rehabilitation, and optimal functioning in ADLs. These needs should be translated into objectives to be met through the referral and service delivery process. A written plan then guides the selection of resources, the referral process, and the evaluation of care. The assessment process and determination of needs are illustrated in the case study of Mrs. Kim and in Table 21–3.

Search for Resources

Although knowledge about community services and functions is essential in helping and advocat-ing for clients and families, most novice profes-sionals do not have this knowledge. Thus, the inexperienced professional needs a systematic approach to finding information quickly and effi-ciently about the range of services available in the community. Consequently, the second step is identifying and locating specific agencies that offer services to meet the client's needs. In order to limit the number of potential agencies, initial determination of the type of agency required and desired by the client should be made.

Determining the Type of Agency The cli-ent's financial status and transportation re-sources will directly influence whether a public or private agency is appropriate. These factors must be discussed in depth with the client, since this information may automatically limit choices. For example, the professional caregiver need not inquire about services of agencies that are too expensive or too distant from home if the client has no transportation.

Locating Suitable Agencies Even after this initial elimination process, locating agencies may seem overwhelming if the caregiver has no plan to follow. Most organizations have a resource file or more experienced team members who can help. Such information is useful, even though it needs periodic updating.

Let us assume, however, that no resource file exists. A recommended first step is to consult major information sources on either a national or local level and begin your own file. There are two valuable sources on the national level. First, the National Health Information Clearinghouse in Washington, D.C., assists consumers and health professionals in locating health resources. They have a toll-free number. Second, *The Ency-clopedia of Associations* is available in the refer-ence section of most libraries. The two most useful sections for health providers are labeled "Social Welfare" and "Health"; both sections list many agencies for the blind, the handicapped, drug abusers, alcohol abusers, and so forth.

On a local level one can contact health de-partments; local, state, and federal government

TABLE 21-3. Mrs. Kim's categories of need

Data	Need Category
Medical diagnosis: multiple sclerosis	**Clinical care** Requires ongoing medical supervision, outpatient clinic visits. Needs hospitalization during exacerbations. Needs to understand purpose of treatment. Family needs information about disease, prognosis, treatment. Needs consistency between hospital and home care.
Disease process has depleted her strength and stamina for extended activities. Can ambulate short distances with leg braces and assistance of one person. Longer distances require use of wheelchair. Spends much time watching television. Complains of having nothing useful to do.	**Rehabilitation** Needs daily walking with assistance. Needs periodic supervision and encouragement of daily exercise program. Needs assessment of living facility for wheelchair access (planning for future). Needs occupational therapy assessment.
Physical limitations prevent some self-care activities of personal hygiene, dressing, and meal preparation. Family cannot provide help with bath or noon meal preparation. Family does most of cooking, all cleaning, laundry, and shopping.	**Optimal functioning in ADL** Needs service agency to provide assistance with bathing, shampoo, and dressing. Needs noon meal preparation. Teach family to give Mrs. Kim opportunities for self-care and help with daily tasks within her capability.
Uses religion as a significant support system, but because of physical and financial limitations has been unable to attend services. States that she is very lonely being at home all day alone.	**Psychological/spiritual needs** Needs a church that is wheelchair accessible and provides transportation. Needs financial support toward handicapped vehicle (discuss with family). Needs friendship, companionship, and mental stimulation during day (assess community resources for visiting companions, social support groups).

SOURCE: Adapted from Friedemann and Scheffer (1990).

offices; local referral centers; chambers of commerce; neighborhood information centers; crisis centers; or hospital social workers or discharge planners, such as home care coordinators. Other printed materials, television, and radio can also be explored. Table 21-4 lists examples of resources available in all areas of the country. The appendix lists selected national and common local agencies that focus on chronic illnesses. It is also a good idea to stay alert to announcements of new agencies at all times and to add them to your file.

Once information on agencies is obtained, it needs to be stored for future reference. For frequently used agencies, memory may suffice in the short term. In some agencies, computers are available to store material for future reference. However, many professionals still use written cards in their resource file. Regardless of the method used, these references should include not only the agency name, address, and phone number but also information about type of agency, funding source, and contact person. In addition, eight areas of assessment need to be explored and noted. These areas are discussed in the next step of the model. The brochure or pamphlet provided by some agencies that describes their services should be filed with the resource material.

Integral to locating resources is establishing professional relationships with other health care

TABLE 21-4.   Examples of local resources
nationwide[1]

- Telephone book, Yellow Pages
  (Explore the categories "Social Service Organiza-
  tions," "Nurses," "Health Maintenance Organiza-
  tions," etc. Also consult the index to the Yellow
  Pages. Letter *I*, for example, lists "Ileostomy Sup-
  plies," "Infant and Toddler Programs," "Information
  Bureaus," and "Invalid Supplies.")
- Chamber of Commerce directories
- Social service directories from the United Fund and
  others
- Advertisements in newspapers
- Television and radio announcements and
  commercials
- Computer databases and information systems

[1]See the Appendix for a listing of selected national agencies that
focus on chronic illnesses.
SOURCE: From Friedemann and Scheffer (1990).

providers. Called *networking,* this is accomplished by contacting key resource individuals
(see Figure 21-2). Networking skills are a most
valuable asset to caregivers. The saying "It's who
you know, not what you know, that counts"
illustrates the importance of personal contacts.
The case study on networking follows Jim Mitchell, a new nurse working with the Visiting
Nurse Association (VNA) to see how he uses
networking.

This case study illustrates the way in which
professional relationships become basic components of networks: New resource persons are
added to the file, and the relationships of old
contacts are reinforced by providing feedback
on a client's progress, acknowledging previous
help, or helping other agency professionals and
their clients in a similar manner.

**Finding Specific Information about Agen-
cies**   Locating resources is only the beginning.
In order to determine if the client's needs and
agency resources are compatible, the caregiver
needs specific information about what services
are provided. The agency's name usually gives a
clue to its function: Vocational Rehabilitation,
Heart Association, Department of Community
Mental Health, and so forth. However, compar-

ing agency services to client needs requires an
eight-area agency assessment (see Table 21-5).
The first three areas should be assessed in the
order indicated; the priority of the others depends on the situation. A brief description of
each assessment area follows.

Eligibility Requirements   Some agencies screen
clients according to medical diagnosis, type of
disability, age (child or adult), and financial status. Eligibility questions *must* be asked first in
order to save time. A client on Medicaid will
not be seen by an agency that does not accept
Medicaid recipients. Such information needs to
be noted for further reference with other clients.

Geographic Location/Accessibility   Physical location affects usefulness of services. Clients may
have transportation problems, be unwilling to
travel long distances, or fear the neighborhood
where the agency is located. Screening agencies
by location saves time and unnecessary work.

Types of Service Provided   Services can generally be categorized as research, education, or
direct care. Most chronic illness problems require the latter. Each need area has corresponding types of agencies (see Table 21-6).
Caregivers have to inquire carefully and in detail
about services. This can be accomplished by
contacting key persons in each agency, former
consumers (clients), or professionals who have
previously worked with the agencies.

Comprehensiveness of Service   The chronically
ill generally need care in more than one area. It
is easier and more efficient for a client and family
to deal with one person or agency to meet three
needs, rather than to deal with three different
agencies. For example, a hospice nurse can meet
the client's personal care and psychosocial needs
and the family's need to deal with grieving. However, comprehensiveness of service does not
mean superiority of services. The caregiver who
is arranging services needs to individually evaluate the quality of each service against comprehensiveness before reaching a decision.

Credentials of the Agency and Its Staff   Credentials imply some level of quality based on standards. The area of credentials is a highly relevant

CASE STUDY
Mr. Mitchell, R.N., B.S.: Networking

March 1993. While attending a workshop on third-party reimbursement of health services and health care reform, Mr. Mitchell neets Mrs. James from the Department of Social Services (DSS), Ms. Kelly from Community Mental Health (CMH), Ms. Stabb from the community hospice program, and Mr. Hadley from the local chapter of the American Diabetes Association. Mr. Mitchell introduces himself to all four agency reprentatives, collects their business cards, and gives them his.

April 1993. Mr. Mitchell receives a new client, Mrs. Jewel, who is a 50-year-old widow. She has diet-controlled diabetes and progressive blindness and lives on a pension and Social Security. She complains of loneliness because she cannot go out of the house. Assessment also indicates that she needs help with meal preparation. The Visiting Nurse Association's resource file contains a resource for meal preparation, Meals on Wheels, whose contact person is Mrs. Hoover. Mr. Mitchell calls her and initiates a referral for Mrs. Jewel. He also remembers the resource people he met at the workshop. He calls Mr. Hadley (Diabetes Association) and reminds him of their meeting the

previous month. Then he goes on to explain Mrs. Jewel's needs. Mr. Hadley recommends that he call three agency contacts: Mr. Jackson at the Guide Dogs for the Blind, Mrs. Hunrich from the Senior Citizen's Visitors Group, and Miss Fuller, who is in charge of "Talking Books" at the library. Figure 21-2 shows the networking system developed by Mr. Mitchell as he goes through the process of linking this client to suitable resources.

May 1993. Another new referral, Mr. Crane, is blind and wants to obtain a guide dog. Mr. Mitchell calls Mr. Jackson (Guide Dogs for the Blind), reminds Mr. Jackson of their last contact, provides updated information on Mrs. Jewel, and explains Mr. Crane's needs. Since Mr. Crane sounds like a good candidate, arrangements are initiated for a direct contact between this client and this agency. The following diagram illustrates the use of Mr. Mitchell's previously developed network for another client.

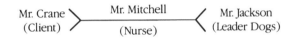

Mr. Crane (Client) — Mr. Mitchell (Nurse) — Mr. Jackson (Leader Dogs)

SOURCE: Adapted from Friedemann and Scheffer (1990).

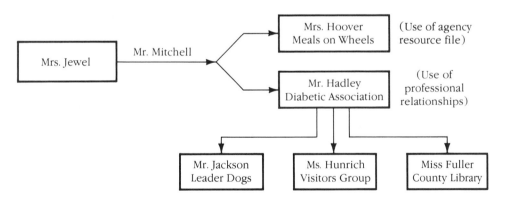

FIGURE 21-2. Mr. Mitchell's Networking

SOURCE: Modified from Friedemann and Scheffer (1990).

issue in home care. Certain terms need to be understood by the caregiver and the client in selecting a quality home care agency (see Table 21-7).

Once the credentials of the agency have been determined, the credentials of the staff need to be considered. Usually, formal educational preparation of professionals is considered

TABLE 21-5. Areas of assessment

- Eligibility requirements
- Geographic location and accessibility
- Types of services required
- Comprehensiveness of service
- Credentials of the agency and its staff
- Philosophy of agency
- Direct cost to the client
- Referral process and contact person

SOURCE: Modified from Friedemann and Scheffer (1990).

a measure of their ability; however, educational credentials do not always represent quality of care. For instance, the alcohol therapist who has only a high school education but was an abuser and now has 15 years of alcohol counseling experience may be more effective than an inexperienced counselor with a master's degree in psychology. Networking and personal contacts greatly enhance decisions about what agencies and which professionals have accomplished the best results for clients.

Philosophy of the Agency A brief assessment of a prospective agency's philosophy, goals for services, and attitude toward clients and families is imperative. Many community agencies are managed by religious, cultural, or philanthropic organizations that may not be compatible with the values and beliefs of the client or the established goals for care.

Direct Costs to the Client Some agencies charge no client fees, being supported by tax revenues or donations. Others accept total or partial payment from third-party payers, such as Medicare, Medicaid, or private insurance. Certain agencies have a sliding fee scale based on the client's ability to pay, and still others, usually privately owned, will charge the client the entire fee for services rendered (Clark, 1984). It is useful to weigh cost carefully against quality of service, even if the client has no financial difficulties and is willing to pay the entire fee.

Referral Process and Contact Person In order to prepare the client, the caregiver needs to in-

quire of the agency what paperwork will be needed and who will be the intake worker. This will be discussed in detail as a major step in progressing through the maze.

Select the Best Match

At this point, the caregiver has assessed the client's needs and identified one or more resources to help solve the client's problem. If only one agency is available, it is obviously the one to contact. But what if there is more than one? What criteria can help the caregiver and the client make the best selection?

Selecting the best agency for the client requires cooperation between caregiver and client. It is very easy for a busy caregiver to assume that professional judgment is enough and therefore

TABLE 21-6. Agencies that meet need categories
(partial listing)

Need	Agency
Clinical care	Hospital
	Medical clinic
	Physician's office
	Nursing home/skilled nursing facility
	Public health department
	Home health agency
Psychological/ spiritual	Counseling agencies
	Alcoholics Anonymous
	Pastoral care services
	Crisis centers and hot lines
	Support groups
	Shelter homes
Rehabilitation	Department of Vocational Rehabilitation
	Association for Retarded Citizens
	Hospital physical therapy/ occupational therapy
	Recreational therapy
Optimal level of ADL	Housing commission
	Meals on Wheels
	Home health care
	Homemakers
	Adult foster home
	Respite care

SOURCE: Modified from Friedemann and Scheffer (1990).

TABLE 21-7.   Terms used for accrediting agencies[1]

Bonded agency	The agency has obtained a bond that acts as an insurance policy. The agency pays a fixed amount of money, similar to a premium for insurance, for the bond. The bond serves simply as a security in case the agency is sued by a client and loses the court case. It does not ensure quality of service.
Certified agency	The agency is eligible to be reimbursed for Medicaid and Medicare service. To qualify, the agency must meet basic federal and state requirements for financial management and standards for patient care. Certification implies some quality.
Accredited agency	Accreditation is granted by special nonprofit groups whose goal is excellence of care. The agency must pass a detailed and careful review of its services, policies, practice, patient records, and management procedures. Accreditation is voluntary and is the best predictor of quality available.

[1]National groups most commonly involved in accrediting for home care: National Homecaring Council, National League for Nursing, American Public Health Association, Joint Commission on the Accreditation of Health Care Organizations.
SOURCE: From Friedemann and Scheffer (1990).

to make decisions *for* instead of *with* the client. This can result in making choices too quickly. The client and family should make the ultimate choice. Participating in the decision says two important things to the client: The decision is his or hers, and the caregiver will help with the referral.

Often caregivers know from experience that one agency gives better care than another. This knowledge should be shared with the client so that, ultimately, a more informed choice can be made. When possible, it is useful to share written agency information, such as what is noted on the resource card, or to give the client a copy of the agency's brochure.

There are effective and ineffective ways of sharing unwritten knowledge about an agency's quality, as shown in the following example:

> INEFFECTIVE: "They are doing a terrible job."
> EFFECTIVE: "I've talked with several people who have used this agency before and were not satisfied. They complained of having to wait a long time and constant staff turnover. This means that you may not see the same person each week."

Information and explanations should be given about all possible agencies and resources. Then the family or client is ready to decide which would work best.

Decision making can sometimes be awkward. When a client is undecided or refuses to make any decision, the caregiver may be asked to assume this responsibility. Depending on the situation, the caregiver might act or refrain from acting on the client's behalf. Care must be taken not to push a client into using a resource on the basis of the caregiver's value system. If the client lacks motivation—for example, by showing reluctance to start needed mental health counseling—decisions should be delayed until feelings of resistance have been worked through so that the client can accept help. It can be difficult for caregivers who want immediate action or solutions to adjust their own pace to that of the client. It is useful to review the treatment goals to be sure they are truly determined by the client.

Initiate the Referral

Assume that the client has selected an appropriate agency and is ready to proceed. This fourth step is achieved by answering four questions: Whom do I contact? How do I contact? What do I ask? What should the client expect?

Whom Do I Contact?   The correct contact person's name can often be learned while collecting information about the agency. But in many situations, the first person the client will see is not the regular contact person but an intake worker who collects preliminary information. It can be helpful if the referring caregiver can share some client data on the telephone to start the referral process.

How Do I Contact? How to make contact may be listed under "referral process" on agency brochures. If the information is not available, a telephone call is needed to find out if the process should be initiated by client or caregiver, if it needs to be done in person, or if it requires that the client be accompanied by the caregiver. When talking to an agency about the needs of a client, the caregiver must respect confidentiality. Either of two measures should be used to assure confidentiality: (1) avoid using the client's name or other identifying characteristics when explaining the client's needs; (2) obtain the client's written permission to communicate personal information.

What Do I Ask? The situation determines what should be asked. The client's eligibility must be confirmed, and the agency's ability to provide the required service and its clear understanding of the client's needs should be determined. It is appropriate to ask when the client can be seen, since time is a prime factor: Is there walk-in service? What is the appointment procedure? Is there a waiting list or waiting period, and if so, how long is it? What is the cancellation policy, if any? If the waiting list is very long, say three to six months, then even a perfect match of client need and agency may be of no help to the client.

What Should the Client Expect? The client should be told that often the purpose of the first visit may be simply to collect information. Preparing the client for the intake process ahead of time decreases frustration for both client and agency. Intake can include forms to fill out, documents that need to be seen regarding medical status or finances, and so forth. The client should be informed as to how long the first interview will probably last and whether or not service will be provided during that first contact.

The first four steps in this model can be carried out by most health professionals without much difficulty. But the next three steps tend to require more sophisticated need–resource linking. These remaining steps will be noted briefly here so that the clinical practitioner or novice community worker has a greater understanding of the process taken by community health nurses and social workers with more experience. The

remaining three steps are assisting the client in using the resource, taking necessary follow-up steps, and evaluating the results.

Assist the Client in Using the Resource

Facilitation is the key work for this step. To help the client make the initial contact successful, the experienced caregiver cannot take any process for granted (see Table 21-8). Any written material the client receives should take into account the client's literacy, language, and visual acuity. If transportation is a stumbling block, and private or public transportation is not readily available, resourcefulness is needed. Acceptable options include local church and volunteer groups and special agencies offering transportation services.

If child or adult care is needed, this can prevent the client or family member from leaving the home. Joint problem solving with the client, done in advance of the actual appointment, will usually lead to a solution. Again, church groups or adult day care organizations may be of assistance. Should cancellation be necessary, knowing how to cancel an appointment enhances the client's acceptability to the agency, since it shows a degree of responsibility. Some clients do not operate under such a value system and do not realize the negative impression they may leave if they fail to cancel. Educating the client

---

TABLE 21-8. Checklist for smooth referrals

1. Does the client have in writing:
    Name and address of the agency?
    Name of the person to contact?
    Date and time of the appointment?
    Directions to get to the agency?

2. Does the client have transportation?

3. Does the client have child or adult care, if needed?

4. Does the client know how and whom to contact if the appointment must be canceled?

5. Can the client effectively explain his or her needs?

6. Does the client fully understand why the referral is being made?

7. Is the client comfortable in making this contact?

SOURCE: Modified from Friedemann and Scheffer (1990).

to agency expectations is an important caregiver task.

When a client is insecure or unable to explain his or her needs, providing an opportunity for role playing can be helpful. If role playing reflects a deficiency in the client's communication skills, roles can be reversed. This allows the caregiver to model skills that enhance communication. Then, by again reversing roles, the client can try out the approach presented by the caregiver. Basic principles in learning as well as experience support the value of this technique. The client may also feel insecure about initiating contact with the agency, which can usually be handled, in advance, by encouraging verbalization of fears followed by problem solving, such as identifying what is needed to increase comfort level. It can sometimes be as simple as bringing a book to read while waiting or asking a friend or relative to come along on the intake visit.

Follow up on the Referral

This step is based on the principle of continuity of care. Even if all the preceding steps have been executed properly, something can still go wrong. Talking to the client shortly after the first contact with the new agency allows the caregiver to ask if the appointment was kept, what happened during the visit, if the visit was satisfactory, and what the client wants to do next. If the appointment was missed, the reasons need to be explored and solutions suggested before another appointment is made. If the client did not understand what happened during the first visit, it needs to be clarified. For example, a rheumatoid arthritis patient may be unclear as to why blood samples are necessary before receiving colloidal gold injections. Knowing the importance of baseline blood values and the need for regular evaluation to ensure that gold is not causing harmful side effects can lead to continued cooperation.

Satisfaction with the outcome of the visit can vary for a number of reasons. Dissatisfaction can be the result of overly high expectations or of the agency's not meeting the client's needs. What the client wants to do next will depend on his or her degree of satisfaction. In reality, few agency services are perfect matches for all needs. Those services that prove ineffective should be terminated quickly. Good and fair services, however, require evaluation of how well clients believe their needs were met.

If use of this resource is to be continued, the caregiver continues the role of liaison by enhancing communication between client and agency staff in order to develop a trusting relationship between them. As trust grows, the need for a liaison decreases and eventually disappears. Closure is frequently accompanied by a final statement of support such as "Here are my name and phone number. Call me if you need help in the future."

Evaluate the Results

With a written plan and mutually acceptable objectives, much of the evaluation can be accomplished throughout the referral and follow-up process. A final evaluation allows for systematic examination of each step of the process and the corresponding outcomes. For unsuccessful referrals, evaluation enables the caregiver to determine what caused the negative outcome. It is important to determine whether client needs were accurately identified, whether the agency screened effectively, and whether an optimal match between client and agency was achieved.

Client participation should be evaluated also: Did the client receive the necessary assistance in making contact with the agency? Did the client feel respected and comfortable? Was follow-up and follow-through complete? Negative feedback in any portion of the evaluation supports client and caregiver in mutually exploring problems and working together to avoid subsequent difficulties.

Any evaluative feedback should be documented on the resource care for future reference. Sharing this information with other professionals (while protecting client confidentiality) can save time and expedite referrals for others. The case study on how Paul S. dealt with the agency maze illustrates the entire process of traveling through the agency maze when more than one person is involved in the need–resource linking process. In this case, the office nurse assumed primary responsibility for following the process through to completion, including evaluation of the extent to which the plan was followed and needs were met.

CASE STUDY
Paul S.: Dealing with the Agency Maze

Paul S., a 50-year-old, was married with three grown children when his wife, Edna, had a radical mastectomy for breast cancer. Now, a year later, Edna has begun chemotherapy because of metastasis.

As a result of stress, Paul sleeps poorly and has become irritable at work. His secretary, Mary, knows Edna's health problems have been emotionally upsetting to Paul. Although Mary had no experience in using community resources, she gained her employer's permission to seek professional assistance for him and then called their family physician's office and described the problem to Ms. Reis, the office nurse and case manager.

Identify Client Needs. Ms. Reis collected the following information about Paul S.:

- He has been sleeping only 3 to 4 hours a night during the past two weeks
- He is short tempered and irritable with his subordinates at work
- He is confused about his wife's condition and how to help her
- He fears his wife's imminent death
- He is receptive to professional help
- He has insurance covering professional mental health counseling and also can afford to pay for counseling services

Ms. Reis realized that Paul's psychological/spiritual needs were approaching a crisis situation requiring rapid intervention. She therefore prioritized stated needs and developed objectives for each of them.

Search for Resources. In addition to known agencies that might be helpful, Ms. Reis checked the office resource file and found a new agency—Counseling for Coping. The brochure describing their services indicated that the agency might be appropriate to meet Paul's needs. Even though she had never used this agency, she knew that new agencies frequently had shorter waiting time.

Select the Best Match. Over the telephone, Ms. Reis shared information about all the identified resources with Mary and discussed which would

best meet Paul's needs. The new resource, a partnership of independent nurse practitioners, seemed most appropriate. Although the agency did not allow third-party reimbursement, it was chosen because it offered the type of service that Paul needed and could see him soon. Ms. Reis suggested that Mary share this information with the Mr. S's family. She provided photocopies of the file cards on all the resources and made a note to herself to call within a couple of days to follow up on the situation.

Initiate the Referral. Mary shared the information with Paul and Edna. Mary called Counseling for Coping and talked directly to Mrs. Davis who not only described the agency services in detail but indicated that she was also the intake worker. An intake interview and problem assessment appointment was made for the next day. Mary obtained directions to the agency and instructions for parking.

Assist the Client in Using the Resource. Mary gave Paul the agency's name, address, and phone number, Mrs. Davis's name, and information on the intake procedure and agency services. Paul kept the appointment and had no problems with expressing his needs; he seemed comfortable seeking help.

Follow up on the Referral. Ms. Reis called Mary the next morning to ask if the agency had been contacted and if Paul had been seen. Mary gave her a progress report.

Evaluate the Results. One week later, Ms. Reis called Mr. S.'s family and found out that Paul was feeling better, was sleeping better, and consequently was more rested. Three weeks later, during an office visit, Ms. Reis took the opportunity to talk to Paul about the service he obtained at Counseling for Coping. He reported that he was very well satisfied with the way they had helped him express his concerns and had helped him understand what to expect in the future. A summary of Paul's comments were recorded on Ms. Reis's office file card, and the information was shared with other nursing and medical personnel.

Summary and Conclusions

There are multiple health care issues affecting resources and care for the chronically ill. Not only has the health care delivery system undergone major change over the past two decades, but longer life expectancies and advanced health care technology have resulted in drastic increases in the incidence of chronic illnesses. While political support for access to health care was on the rise in the 1960s and 1970s, it has since decreased largely because of cost-containment efforts. Funding for programs and services addressing the needs of the chronically ill has diminished as a result of federal budget cuts. Efforts in the 1990s refocused attention on access to comprehensive health care services as a right of citizenship; however, the extent to which the multiple service needs of community-based chronically ill clients will be addressed within health care reform proposals remains unclear.

The needs of the chronically ill were described, and many of the community resources required to meet these needs were noted. Resources and agencies can be public or private, official or voluntary, and these classifications provide information as to the type of service offered and the source of funding.

Rapid changes in the health care delivery system have resulted in several positive effects on client and professionals alike. Increased awareness of the needs of the chronically ill has encouraged better educational preparation of caregivers and has increased coordination of health services. New delivery systems have been developed, such as HMOs and combined service agencies, providing both support and basic services. As a result, clients have more choices with respect to kinds of services. This enhances both the quality of life and the client's autonomy.

Unfortunately, there are also negative effects. Unresolved issues include fragmentation and duplication of services, lack of communication among agencies, and political changes that have resulted in the closure of some agencies and the infringement of competition and profit making on quality of service. Any of these can result in the client's not receiving the necessary service and feeling overwhelmed by the system. The professional can also be overwhelmed, frustrated, and confused by the system.

To assist the caregiver in restoring a sense of control, a model for dealing with the agency maze was presented. This seven-step model can be used with the chronically ill and generalized to other populations that need community resources.

In the future, ongoing research in chronic illness will help document and validate the health care and service needs of these clients. Advocacy organizations will increase public awareness and provide political pressure to ensure recognition of the needs of special groups such as the elderly. The referral process will also continue to change. As more agencies like On Lok and ACCESS develop, health care for the chronically ill will become more coordinated and comprehensive.

In addition, computer technology will make information collection and resource retrieval a much more manageable task. Computerized locating services are becoming available locally, regionally, nationally, and internationally. However, no matter how sophisticated computer searching or system reorganization becomes, the chronically ill and their families will still require the assistance of skilled professionals. Understanding the model presented in this chapter and gaining experience in using it will be a valuable asset for the caregiver in any setting.

STUDY QUESTIONS

1. Explain how demographic changes within the population are related to chronic illness.
2. Give three examples of needs a chronically ill person may have in each category:
   - Clinical care
   - Psychological/spiritual
   - Rehabilitation
   - Optimal functioning (ADLs)

Use as examples the following individuals:
   - A young child with epilepsy
   - A woman with leukemia
   - An elderly man with leg ulcers
3. Discuss how fragmentation, poor agency communication, costs of services, and politics can affect one of the individuals listed above.

4. Explore your own community to identify agencies that can serve one of the above clients to meet his or her clinical needs, psychological/ spiritual needs, rehabilitation needs, or ADL needs.

References

American Nurses' Association (1988). *Nursing case management.* Kansas City, MO: American Nurses' Association.

Anthony, W., & Lieberman, P. (1986). The practices of psychiatric rehabilitation. *Schizophrenia Bulletin, 12,* 542.

Berkowitz, G., Halfon, N., & Klee, L. (1992). Improving access to health care: Case management for vulnerable children. *Social Work in Health Care, 17,* 101.

Calahan, D. (1992). Reforming the health care system for children and the elderly to balance cure and care. *Academic Medicine, 67,* 219.

Caton, C. (1981). The new chronic patient and the system of community care. *Hospital and Community Psychiatry, 32,* 475.

Centers for Disease Control and Prevention (1993). *Health Data on Older Americans: United States, 1992,* Publication No. PHS 93-1141. Hyattsville, MD: U.S. Department of Health and Human Services.

Clark, M. D. (1984). *Community nursing: Health care for today and tomorrow.* Reston, VA: Reston.

Clinton, W. J., and Gore, A. (1992). *Putting people first: How we can all change america.* New York: Times Books.

Department of Health and Human Services (DHHS) (1993). *Health care financing review: Medicare and Medicaid statistical supplement.* Baltimore: Health Care Financing Administration.

Dimond, M. (1991). Health care and the aging population. In B. Spradley (Ed.), *Readings in community health nursing.* Philadelphia: J. B. Lippincott.

Eggert, G., Bowlyow, J., & Nichole, C. (1980). Gaining control of the long term care system: First returns from the ACCESS Project. *The Gerontologist, 20,* 356.

Fee, E., & Fox, D. (1992). *AIDS: The making of a chronic disease.* Berkeley, CA: University of California Press.

Friedemann, M. L., & Scheffer, B. (1990). The agency maze. In I. Lubkin (Ed.), *Chronic Illness: Impact and intervention* (2nd ed.) Boston: Jones and Bartlett.

General Accounting Office (GAO) (1990). *Home visiting: A promising early intervention strategy for at-risk families,* Publication No. GAO/HRD 90-83. Washington, D.C.: U.S. General Accounting Office.

Gore, A. (1993). *The Gore report on reinventing government.* New York: Times Books.

Haddad, A., & Kapp, M. (1991). *Ethical and legal issues in home health care.* Norwalk, CT: Appleton & Lange.

Jacobs, P. (1991). *The economics of health and medical care.* Gaitherburg, MD: Aspen Publishing.

Knollmueller, R. (1988). Case management: What's in a name? *Nursing Management, 20,* 38.

Lewis, I. (1983). Evolution of federal policy on access of health care: 1965-1980. *Bulletin of the New York Academy of Medicine, 59,* 9.

Maraldo, P. (1990). The nineties: A decade in search of meaning. *Nursing and Health Care, 11,* 11-14.

Moon, M. (1987). The elderly's access to health care services: The crude and subtle impacts of Medicare changes. *Social Justice Research, 1,* 361.

Office of Technology Assessment (OTA) (1990). *Health care in rural America,* Publication No. OTA-H-434. Washington, D.C.: U.S. Congress, Office of Technology Assessment.

Palmer, H., & Vogel, R. (1985). *Long term care: Perspectives from research and demonstrations.* Rockville, MD: Aspen.

Preston, K. (1992). Access to home health care: Negotiating with the gatekeepers. *Journal of the Home Health Care Practitioner, 4,* 61.

Rucklin, H. S., Norris, J. N., & Eggert, G. M. (1982). Management and financing of long-term care services: A new approach to a chronic problem. *New England Journal of Medicine, 306*(2), 101-105.

Smith, W. (1987). *Cancer.* New York: Facts on File Publishers.

Stanhope, M., & Lancaster, J. (1992). *Community health nursing: Process and practice for promoting health.* St. Louis: Mosby-Year Book.

Stroul, B. (1989). Introduction to the special issue: The community support systems concept. *Psychosocial Rehabilitation, 12,* 5.

Wasik, B., Bryant, D., & Lyons, C. (1990). *Home visiting.* London: Sage Publications.

Werley, N., Drago, L., & Hadley, T. (1990). Improving the physical health–mental health interface for the chronically mentally ill: Could nurse case managers make a difference? *Archives of Psychiatric Nursing, 4,* 108.

CHAPTER 22

Financial Impact

Timothy Philipp

Introduction

For nearly thirty years, the rise in health care costs has been a growing crisis in this country. Concerns over increasing costs first gained national prominence shortly after the introduction of Medicare and Medicaid in 1966. These government health programs alleviated recognized barriers to access by using public funds to subsidize the health care needs of the elderly and the poor.

Numerous factors have contributed to the rising costs of health care, including changing demographics, increasing personal income, and malpractice and defensive medicine costs. In addition, many causes gain recognition and popularity during political contests or as a result of activism over health problems such as AIDS. Most economists believe that these factors are not as significantly related to the sharp cost increases of the past 30 years as are the new and expensive technologies interacting with increased third-party payments (Congressional Budget Office, 1992a; Feldstein, 1993). However, current trends point to the increasing importance of demographic changes as our baby boomers begin to reach retirement age in the year 2010 and our old and very old populations grow in numbers (*Aging America,*

1991; American Association of Retired Persons, 1992).

Historically, Americans have come to expect a great deal. We have built an acute care system that offers the finest and the newest in technology. Yet our criticisms of this system arise from a growing dissatisfaction over navigating more complex and disjointed services, limited access, and rising costs that limit access (American Hospital Association, 1992; Folland, Goodman, & Stano, 1993). It is the *unaffordability* of health care that has entrenched us in a two-tier system of delivery based on ability to pay. Wealth and health insurance provide access and financial protection to many. However, many other Americans have inadequate or no health insurance to deal with the financial burden of illness. In fact, the number of underinsured and uninsured is expected to grow. This is proving unacceptable, since increasingly the public has communicated to its political leaders that medical care is a right, not simply a privilege.

Gauging Health Care Costs

Several economic or financial measures are commonly used to gauge health care expenses. These measures include total costs, a percent of the

Gross Domestic Product (GDP),[1] and per capita costs. The continued upward trend in these measures is important to politicians and policymakers in identifying the current crisis in health care.

Total Costs   The Congressional Budget Office (CBO) reports that over the last three decades, total health care costs, adjusted for general inflation, have increased sixfold, from $121 billion to $751 billion. These costs have risen at least twice as rapidly as those of general goods and services in everyday use (CBO, 1993).

Gross Domestic Product   The GDP reflects our country's overall economic output or capacity. Comparing total health care costs to the GDP shows what portion of our domestic economy is ascribed to the production of health care. Over the past three decades, costs of health care have steadily increased as a percent of GDP (see Figure 22–1). Expenditures in 1991 accounted for more than 13 percent of the GDP, up a full percent from 1990 and four times greater than the "growth rate" in the general economy for the same period (Letsch, 1993).

Per Capita   Per capita expenditures reflect average health care costs per person. This measure is particularly useful for group comparisons based on socioeconomic and geographic differences, although such data are based on averages and can be misleading. Since 1960, per capita expenditures, adjusted for general inflation, have increased fivefold (CBO, 1993).

Like the GDP, per capita costs in the United States have risen faster than in other industrial nations and are projected to continue to do so (CBO, 1992a). The elderly are often singled out for examination because they are more likely to suffer from chronic illnesses that have higher health care utilization rates. Based on the 1987 National Health Expenditures Survey (NHES), persons 65 and older spent more than four times the per capita than their younger counterparts, with Medicare funds accounting for 44 percent of their total per capita spending (*Aging America,* 1991; American Association of Retired Persons (AARP), 1992).

The most current aggregate data available come from 1991. That year health care expenditures totaled $751.8 billion, with most of the costs associated with hospitalization, physicians, drugs, and nondurable medical good and services.

Problems and Issues of Rising Health Care Costs

Despite several decades of cost-containment efforts, the amount spent on health care continues to outpace general inflation.[2] Politicians, policymakers, and academicians point to these rising costs as a growing crisis because health care is becoming increasing unaffordable, these costs are consuming larger and larger portions of the federal budget, and they will continue to contribute significantly to the federal deficit in the late 1990s.

To more fully explain the pattern and trends in health care expenditures and how, in part, the crisis has come to be identified, three areas will be addressed: how health care is paid for, where this money goes, and the amount of money spent.

---

[1]Historically, the Gross National Product (GNP) was the accepted basis for cost comparisons. The GNP represented the value of *all* final goods and services produced. However, because of the changes in the world economy, the GDP has become the accepted measure for comparison, since it reflects only domestic output and not sources from abroad.

[2]This section is based on information released in 1993 from 1991 data, the most current year aggregate data available. Includes notes from classical 1987 NHES data. Additional data can be obtained by writing to (a) Congressional Budget Office, 2nd & D Streets, S.W., Washington, D.C. 20515; (b) Agency for Health Care Policy and Research, Department of Health and Human Services, Executive Office Center, 2101 E. Jefferson Street, Rockville, MD 20852; (c) Health Care Financing Administration, 200 Independence Avenue, S.W., Washington, D.C. 20201; (d) Prospective Payment Commission, 300 7th Street, S.W., Suite 301B, Washington, D.C. 20024.

Percent

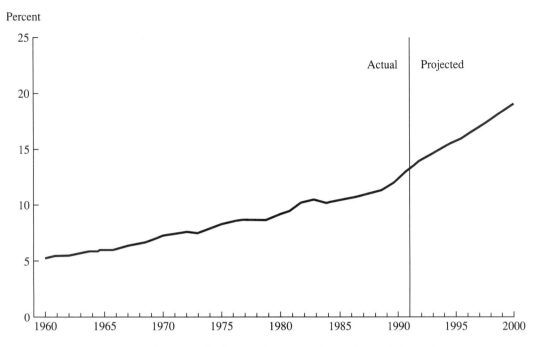

FIGURE 22-1.   National Health Expenditures as a Percentage of Gross Domestic
Product,[1] 1960-2000

[1]GDP is equal to gross national product minus net property income from abroad. Using GDP for international comparisons of spending for health eliminates variations that arise from differences in the rate of foreign transactions in different economies.

SOURCE: Congressional Budget Office (CBO) calculations are based on data from the Health Care Financing Administration, Office of the Actuary, 1992, and CBO baseline data for gross domestic product (GDP), January 1993.

Paying for Health Care

There are three primary sources of payment: public sources, private insurance, and direct or out-of-pocket expenditures by consumers (See Figure 22-2 and Tables 22-1 and 22-2).

Public Sources Since the introduction of Medicare and Medicaid in the mid 1960s, the federal government has become the single largest payor for health care. Federal disbursements have increased from 9 percent in 1960 to 31 percent of the total personal health expenditures in the country.[3] Combined with state and local governments, all governments account for 44 percent of total personal health care spending (Letsch, 1993).

Currently, health care consumes more than 14 percent of the Federal budget. However, it is estimated that health spending will increase to nearly 24 percent of the total federal budget by 1998 (CBO, 1993). This continued rise has led to government attempts to limit further growth in costs.

Congress attempts to hold down health care costs by avoiding the expansion of benefits and

[3]Personal health care expenditures account for 88 percent of total health care spending and reflect the costs of individual care. Other costs for research, construction, program administration, and public health activities make up the balance of total costs. The proportion of these costs has remained constant over the past three decades.

TABLE 22-1. National health expenditures, by source of funds, billions of dollars, selected calendar years 1960–1991

Source of Funds	1960	1970	1980	1985	1988	1989	1990	1991
NATIONAL HEALTH EXPENDITURES	$27.1	$74.4	$250.1	$422.6	$546.1	$604.3	$675.0	$751.8
Private funds	20.5	46.7	145.0	248.0	319.0	351.0	390.0	421.8
Consumer payments	19.2	42.3	132.9	228.6	293.8	323.3	358.7	388.6
Out-of-pocket payments	13.4	25.6	59.5	94.4	118.5	126.2	136.5	144.3
Private health insurance	5.9	16.7	73.4	134.2	175.3	197.1	222.2	244.4
Other private funds	1.3	4.4	12.1	19.4	25.2	27.7	31.3	33.2
Public funds	6.7	27.7	105.2	174.6	227.1	253.3	285.1	330.0
Federal funds	2.9	17.7	72.0	123.5	156.6	175.0	194.5	222.9
Medicare	–	7.6	37.5	72.0	90.5	102.6	110.7	122.8
Medicaid	–	2.9	14.5	23.1	31.0	35.4	42.8	55.9
Other federal	2.9	7.3	19.9	28.3	35.2	36.9	41.0	44.2
State and local funds	3.7	9.9	33.2	51.2	70.5	78.3	90.5	107.1
Medicaid	–	2.5	11.6	18.6	23.9	26.8	32.7	44.6
Other state and local	3.7	7.5	21.6	32.6	46.6	51.5	57.9	62.4
Total Medicaid	–	5.3	26.1	41.8	54.9	62.2	75.5	100.5

Growth (average annual percent change from previous period shown)

Source of Funds	1960	1970	1980	1985	1988	1989	1990	1991
NATIONAL HEALTH EXPENDITURES	–	10.6%	12.9%	11.1%	8.9%	10.7%	11.7%	11.4%
Private funds	–	8.6	12.0	11.3	8.8	10.0	11.1	8.2
Consumer payments	–	8.2	12.1	11.5	8.7	10.0	10.9	8.4
Out-of-pocket payments	–	6.7	8.8	9.7	7.9	6.5	8.2	5.7
Private health insurance	–	11.0	15.9	12.8	9.3	12.4	12.7	10.0
Other private funds	–	13.3	10.7	10.0	9.0	10.2	12.9	6.0
Public funds	–	15.3	14.3	10.7	9.2	11.5	12.5	15.7
Federal funds	–	19.8	15.0	11.4	8.3	11.7	11.1	14.6
Medicare	–	–	17.3	13.9	7.9	13.4	7.9	10.9
Medicaid	–	–	17.6	9.8	10.2	14.4	20.8	30.6
Other federal	–	9.6	10.6	7.3	7.5	5.0	11.0	7.8
State and local funds	–	10.2	12.8	9.0	11.3	11.1	15.6	18.3
Medicaid	–	–	16.8	9.8	8.7	12.2	21.9	36.6
Other state and local	–	7.1	11.2	8.6	12.7	10.6	12.3	7.9
Total Medicaid	–	–	17.3	9.8	9.5	13.4	21.3	33.2

SOURCE: From the Health Care Financing Administration, Office of the Actuary (1992).

beneficiaries to existing programs and by limiting new programs. History has demonstrated that some expansions are very costly, such as the addition of both end stage renal disease (ESRD) and disabled patients to Medicare, since they incur higher costs than do other Medicare recipients (CBO, 1993; Iglehart, 1993). The more recent debate in Congress over coverage for catastrophic illness, prescription drugs, and long-term care illustrates Congress's apprehension over adding new benefits or programs because of their associated costs. Ultimately, the Catastrophic Health Protection Act, which represented the largest expansion in Medicare since its inception, was repealed as a consequence of serious voter discontent over who should pay (Philipp & Biordi, 1990).

Yet another important and more visible means Congress has used in attempting to limit the growth of health care spending is budget

Percent

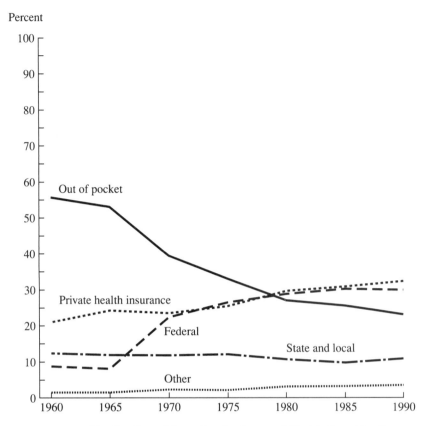

FIGURE 22-2. Distribution of Spending for Personal Health Care,[1] by Source of Payment, 1960–1990

[1]Personal health care expenditures are equal to national health expenditures minus spending for public health, research, construction, and administrative costs.

[2]The "Other" category includes philanthropy and industrial in-plant spending for health.

[3]Data are plotted at five-year intervals.

SOURCE: Congressional Budget Office calculations are based on data from the Health Care Financing Administration, Office of the Actuary, 1992.

control and changes in benefits and financing mechanisms. Most notable is Medicare's Prospective Payment System (PPS) based on Diagnostic Related Groups (DRGs). Implemented a decade ago, the PPS shifted the financial risks of treating Medicare inpatients to hospital providers by moving away from a cost-based reimbursement practice to a predetermined payment—that is, a capitated, per-case payment based on the patient's diagnosis. As a result, the annual rate of

increase in hospital costs for the elderly has declined and is now less than the rate of increase for their younger counterparts (CBO, 1993).

Medicaid Unlike Medicare, Medicaid programs are designed and operated by individual states, with the financing shared by both the state and federal governments. Medicaid represents only one-third of federal health spending, yet increases in Medicaid expenditures account for

TABLE 22-2.   National health expenditures, by source of funds and type of expenditure, billions of dollars, calendar year 1991

| Type of Expenditure | Total | Private | | | | | Government | | |
		All Private	Consumer Total	Out of Pocket	Private Insurance	Other[1]	Total	Federal	State/Local
NATIONAL HEALTH EXPENDITURES	$751.8	$421.8	$388.6	$144.3	$244.4	$33.2	$330.0	$222.9	$107.1
Health services and supplies	728.6	412.7	388.6	144.3	244.4	24.1	315.9	212.0	103.9
Personal health care	660.2	377.0	353.5	144.3	209.3	23.4	283.3	204.1	79.1
Hospital care	288.6	126.0	111.4	9.9	101.5	14.7	162.6	119.1	43.5
Physician services	142.0	92.5	92.5	25.7	66.8	0.1	49.4	39.0	10.4
Dental services	37.1	36.0	36.0	19.9	16.1	–	1.1	0.6	0.5
Other professional services	35.8	27.5	23.0	9.7	13.3	4.4	8.4	6.4	2.0
Home health care	9.8	2.7	2.0	1.2	0.7	0.7	7.1	5.7	1.3
Drugs and other medical nondurables	60.7	53.3	53.3	44.3	9.0	–	7.3	3.6	3.7
Vision products and other medical durables	12.4	8.8	8.8	7.7	1.2	–	3.5	3.1	0.4
Nursing home care	59.9	27.6	26.5	25.8	0.6	1.1	32.3	19.5	12.8
Other personal health care	14.0	2.4	–	–	–	2.4	11.6	7.0	4.6
Program administration and net cost of private health insurance	43.9	35.7	35.1	–	35.1	0.6	8.1	5.2	3.0
Government public health activities	24.5	–	–	–	–	–	24.5	2.7	21.8
Research and construction	23.1	9.1	–	–	–	9.1	14.0	10.9	3.2
Research[2]	12.6	0.9	–	–	–	0.9	11.7	10.2	1.5
Construction	10.6	8.2	–	–	–	8.2	2.4	0.7	1.6

[1]Includes funding through philanthropy and other nonpatient revenues, business spending for industrial in-plant health services, and privately financed construction.

[2]Research and development expenditures of drug companies and other manufacturers and providers of medical equipment and supplies are excluded from "research" expenditures but are included in the expenditure class in which the product falls.

SOURCE: From the Health Care Financing Administration, Office of the Actuary (1992).

much of the recent increases in total federal health spending. Because of differences among states for income eligibility, Medicaid provides medical services to only about one-half of the nation's poor, approximately 6 percent of the total population (CBO, 1992a).[4] Although origi-

[4]Medicaid eligibility is largely determined by income and includes the following categories: persons receiving Aid to Families with Dependent Children (AFDC) or Supplemental Security Income (SSI), persons qualifying for cash assistance programs, and medically needy individuals after their income has been spent down.

nally designed to provide comprehensive health coverage at no personal expense to the categorically needy, a growing and significant portion of the Medicaid budget goes to pay for long-term nursing home services.

Medicare Medicare and the *elderly* are nearly synonymous terms, since Medicare covers the majority of individuals over age 65, although, as mentioned, individuals with ESRD and the disabled are also covered (*The Medicare Handbook*, 1993). Growth in the elderly segment of the population and the disparity between its per capita costs and that of the general population show that aging is directly associated with the rise in health care expenditures. In 1900, only 4 percent of the population was 65 years of age or older, but it is projected that this cohort will reach 22 percent of the total population by the year 2030 (*Aging America,* 1991).

Medicare accounts for more than half of federal health care spending (Letsch, 1993). Interestingly, the Medicare program is highly efficient, with 98 percent of all expenditures going for benefits. This efficiency is one of the major arguments for single-payer health insurance.

Private Health Insurance Business is the major supplier of health insurance. About three-fourths of the population under age 65 has some form of private health insurance, mostly employment-based. Unfortunately, having insurance isolates the consumer from the true cost of health care. In fact, the widespread availability of insurance is linked to the increased use of health care services and therefore to increased total costs. Covered individuals generally have higher incomes, are highly skilled, have stable jobs, work for larger companies, and are older in age. Those likely not to have insurance have the opposite characteristics. Since employers pay a large fraction of the insurance premiums (usually 75 to 80 percent), having insurance often leads to quiet tradeoffs for employees: lower wages, less generous nonmedical benefits, and fewer job opportunities (CBO, 1992a).

Generally, employees share insurance costs through payment of the smaller share of premium costs (around 20 to 25 percent) as well as through deductibles and copayments. Deductibles represent a fixed dollar amount that needs to be paid before the insurance picks up all or part of additional cost. They can lower insurance administration costs and premium costs and, perhaps most important, provide incentives for the consumer to price-shop. However, when they are too high (relative to one's income), they act as a deterrent to seeking care. Coinsurance, or copayments, represents the portion paid by the consumer after the insurance company has paid. Typically, insurance companies pay 80 percent of what are referred to as reasonable charges,

leaving the consumer responsible for the remaining 20 percent. Coinsurance allows the consumer to share the financial burden and may provide some incentive to be a prudent consumer.

Private health insurance accounts for 32 percent of the total money spent on personal health costs. Insurance companies can have very high program costs, that is, if one compares their revenue from premiums to total benefits paid. Program costs plus the costs associated with the vast amount of paperwork involved are important concerns for future health care reform and cost control.

To further reduce the financial risk associated with health care, many elderly Americans carry supplemental private health insurance in addition to their Medicare coverage. Often referred to as Medigap policies, these plans are individually purchased or part of employee-sponsored retiree plans. Medigap plans typically cover the deductibles and copayments of Medicare services plus some uncovered services, particularly prescription drug costs (Chulis et al., 1993). Medigap coverage is considered important by many elderly because they spend over twice as much as their younger counterparts do on insurance, prescription drugs, and medical supplies, with health insurance being their major expense (*Aging America,* 1991). (See Table 22-3.)

Out-of-Pocket Expenses Out-of-pocket dollars represent the amount of money individuals directly pay in deductibles and copayments for hospitals and nursing homes, for dental and medical care and other professional services, and for vision care, drugs, and other nonmedical durables. Interestingly, for care with high financial risks such as hospitalization, out-of-pocket costs are relatively small; for items with low financial risk such as drugs and medical nondurables, out-of-pocket costs are high (CBO, 1993; Letsch, 1993). For the elderly and chronically ill who use many drugs, these expenses can seem exorbitant. One notable exception to the ratio of cost and out-of-pocket expenses is long-term care, where private insurance has little impact and the costs are nearly evenly split between state

TABLE 22-3. Health care expenditures of consumer units, by type of expenditure and age of reference person, 1989

Type of Expenditure	Age of Reference Person			
	Under 65	65+	65-74	75+
Number of units (thousands)	75,496	20,322	11,848	8,474
	Amount of Expenditures			
Health care, total	$1,211	$2,135	$1,981	$2,351
Health insurance	428	943	939	950
Medical services	518	632	555	738
Drugs and supplies	264	560	487	662
Drugs	189	428	402	465
Medical supplies	75	132	85	197
	Percent Distribution			
Health care, total	100.0	100.0	100.0	100.0
Health insurance	35.3	44.2	47.4	40.4
Medical services	42.8	29.6	28.0	31.4
Drugs and supplies	21.8	26.2	24.6	28.2
Drugs	15.6	20.1	20.3	19.8
Medical supplies	6.2	6.2	4.3	8.4

SOURCE: From U.S. Department of Labor, Bureau of Labor Statistics (1990, November 20). Also, unpublished data from the 1989 Consumer Expenditure Survey.

Medicaid programs and individuals who pay out of pocket.

With the rise in government and private insurance outlays to nearly 82 percent of total health care costs in 1991, out-of-pocket expenses for personal health expenditures have decreased markedly over time, further isolating individuals from the true cost of health care. Unlike other purchases in our lives, such as cars, housing, and entertainment, health care consumers in general are so isolated from the true costs involved that they do not consider the real financial outlay of major medical care. This trend dampens the effects of a competitive marketplace for health care (CBO, 1992a).

Most people spend out-of-pocket health care dollars only on over-the-counter and insurance costs (including premiums, deductibles, and co-insurance). Despite this decline, out-of-pocket expenses as a proportion of income have re-mained relatively constant (4.6 percent) for Americans in households not headed by an elderly person. For households headed by an elderly person, these costs are a considerably higher percent (11 percent) of income (CBO, 1993). Ultimately, all health care expenses come out of the consumer's pocket in the form of direct payments, higher premiums and taxes, or lower wages or fewer nonmedical benefits.

Health Care Spending

Health care and the national economy are critically linked. Yet the increasing cost of health care negatively affects businesses and the economy in general. If the economy grows faster than health care costs, the nation is able to support these increasing expenses. But if the economy shows weak growth, the reverse is true (Ginzberg, 1990). Unfortunately, rising health care expenditures have generally outpaced the increase in general inflation. Currently, as determined by the GDP for 1991, health care expenditures are outstripping our economic output at a 4 to 1 rate (Letsch, 1993).

Since 1961, overall health care expenditures, adjusted for general inflation, have increased sixfold, although the amount of increase varies for different services. For example, from 1961 to 1991, hospital costs rose sevenfold, physician costs sixfold, and drugs and other medical nondurable products and services threefold (CBO, 1993). More recently, the costs for nursing homes and home health care have been increasing at a faster rate than has the rise in other major health categories (Letsch, 1993).

Statistics demonstrate that as our population ages we will witness a proportional increase in health care spending, since chronic illness increases with age, and the chronically ill are the largest users of health care dollars (*Aging America*, 1991; Mendelson & Schwartz, 1993).

The question of how to determine an appropriate level for health care costs in terms of the GDP is often asked, but remains without a definitive answer. In 1990, the United States spent nearly twice as much of its GDP on health care than was spent in the United Kingdom or Japan, and 1.5 times as much as was spent in Germany and Canada (CBO, 1993). Given that current existing programs do not change, these costs are expected to rise to 32 percent of the GDP by year 2030 (Burner, Waldo, & McKusick, 1992). These trends are alarming and should serve as an important impetus for political action for health care financing reforms.

The outlay of money can also be viewed from a per capita basis. Since per capita data reflect the average expenses for health care, one needs to ask if everyone spends that amount. Berk and Monheit (1992) show that the distribution of spending is heavily skewed. In 1987, the top 1 percent of persons with health expenditures accounted for 30 percent of total health expenditures, and the top 5 percent of such persons accounted for over half of the total expenditures. Wicker (1991) reported similar concentrations of expenditures while examining Ohio Blue Cross/Blue Shield 1989 insurance

claims. Berk and Monheit (1992) show further that top spenders are disproportionately elderly or black Americans, since nearly half of the top spenders were elderly and 16 percent were blacks. In contrast, the 50 percent of Americans spending the fewest dollars accounted for only 3 percent of the total health expenditures. The concentration of spending will have important implications for policymakers attempting to control rising health care costs.

Where Health Care Money Goes

It is estimated that chronically ill persons consume 80 percent of health care resources (Evans, 1983) and that currently 80 percent of all illnesses arise from chronic conditions (Henry, 1991). Persons with either a disability or disabling conditions report higher health care costs—as much as five times that of persons with no limiting conditions (Rice & LaPlante, 1992). In fact, the longer a person lives, the more susceptible that person becomes to functionally limiting chronic conditions and thus to greater utilization of health care services (*Aging America*, 1991). Further, the current focus on rising costs and health care reform has brought a renewed focus on the fact that health care expenses are extremely high for persons in the last year of life (CBO, 1992a; Lubitz & Riley, 1993; Lubitz & Prihoda, 1984).

Hospitals Hospitals, including inpatient and outpatient services, accounted for 44 percent of personal health care spending in 1991. (See Table 22-4). Public funds paid for more than half this amount, and private health insurance covered more than a third (Letsch, 1993). Since 1961, hospital spending has increased sevenfold (CBO, 1993).[5]

The utilization of hospital services shifted substantially during the 1980s to fewer inpatient days and a growth in less expensive out-patient services. Despite this shift, hospital costs continue to rise and are expected to continue to grow at a rate of 11 percent annually (CBO,

[5]Increase adjusted for inflation.

TABLE 22-4. National health expenditures, aggregate amounts and average annual growth, billions of dollars, selected calendar years 1960-1991

Spending Category	1960	1970	1980	1985	1988	1989	1990	1991
NATIONAL HEALTH EXPENDITURES	$27.1	$74.4	$250.1	$422.6	$546.1	$604.3	$675.0	$751.8
Health services and supplies	25.4	69.1	238.9	407.2	526.2	583.6	652.4	728.6
Personal health care	23.9	64.9	219.4	369.7	482.8	530.9	591.5	660.2
Hospital care	9.3	27.9	102.4	168.3	212.0	232.4	258.1	288.6
Physician services	5.3	13.6	41.9	74.0	105.1	116.1	128.8	142.0
Dental services	2.0	4.7	14.4	23.3	29.4	31.6	34.1	37.1
Other professional services	0.6	1.5	8.7	16.6	23.8	27.1	30.7	35.8
Home health care	0.0	0.1	1.3	3.8	4.5	5.6	7.6	9.8
Drugs and other medical nondurables	4.2	8.8	21.6	36.2	46.3	50.5	55.6	60.7
Vision products and other medical durables	0.8	2.0	4.6	7.1	10.1	10.4	11.7	12.4
Nursing home care	1.0	4.9	20.0	34.1	42.8	47.5	53.3	59.9
Other personal health care	0.7	1.4	4.6	6.4	8.7	9.8	11.5	14.0
Program administration and net cost of private health insurance	1.2	2.8	12.2	25.2	26.9	33.8	38.9	43.9
Government public health activities	0.4	1.4	7.2	12.3	16.6	18.9	22.0	24.5
Research and construction	1.7	5.3	11.3	15.4	19.8	20.7	22.7	23.1
Research	0.7	2.0	5.4	7.8	10.3	11.0	11.9	12.6
Construction	1.0	3.4	5.8	7.6	9.5	9.7	10.8	10.6
National health expenditures per capita[1]	$143	$346	$1,064	$1,711	$2,146	$2,352	$2,601	$2,868
Gross domestic product (GDP), billions of dollars	$513	$1,011	$2,708	$4,039	$4,900	$5,251	$5,522	$5,677
National health expenditures as percent of GDP	5.3%	7.4%	9.2%	10.5%	11.1%	11.5%	12.2%	13.2%

1993). Direct payments by consumers for hospital services have steadily declined since 1960 and are now only 3.4 percent of total hospital expenditures.

Physicians Physician services accounted for 21.5 percent of personal health care spending in 1991, a sixfold increase since 1961,[6] although direct payments to physicians by consumers have declined substantially over this time span. Public funds, mainly Medicare, accounted for more than a third of payments received by physicians, with private health insurance accounting for nearly half in 1991 (Letsch, 1993)—the reverse of how hospital care is financed.

Physicians play an important role in the use of most health care services, particularly expensive services, via their orders or prescriptions, which account for more than 70 percent of the total personal health expenditures. Physician costs are expected to continue to grow at a rate of 10 percent annually (CBO, 1993; Letsch, 1993).

Drugs and Other Nondurable Medical Goods
Prescription and over-the-counter drugs and

[6]Increase adjusted for inflation.

TABLE 22-4. *Continued*

Spending Category	1960	1970	1980	1985	1988	1989	1990	1991
Growth (average annual percent change from previous period shown)								
NATIONAL HEALTH EXPENDITURES	–	10.6%	12.9%	11.1%	8.9%	10.7%	11.7%	11.4%
Health services and supplies	–	10.5	13.2	11.3	8.9	10.9	11.8	11.7
Personal health care	–	10.5	13.0	11.0	9.3	10.0	11.4	11.6
Hospital care	–	11.7	13.9	10.4	8.0	9.6	11.1	11.8
Physician services	–	9.9	11.9	12.1	12.4	10.4	11.0	10.2
Dental services	–	9.1	11.9	10.1	8.2	7.5	7.7	8.8
Other professional services	–	9.6	19.1	13.8	12.6	13.8	13.5	16.7
Home health care	–	14.5	25.2	23.3	5.6	24.4	34.4	29.0
Drugs and other medical nondurables	–	7.6	9.4	10.8	8.6	9.1	10.3	9.0
Vision products and other medical durables	–	9.6	8.5	9.4	12.4	2.8	12.6	5.4
Nursing home care	–	17.4	15.2	11.3	7.8	11.1	12.3	12.4
Other personal health care	–	7.1	12.8	6.9	11.1	11.8	17.4	21.9
Program administration and net cost of private health insurance	–	9.0	16.0	15.5	2.2	25.7	15.3	12.7
Government public health activities	–	13.9	18.0	11.3	10.4	14.3	16.0	11.6
Research and construction	–	12.1	7.8	6.4	8.8	4.2	9.6	2.1
Research	–	10.9	10.8	7.4	9.9	6.2	8.0	6.1
Construction	–	12.8	5.6	5.4	7.7	1.9	11.5	– 2.2
National health expenditures per capita	–	9.3	11.9	10.0	7.9	9.6	10.6	10.3
Gross domestic product	–	7.0	10.4	8.3	6.7	7.2	5.2	2.8

¹Per capita figures are derived using July 1 Social Security area population estimates.

SOURCE: From the Health Care Financing Administration, Office of the Actuary (1992).

other nondurable medical goods, such as bandages, accounted for about 9 percent of personal health expenditures in 1991, with prescription drugs representing the largest portion of these expenditures (Letsch, 1993). The elderly, who represent only 12 percent of the population, consume one-third of all outpatient prescription drugs purchased in this country, about 4 times what persons under age 65 consume (*Aging America*, 1991). It should be noted that medication regimens are often used to manage many chronic diseases of the elderly, such as hypertension, diabetes, and various heart ailments (AARP, 1992).

Third-party payers, mostly private insurance and Medicaid, accounted for nearly half of the payments for prescription drugs between 1990 and 1991. In fact, Medicaid prescription costs grew nearly 25 percent between 1990 and 1991, the highest growth rate in 20 years (Letsch, 1993). Rapidly rising costs in prescription drugs will be a problem for public and private insurers, the elderly, and the chronically ill. One response has been the implementation of mail-order programs to control costs.

Overall, spending for all drugs and nondurable items has risen less rapidly than spending for hospital care and physicians, having only tripled during the past three decades.[7] Historically, insurers paid little of these costs. Since 1960, even though direct payments declined for prescription drugs, costs for most other drugs and nondurable medical goods were paid by consumers through direct payments, accounting for nearly one-third of their total out-of-pocket expenses (CBO, 1993).

Nursing Homes The use of nursing home care is substantial and growing, but these facilities are financed differently than hospitals, physicians, and drugs. Medicare pays only for medically focused care, not custodial care (*The Medicare Handbook*, 1993), and there is a lack of private long-term care (LTC) insurance for the elderly. Yet many persons in nursing homes need only custodial care, since not all chronic illness and impairments in activities of daily living (ADLs) have an associated ongoing medical need. On the other hand, Medicaid is very liberal in nursing home coverage, since it does not restrict payment only to recovery from serious illness (*Aging America*, 1991). The major health concern of elderly Americans is financial protection against the high cost of LTC.

Nursing home care accounted for about 9 percent of personal health expenditures in 1991.[8] Slightly over half was paid out of pocket by consumers, with Medicaid paying most of the rest. Currently, nursing home expenditures are rising at a faster rate than the rise in total health care expenditures (Letsch, 1993). The lack of private insurance among the elderly, along with the substantial use of Medicaid support for this cohort and younger age groups, has implications for the structure, delivery, and financing of LTC.

It is interesting to note that age is directly related to nursing home use. Five percent of persons aged 65 or older were in nursing homes at any given time during 1985, with numbers of resident days increasing proportionately with age. The average nursing home resident is an 80-year-old white widow with several chronic conditions. Typically, she has been a resident for 18 months after being discharged from a hospital or other facility (*Aging America*, 1991).

It is projected that 9 million will need nursing home care by the year 2000 and 18 million will need it by the year 2040 (*Aging America*, 1991). Kemper and Murtaugh (1991) estimate that 45 percent of persons aged 65 in 1990 will use nursing home services sometime during their lives, and long-term use (five years or more) is expected to increase. It is well to remember that the elderly are concentrated in nine states, so there could be a disproportionate problem.

There are a substantial number of individuals aside from the elderly who use nursing homes. Based on 1986 mortality data, 29 percent of persons aged 25 and over were nursing home residents at some time in their lives (Kemper & Murtaugh, 1991). Most of these persons had a cumulative total use ranging between one year and five years. The probability of nursing home use is greater for women than for men, for whites than for blacks, and for nonmarried than for married individuals (Kemper & Murtaugh, 1991). In spite of the need for this growing use of nursing homes, no one knows how to pay for it, and Medicaid liability continues to rise, putting the burden on individual states. It is conceivable that we could end up with 50 different views and 50 different solutions.

Home Care It has been argued that home health services are a low-cost alternative to continued hospitalization or care at a skilled nursing facility. Here, home health services are defined as primarily medical in nature and not custodial. Although not currently a major expenditure category, the rise in home health care spending is dramatic: 35 percent from 1989 to 1990 and 29 percent from 1990 to 1991 (Letsch, 1993). These costs are increasing more rapidly than any other health category and reflect a shift from costly inpatient stays to home treatment. The CBO expects that the growth rate in home health care costs will taper off to 12 percent as the health industry expands and matures by year 2000, and that costs will exceed $35 billion by then (CBO 1992a).

---

[7]Increase adjusted for inflation.

[8]Increase adjusted for inflation.

Impact of Rising Costs on Individuals

The continued rise in the cost of health care negatively affects the nation and its citizens by limiting the availability of health insurance for some and preventing adequate coverage for others. Currently, it is estimated that about 37 million Americans have no health insurance. What is alarming is that a large percentage of these persons are employed.

Low income is a special risk factor because it is coupled with a high incidence of death from chronic conditions like heart disease. In fact, there is an inverse relationship between cancer and family income. HIV and tuberculosis also disproportionately affect the poor (*Healthy People 2000,* 1991).

Employed but Uninsured With the rise in costs to employers and changes in the economy from industrial to service industries that offer low-paying jobs and no health benefits, more people are forced to forego health coverage (Levit, Olin, & Letsch, 1992). Nearly 80 percent of uninsured persons are employed or dependents of employed persons, pointing out the importance of employer-sponsored health insurance. By the year 2000, the number of people under age 65 who fall into the category of employed but uninsured is expected to rise to 40 million (CBO, 1992b).

There are several reasons that these individuals are uninsured. Employers may not offer insurance, and if they do, low wages may prevent employees from paying their share of the premium. Often coverage is offered only to full-time employees, but an increasing number of jobs are part-time. Coverage may be limited to the employee, with no family benefits available. Another reason contributing to the lack of coverage is that insurance companies increasingly exclude high-risk people, refuse coverage for pre-existing conditions, or set dollar limits for care of such conditions when underwriting policies (CBO, 1992a).

Employed individuals who are uninsured are concentrated in certain groups: They work for small businesses of 100 or fewer employees,

have incomes no more than twice the poverty level, or are single-parent families. This group comprises primarily young adults, children, and black Americans (CBO 1992b).

In addition, health insurance provided by small business firms of 100 or fewer employees has been declining since 1989. These small businesses strongly oppose being mandated to provide health insurance coverage because of the adverse financial impact on their businesses (Sullivan et al., 1992).

The lack of health insurance has serious consequences, since no coverage often translates into an inability to pay. The resulting debts are often transferred to others through "cost-shifting," that is, higher premiums or higher service costs. For many individuals, the lack of coverage serves as a deterrent to seeking health care, limits access through denial of services by providers, and carries great financial risks for less than catastrophic events. Yet the lack of insurance should not be equated with no health care. Studies show that these people receive health care, albeit somewhat less than individuals with coverage (CBO, 1992b).

Uninsured Children Children under the age of 18 comprise 33 percent of those without coverage. Most of these children live in families where at least one parent is employed full-time and is covered by an insurance-based health plan (Oberg, 1990). This last point is important because insurance benefits may just cover the employee, or if family coverage is available to the employee for additional premiums, the employee may be unable to afford his or her share of the premium.

Children from near-poor families are more impacted than others when it comes to health care. They are more likely to fall through the Medicaid safety net than are children in poor families who qualify for federally sponsored health care programs (Levit, Olin, & Letsch, 1992). Poor minority children and those without health insurance have diminished access to the health care system, receive fewer health care services, and are more likely to have adverse health outcomes (Cartland & Yudkowsky, 1992; Aday et al., 1993).

The Poor and Near-Poor Income is recognized as the single most important factor for a nonelderly family's decision to purchase or not purchase health coverage (Levit, Olin, & Letsch, 1992). For more than a decade, the number of people at or near the poverty level has increased, yet the percent of those with insurance coverage has decreased. Although the poor need health care as much as the rest of the population, they cannot pay what they do not have. Uninsured Americans living below the federal poverty level account for 35.6 percent of uncovered persons (Oberg, 1990).

The Elderly Poor Aside from families, there are also a number of elderly who are classified as poor. Less than 3 percent of the elderly poor lack health coverage for acute care, since Medicare provides coverage for this age group. However, 12 percent of all the elderly have incomes below the poverty level, and an additional 28 percent are near that level and cannot afford supplemental insurance.

Most of the elderly poor are women, the very old (85 and over), or minorities. Those who live alone tend to have lower incomes than older couples. The likelihood of living alone increases with age. Unfortunately, because of differences among states for eligibility requirements, most poor and near-poor elderly are not covered by Medicaid (*Aging America,* 1991).

Older people, poor or otherwise, have a high prevalence of chronic illness that may lead to varying degrees of disability and functional impairment. They also have greater limitations in one or more ADLs, which serve as an important indicator of the need for long-term care (*Aging America,* 1991).

Chronic Illness and Costs

As persons grow old, acute conditions become less frequent and chronic conditions become more prevalent. In fact, the incidence of most chronic diseases increases with age, with most of those over age 65 having one or more such conditions. The leading chronic conditions are arthritis, hypertension, hearing impairment, and heart disease (see Figure 22-3). Most visits by the eld-

erly to the hospital or to physicians are for chronic conditions related to cancer, circulatory, digestive, or respiratory disorders, or for those of the nervous or musculoskeletal systems (*Aging America,* 1991).

For the disabled elderly who live in the community, there are indirect costs of care that are not covered by Medicare or other health insurance. Spouses, children, other relatives, and friends provide as much as 75 percent of needed hands-on assistance, often unpaid, to the elderly with chronic disabling conditions (see Chapter 12, on family caregivers).

Chronic conditions vary by sex and race. Men suffer more acute, life-threatening conditions such as coronary heart disease, which shorten their life span, while women suffer more chronic conditions such as arthritis and osteoporosis, which cause physical limitations. More elderly blacks report their health as fair or poorer than do elderly whites, and they have higher incidences of diabetes, hypertension, and arthritis (*Aging America,* 1991).

Heart disease is the leading diagnosis requiring short-stay hospitalization for elderly individuals, and it is also the leading cause of death among them. In fact, heart disease, cancer, and cerebral vascular accidents (CVAs) account for 70 percent of the mortality among the elderly, 20 percent of their visits to physicians, 40 percent of all hospital days, and 50 percent of all days spent in bed (*Aging America,* 1991). As Table 22-5 shows, some prevalent chronic conditions are associated with significant economic costs.

While it is well recognized that the prevalence of chronic conditions varies, more recent research has shown (1) that there is a disjunction between the prevalence of conditions and their impact in terms of physical and social disability, and (2) that certain combinations of conditions lead to greater impact. To illustrate, research shows that some high-incidence conditions, such as arthritis, may have low or moderate impact, like a low or occasionally moderate degree of disability, and low-incidence conditions, such as osteoporosis, may have moderate to high impact for afflicted persons (Verbrugge, Lepkowski, & Imanaka, 1989).

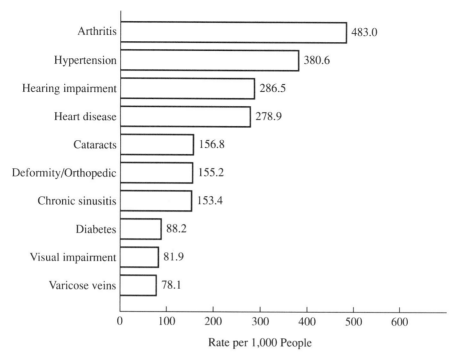

FIGURE 22-3. The Top Ten Chronic Conditions for People 65+, 1989

SOURCE: From the National Center for Health Statistics (1990, October).

Further, since many elderly persons suffer from multiple chronic conditions, it is imperative not to confine our attention as caregivers and policymakers only to single diseases. As the number of chronic conditions increases in older people, disability rises rapidly. Certain combinations of chronic conditions lead to a greater degree of disability; that is, they are termed as giving extra propulsion to disability (Verbrugge et al., 1989). These combinations are cardiovascular disease with hip fracture, diabetes, or osteoporosis; hip fracture with osteoporosis or atherosclerosis; visual impairment with osteoporosis; or ischemic heart disease with cancer. As you can see, the synergism typically stems from uncommon pairs with exacerbating effects. Simple and multiple conditions often are associated with long-term and growing financial risks.

The 1980 National Medical Care Utilization and Expenditure Survey Data showed that dis-

ability and disabling comorbidities[9] lead to substantial financial burden (Rice & LaPlante, 1992). Rice and LaPlante showed that per capita expenditures were 1.5 times greater for people reporting one disabling chronic condition and 5 times greater for persons reporting two such conditions than for persons reporting no such conditions. In addition, the incidence of comorbidity and related costs vary by age. Comorbidity rates for noninstitutionalized people under age 65 are less than for the elderly. Likewise, where single or multiple conditions exist, younger age groups have lower costs than older people (Rice & LaPlante, 1992).

Adults: Ages 25 to 64   There are a number of chronic conditions associated with risk factors

[9]*Comorbidity* is defined as the coexistence of multiple diseases and chronic conditions.

TABLE 22-5.   Costs of treatment for selected preventable conditions[1]

Condition	Overall Magnitude	Avoidable Intervention[2]	Cost per Patient[3]
Heart disease	7 million with coronary artery disease 500,000 deaths/year 284,000 bypass procedures/year	Coronary bypass surgery	$30,000
Cancer	1 million new cases/year 510,000 deaths/year	Lung cancer treatment	$29,000
		Cervical cancer treatment	$28,000
Stroke	600,000 strokes/year 150,000 deaths/year	Hemiplegia treatment and rehabilitation	$22,000
Injuries	2.3 million hospitalizations/year 142,500 deaths/year 177,000 persons with spinal cord injuries in the United States	Quadriplegia treatment and rehabilitation	$570,000 (lifetime)
		Hip fracture treatment and rehabilitation	$40,000
		Severe head injury treatment and rehabilitation	$310,000
HIV infection	1–1.5 million infected 118,000 AIDS cases (as of January 1990)	AIDS treatment	$75,000 (lifetime)
Alcoholism	18.5 million abuse alcohol 105,000 alcohol-related deaths/year	Liver transplant	$250,000
Drug abuse	Regular users: 1–3 million, cocaine 900,000 IV drugs 500,000, heroin Drug-exposed babies: 375,000	Treatment of drug-affected baby	$63,000 (5 years)
Low birth weight baby (LBWB)	260,000 LBWB born/year 23,000 deaths/year	Neonatal intensive care for LBWB	$10,000
Inadequate immunization	Lacking basic immunization series: 20–30%, aged 2 and younger 3%, aged 6 and older	Congenital rubella syndrome treatment	$354,000 (lifetime)

[1]Data compiled from various sources by the Office of Disease Prevention and Health Promotion.
[2]Examples (other interventions may apply). *Note:* The term "avoidable" indicates that preventive interventions would lower the number of these disorders.
[3]Representative first-year costs, except as noted. Not indicated are nonmedical costs, such as lost productivity to society.
SOURCE: Adapted from *Healthy People 2000* (1991).

related to life-style. These conditions include cerebral vascular accidents (CVAs), chronic liver disease with or without cirrhosis, nonfatal heart attacks, and hypertension that is associated with heart attacks or strokes. For instance, about 30 percent of all adults have high blood pressure, and most do not have it under control (*Healthy People 2000,* 1991).

Preventing some chronic disease often depends on individual decisions to quit smoking,

CASE STUDY
Cycle of Impoverishment

Mr. C., a middle-class father of two, had been an electrician all his adult life. At age 42, he began experiencing some pain and stiffness in his joints, making the execution of his job duties very difficult. He visited his doctor, who diagnosed his condition as rheumatoid arthritis. His disease progressed rapidly, affecting his hips, hands, knees, and neck. Hospitalization, treatment, and medication resulted in mounting medical bills. His insurance covered most of these costs. His illness forced him to use all his allotted sick time, which severely affected his income.

Within nine months, he was entirely unable to work. He was subsequently laid off. Losing his job meant losing his medical insurance, even though his medical bills continued to mount. Costly gold salt injections were prescribed. His wife was forced to work, but her salary was only a fraction of what he had been earning. Medical and hospital bills consumed the "nest egg" of $100,000 within two years after he lost his job. The family had to apply for Medicaid to meet medical expenses. This meant that they had to deplete their real property so that they would be eligible.

SOURCE: From Neifing (1990).

use alcohol only in moderation, reduce saturated fat intake, achieve weight control, and increase physical activity. In contrast to the elderly who are retired, the indirect costs of chronic disease among adults is significant in terms of lost income, and these adults frequently run the risk of losing their health insurance, too. The case study of Mr. C. illustrates these impacts.

Children and Chronic Illness Few studies have examined the cost of chronic illness in the pediatric population. Perrin et al. (1993) reported on utilization and costs for 10 chronic childhood illnesses. The data showed a greater use of health services and greater service costs for children with chronic illness than for their able-bodied counterparts.

Using 1988 NHES data on child health, researchers estimated that 28 million children are affected by chronic conditions. The most prevalent conditions include respiratory allergies, repeated ear infections, and asthma (Newacheck & Taylor, 1992). Single chronic conditions predominate, although some children have two and three comorbidities.

Severity of the illness and its effect on the child's health and use of services was determined. The majority reported mild condi-

tions, but there were 5 percent with severe conditions. Children reported as having severe conditions, although small in number, accounted for 21 percent of physician contacts and 33 percent of hospital days (Newacheck & Taylor, 1992).

Mental retardation, learning disorders, emotional and behavioral problems, and vision and speech impairments are more prevalent among children living in poverty than among those at higher socioeconomic levels (*Healthy People 2000,* 1991). Chronic physical conditions, such as hearing and speech impairment, are on the rise. Again, low-income children are at greater risk for health problems, are more likely to lack health insurance, and are at greater risk of being underserved.

Compared to adults, chronic illnesses in children may lead to different and sometimes substantial indirect costs. Loss of income results when parents take time off from work or need to quit a job to care for a child. On the other hand, parents with employer-provided insurance may forgo career advances and job changes in order to maintain health insurance benefits. A change in job may result in the sick child being excluded from his or her parents' new health insurance. Other indirect costs arise from child care, transportation, and lodging costs when the family must travel to pediatric centers for specialized care that is not available in adult acute care facilities (Perrin et al., 1993).

Finally, chronic illness occurring early in life can exhaust or cap the lifetime expenditures allowed with most health insurance coverage. Although most children will never reach these financial limits, their improved survival rates will lead to greater utilization and therefore costs. Although the prevalence of chronic childhood diseases remains steady, the prevalence of adults with these diseases will increase as these children grow into adulthood. Current providers, including physicians, are not prepared or trained to treat these individuals.

Specific Chronic Conditions

Discussing the financial implications of all chronic conditions is impossible in one chapter. However, two are discussed here to demonstrate the impact of chronic conditions on health dollars. These are the cognitive disorders, including Alzheimer's disease, which affects primarily the elderly, and diabetes mellitus, which impacts individuals throughout the life cycle.

Cognitive Disorders   According to the Alzheimer's Association (1992), more than half of all nursing home residents are victims of Alzheimer's disease or other dementias. In 1985, 63 percent of older nursing home residents were disoriented or had memory impairment severe enough that their ability to perform ADLs was affected. Although Alzheimer's disease was common, nearly half of these individuals were diagnosed with senile dementia or chronic organic brain syndrome (*Aging America,* 1991).

Alzheimer's is the leading cause of cognitive impairment in old age and, along with other organic mental disorders, affects 1 in every 10 older adults living in the community. The incidence of Alzheimer's increases with age, so that by the time this cohort reaches age 85, 47 percent will have this diagnosis (*Aging America,* 1991). It is anticipated that the number of cases of dementia, regardless of cause, will increase to 7.4 million by the year 2040 (Coughlin & Liu, 1989).

The annual cost for keeping a person with Alzheimer's disease at home is estimated to be $18,000, with families covering most of these expenses. This figure does not reflect the free care given by family members, which can add an additional $36,000 per year (Alzheimer's Association, 1992; Weinberger et al., 1993). For comparison, the annual expenditure by public funds or private insurance for one of these patients at a nursing home varies from $36,000 to as high as $56,000. Should the person require hospital inpatient service, costs will be much higher because of greater care needs (Hay & Ernst, 1987; Welch, Walsh, & Larson, 1992).

Alzheimer's is an expensive disease requiring a great deal of formal and informal services. Many of these services, like nursing home care, adult day care, respite care, custodial care by family, and financial and legal services are not covered by health insurance. Alzheimer's disease is not rapidly fatal, but has an expected duration of about eight years, often requiring several years of long-term care. These patients do not meet the strict eligibility requirements for home care provided by Medicare or home care provided by other third-party payers, even though they would benefit from the services of home health aides, companions, and respite care (Weinberger et al., 1993).

Diabetes Mellitus   Diabetes mellitus (DM) is one of the most prevalent chronic conditions. It affects 14 million Americans (Bransome, 1992), with 650,000 newly diagnosed cases being identified each year. Diabetes ranks as the sixth cause of all deaths; it directly causes 37,000 deaths annually and contributes to 100,000 others each year (*Healthy People 2000,* 1991).

Diabetics are admitted to the hospital twice as often as the general population and stay there longer (Bransome, 1992). In 1987, health care costs for this disease alone were estimated at nearly $10 billion in direct costs, mostly for inpatient care. Indirect costs, which result from a loss of productivity and income, were mostly attributed to premature death (American Diabetes Association, 1991; Knollmueller, 1992; Bransome, 1992).

Diabetes is associated with a lot of comorbidity, the "hidden" burden of chronic complications. Diabetics are 22 times more likely to develop skin ulcers and gangrene, are 15 times more likely to have peripheral vascular disease, have 10 times the incidence of atherosclerosis, and are 6 to 10 times more likely to develop heart disease and CVAs then any other segment of the population. Diabetics experience more serious complications, such as renal disease and kidney failure, blindness, amputations, and cardiac disorders, during their shortened life span than do others. When a pregnant woman is diabetic, there is a threefold increase in the risk for congenital malformations and perinatal mortality (*Healthy People 2000,* 1991; American Diabetes Association, 1991).

In spite of its insidious nature and the fact that the incidence of DM increases with age (Helms, 1992), there is inadequate reimbursement for outpatient diabetes education, including training in self-care. Currently, Blue Cross of Maine is taking a step in the right direction by providing such funding for preventive care (Bransome, 1992).

Impact of Rising Costs on the Nation

Increasing health care costs negatively impact the nation in two important ways. First, increased health care costs have led to higher premiums, a cost borne primarily by employers. However, employees indirectly carry these costs through limited growth or reduction in future cash wages and benefits. Consumers pay, too, through higher price tags for products. For example, nearly $1,000 of each new car purchase goes to pay automotive employees' health care benefits. More alarming, increased costs have resulted in more and more employers' not offering health care coverage.

Second, increased costs for government-sponsored health insurance consume larger portions of the budget. These increased costs preempt resources from other government programs and investments and contribute to the growth in the federal deficit. Without a change in benefits or financing, CBO (1992a) projects that federal health spending will be the major reason for the increasing federal deficit by the late 1990s. As the government borrows money,

less money is available from private savings for investment purposes, a serious concern for both economists and business people.

The federal government has attempted to control rising health care costs in both Medicare and Medicaid programs through changes in financing mechanisms, benefits, and cost-sharing provisions. Part A of the Medicare Trust Fund, which pays hospitalization benefits, is projected to be insolvent by the year 2002. To avoid this, payroll deductions need to double and current benefit levels need to be cut in half (Burner, Waldo, & McKusick, 1992). Medicare physician costs (Part B benefits) are rising also, and this will lead to continued increases in beneficiary premiums. Such outcomes have negative consequences for the elderly and the poor, who experience a greater incidence of chronic illness and conditions.

Solutions to Rising Health Care Costs

Americans are faced with difficult decisions regarding the nature of their health care delivery system and the growing personal and public inability to gain access to or pay for health services. For more than two decades, efforts to control rising costs have largely come from government legislation. Federal, state, and local governments have a vested interest in controlling costs, having become major purchasers of health care. During the 1970s, government regulations attempted to control the growth of providers and services by various means. The 1980s reflected a different political agenda with an emphasis on competition, managed care, and a radical change in financing mechanisms. The success of future cost control measures must link financing mechanisms with redefined national goals that address the important issues of entitlement; right to adequate, affordable health care; limited resources; and changing health care needs.

Managing Chronic Conditions

About 80 percent of all costs for illness in the United States are attributed to chronic conditions. Further, chronic conditions, rather than acute illness, claim the most lives in this country (Henry 1991, 1993). Despite this, our health care delivery system continues to focus on treating the acute care patient population. The growing dissatisfaction with this fragmented and highly specialized delivery system is giving rise to "integrated health care systems" that are proposed to be more cost-effective. Because of their structure these systems would be more appropriate to the care of the chronic population (American Hospital Association, 1992; Knowles, 1992).

The recognition of chronic illness as a dominant model will develop incrementally over time. Some examples include the geriatric centers and chronic care and disability units found in many hospitals, and the fellowships focused on chronic illness and disabilities appearing in medical schools.

One important trend occurring in chronic care today is the development of the National Chronic Care Consortium. Involving 20 community-based networks across the nation, these providers are implementing programs that provide acute and long-term care within a chronic care service delivery system that coordinates all services (not just the traditional medical ones) and correlates funding to better meet the needs of the chronically impaired while containing costs (Bowe, 1992).

Within our current system, multiple providers and payers inhibit our ability to gather reliable and complete financial information about all illnesses. By coordinating both services and funding, not only should there be better patient outcomes and lesser costs, but we should gain better information about the lifetime costs of chronic care.

Health Prevention

The importance of prevention in reducing health care expenditures cannot be overemphasized. Much of the economic burden of illness can be averted through appropriate preventive activities. For example, knowledge about hypertension and the importance of receiving early treatment and thereby achieving adequate control have greatly increased over the past two decades (Oparil, 1993).

Other activities that prevent illnesses also need to be emphasized. Immunizations represent a cost-effective intervention when compared to the expenses associated with treatment, rehabilitation, and maintenance of afflicted individuals. Early and comprehensive prenatal care reduces the incidence of infant mortality and low-birth weight infants, who experience greater health care risks (*Healthy People 2000,* 1991). Greater savings from immunizations and prenatal care will be realized when these services are more affordable, if not freely available, and when there is identification and greater participation among groups less likely to use these services.

Unhealthy life-style behaviors are associated with many significant life-threatening, debilitating, and costly chronic conditions, including CVAs, heart disease, and certain cancers. Equally important, many life-style factors, such as tobacco and alcohol consumption or diet and activity patterns, contribute to higher mortality rates in the United States. These factors lead to significant indirect costs secondary to lost income (McGinnis & Foege, 1993) and higher direct costs. For instance, smoking increases lifetime health care expenditures by $100,000 (Fries, 1993).

Current trends point to changing beliefs and practices toward healthier life-style behaviors. For example, there has been a decline in this country in cigarette use and hard alcohol consumption; increased attention given to smoke-free environments, designated drivers, and safe sexual activity; mandatory seat belt laws; and a growing emphasis on weight and stress reduction in our daily lives (*Healthy People 2000,* 1991). Healthier life-styles generate cost savings directly by averting the need to treat illness earlier than necessary, and indirectly by allowing many individuals to remain productive in the work force for a longer period of time.

Employers are also getting involved. They are recognizing the importance of prevention and health promotion in generating savings on their health insurance premium costs (Fries, 1993). Resulting changes in life-style among employees suggest greater personal responsibility in managing one's own health. In general, effective prevention and health care will require such shared responsibility and effort between health providers, employers, and clients.

The importance of preventive health care is receiving greater emphasis in the 1990s. Two recent initiatives supported by the Department of Health and Human Services are *Healthy People 2000* and Healthy Communities 2000 (Knollmueller, 1992), which focus on health promotion, health protection, and preventive services aimed at reducing the incidence of selected chronic and disabling diseases, their complications, and subsequent health care costs (Knollmueller, 1992). These two initiatives establish a springboard for future development and implementation by interested parties. The continued focus on prevention is likely to increase in the future.

Health Care Reform

State Plans   Many states across the nation are experiencing runaway health care costs that are forcing them to examine needed changes in their health care delivery systems. These states recognize that cost is inextricably linked to issues of access (and consequently insurance) and quality. Actions they have taken will have an important influence on larger changes at the national level. Hawaii has developed a system of near-universal access and mandated changes in employer-based insurance provisions. Minnesota has legislated insurance reforms and implemented a state-subsidized health care plan that provides progressive access to low-income and working poor persons. The states of Florida and Washington are expanding access and containing costs through a managed-competition model. Maryland is effecting broad insurance market reforms and cost containment by regulating physician fees (Thompson, 1993; Dukakis, 1992; Miles et al., 1992).

Federal Reform: The Clinton Plan   Health care reform is also considered at the national level. The President plays an important role in setting the national agenda in and directing congressional and policy efforts toward reforming health care (Philipp & Biordi, 1990). In 1994, Clinton submitted a major health reform plan to Congress that represented an involved and complex change to the health care system.

To finance the reform, Clinton planned to rely mainly on savings coming from Medicare program revisions and additional revenues to be raised from "sin taxes" on tobacco products. Critics argued that changes in the Medicare program would be opposed by some members of Congress and many elderly individuals (Goodgame, 1993). Opposition from the elderly can be formidable, as is apparent from the repeal of the Catastrophic Health Protection Act in 1989, which was largely due to senior citizen complaints over the increased premiums and cost-sharing provisions of the act (Philipp & Biordi, 1990). Still others note that revenues generated from sin taxes are opposed by states supporting the tobacco industry and by that industry's strong lobby (Pallarito, 1993). Further, since increasing taxes adversely affect total sales, the revenues gained from these taxes decline as consumers buy less.

Other formidable opposition came from small businesses, who under the proposal would have been mandated to provide health insurance to employees. Small businesses fear that they cannot afford these additional expenses and that this will negatively impact future hiring, wages, and work force retention (Quinn, 1993).

The Clinton plan contained other proposed system changes—malpractice reform; attacking fraud and abuse; managed care and cooperative purchasing groups; and standardization of information, paperwork, and insurance claims (Health Care: A Proposal, 1993; Peck, 1993). Critics point out that health care providers lack the computerized information systems necessary to implement the proposed health security cards and that a National Health Board and 50 state Health Care Alliances (cooperative purchasing groups) would add layers of bureaucracy and additional costs to the system (Goodgame, 1993).

Federal Reform: Congressional Plans   At least six other major health care bills were submitted to Congress in 1993 and 1994. These bills address health reform in a multitude of ways:

single payor, managed competition, universal access, standardization of benefits, employer-based insurance mandates, cost control provisions, and insurance reforms (Health Care: A Proposal, 1993; Goodgame, 1993; Peck, 1993; White, 1993). Differences among them largely reflect the philosophical differences among the many members of Congress.

Issues of Health Care Reform Plans Although there are many beneficial provisions offered in the proposed reform bills, financing issues are likely to be the center of any debate. Historically, many Americans have opposed government intervention and "big government" programs. In fact, our government has been criticized for *overestimating* savings and *underestimating* program costs. Further, Americans may not want to pay for health care reform. As Jane Bryant Quinn (1993) notes, "Americans want universal coverage as long as it won't cost too much." As the debate over health care develops, the real issues are likely to be not how much it costs or how will we pay for it, but rather who should pay.

Others also have taken leadership in health care reform and cost control. For instance, former Governor Lamm of Colorado (1990) points to the need for broad-view changes in financing, composition, and efficacy of health care services. He proposes that rising costs need to be controlled by linking the financing mechanism to policy decisions that consider whether benefits exceed costs, and that any health plan should be based on the greatest good for the greatest number. Most important, Lamm views reform as a means to achieve universal access to basic health care services. He also feels that although some forms of technology can lead to savings, such as lithotripsy, most add to rather than reduce costs; too many technologies are beneficial only at the margin. Perhaps worse, these expensive technologies consume resources that can not be used elsewhere, such as for basic services (Lamm, 1990).

Looking Ahead

As we look to reform of our current health care system, we must not lose sight of our evolving future, which will be a different system than the one we know today. Goldsmith (1992a, 1992b) notes that rapid advances in diagnostic and therapeutic technologies have allowed health care workers to detect certain chronic diseases before acute symptoms require hospitalization, allowing patients to receive earlier treatment on an ambulatory basis that can be managed more inexpensively. Goldsmith predicts that future changes from advances in genetics and immunology will allow health care workers to predict chronic disease risk before persons experience presenting symptoms.

Genetics is a particularly important area of study. We already know that a great number of chronic illnesses originate in our genome, as evidenced by the occurrence of diseases in multiple family generations (Goldsmith, 1992a, 1992b). We are witnessing advances in genetic and immunological discoveries in breast, ovarian, and prostate cancer; diabetes; Huntington's chorea; cystic fibrosis; and Alzheimer's disease. As we develop inexpensive diagnostic tests, monitoring and early detection will ultimately prove to be less expensive than current diagnosing and treatment after the symptoms present (Goldsmith, 1993).

Along with current reform efforts and future medical advances, we must come to grips with the reality of our limited resources and the potential for deliberate, open, and sensible rationing of health care—a concept difficult for both health professionals and lay people to accept. Governor Lamm reminds us that we cannot do everything for everybody and that an explicit decision to fund some health services implies an implicit decision not to fund other services. This decision process is, in essence, rationing (Lamm, 1990).

Yet others note that rationing is already implicitly achieved by restricting access to health care services (White, 1990). The State of Oregon's plan to expand Medicaid coverage to all Oregonians, including the uninsured poor, requires that there must be rationing of services covered. The plan is not without controversy. In order to expand the number of recipients, Oregon has developed a priority list of health services. Items high on the priority list are prevention and primary care services, and items low on the list are services that were found to have only marginal effectiveness. The obvious trade-off is that there is greater access to effective care in an affordable manner for all, but a cutback in the least efficient treatment and tests (White, 1990; Thorne, 1993). This approach is cost-effective because it focuses limited financial resources on interventions that provide the greatest good to the greatest number of people. Successful experimentation in Oregon will likely have a broad impact on future health care reform efforts.

Summary and Conclusions

One must ask if this nation can devote ever increasing resources and money to the health care industry. Proponents highlight that we have the finest system in the world. Opponents criticize that it is a "nonsystem": highly fragmented, lacking coordination, lacking universal coverage, and too focused on acute care. As we come to grips with our inability to afford the current system, we are increasingly likely to move toward a new and different system.

The nature of acute illness, on which our health system was built, is not the same today. About 80 percent of all illnesses are attributed to chronic conditions rather than acute illness, and these chronic conditions claim the most lives in this country (Henry, 1991).

It is important that nurses expand their knowledge beyond the clinical and psychosocial elements of patient care and into new arenas, including health care financing, economics, and insurance (Wieseke & Bantz, 1992; Campbell, 1992). Patients are increasingly faced with serious financial forces and decisions about their health care. Further, patients lack a fundamental understanding of health care delivery, costs, financing, and insurance (Garnick et al., 1993). Nurses serve an important role in supporting and educating patients through their shared concerns, as well as in examining their own beliefs and practices so they can provide more cost-effective, quality care.

Nurses are increasingly affected, often indirectly, by the same economics of health care. Health care providers' profits and losses influence decisions about acquisitions of equipment used by nurses, budgets for nursing education departments, operational budgets that influence salaries, and increases and decreases in allotted nursing care hours. The future of nursing is in our ability not only to self-examine and change but to be leaders and innovators in a changing health care system. We must look beyond the clinical and become more involved in the operational, financial, and political decisions of our employers and our governments.

STUDY QUESTIONS

1. Name three key factors that led to the rise in health care costs over the past 30 years?
2. Identify the three primary sources of payment for health care, and discuss the shifts in payment and their impact on government in financing health care.
3. Describe out-of-pocket expenses and their implications for the elderly and chronically ill population.
4. If the production of health care is an important part of our national economy, how does the rising cost of health care have a negative impact on business and the economy in general?
5. Describe some of the substantial indirect cost sources associated with chronic illness.

6. Discuss the role of prevention and health promotion in curbing the rise in health care costs.
7. Discuss the process of rationing in health care and identify nursing's role in shaping this future.
8. Identify three major provisions in current health care reform legislation and their long-term effects in curbing the rise in health care costs.
9. Recognizing the importance of science and technology on medicine, nursing, and health care services, discuss current changes and how these will affect health care delivery and future health expenditures.

References

Aday, L., Lee, E., Spears, B., Chung, C., Youssef, A., & Bloom, B. (1993). Health insurance and utilization of medicare care for children with special health care needs. *Medical Care, 31*(11), 1013-1026.

Aging America: Trends & Projections (1991). Washington, D.C.: U.S. Senate Special Committee on Aging.

Alzheimer's Association (1992). *Statistical data on Alzheimer's disease.* Chicago: Alzheimer's Disease and Related Disorders Association.

American Association of Retired Persons (AARP) (1992). *A profile of older Americans.* Washington, D.C.: AARP.

American Diabetes Association (1991). *Diabetes: 1991 vital statistics.* Washington, D.C.: American Diabetes Association.

American Hospital Association (1992). *A healthier America: Reforming our health care system.* Chicago: American Hospital Association.

Berk, M., & Monheit, A. (1992). The concentration of health expenditures: An update. *Health Affairs,* 11(4), 145-149.

Bowe, J. (1992). Multi-dimensional care: Geriatric networks overcome fragmentation. *Contemporary Long Term Care, 15*(9), 42-44.

Bransome, E. (1992). Financing the care of diabetes mellitus in the US. Background, problems, and challenges. *Diabetes Care, 15*(Supplement 1), 1-5.

Burner, S, Waldo, D., & McKusick, D. (1992). National health expenditures projections through 2030. *Health Care Financing Review, 14*(1), 1-28.

Campbell, B. (1992). Assessment of attitudes toward cost-containment needs. *Nursing Economics, 10*(6), 397-401.

Cartland, J., & Yudkowsky, B. (1992). State estimates of uninsured children. *Health Affairs, 11*(4), 144 +.

Chulis, G., Eppig, F., Hogan, M., Waldo, D., & Arnett, R. (1993). Health insurance and the elderly. *Health Affairs,* 12(1), 111-118.

Congressional Budget Office (CBO) (1992a, October). *Projections of national health expenditures.* Washington D.C.: CBO.

——— (1992b, October). *Economic implications of health care costs.* Washington D.C.: CBO.

——— (1993, June). *Trends in health spending: An update.* Washington D.C.: CBO.

Coughlin, T., & Liu, K. (1989). Health care costs of older persons with cognitive impairments. *The Gerontologist, 29*(2), 173-182.

Department of Labor, Bureau of Labor Statistics (1990, November 20) *Consumer expenditures in 1989.* Press release USDL: 90-616.

Dukakis, M. (1992). The states and health care reform. *New England Journal of Medicine, 327*(15), 1090-1092.

Evans, R. (1983). Health care technology and the inevitability of resource allocation and rationing decisions. *Journal of the American Medical Association, 249,* 2047-2053.

Feldstein, P. (1993). *Health care economics* (4th ed). Albany: Delmar Publishers.

Folland, S., Goodman, A., & Stano, M. (1993). *The economics of health and health care.* New York: Macmillan.

Fries, J. (1993). Reducing need and demand. *Healthcare Forum Journal, 36*(6), 18-20, 22.

Garnick, D., Hendricks, A., Thorpe, K., Newhouse, J., Donelan, K., & Blendon, R. (1993). How well do Americans understand their health coverage. *Health Affairs, 12*(3), 204-213.

Ginzberg, E. (1990). High-tech medicine and rising health care costs. *Journal of the American Medical Association, 263*(13), 1820-1822.

Goldsmith, J. (1992a). The reshaping of healthcare. Part 1. *Healthcare Forum Journal, 35*(3), 19-27.

——— (1992b). The reshaping of healthcare. Part 2. *Healthcare Forum Journal, 35*(4), 34-41.

——— (1993). Technology & the end to entitlement. *Healthcare Forum Journal, 36*(5), 16-23.

Goodgame, D. (1993). Ready to operate: Clinton's plan would cover everyone. Here's how it would work and what it will cost you. *Time, 142*(12), 54-58.

Hay, J., & Ernst, R. (1987). The economic costs of Alzheimer's disease. *American Journal of Public Health, 77*(9), 1169-1175.

Health care: A proposal for reform. (1993). *Human Resource Executive, 7*(11), 29-43.

Healthy People 2000. National health promotion and disease prevention objectives. (1991). Washington, D.C.: Department of Health and Human Services, Public Health Service.

Helms, R. (1992). Implications of population growth on prevalence of diabetes. *Diabetes Care, 15*(Supplement 1), 6-9.

Henry, W. (1991). Chronic care needs to be a higher priority. *Hospitals, 65*(4), 68.

——— (1993). Managing chronic health conditions is a critical need ignored by many. *Trustee, 46*(3), 20-21.

Iglehart, J. (1993). The end stage renal disease program. *New England Journal of Medicine, 328*(5), 366-371.

Kemper, P., & Murtaugh, C. (1991). Lifetime use of nursing home care. *New England Journal of Medicine, 324*(9), 595-600.

Knollmueller, R. (1992). Prevention and home care: Not strange bedfellows. *Caring,* 11(12), 4-6, 8, 11.

Knowles, E. (1992). Integrated care: A look inside tomorrow's hospital. *Hospitals, 66*(8), 47-51.

Lamm, R. (1990). High-tech health care and society's ability to pay. *Healthcare Financial Management, 44*(9), 21-30.

Letsch, S. (1993). National health care spending in 1991. *Health Affairs, 12*(1), 94-110.

Levit, K., Olin, G., & Letsch, S. (1992). Americans' health insurance coverage, 1980-91. *Health Care Financing Review, 14*(4), 31-39 +.

Lubitz, J., & Prihoda, R. (1984). The use and costs of Medicare services in the last 2 years of life. *Health Care Financing Review,* 5(3):117-131.

Lubitz, J., & Riley, G. (1993). Trends in Medicare payments in the last year of life. *New England Journal of Medicine, 328*(15), 1092-1096.

McGinnis, J., & Foege, W. (1993). Actual causes of death in the United States. *Journal of the American Medical Association, 270*(18), 2007-2212.

The Medicare Handbook (1993). Baltimore: Department of Health and Human Services, Health Care Financing Administration.

Mendelson, D., & Schwartz, W. (1993). The effects of aging and population growth on health care costs. *Health Affairs,* 12(1), 119-125.

Miles, S., Lurie, N., Quam, L., & Caplan, A. (1992). Health care reform in Minnesota. *New England Journal of Medicine, 327*(15), 1092-1095.

National Center for Health Statistics (1990, October). Current estimates from the National Health Interview Survey, 1989. *Vital and Health Statistics Series,* 10(176).

Neifing, T. (1990). Financial impact. In I. Lubkin (Ed.), *Chronic illness: Impact and interventions* (2nd ed.). Boston: Jones and Bartlett.

Newacheck, P., & Taylor, W. (1992). Childhood chronic illness: Prevalence, severity, and impact. *American Journal of Public Health, 82*(3), 364-370.

Oberg, C. (1990). Medically uninsured children in the United States: A challenge to public policy. *Journal of School Health, 60*(10), 493-500.

Oparil, S. (1993). Antihypertensive therapy: Efficacy and quality of life. *New England Journal of Medicine, 328*(13), 959-961.

Pallarito, K. (1993). A tug of war over taxes. States, feds looking at same revenue sources to finance their healthcare agendas. *Modern Healthcare, 23*(29), 24-26.

Peck, P. (1993). A summary of the health security act of 1993. *Internal Medicine News & Cardiology News, 26*(20), 19.

Perrin, J., Shayne, M., & Bloom, S. (1993). *Home and community care for chronically ill children.* New York: Oxford University Press.

Philipp T., & Biordi, D. (1990). Financial ruin or financing catastrophic health coverage: Who pays? *Journal of Professional Nursing, 6*(2), 94-102.

Quinn, J. B. (1993). Paying for universal care. *Newsweek, 122*(22), 59.

Rice, D., & LaPlante, M. (1992). Medical expenditures for disability and disabling comorbidity. *American Journal of Public Health, 82*(5), 739-741.

Sullivan, C., Miller, M., Feldman, R., & Dowd, B. (1992). Employer-sponsored health insurance in 1991. *Health Affairs, 11*(4), 172-185.

Thompson, R. (1993). States advance their own plans. *Nation's Business, 81*(8), 52-54.

Thorne, J. (1993). As the nation waits, Oregon moves forward. *American College of Surgeons Bulletin, 78*(3), 8-14.

Verbrugge, L., Lepkowski, J., & Imanaka, Y. (1989). Comorbidity and its impact on disability. *The Milbank Quarterly, 67*(3-4), 450-479.

Weinberger, M., Gold, D., Divine, G., Cowper, P., Hodgson, L., Schreiner, P., & George, L. (1993). Expenditures in care for patients with dementia who live at home. *American Journal of Public Health, 83*(3), 338-341.

Welch, G., Walsh, J., & Larson, E. (1992). The cost of institutional care in Alzheimer's disease: Nursing home and hospital in a prospective cohort. *American Geriatrics Society, 40*(3), 221-224.

White, J. (1990). Rationing healthcare: Is it time? *Health Progress, 71*(10), 10-12, 23.

——— (1993). Clinton's health plan: Politics and state responsibility. *Health Progress, 74*(9), 12-15.

Wicker, T. (1991, July 21). Code blue on insurance. *The New York Times,* pp. 4-17.

Wieseke, A., & Bantz, D. (1992). Economic awareness of registered nurses employed in hospitals. *Nursing Economics, 10*(6), 406-412.

Bibliography

American Diabetes Association (1988). *Direct and indirect costs of diabetes in the United States in 1987.* Washington, D.C.: American Diabetes Association.

Bergman, R. (1993). Quantum leaps. *Hospitals and Health Networks, 67*(19), 28-35.

Bove, V. (1992). Health care costs tied to many issues. *Physician Executive, 18*(5), 23-29.

Congressional Budget Office (1991, April). *Rising health care costs: Causes, implications, and strategies.* Washington D.C.: CBO.

Cronin, C., & Milgate, K. (1992). Organized systems of care. *Health Progress, 73*(8), 22-28.

Enthoven, A., & Nichols, S. (1993). Managed competition: Point, counterpoint. *Health Systems Review, 26*(3), 24-29.

Friedman, E. (1993). Managed care: Where will your hospital fit in? *Hospitals, 67*(7), 22-27.

Hurst, J. (1991). Reforming health in seven European countries. *Health Affairs, 10*(3), 7-21.

Jones, W., Peilly, B., & Broyles, R. (1992). Cost containment, access, and American health financing: Getting beyond the shell game. *Journal of Health and Human Resources Administration, 4*(3), 290-306.

Kassirer, J. (1992). A look at ourselves—an overview of the American health care system. *New England Journal of Medicine, 326,* 945-946.

Lee, P., Soffel, D., & Luft, H. (1992). Costs and coverage. Pressures toward health care reform. *Western Journal of Medicine, 157*(5), 567-583.

Levit, K., & Cowan, C. (1992). The burden of health care costs: Business, households, and governments. *Health Care Financing Review, 12*(2), 127-137.

Newhouse, J. (1993). An iconoclastic view of health cost containment. *Health Affairs, 12* (supplement), 152-171.

Pauly, M. (1993). U.S. health care costs: The untold true story. *Health Affairs, 12*(3), 152-159.

Pedelmeier, D., & Fuchs, V. (1993). Hospital expenditures in the United States and Canada. *New England Journal of Medicine, 328*(11), 772-778.

Scheiber, G., Poullier, J., & Greenwald, L. (1991). Health care systems in twenty four countries. *Health Affairs, 10*(3), 22-39.

Starr, P. (1992). *The logic of health-care reform: Transforming American medicine for the better.* Knoxville: Whittle Communications.

Sullivan, C., & Rice, T. (1991). The health insurance picture in 1990. *Health Affairs, 11*(2), 104-115.

CHAPTER 23

Social/Health Policy

Carolyn Lewis • Christine Elnitsky

Introduction

As new proposals for health care reform prolifer-ate in today's political arena, chronic illness must be viewed from the perspective of forces that drive policy changes. Prior to the turn of the century, most policy focused on acute illness. However, with increasing prevalence of chronic conditions and disability, strategies need to change so that acute illness is supplanted as a major challenge to policymakers.

Wilson and Drury's (1984) review of illness trends from 1960 to 1980 found 15 chronic ill-nesses had an increased average prevalence of 50 percent or more among them. This was found true not just in individuals over age 65 but in those aged 45 to 64. The total increase of chronic conditions and disabilities more than doubled from 4.4 percent to 10.8 percent during that time. Consequently, the central concern of social/health policy needs to change in reaction to these trends.

Concept of Social/Health Policy

To better grasp the concept of social/health pol-icy, one must first understand what is meant by *public policy*. In 1970, public policy was defined as "a projected program of goals, values, and practices" (Lasswell & Kaplan, 1970, p. 71).

Later, Dye (1987, p. 2) stated, "public policy is whatever governments choose to do or not to do." These two views differ widely and do not serve to clarify. A more workable definition of public policy, as adapted from the views of these authors, is this:

> Any action by the government on a local, state, or national level that is in response to demands of society to achieve desired out-comes on their goals, values, and practices.

In practice, public policy is either proactive or reactive. *Proactive policy* is based on specific data that guide the decision-making process prior to a crisis situation. *Reactive policy* is for-mulated in response to a crisis situation, often omitting critical analysis prior to the situation.

Social and health policies are subsets of pub-lic policy, although the two terms are often used interchangeably. Social policy addresses the intrasocietal relationships among individuals, groups, and society as a whole. Health policy is, in actuality, a subset of social policy that addresses how and by whom health care is de-livered and financed; it also deals with the envi-ronmental influences on the nation's health, with social issues only considered insofar as they influence people's health (Vail, 1990).

An example of a public policy decision that deals with both social and health policy is the

Catastrophic Coverage Act of 1988. This legislation was originally intended to shield Medicare beneficiaries from the high costs of hopsitalization (Schauffler, 1993) and thus was health policy legislation addressing health care financing for this population. However, the new benefits that were added required beneficiaries to pay additional premiums based on their incomes. Both elderly beneficiaries and grass-roots organizations lobbied against the new act because the long-standing social contract that promised to cover virtually all elderly (Dye, 1987) would now be subject to means testing (Schauffler, 1993). Means testing would have altered the contract between American society and its elderly. In the end, it was the lack of support from both Medicare beneficiaries and grass-roots organizations, as well as disagreements over financing methods, that contributed to the repeal of the act in 1989 (Schauffler, 1993).

Historical Perspective of Social/Health Policy

The management of chronic illness through appropriate health policy has been a growing problem for several decades and has impacted health care policy decision making. In the 1920s, public health officials and scientists first noted the increasing numbers and significance of chronic illnesses. By the 1930s, chronic illnesses were recognized as the most frequent reason for hospital admissions among adults (Fox, 1989). During this same period, the federal government and some state governments, along with some voluntary agencies, began to focus policy decisions on the growing magnitude of the problem of chronic illness.

In the late 1940s, health care providers began responding to the health needs of patients with those chronic illnesses that had been identified in the 1930s. However, since the definition of chronic illness was vague (see Chapter 1, on what is chronicity, Table 1–1), concerted effort at policymaking was difficult. For example, tuberculosis and mental illness were often not included as chronic conditions. The vagueness that existed in reference to a number of chronic con-

ditions often became a political ploy to obtain more support for public budgets and to influence legislation (Fox, 1989).

From World War II until the early 1960s, rapid increases in population, scientific knowledge, and medical technology occurred (Yura & Walsh, 1988). During this period, many coalitions, formed to respond to the increased prevalence of chronic illnesses, struggled to influence policy. However, instead of policies specifically addressing the health care and financing needs of those with chronic conditions, most policy decisions continued to support research aimed at the treatment and cure of acute illness.

Even in the 1960s, health policy dealing with chronic illnesses continued to be far from secure. New problems, such as the deinstitutionalization of the chronically mentally ill, emerged. Aviram (1990) defines deinstitutionalization as ". . . the discharge of large numbers of patients from mental hospitals into the community and the avoidance of and decrease in hospitalization of mentally ill people . . ." (p. 70). The passage of the Community Mental Health Centers Construction Act of 1963 and its amendments of 1975 resulted in the rapid discharge of mentally ill patients during the late 1960s and 1970s into communities unable to plan and implement treatment and services for them. In fact, deinstitutionalization served to place an excessive burden on families and communities while failing to provide adequate treatment programs for the discharged patients (Stuart & Sundeen, 1991).

One of the most significant examples of public policy was the expansion of the Social Security Act in 1965. The addition of Medicare and Medicaid to the Social Security Act provided medical coverage to many Americans through increased benefits to the blind, to the dependent, to aged people, and to children of deceased beneficiaries (Smith, 1990). In essence, these legislative acts were probably the first significant social/health policy developments because they established a limited form of coverage for the chronically ill.

Cost containment has dominated health policy debates since the early 1970s (Schauffler, 1993). By the late 1970's, chronic illnesses were covered by third-party reimbursement. Yet reimbursement was prohibited for preventive services by the largest publicly financed health care program in the United States, namely, Medicare (Schauffler, 1993). Over 30 Medicare preventive service bills were introduced in Congress between 1965 and 1970, but all failed (Schauffler, 1993).

Additional cost containment legislation was instituted in the 1970s that affected Medicare benefits, including (1) limiting the frequency of payment for certain services and (2) adding beneficiary copayments and deductibles (Schauffler, 1993). However, many health promotion and disease prevention services remained uncovered by most public and private health insurance (Mockenhaupt & Muchow, 1994). Some authors suggest that hospital care continues to dominate the American health care system "at the expense of essential developments in primary health care" (Smith, 1990, p. 487).

Current Policies

Medicare and Medicaid, which comprise the current health policy of the federal government, have already been mentioned several times. Therefore, additional information on both is appropriate.

Medicare Medicare is a federal program that covers approximately 30 million Americans and represents 17 percent of the total national spending on personal health care (Steuerle, 1993). Medicare provides coverage to those aged 65 and over and to certain categories of the disabled. It provides physician services, hospital care, and, in some cases, a limited number of days in skilled nursing facilities (Reinhardt, 1992). Since many older recipients of Medicare find themselves inadequately protected, they purchase additional coverage, known as Medigap policies, that supplements Medicare.

In 1983, Medicare implemented distinct fees for 500 Diagnostic Related Groups (DRGs) in an effort to decrease hospital costs incurred from unnecessary hospital stays and treatment. Unfortunately, even this effort has not controlled such costs. Since Medicare's beginnings, fees for physicians were based on *customary, prevailing,*

and *reasonable* (CPR) charges. Since physicians are not reimbursed for their total fees under DRGs, many refuse to take Medicare patients (Steuerle, 1993).

Congress passed a *resource-based relative value scale* (RBRVS) founded on the relative cost of performing certain procedures from a nationwide standard fee schedule in January of 1992. An argument against the RBRVS scale is the difficulty in determining if a service that is twice as costly as another is worth twice as much (Reinhardt, 1992).

Medicaid Medicaid is also a federally financed program, but it is state administered. It provides health care coverage for many unemployed or underemployed individuals, including a number who are chronically ill. It covers some 24 million low-income Americans of all ages. Medicaid coverage has decreased from 60 to 46 percent since the program began in 1965, with half of Medicaid expenditures used for financing long-term care for the elderly (National Leadership Commission on Health Care, 1989).

Coverage provided by Medicaid varies from one state to another, and there are vast disparities in income eligibilities. Since compensation rates are set by the state governments, coverage for health care is usually far below that provided by Medicare, and services differ among the states.

Policy Problems and Issues Affecting Chronic Illness

Americans see health care as a basic human need that is essential for people to function in society. It follows, therefore, that society has an obligation to provide policy not only for acute conditions but for the chronically ill so their health care needs are adequately addressed. In today's climate of growing unemployment, economic instability, changing demographic characteristics, and a rapidly changing health care system, the interdependence of these factors with the social and political forces drastically affects health policy's impact on the chronically ill.

Currently, the struggles for health policy continue to address ways of financing long-term health care and cost containment for chronically ill people. According to Fox (1989), "For six decades Americans have, hesitantly and amid political turmoil, created public and private policy to pay most of the costs of managing the growing burden of chronic illness and disability" (p. 280).

Political Issues and Forces

There are three major areas of concern in today's health care crisis that impact policy for acute and chronic health care: escalating costs, limited access, and quality of care. These problems present a clear and compelling case for change.

Escalating Health Costs   The most propelling factor driving health care policy reform is its cost, which directly affects both access to care and quality of care. During the 1960s and early 1970s, there was a rapid explosion of new technologies and concomitant increases in health care expenditures. The drive to cost containment became a consequence of these escalating health expenditures.

Between 1970 and 1990, health care expenditures in the United States increased exponentially compared to national income increases (see Chapter 22, on financial impact). In fact, the health care share of the Gross Domestic Product (GDP) grew from 7.3 percent to 12.3 percent in the same 20 years. During that period of time, it was accurately predicted that the share of the GDP for health care would rise to 14 percent per year by 1992 and continue to rise to 16 percent by the year 2000 (Steuerle, 1993).

Steuerle (1993) also accurately estimated that total health care expenditures in the United States would exceed $700 billion per year by 1992, with money coming from individuals (out-of-pocket); employers' and employees' share of private health insurance; other private sources; Medicare, Medicaid, and other public programs; federal tax subsidies; and state tax subsidies (see Figure 23-1).

In today's health care system, individuals with chronic illnesses or their families are often responsible for a major part of their health care costs. Steuerle (1993) estimates that the average health care costs per household in the United

States is $8,000 per year, with approximately a third paid directly by individuals or families. Frequently, people with a chronic illness are excluded from private sector insurance plans. According to the Congressional Office of Technology Assessment, in the spring of 1988, of the 30 conditions that were cited as causes for denial of insurance coverage, all but one were considered to be a chronic illness (Lee, Soffel, & Luft, 1992).

Cost Containment   Attempts have been made by both the private and public sectors at a variety of cost-containment efforts. According to the National Leadership Commission on Health Care (1989), factors driving cost increases in health care, especially in long-term care, include inflation in medical care prices; the aging of the population; greater demands for access and quality, which increase use of inappropriate care; the oversupply of physicians; the practice of defensive medicine; and expensive new technologies.

The current system of fee-for-service medicine, along with third-party reimbursement, rewards providers for dispensing more service regardless of benefits or appropriateness (Enthoven, 1988). It is interesting to note that if reimbursement policies included incentives to prevent disease and to treat acute illness in less costly settings, and if there were changes in how physicians' services are paid, care for chronic illness could be met without substantial increases in cost (Fox, 1989).

In the authors' opinion, providing health care for those who cannot afford to purchase it inevitably requires financial resources from those who can pay. The need for adequate financial coverage is a problem that policy has not adequately addressed. Unfortunately, individuals who are either uninsured or underinsured tend to delay seeking help until they are extremely ill, creating more of a burden on the health care system.

Access   As the goals of our nation's health care programs are restructured, the priority given to access and quality of care for the chronically ill patient becomes important. In fact, access to health care is so interrelated to cost and quality

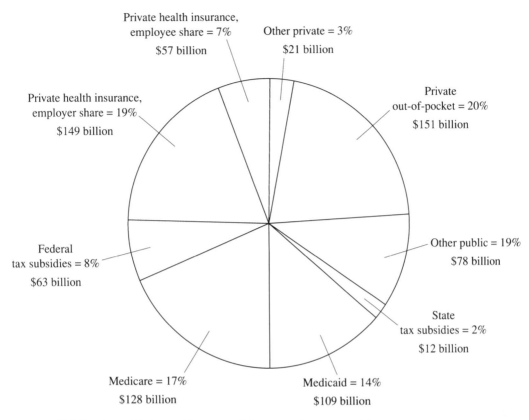

Private health insurance, employee share = 7%
$57 billion

Other private = 3%
$21 billion

Private out-of-pocket = 20%
$151 billion

Private health insurance, employer share = 19%
$149 billion

Other public = 19%
$78 billion

Federal tax subsidies = 8%
$63 billion

State tax subsidies = 2%
$12 billion

Medicare = 17%
$128 billion

Medicaid = 14%
$109 billion

FIGURE 23-1.   Estimated Sources of Financing for U.S. Health Care Expenditures, Fiscal Year 1992

SOURCE: From Steuerle, E. C. (1993). The search for adaptable health policy through finance-based reform. In R.B. Helms (Ed.), *American health policy: Critical issues for reform* (p. 336). Washington, D.C.: The American Enterprise Institute Press.

of health care that interrelated solutions must be sought (National Leadership Commission on Health Care Reform, 1989). Access to health care increased in the 1960s and early 1970s, with the institution of third-party reimbursement, Medicare, and Medicaid paying for services rendered.

Our current system of health care accommodates the chronically ill person in a fragmented way in spite of the fact that the chronically ill need a continuum of services as their illnesses shift between acute and long-term care. Full access to needed services is not available, making quality of care difficult to address. The issue of access versus quality of care often finds patient

advocate groups in direct conflict with those who pay for patient care (Benjamin, 1988).

Impact on Quality of Care   Another political force shaping today's health care policy reforms are special interest groups and professional organizations interested in seeing that individuals within their areas of concern receive quality care. Kalisch and Kalisch (1987) defined a special interest group as "an association of people concerned with protecting and promoting shared values through the use of political power." Special interest groups demonstrate their power collectively by learning about and understanding issues and articulating this knowledge to legislators. A few examples of special interest groups that influence health care policy changes include The American Nurses' Association (ANA), the American Medical Association (AMA), the American Federation of Labor–Congress of Industrial Organizations (AFL-CIO), and the American Association of Retired People (AARP).

Many special interest groups have full-time lobbyists monitoring governmental activities for their organizations, so that action to promote their interests can be initiated and attempts can be made to block actions that would negatively affect their concerns. Regardless of the type of special interest group, access to legislators and knowledge of the political process is a key to influencing policy decisions (DeVries & Vanderbilt, 1992).

Social Issues and Forces

Social issues affecting policy that impact chronically ill individuals include the social components of increased health care costs, the aging of our population, the acquired immune deficiency syndrome (AIDS) epidemic, the deinstitutionalization of the mentally ill, the increasing prevalence of disability across all age groups, and the provisions for long-term care.

Health Care Costs   Health care costs are a social as well as a political issue. Today's political environment finds many opposing forces, not only in health care but in environmental regulation, social and welfare reform, housing, and so forth. Fiscal budgets, with scarce money resources, are influenced by both the numbers and the political persuasions of people competing for these limited funds (Steuerle, 1993; DeVries & Vanderbilt, 1992; Fox, 1990).

Indirect costs of illness will rise significantly as the number of individuals with functional limitations associated with chronic illnesses increases. Lubeck and Yelin (1988) point out the importance of measuring these indirect costs in an effort to provide accurate information to policymakers who are determining the allocation of scarce resources. They have developed a basic health status tool that measures the loss of capacity to function rather than focusing on expenses

incurred for medical services. This tool measures work-related, social, and leisure activity as well as the person's ability to perform these activities over time.

The Aging of Our Population   The number of elderly in the population is expected to grow from 30.3 million in 1988 to twice that number by the year 2025. By that year, one in every five persons will be over 65 years of age, with one-third that number over 85 years of age (National Leadership Commission on Health Care, 1989). American policy must be prepared to meet the support, housing, and health care needs of this enormous group of elderly.

The AIDS Epidemic   Until recently, there was a poor understanding of the long-term care requirements of AIDS (Benjamin, 1988). Most people who determine health policy perceive AIDS as the end stage of "a chronic disease that is spreading most rapidly among the disadvantaged, especially among Blacks and Hispanics" (Fox, 1990, p. 34). In fact, by 1988, the cumulative total of cases per 100,000 was three times higher among African-American men and two times higher among Hispanic men than among white men. In the pediatric population, the cumulative rates were four times higher among African Americans and two times higher among Hispanics (CDC, 1989).

Policy related to AIDS needs to be based on prevention because prevention is proving to be the most cost-effective intervention. For example, in the homosexual population where prevention is addressed, the incidence of AIDS is decreasing, even though it is increasing in the heterosexual population (Fox, 1990). However, the increased incidence of AIDS and the cost involved in its treatment have an adverse financial impact on policy geared to assisting the elderly and other chronically ill individuals.

Important similarities exist between the care needs of the AIDS population and those of the frail elderly. Both populations experience health conditions that are chronic, possibly debilitating, and terminal. Both populations are characterized by relatively brief episodes requiring hospitalization and longer periods where care can be provided in nursing facilities or at home (Fox, 1990).

Both populations require personal care and support services from their communities, since most of their time is spent there (Benjamin, 1988; Fox, 1990); unfortunately, support services that are often in short supply. In addition, both populations depend on friends and family (see Chapter 12, on the family caregiver), nonprofessional support persons who may themselves be vulnerable to illness and dependency (Benjamin, 1988).

Attempts to meet both the acute and chronic health care needs of both populations often fail to consider complex issues related to the development and implementation of services based on need. Currently, assistance is based on "controlling the utilization of hospital care; limiting the role of nursing home care; expanding the availability of home- and community-based services and of hospice care; and developing case management as a mechanism to coordinate the delivery of care" (Benjamin, 1988, p. 418). Policy must be expanded so it not only deals with the acute and chronic health care needs of individuals but emphasizes prevention and lifestyle changes.

Deinstitutionalization   In the 1960s, it was believed that clients' conditions would improve, care would be more humane, and costs would decrease if the mentally ill were cared for in communities. In fact, the desire for deinstitutionalization was driven by concerns over inhumane custodial treatment and a growing interest in freeing patients from hospitalization while offering a less restrictive treatment alternative. The release of so many individuals who required ongoing mental care created a further demand for services, but no concurrent growth in the number of community-based health centers was forthcoming. Thousands of people were discharged into areas unprepared to care for them.

Even today, in addition to their health care needs, this population faces problems in housing, employment, rehabilitation, and financing (Aviram, 1990). Some estimate that about one-third of the homeless are persons with mental illness. Some 30 years following the advent of deinstitutionalization, many individuals still emphasize the need to establish a comprehensive system of community care and treatment (Aviram, 1990).

The release of the mentally ill into communities is comparable to the current emphasis on limiting the utilization of hospital-based care for chronic conditions. It is felt by some that there is a potential for cost savings when fewer days of hospital care of the chronically ill patient are associated with increased community-based care. However, one must question if there will be a repeat of the problems that plagued deinstitutionalization, or if communities will be prepared to meet the needs of patients discharged from hospitals in a more acute state.

Disability and Impairment   There are a growing number of individuals with disabilities or impairments (see Chapter 24, on rehabilitation). For instance, 10 to 15 percent of American children have chronic illnesses, and an increasing proportion of them have some degree of activity limitation (Newacheck & McManas, 1988). A major factor that has contributed to the increased prevalence of childhood disability is the increasing survival rates of low-birth-weight babies and their residual chronic illnesses. Chronically ill children with activity limitations use more health care services, such as hospital-based services and those provided by nonphysician health professionals, than other children (Newacheck & McManas, 1988). Total charges for health services per affected child showed a threefold increase in 1986 compared to 1980.

Disabled people are present in all social classes and status groups in American society. As many as 1 in 11 Americans of working age identify themselves as having a disability. Research suggests that two to eight times as many disabled or functionally impaired persons are cared for in the community as are institutionalized (Ford et al., 1991). It is interesting to note that while functional impairment and mental health impairment increase the chances of being institutionalized, multiple chronic conditions do not (Ford et al., 1991).

Long-Term Care   Long-term care is supportive care (such as nursing, medical, or rehabilitative) needed by individuals with physical or mental impairments over an extended period of time. Unfortunately, it can be very expensive. Scientific and technological advances of the 20th century allow more people to survive birth, injury, and chronic illness. However, the resultant increase in longevity is accompanied by a continuously rising number of individuals with chronic disabilities.

It is estimated that by the year 2000, at least 40 percent of those in need of long-term care secondary to chronic conditions will be under 65 years of age (National Leadership Commission on Health Care, 1989). It goes without saying that as people live longer, they remain eager to maintain their independence while they cope with chronic illness (Fox & Willis, 1989).

Currently, the majority of residents in long-term care facilities suffer from multiple chronic illnesses and confront multiple losses: physical, self-concept, role performance, family and social relationships, independence, and financial. These individuals are disproportionately very old, female, and white, and their health problems tend to restrict their ability to care for themselves. (Fox & Willis, 1989).

Since the introduction of Medicare and Medicaid, the rate of long-term care facility use has gone from 2.5 percent to 5 percent among the over-65 age group. Current projections indicate that by 2000, the number of nursing home residents over the age of 65 will increase from the 1985 figure of 1.3 million to 2.0 million. This number is expected to more than double to 4.6 million by 2040 (National Leadership Commission on Health Care, 1989).

Unfortunately, Medicare focuses on covering acute care, and many services remain outside its usual scope. The nursing home benefit covered by Medicare is restricted to 100 days and must follow acute hospitalization, leaving most long-term care of chronically ill patients uncovered. In addition, beneficiaries are now required to pay co-payments and share the costs of their care.

Although Medicaid supplements Medicare, benefits for those who are eligible occurs only after Medicare benefits have been exhausted and the patient is impoverished. Medicaid benefits, which vary from state to state, are less than costs. The elderly in long-term care facilities who have exhausted their financial resources and Medicare benefits may be faced with discharge from the institution (Burgess & Ragland, 1983). In addi-

tion, many skilled nursing facilities do not take Medicaid because of the low reimbursement schedule.

It can thus be seen that chronic illness is often accompanied by uncertainty and often by the loss of financial security, creating a feeling of loss of control. This perception of powerlessness can lead to a cycle of lowered self-esteem, depression, isolation, loneliness, and eventually death (Bruss, 1988; Miller, 1992). The case study of M. B. shows how being in a long-term facility can adversely impact an individual.

Solutions and Interventions

To plan for solutions in health care reform, especially for those with chronic conditions, is difficult considering the present political climate. Given the ongoing improvements in medical technology and a concomitant increase in life expectancy, there is a coinciding, substantial rise in the number of individuals with chronic disease. Although policy research seeks solutions for organizing, financing, and delivering acute and long-term care services, no satisfactory conclusions have as yet been reached.

Several proposed solutions that seek to provide expanded access, cost containment, and a more comprehensive method of financing health care are presented briefly. Health providers can be more effective in influencing policy by becoming activists through gaining knowledge about health care issues and educating both legislators and the general public. In addition, the authors suggest a systems theory approach as a method that could be useful in achieving activism. The authors also take the liberty of making several suggestions for policy reform.

Proposed Solutions to Meet Policy Needs

The problems of financing health care have catalyzed a national movement toward reform. Financing is not only of major interest to policymakers, but paying for health care, acute or chronic, is an increasing concern of most Americans. Much of the public's misgivings about our present health care system arise from

CASE STUDY
A Long-Term Care Resident in a Nursing Home

M. B. was an 82-year-old male widower, "involuntarily" admitted to a long-term care facility following surgery for a left hip fracture. Following hospitalization, hip pinning, and recovery from this acute condition, the hospital social worker on his case was given the task of arranging his discharge planning.

The only family members M. B. had were two adult children living out of state. Relations with his family were estranged. His rehabilitation, level of dependence, and continuing need for care required admission to a long-term facility because there was no one to care for him at home. M. B. also had a long history of various chronic illnesses, including arteriosclerotic heart disease, chronic

obstructive pulmonary disease, and congestive heart failure. Treatment for these illnesses required a complex daily regimen of medications.

During the one year of his residence in the facility, M. B. complained that his home and personal belongings and other financial resources were being exhausted. In his perception, the system was "stealing my (his) identity."

M. B. exhibited severe depression and adapted poorly to life in the long-term care facility. Therapeutic interactions and antidepressant prescriptions were unsuccessful. M. B. died two weeks later after he developed complications of his congestive heart failure even though it was felt the complications were not severe.

---

the inequitable manner in which health care costs are funded.

Government involvement is an outgrowth of our present fragmented system and the presence of millions of Americans who are either uninsured or underinsured. The National Leadership Commission on Health Care (1989) stated that approximately 37 million Americans have no health insurance and that approximately 75 percent of these individuals are employees or dependents of employees; most in this group are in jobs where health insurance is not offered.

Many individuals with acute or chronic conditions who have insurance find themselves paying higher premiums for coverage. A variety of cost-containment and financing measures have been attempted by both private and public sectors, but these attempts have been unsuccessful in decreasing costs.

In the early 1980s, the predominant health insurance arrangement was conventional "indemnity" plans purchased by employers as a benefit (Weiner & Lissovoy, 1993). About 90 percent of working Americans and their dependents were covered by these plans. Under this system, the insured could choose any provider, and physicians and hospitals had few constraints. Insurance companies paid all bills submitted to them on a retrospective basis known as "fee-for-

service." Generally, providers determined the rates and terms of reimbursement. Both Medicare and Medicaid are structured along the lines of this traditional model.

However, with the growing number of individuals who are not covered by any plan, and with the escalation of health care costs, attention is now directed at other methods of attaining coverage. These methods are addressed briefly, but the reader is encouraged to explore them in greater depth.

Consumers of health care need to be educated in the selection of services in the least costly settings. Merely being presented with health care plans is not enough to achieve the needed results of lowered costs. A solution may require the creation of competition among providers. Consumers must be offered a choice that will provide for their health care needs as well as the delivery of a basic quality of care. An environment needs to be created to reward providers for both quality and economy, and might benefit from being managed by a third party or sponsor (Kronick, 1993). Consumers must decide, should such an approach be implemented, if they are willing to limit the many choices that now exist.

Approaches for Funding Health Care Two systems have been considered in recent years for covering the costs of health care, both emphasizing the responsibility of employers. The first, called "pay-or-play," was heralded in 1993 as the financial means of extending health care coverage to all consumers. In 1994, the emphasis shifted to "employer mandates" as the best way of financing health care. The entire area of financial approaches continues to be volatile, and a final solution to this issue remains undecided.

In the pay-or-play system, employers would either have to purchase insurance for all their employees (play) or be assessed a tax (pay) (Steuerle, 1993). Employers who "played" would receive a tax credit for the sum they spent on insurance. The tax paid by employers who did not participate would help finance an insurance plan managed by the government (Sharp, 1992). Opponents of this system argue that it would be unfair to employers, and that unemployed or retired people would not be covered. In addition, moving from a private to a public plan could be very time consuming and could require a constant adjustment of insurance policy charges and the withholding rate (Steuerle, 1993).

The emphasis on employer mandates differs from the pay-or-play approach. Under this system, employers would pay most of the costs of health care coverage, with employees contributing a lesser amount. Changing employment or the onset of a chronic condition would not impact adversely on coverage. Opponents of the employer mandate argue that the system would add an unfair burden on small businesses. Others believe that under this system, spreading the health care costs of the unemployed and uninsured onto the business community would be unfair (Zuckerman, 1993).

Managed Care By 1990 a variety of new health care delivery systems had developed, and traditional indemnity health insurance policies no longer covered the majority of American consumers. These new systems have become known as "managed care" or "alternative delivery systems" (Weiner & Lissovoy, 1993). (See Chapter 20, on nursing case management.) The criterion that distinguishes managed care plans from prior ones is the use of practice controls on the provider's patterns of billing.

Managed care is a term used for all types of integrated delivery systems and often refers to the utilization control methods that are employed in various settings to manage the practices of physicians, hospitals, and others. These methods may include a mandatory second opinion before surgery, pre-admission approval, certification of treatment plans for non-emergency services, and case managers to monitor the care of particular patients (Weiner & Lissovoy, 1993). In other words, "The patients's treatment must be authorized before it is delivered, with approval based on proprietary protocols for care" (Finkel, 1993), not on fee for service.

Managed care proponents contend that costs are controlled by regulating the types and frequency of visits. Finkel (1993) contends that managed care "neither can nor will contain overall health care spending." Unfortunately, Finkel's contention has proven true. Managed care has not proven to be cost effective and has dramatically added to fragmentation of care and an inefficient system.

Health Maintenance Organizations The health maintenance organization (HMO) is a type of managed care chosen by 5 percent of Americans in 1980 (Weiner & Lissovoy, 1993). An HMO is defined as "a prepaid organized delivery system where the organization and the primary care physicians assume financial risk for the care provided to its enrolled members" (Weiner & Lissovoy, 1993). Typically, the physician or organization is paid on a capitation (per head) basis. In this closed network, members must obtain care from within the system if it is to be reimbursed.

HMO savings, which come from elimination of unnecessary hospital admissions, decreased length of stay, and controlled hospital costs, have merely shifted the expenses to diagnostic service and outpatient costs (Finkel, 1993). In addition, the HMO industry is finding the need to deal with complaints of dissatisfaction from both patients and physicians: Patients complain about difficulty in seeing the same physician, and physicians complain of not getting to know their patients.

Preferred Provider Organizations Another type of managed care plan is the preferred provider organization (PPO). The PPO acts as a broker channeling consumers to in-plan providers by the use of incentives and disincentives related to benefit coverage. Providers agree to imposed practice controls in return for patient referrals. A successful PPO identifies efficient health care providers who furnish quality care at a reasonable cost (Finkel, 1993). Under the PPO system employers can assure recipients that all are receiving the same access to and quality of care. However, the employer cannot assure the recipient that the quality of care within the PPO is the same as the quality of care outside the PPO (Finkel, 1993).

Managed Competition Managed competition is a different health care system model that integrates many features of managed care. In this type of system, independent integrated managed care plans would compete with one another in a market system closely regulated by the federal government. In other words, the health plan itself would be "managed" (Weiner & Lissovoy, 1993). This model proposes to control health care spending and ensure access by encouraging providers and insurance companies to merge and form community-based health partnerships. Managed competition would be promoted "among health care plans, insurance and Medicaid reform, and tax code changes" (Sharp, 1992). Such a plan would be subjected to national and state budgets, and prepaid HMOs would become a favorite among the plans offered to consumers.

Although managed competition allows insurers to compete, thus possibly controlling or lowering health care costs, one must question what this will do to quality of care. Most physicians would be unwilling to quote a set fee for care without first knowing the patient's symptoms, since costs in the past were determined by the patient's acuity. Will health care be purchased on the basis of value and will contracts be given to providers who deliver the best care for the best price? Or will price be the only consideration? Many experts in health care contend that a cost discipline needs to be built into efforts to improve access to care, and could best be achieved through incentives rather than government control (Meyer, 1993).

Government-Based Approach: Single Payer
Many individuals favor a single-payor health care system that provides universal access through a health insurance system administered by the government. Under this system, savings would occur through an expanded program and cost controls on provider reimbursements. This approach anticipates that the savings on insurance administrative costs would provide enough funds to cover the uninsured or underinsured. The system would use a single, public payor as the administrator. One argument in favor of this system is the low administrative costs of the Medicare system compared to the costs of private insurance plans (Sharp, 1992).

Under a single-payer system, private fee-for-service care would be allowed via contract with the payor. However, the nonprofit prepaid groups with salaried physicians would be preferred; more funds would be received by prepaid group practices that maintain a high percentage of elderly and chronically ill enrollees (Bosenheimer, 1993). The single-payer program is currently in use in Canada.

Private Sector Approach There is a reluctance among many Americans to make radical changes in our health care system which they consider one of the best in the world. The authors believe that these individuals feel that the current system of coverage and financing should remain with some changes. Modification of our current system could be accomplished by simplifying forms in use or using a universal form, by continuing coverage even in the face of a chronic illness, or by continuing coverage even if there is a loss of employment.

Policy as a Systems Approach

Knowledge alone is inadequate if health providers are to participate in the development of meaningful health care policy. Providers must be actively involved in the process of developing and planning for health care if they value choice and quality. They must share the responsibility, with consumers, of seeing that there is satisfactory financing and access for all.

A systems approach is one method of achieving activism. Social policy may be approached

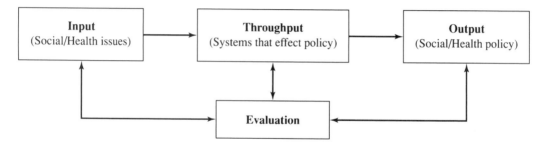

FIGURE 23-2. Open-System Approach to Social/Health Policy

as an open system that is always in an evolutionary state (see Figure 23-2). This approach was first described by Easton (1957) in relation to political systems, and it has been modified numerous times by public policy scholars and by various authors. The first stage, *the issues at hand,* is the inputs or demands on the political system. The second stage, *throughput,* is the activities of special interest groups and their specific issues struggling to influence policy. The third stage, *output,* is the decisions or actions that emerge from the political system in the form of social/health policy. Included in this third stage is the implementation of policy, which is essentially the end product of the throughput stage.

The fourth stage involves *evaluation,* which is of extreme importance yet is often overlooked (Dye, 1987). Evaluation can occur at the end of each stage so modifications can be made, but should also be done at the completion of the other three stages to determine the impact or effectiveness of *actions* on the policy that results.

The case study dealing with legislation on prescriptive authority for nurse practitioners is one example of the use of systems theory to achieve constructive change in health policy.

Education

Education regarding chronic illness for future health care providers is becoming a more important area of curriculum. In the opinion of the authors, it should be mandatory for health care curricula to include the epidemiological trends of chronic illness, to identify political and social

forces, and to encourage students to become familiar with possible intervention strategies, so that, as future practitioners they can effectively address the trends and needs from which policy can emerge.

However, education is not limited to those in school. Practicing professionals need to become knowledgeable on a subject or subjects, thereby becoming experts. As experts they can educate legislators, become community activists to increase public awareness of health issues, and contribute to health political action in other ways. In other words, becoming cognitive of the problems, issues, and trends allows health care providers to predict and plan for future needs, and it allows them to educate the public on the problems and issues that exist, including those of the chronically ill.

Education of Legislators Knowledgeable health care providers can educate legislators to ensure effective health care policy. The impact of the increasing prevalence of chronic illness must be understood before effective policies can emerge. The general public must also be educated so they can articulate to legislators their concerns about the need for a rational policy.

Policy makers must (1) know value preferences and the impact of these values on society; (2) be familiar with existing and potential alternative policies and understand their impact; (3) know the benefits to society that alternatives will achieve; and (4) be able to select the most appropriate policy, current or alternative, that will achieve the greatest impact and meet particular needs (Dye, 1987). For this decision-making process to occur, an educative component is

CASE STUDY

Social/Health Policy as an Open System: Legislation on Prescriptive Authority for Nurse Practitioners (An example of legislation in a U.S. East-Coast state)

Access to health care for all citizens was an issue of concern to nurses (Stage I). The state nurses' association began to formulate a plan in collaboration with the state nurse practitioner group (Stage II). A patron to sponsor the legislation was identified in the state legislature, and the bill was presented before the General Assembly. Unfortunately, the bill did not carry (Stage III). A thorough evaluation of the failure of the legislation indicated that state legislators and the general public lacked knowledge on the issue. (Stage IV).

The situation was critically analyzed, and changes were implemented as appropriate. A plan was initiated to educate the state legislators and the general public about the role of nurse practitioners (Stage II). A nurse was assigned to each state legislator and charged with the responsibility of educating that one individual on the issue and how the extended role of nurse practitioners would increase access to health care. Also, information pamphlets were prepared and distributed on the advance practice roles of nurse practitioners. These educational efforts were continued until the next session of the General Assembly.

The coalition building through education on this issue was effective. The legislation carried in the next session with only four dissenting votes (Stage III).

---

necessary in order that policy can achieve maximum social gain.

Public Education Nurses historically have been advocates on behalf of their clients. In today's climate, it is not uncommon to see nurses assuming a major role in education of the general public on health care issues. Through education, the public gains an understanding of the need for health care reform and prompts action as a public policy process. Nurses expedite this process not only through public education but by testifying at public hearings and sharing their expertise on health care issues with others (DeVries & Vanderbilt, 1992).

Public Support

Most of the reforms now being proposed for health care, including those for chronic illness, cannot possibly succeed without a substantial level of public support. There exists a major gap between the public's view of the health care crisis and the way the crisis is viewed by experts (Yankelovich & Immerwahr, 1991). The public perception is that the driving forces behind rising health care costs are human and moral in nature: greed and waste. Experts and political leaders see the causes as technical and structural in nature: technological and medical advances and increasing numbers of chronically ill individuals. The gap between these perceptions must be addressed before the nation can solve its health care crisis (Yankelovich & Immerwahr, 1991).

Given this basic difference of opinion, it is not surprising that limited public support exists for solutions that have been proposed to address the crisis in chronic illness. Yankelovich and Immerwahr (1991) recommend that proposed reforms be debated openly in an effort to provide information to, as well as educate, the general public. The perception gap between legislators and the general public on the problems and issues related to chronic illness can only be closed through education. Nurses can assist in bridging this gap and achieving public support by testifying at public hearings, sharing professional views with legislators, and making recommendations for legislative proposals that relate to chronic illness.

Future Policy Direction

The historical, political, and social forces previously identified, and the problems and issues of the chronically ill, impact future policy. Rational policies should be based on principles that are widely accepted and that meet the needs of the chronically ill. They should be comprehensive and include a full range of health and social services to provide a continuum from community-based care to institutional care (Lewis, 1993).

A policy that utilizes a special-needs approach to disability has a short-run perspective. A universal policy is needed that recognizes the entire population as being at risk for chronic illnesses and disabilities (Zola, 1989). Disease progression should be considered a universal approach; an important caveat to this perspective is the changing nature of disability—that is, the awareness that health care needs change (Zola, 1989).

Will a universal policy cover the spectrum of specific individuals' health care needs as their chronic illnesses progress over their life spans? And will a universal policy cover all individuals regardless of age if they have chronic illnesses? Until recently, there was a failure of policy to understand the chronic care requirements of most disease trajectories. These must be considered in the future if policy is to be effective.

Many uncertainties about the current climate of health care reform make predictions or recommendations about future policy difficult. Ideally, social/health policy for the chronically ill should rest exclusively on the application of altruistic and ethical principles (see Chapter 19, on nursing ethics). To date, this has not occurred. Future policy on chronic illness must focus in four areas: surveillance, prevention, research, and financing.

Surveillance　Attention to prevalence and incidence of chronic illnesses and projection of numbers into the future will be vital for planning proactive strategies to meet the health care needs of the chronically ill. The authors' greatest fear is that, although statistics are available, nothing is being done with the information, and this might continue until reform in health policy becomes so critical that action is imperative, and we end up with reactive policy.

Prevention　Prevention policy is expanding to include educating the general public about healthy life-styles so that they can become integrated throughout their life spans. Such education can delay the onset of chronic illnesses as well as reduce the number of people who acquire these illnesses. A new paradigm is emerging, and the medical model is changing to one of prevention, which is the most cost-effective intervention. Health professionals are major players in this model and recognize that prevention can be integrated into people's life-styles at a much earlier age. But the role of health professionals is only part of the solution. More consumers are taking more responsibility for maintaining healthy life-styles for prevention, and many now consider this almost a moral obligation.

Research　Research is the means for appropriate planning to occur. In the past, research focused on cost containment as opposed to outcome-based studies (see Chapter 17, on research).

> While a good deal of research is conducted on various medical technologies, not enough has been done on their effectiveness in common settings or in very specific circumstances. In other words, whether a technology works does not necessarily answer the question whether it makes a difference in the end results. (National Leadership Commission on Health Care 1989, Appendix C)

The government, via the Institutes of Health, provides funding for much of the research done in health care. It becomes imperative for the institutes to include more research dollars to study the long-term effects of chronic illness, including such factors as illness' impact on functional well-being, on chronically ill individuals' access to health care services, and on the availability of health care services for this population.

Finances　Financing health care for persons with chronic illnesses is the most difficult policy area currently being considered. Meeting the needs of the chronically ill is expensive and will become more so as increasing numbers of people live longer. A sane and sound policy dealing with the financial burden faced by the chronically ill person requires knowledge of health status, specific demographics (such as rural versus urban), and the specific chronic condition.

Summary and Conclusions

Current health policy has not solved the problems of access, costs, and quality of care for all Americans, including the chronically ill. Defining the dimension of the problems that exist and identifying various approaches to organizing, financing, and delivering acute and long-term care services continue to be a major focus for health care policy reform. The chronically ill person who continues to absorb an ever-growing proportion of our public and private resources must be given attention.

The intent of this chapter has been to allow the reader to recognize some of the social and political issues that are driving policy reform. The problems of reform arise from a combination of social, historical, political, and technolog-

ical factors. Simple solutions are unlikely unless the driving forces are addressed. The prospect of reform is exciting and is presently energizing the policy arena to take action. Every American must become actively involved, since Americans place a high premium on health care, which they regard as a fundamental right. Providers must realize that they are competing in a market that continues to demand both quality and access, with consumers demanding cuts in cost. The political dynamics of the issues must be understood by providers, and there must be a response to consumer demands.

In the presence of widespread disagreement on the financing of health care, the creation of a mechanism more equitable and more efficient to all Americans, including those with chronic illnesses, has yet to be accomplished. In the meantime, millions of Americans continue to go without needed health care, and billions of dollars are spent each year on health care that in no way provides adequate coverage to all Americans.

STUDY QUESTIONS

1. Who is at risk for chronic illness or disability?
2. Describe the trends in prevalence of chronic illness and how these trends are significant in relation to health policy.
3. Describe social/health policy's relation to public policy.
4. How did social/health policy's relationship to chronic illness change following World War II?
5. Explain the significance of the Social Security Act of 1965.
6. What was the goal of health policy in the late 1970s?
7. Describe the major political issues affecting health policy for the chronically ill.
8. Define special interest groups and describe their significance to chronic illness.
9. Name and describe the major social issues affecting health policy for the chronically ill.
10. Compare managed care and managed competition.
11. In what ways can education influence social/health policy of chronic illness?
12. Explain the systems approach to social/health policy. When should the evaluation stage occur?
13. List four areas of focus that future health policy for chonic illness must consider.

References

Aviram, U. (1990, February). Community care of the seriously mentally ill: Continuing problems and current issues. *Community Mental Health Journal, 26*(1), 69–86.

Benjamin, A. E. (1988). Long-term care and AIDS: Perspectives from experience with the elderly. *The Milbank Quarterly, 66*(3), 415–439.

———(1993). An historical perspective on home care policy. *The Milbank Quarterly, 71*(1), 129–166.

Bosenheimer, T. A. (1993, June). Yes, for single payer. *Networks, 5*(23), 3.

Brant, B. J., & Osgood, D. W. (1990). The suicidal patient in long term care institutions. *Journal of Gerontological Nursing, 16*(2), 15–18.

Bruss, C. R. (1988). Nursing diagnosis of hopelessness. *Journal of Psychosocial Nursing and Mental Health Services, 26*(3), 28-31.

Burgess, W., & Ragland, E.C. (1983). *Community health nursing: Philosophy, process, practice.* Norwalk CT: Appleton-Century-Crofts.

DeVries, C. M., & Vanderbilt, M. W. (1992). *The grassroots lobbying handbook: Empowering nurses through legislative and political action.* Washington D.C.: American Nurses' Association.

Dye, T. R. (1987). *Understanding public policy* (6th ed.). Englewood Cliffs, NJ: Prentice-Hall.

Easton. D. (1957). An approach to the analysis of political systems. *World Politics, 9,* 383-400.

Enthoven, A. (1988). Managed competition of alternative delivery systems. *Journal of Health Politics, Policy and Law, 13,* 305-322.

Finkel, M. L. (1993, Spring). Managed care is not the answer (Commentary). *Journal of Health Politics, Policy, and Law, 18*(1), 105-111.

Ford, A. B., Roy, A. W., Haug, M. R., Folmar, S. J., & Jones, P. K. (1991). Impaired and disabled elderly in the community. *American Journal of Public Health, 81*(9), 1207-1209.

Fox, D. M. (Ed.) (1989). Policy in epidemiology: Financing health services for the chronically ill and disabled 1930-1990. *The Milbank Quarterly, 67*(2), 257-283.

——— (1990). Chronic disease and disadvantage: The new politics of HIV infection. *Journal of Health Politics, Policy and Law, 15*(2), 341-355.

Fox, D. M., & Willis, D. P. (1989). Introduction. *The Milbank Quarterly, 67*(2, part 1), 1-12.

Hadley, J. P., & Langwell, K. (1991). Managed care in the United States: Promises, evidence to date and future directions (Review). *Health Policy, 19,* 91-118.

Kalisch, P. A., & Kalisch, B. J. (1987). *The changing image of the nurse.* Menlo Park, CA: Addison-Wesley.

Kronick, R. (1993). Managed competition—why we don't have it and how we can get it. In R. B. Helms (Eds), *American health policy: Critical issues for reform* (pp. 44-63). Washington, D.C.: AEI Press.

Lasswell, H. D., & Kaplan, A. (1970). *Power and society.* New Haven: Yale University Press.

Lee, P. R., Soffel, D., & Luft, H. S. (1992). Costs and coverage: Pressures toward health care reform. *Western Journal of Medicine, 157*(5), 576-583.

Lewis, C. K. (1993). *The relationship of health status, population characteristics, and specific chronic health conditions of the frail rural elderly to the availability/utilization of community-based services with implications for future policy.* Fairfax, VA: George Mason University.

Longer, C. R. (1988). Nursing diagnosis of hopelessness. *Journal of Psychosocial Nursing and Mental Health Services, 26*(3), 28-31.

Lubeck, D. P., & Yelin, E. H. (1988). A question of value: Measuring the impact of chronic disease. *The Milbank Quarterly, 66*(3), 444-462.

Meyer, J. A. (1993). Innovations and Impediments in private sector initiatives. In R. B. Helms (Ed.), *American health policy critical issues for reform* (pp. 213-224). Washington D.C.: AEI Press.

Miller, J. F. (1992). *Coping with chronic illness: Overcoming powerlessness.* Philadelphia: F. A. Davis.

Mockenhaupt, R. E., & Muchow, J. A. (1994). Disease and disability prevention and health promotion for rural elders. In J. A. Krout (Ed.), *Providing community-based services to the rural elderly.* Beverly Hills, CA: Sage.

National Leadership Commission on Health Care. (1989). *For the health of a nation: A shared responsibility.* Ann Arbor, MI: Health Administration Press Perspectives.

Newacheck, P. W., & McManas, M. A. (Eds.) (1988). Financing healthcare for disabled children. *Pediatrics, 81*(3), 385-394.

Reinhardt, U. E. (1992, Winter). The United States: Breakthroughs and waste. *Journal of Health Politics, Policy and Law, 17*(4), 637-666.

Schauffler, H. H. (1993). Disease prevention policy under Medicare: A historical and political analysis. *American Journal of Preventive Medicine, 9* (2), 71-77.

Sharp, N. (1992, November 23). Major themes in healthcare reform (Washington Correspondent). *The Nursing Spectrum,* p. 13.

Smith, J. P. (1990). The politics of American health care. *Journal of Advanced Nursing, 15,* 487-497.

Steuerle, C. E. (1993). The search for adaptable health policy through finance-based reform. In R. B. Helms (Ed.), *American health policy: Critical issues for reform* (pp. 334-361). Washington, D.C.: AEI Press.

Stuart, G. W., & Sundeen, S. J. (1991). *Principles and practice of psychitric nursing* (4th ed.). St. Louis: Mosby.

Vail, J. D. (1990). Health Policy. In J. Dienemann (Ed.), *Nursing administration strategic perspectives and application.* (pp. 71-92). Norwalk, CT: Appleton & Lange.

Weiner, J. P., & Lissovoy, G. D. (Eds.). (1993, Spring). Razing a tower of Babel: A taxonomy for managed care. *Journal of Health Politics, Policy and Law, 18*(1), 75-103.

Wilson, R. W., & Drury, T. F. (1984). Interpreting trends in illness and disability: Health statistics and health status. *Annual Review of Public Health 5,* 83-106.

Yankelovich, D., & Immerwahr, J. (1991). A perception gap. *HMO, Third Quarter,* pp. 11-14.

Yura, H., & Walsh, M. B. (1988). *The Nursing process: Assessing, planning, implementing, evaluating* (5th ed.). Norwalk, CT: Appleton & Lange.

Zola, I. K. (1989). Toward the necessary universalizing of a disability policy. *The Milbank Quarterly, 67* (Suppl. 2, part 2), 401-429.

Zuckerman, S. (1993). Commentary on part II. In R. B. Helms (Ed.), *American health policy critical issues for reform* (pp. 201-205). Washington, D.C.: AEI Press.

Bibliography

Anderson, J. M. (1990). Home care management in chronic illness and the self-care movement: An analysis of ideologies and economic processes influencing policy decisions. *Advances in Nursing Science 12*(2), 71-83.

Bicknell, W. J., & Parks, C. L. (1989). As children survive: Dilemmas of aging in the developing world. *Social Science Medicine 28*(1) 59-67.

Burnside, I. (1988). *Nursing and the aged: A Self-care approach* (3rd ed.). New York: McGraw-Hill.

Butler, R. N., Brame, J. B., Kahn, C., McConnell, S., Myers, R. J., Pollack, R., & Rowland, D. (1992). Health care for all: Long-term care, the missing piece. A roundtable discussion: Part 3. *Geriatrics 47*(11), 53-54, 57-61.

Robertson, I. (1987). *Sociology* (3rd ed.). New York: Worth Publishers.

Ruggie, M. (1990, Spring). Retrenchment or realignment? U.S. mental health policy and DRGs. *Journal of Health Politics, Policy and Law, 15*(1), 145-165.

Scotch, R. K. (1988). Disability as the basis for a social movement: Advocacy and the politics of definition. *Journal of Social Issues, 44*(1), 159-172.

Taft, L. B. (1985). Self-esteem in later life: A nursing perspective. *Advances in Nursing Science, 10,* 77-84.

Warner, D. C. (1991). Nursing and public policy: What is the high ground? *Journal of Nursing Administration 21*(5), 52-57.

Yurick, A. G., Robb, S. S., Spier, B. E., & Ebert, N. J. (1984). *The aged person and the nursing process* (2nd ed.). Norwalk, CT: Appleton-Century-Crofts.

CHAPTER 24

Rehabilitation

Pamala Larsen

Introduction

Health care professionals have generally regarded rehabilitation as a service provided to individuals with sudden, traumatic injuries. Victims of accidents resulting in catastrophic injuries have benefited from rehabilitative services and have increased their independence and quality of life.

However, the increased incidence of chronic conditions, such as cancer, cerebral vascular accidents, cardiac diseases, neurological diseases, and pulmonary diseases, is a major factor in the health care system today. Chronic illness and its accompanying disability are impacting society. Modern technology has provided the means to keep the chronically ill person alive through the acute phase of illness. However, the problem now is how to provide a different, ongoing level of care that increases independence, prevents complications, and maintains an optimal quality of life after the acute phase of illness. What can be done to increase successful client outcomes? Rehabilitation is an effective approach in creating positive long-term outcomes for the chronically ill individual.

The goal of rehabilitation has often been defined as restoration to a former capacity of self. However, with a number of chronic diseases, this

is not a realistic goal. Permanent disabilities may occur, and the goal becomes to help the individual accept, adjust to, and compensate for the existing deficits, and to establish an optimal level of functioning. A better stated goal of rehabilitation, therefore, is to achieve the highest level of independence possible. For some, that may include returning to previous employment and functioning in the same job prior to illness. For others, the highest level of independence may be feeding oneself unassisted, being able to use a "sip and puff" wheelchair, or being able to stay in one's home with some assistance. For each rehabilitation client, the specific goals will be different, but for all, the overall goal is to remain as independent as possible in a setting of the client's choice.

The Philosophy of Rehabilitation

Rehabilitation is a philosophy of care as much as it is a set of techniques (Williams, 1984); a number of concepts are part of this philosophy. Basic to this philosophy is the concept of the dignity and worth of each person, whether disabled or able-bodied. In other words, each individual is of value and brings different talents to life.

Another component of the philosophy is that increased independence of clients will increase quality of life. That is, self-care is an integral part of us. By increasing self-care and independence, quality of life is enhanced.

Resocialization, a key aspect of rehabilitation, is the process by which individuals are reintegrated into society after a condition or situation alters their previous roles. Within a rehabilitation setting, resocialization is a continuing goal. Rehabilitation professionals are continually trying to reintegrate the disabled or chronically ill individual into society. This reintegration may be physical, social, emotional, or vocational, but, again, the resocialization process looks at *all* aspects of an individual's life.

As rehabilitation is a comprehensive process involving all components of an individual's life, a team concept of care is essential. No one discipline can provide all the expertise necessary in rehabilitation. Therefore, a team of professionals is necessary. Participation of the client and family in the team rehabilitation process is crucial to its success. It is expected that the client and family will attend team meetings, assist in goal setting, and be active participants in care.

With chronic illness replacing acute and infectious diseases as the premier health problem, the types of clients served by rehabilitation services has increased. There are a number of chronic conditions that may benefit from rehabilitation services. A partial list includes neuromuscular diseases such as multiple sclerosis or Parkinson's disease; cancer; cardiac and pulmonary conditions; musculoskeletal conditions such as rheumatoid arthritis or osteoarthritis; trauma including spinal cord or traumatic brain injuries; burns; cerebrovascular accidents (CVA); and orthopedic conditions such as disk disease, joint replacements, and fractures. Although the above mentioned conditions are dissimilar in a many ways, they are similar in their ability to affect function, cause disability, and decrease independence.

Rehabilitation versus Vocational Rehabilitation

A distinction is made between the terms *rehabilitation* and *vocational rehabilitation*. Although vocational placement or retraining may be an important part of the total rehabilitation proc-

ess for some clients, it may be inappropriate for others. However, the terms *rehabilitation* and *vocational rehabilitation* are often used interchangeably.

Vocational rehabilitation is just *one* component of the rehabilitation process. An act of Congress in 1920 established "rehabilitation services" (Athelstan, 1982). That original act defined rehabilitation as "the rendering of a disabled person fit to engage in a remunerative occupation" (p. 163). Certainly, work provides a sense of contribution to society and personal accomplishment, and for many individuals, work is a major part of their identity.

The vocational emphasis of rehabilitation programs was reaffirmed when medical rehabilitation research and training centers were placed under the Office of Vocational Rehabilitation in 1961 (Athelstan, 1982). This compounded the idea that rehabilitation was the same as vocational rehabilitation. However, for the increased numbers of chronically ill elderly in our society, vocational rehabilitation may not be appropriate. Though they are excellent candidates for rehabilitation, employment is not a goal.

Definitions

Rehabilitation There are a number of terms that are specific to rehabilitation that need to be defined before relating them to chronic illness. Many authors have defined rehabilitation (see Table 24-1), and there is considerable overlap between each definition. All definitions, however, consider the *wholeness* of the person, not just the physical component.

Impairment, Disability, Handicap In their publication, *International Classification of Impairments, Disabilities, and Handicaps* (ICIDH), the World Health Organization (WHO) defines the terms *impairment, disability,* and *handicap* (see Table 24-2). The ICIDH definitions are currently the ones used by rehabilitation professionals, primarily because they are clear. Because each definition is distinct and independent, a person can be impaired without being disabled, and disabled without being handicapped.

TABLE 24-1.   Definitions of rehabilitation

Source	Definition
National Council on Rehabilitation (1944)	Restoration of the handicapped to the fullest physical, mental, social, vocational, and economic usefulness of which they are capable
Rusk (1965)	Ultimate restoration of a disabled person to his or her maximum capacity—physical, emotional, and vocational
Krusen, Kottke, and Ellwood (1971)	The process of decreasing dependence of the handicapped or disabled person by developing, to the greatest extent possible, the abilities needed for adequate functioning in the individual situation
Stryker (1977)	A creative process that begins with immediate preventive care in the first stage of an accident or illness, continues throughout the restorative phase of care, and involves adaptation of the whole being to a new life
Emener, Patrick, and Hollingsworth (1984)	A process of helping handicapped individuals move from positions of dependency in their community toward positions of independency in a community of their choice
DeLisa, Martin, and Currie (1988)	The development of a person to the fullest physical, psychological, social, vocational, avocational, and educational potential consistent with his or her physiological or anatomical impairment and environmental limitations
Dittmar (1989)	The process by which an individual's movement toward health is facilitated
Hickey (1992)	A dynamic process through which a person achieves optimal physical, emotional, psychological, social, and vocational potential and maintains dignity and self-respect in a life that is as independent and self-fulfilling as possible

Impairment Impairment is defined as any loss or abnormality of psychological, physical, or anatomical structure or function (WHO, 1980). Impairment reflects change at the organ level. However, even serious impairments may not affect an individual's ability to function in his or her activities of daily living and thus may not produce a disability.

Disability If the impairment is severe enough to cause a change in functioning, then it is termed a disability, and it affects the individual at the person level. A disability is any restriction or lack (resulting from an impairment) of an ability to perform an activity in the manner or within the range considered normal for a human being (WHO, 1980). Rehabilitation techniques are designed to assist individuals in adapting to and compensating for disability.

The definition of disability as defined by the Americans with Disabilities Act of 1990 (ADA)

concurs with the ICIDH definitions. The ADA defines disability as an impairment that limits one or more major life activities (PL 101-36). This gives further credence to the fact that chronic diseases, disability, and rehabilitation are interrelated.

Handicap Handicap indicates a disadvantage for a given individual resulting from an impairment or a disability that limits or prevents the fulfillment of a role that is normal for that individual (WHO, 1980). Thus, handicap becomes an issue at the societal level. There are no handicapped individuals, but only handicapping societies that affect individuals (Brummel-Smith, 1990). Within a rehabilitation philosophy, all three levels—organ, person, and society—are addressed.

The broad-based definitions of impairment and disability by the ICIDH are all-inclusive of chronic disease. Impairment and disability are

TABLE 24-2. Definitions of impairment, disability and handicap

Impairment	Any loss or abnormality of psychological, physical, or anatomical structure or function
Disability	Any restriction or lack (resulting from an impairment) of an ability to perform an activity in the manner or within the range considered normal for a human being
Handicap	A disadvantage for a given individual resulting from an impairment or a disability that limits or prevents the fulfillment of a role that is normal for that individual

SOURCE: From World Health Organization (1980). *International Classification of Impairments, Disabilities, and Handicaps.* Geneva: World Health Organization. Used with permission.

inherent in every chronic disease. Certainly, chronic disease causes a "restriction to perform an activity," and usually several activities are affected, thus making the chronically ill person an excellent candidate for rehabilitation.

Chronic Illness In 1956 the Commission on Chronic Illness defined chronic illness as

> . . . all impairments or deviations from normal which have one or more of the following characteristics: are permanent, leave residual disability, are caused by non-reversible pathological alteration, require special training of the patient for rehabilitation, and may be expected to require a long period of supervision, observation, or care (Mayo, 1956)

This landmark work in defining chronic illness was perhaps the earliest attempt at identifying the prevalence and impact of chronic illness. Interestingly enough, although rehabilitation was mentioned as an option for the chronically ill in this definition, these services usually have not been considered for such clients. Again, rehabilitation services have been reserved for the traumatically injured.

Likewise, Strauss and associates (1984) framework for viewing chronic illness provides additional support for considering persons with chronic illness as rehabilitation candidates. They addressed the multiple problems of living daily with chronic disease. These problems are

1. The prevention of medical crises and their management once they occur
2. The control of symptoms
3. The carrying out of prescribed regimens and the management of problems attendant on carrying out the regimens
4. The prevention of, or living with, social isolation caused by lessened contact with others
5. The adjustment to changes in the course of the disease, whether it moves downward or has remissions
6. The attempts at normalizing both interaction with others and style of life
7. Funding—finding the necessary money—to pay for treatments or to survive despite partial or complete loss of employment
8. Confronting attendant psychological, marital, and familial problems (p. 16).

In summary, both classic definitions and frameworks for viewing chronic illness support the use of rehabilitation. Rehabilitation is specifically mentioned by Mayo (1956), and Strauss et al. (1984) list the countless problems of chronic illness experienced by the clients that rehabilitation professionals work with daily.

Historical Perspective

The history of rehabilitation reflects society's apathy and insensitivity toward the young, old, poor, mentally impaired, and physically disabled, all of whom are at a disadvantage when compared with the general population. Primitive people, using the philosophy that only the fit should survive, abandoned the disabled and old. Even after such practices had stopped, it was many centuries before people in disadvantageous positions received more than alms. The current standards for the care of the disadvantaged still contain an element of apathy and insensitivity toward those individuals (Stryker, 1977).

The evolution of rehabilitation for the physically disabled is associated with the increase in social consciousness. Marine hospitals, where the disabled could receive care, were established in England as early as 1588 (Stryker, 1977). In 1601 efforts were made to help the disabled through the passage of the Poor Relief Act in England. This law outlawed begging, classified dependent people, and attempted to assist both the poor and the disabled. Our present welfare system is a legacy of that law.

When the Pilgrims came to America, they brought with them the philosophy of establishing almshouses. Although the care was poor, these facilities provided for the aged, insane, blind, deaf, alcoholics, prostitutes, and other citizens without resources, and began a new age of social responsibility (Dittmar, 1989).

The 1800s generated interest in rehabilitation. Physical restoration was used in the training and care of crippled children. The field of occupational therapy was born. The first medical social service department was established at Bellevue Hospital in New York City, and Lillian Wald began the first visiting nursing service (Dittmar, 1989).

War continued to influence the growth of rehabilitation. The return of injured soldiers provided the impetus for the establishment in 1918 of a national rehabilitation program for veterans of World War I. This first program, however, concentrated only on the physical aspects of disability. The disabled veterans of World War II were privy to a more comprehensive program that included both physical and psychosocial rehabilitation. During this time, Dr. Howard Rusk demonstrated to the Army that rehabilitation rather than convalescence was essential for recovery (Kottke, Stillwell, & Lehmann, 1982).

Dr. Rusk's pioneering work provided the impetus for the establishment of the American Academy of Physical Medicine and Rehabilitation in 1938 and the development of rehabilitation medicine as a board-certified specialty in 1947 (DeLisa, Martin, & Currie, 1988). In 1974, the Association of Rehabilitation Nurses was formed, followed closely by the establishment of rehabilitation as a specialty of nursing by the American Nurses' Association (Dittmar, 1989).

Other societal forces continue to expand rehabilitation practice. Industrial and vehicular accidents and trauma from leisure and sporting activities have increased the number of disabled persons. Additionally, advances in medicine and science have lengthened the life span of those with traumatic injuries and chronic disease, providing potential candidates for rehabilitation.

Public Policy and Rehabilitation

Reimbursement Reimbursed rehabilitation services provided to the chronically ill person vary greatly under Medicare, Medicaid, and private insurance. It is essential that health care professionals be knowledgeable of financing restrictions on rehabilitation.

Medicare Medicare was designed as a federal program to provide health care for persons over the age of 65 and for disabled persons. Since a number of our country's chronically ill are over age 65, Medicare benefits and payments are of importance to rehabilitation professionals.

Rehabilitation facilities are reimbursed under the Tax Equity and Fiscal Responsibility Act (TEFRA) of 1982 (Ross, 1992). Originally, TEFRA was to be a bridge to use of the Diagnostic Related Groups (DRG) system, but TEFRA regulations currently remain in effect. Rehabilitation facilities are reimbursed at a flat rate for each Medicare discharge, regardless of diagnosis, length of stay, or services required. Each year a small increase is applied to the cost of each discharge. These increases have varied from 0.5 percent to 5.5 percent (NARF, 1991). However, one half of the rehabilitation units in the country are receiving less from Medicare than what their costs are (Ross, 1992). It is unclear what the future for rehabilitation is under Medicare reimbursement.

Medicaid Medicaid is a health care entitlement program for the poor funded by both the federal and state governments and administered by the various states. Coverage for acute rehabilitation services varies from state to state. Like Medicare, reimbursement to the rehabilitation facility for services is generally considerably less than the cost of care (Ross, 1992).

Workers' Compensation Workers' compensation is a program to compensate workers for on-the-job injuries. It is mandated by law in all 50 states, although each state varies as to procedure and who is covered (Norton, 1990). Both inpatient and outpatient medical rehabilitation services are reimbursed at 100 percent. In addition, injured workers receive a portion of their average weekly wage (Cuddihy, personal communication, 1993).

When the injured worker is deemed medically stable, or when no more significant medical improvement can be reasonably expected, an impairment rating is given the worker by a physician (Cuddihy, 1993). At that time a lump sum payment or settlement may be negotiated between the insurance carrier and the injured worker based on the degree of disability (Norton, 1990).

At present, laws in each state vary as to whether employers are required to retain the injured worker as an employee after rehabilitation. However, under the provision of the ADA, it will be mandatory for employers to make "reasonable accommodations" for injured workers to return to their work setting (Cuddihy, 1993).

Private Insurance Private insurers are coming under more pressure to contain costs. As a result, companies have implemented strict utilization review and catastrophic case management programs. Often case managers are nurses who can justify services or choose to decline services for a client. Regular communication is needed with the case manager about client needs, client progress, and anticipated length of stay. Insurance companies vary in their method of providing financial restitution to rehabilitation facilities. Insurance companies frequently reimburse facilities at a flat rate per day.

Vocational Rehabilitation   State vocational rehabilitation agencies are the main source of vocational services for persons with chronic diseases or disabilities. These agencies, under the Rehabilitation Services Administration of the federal government, are financed primarily by the federal government, with a smaller percentage coming from each state. The purpose of these agencies is to provide vocational evaluation and to coordinate restorative and training services for employment and job placement.

Clients may also receive vocational rehabilitation services from private rehabilitation companies. The private rehabilitation industry has grown rapidly in recent years. These companies may be contracted by insurance companies to evaluate clients, coordinate medical services, retrain clients, and perform job analysis and job placement. With increasing health care costs, insurance companies have sought to reduce their expenses by employing private rehabilitation companies or even having their own in-house rehabilitation services (Athelstan, 1982).

A summary of federal legislation providing vocational rehabilitation is given in Table 24-3.

Americans with Disabilities Act   The Americans with Disabilities Act of 1990 provides disabled individuals physical and vocational access to the private sector of business, industry, and education. Prior legislative efforts, the Rehabilitation Act of 1973 and its amendments were concerned only with access to businesses, organizations, and institutions that received federal financial assistance; the private sector did not have to provide accessibility to the disabled. The ADA makes compliance to equal access mandatory for the private sector (Watson, 1990).

In addition, the ADA provides a less cumbersome definition of disability. Past definitions within public policy have been disease oriented. The ADA defines three categories of disability that are protected:

1. A physical or mental impairment that substantially limits one or more of the major life activities of an individual
2. A record of such an impairment
3. Being regarded as having such an impairment (PL 101-336)

The ADA consists of four major titles that address access to employment, public services, public accommodations and services offered by

TABLE 24-3. Legislation providing vocational rehabilitation

Legislation	Purpose
Smith-Sears, 1918 (PL 65-178)	Authorized Federal Board for Vocational Education to administer a national vocational rehabilitation service to disabled veterans of World War I.
Smith-Fess, 1920 (PL 66-236)	Provided vocational rehabilitation services to people disabled in industry and otherwise.
Social Security Act, 1935 (PL 74-271)	Provided permanent authorization for the civilian vocational rehabilitation program.
Welsh-Clark, 1943 (PL 78-16)	Provided vocational rehabilitation for disabled veterans of World War II.
Hill-Burton, 1954 (PL 83-565)	Provided greater financial support, research and demonstration grants, state agency expansion and grants to expand rehabilitation facilities.
Vocational Rehabilitation Act, 1965 (PL 89-333)	Expanded and improved vocational rehabilitation services.
Rehabilitation Act, 1973 (PL 93-112)	Expanded services to the more severely handicapped by giving them priority; affirmative action in employment and nondiscrimination in facilities.
Rehabilitation Amendments, 1986 (PL 99-506)	Emphasis on functional assessments; new initiative on rehabilitation engineering and technology.

private entities, and telecommunication relay services (see Table 24-4). Throughout each of the titles, the term *reasonable accommodation* for the disabled individual is used extensively. However, it is not clearly defined in the act. The following two examples in the ADA relate to this term and provide some assistance in the definition:

1. Making existing facilities used by employees readily accessible to and usable by individuals with disabilities

2. Job restructuring; part-time or modified work schedules; reassignment to a vacant position; acquisition or modification of equipment or devices; appropriate adjustment or modifications of examinations, training materials or policies; provision of qualified readers or interpreters; and other similar accommodations for individuals with disabilities (PL 101-336)

The ADA constitutes civil rights protection for the disabled individual with access to the private sector guaranteed by law. For those affected by chronic disease, this law has far-reaching effects. With disability defined as an impairment that limits one or more major life activities, all chronic diseases, with their effects on life activities, are included under the law. The chronically ill now have physical and vocational access to the private sector under the ADA.

Problems

Providing rehabilitation services for clients is not without its problems and issues. Primary among these are economics, lack of interest by health care professionals in rehabilitation and chronic illness, and inadequate documentation of rehabilitation outcomes. Other issues include impact of the experience on the client and family, client and family compliance with the treatment regime, increasing substance abuse among the chronically ill, and lack of consensus on the rehabilitation potential of a client.

Impact of Economics

Rising health care costs have made cost containment of health care a major social and political problem in the United States today. Over the last 20 years, health care costs have continued to significantly impact the nation's Gross Domestic Product (GDP), formerly called the Gross National Product (GNP). The cost of health care insurance alone has skyrocketed, and as a result, more than 30 million Americans have no health insurance and millions more have inadequate coverage (Andreoli & Musser, 1985).

TABLE 24-4. The Americans with Disabilities Act

TITLE 1: Employment	Employers cannot discriminate against a qualified disabled job applicant or employee in any manner related to employment and benefits. Employers must make their existing facilities accessible and usable by individuals with disabilities. Accommodations in all aspects of job attainment and performance are required in order to place individuals on an equal plane with the nondisabled.
TITLE 2: Public Services	Qualified disabled individuals must have access to all services and programs provided by state or local governments. Public rail transportation must be made accessible to disabled individuals and supplemented with a paratransit system.
TITLE 3: Public Accommodations and Services Operated by Private Entities	Vitually every entity open to the public must now be made accessible to the disabled. A study is to be conducted concerning accessibility of over-the-road transportation.
TITLE 4: Telecommunications Relay Services	Telephone companies are required to furnish telecommunications devices to enable hearing- and speech-impaired individuals to communicate by wire or radio.

SOURCE: Reprinted from Watson, P. (1990). The Americans with Disabilities Act: More rights for people with disabilities. *Rehabilitation Nursing, 15*(6), 326. Published by the Association of Rehabilitation Nurses, 5700 Old Orchard Road, First Floor, Skokie, IL 60077-1057. Copyright © 1990 Association of Rehabilitation Nurses. Used with permission.

The provision of care to chronically ill or disabled persons has become a societal issue. The chronically ill person with insurance is seeing reduced funding for a number of services as health care costs escalate. The individual without insurance is in a quandary as to what to do. How does our health care system provide ongoing, cost-conscious services to someone who may be chronically ill for decades?

A basic question is What is the economic cost of dependency? What if, as a society, we choose to do nothing and allow the chronically ill to become and remain dependent? It is somewhat easy to add up the costs of acute services for a chronically ill person, but the larger issue is the maintenance costs of keeping that person alive and healthy for years. How much does it cost the individual, family, health care system, and society to keep that person dependent? To increase independence of the chronically ill person is to increase activity. Limitation of activity has a significant societal impact because it has high economic costs of dependency, maintenance, and loss of productivity. However, health care in general has been more focused on the pathology of disease and the "curing" aspect of disease. Dependency from disability has not been a concern. An informal motto of health care has been "To cure is to succeed; to care, restore or perhaps maintain function, is to fail."

Rehabilitation has failed to document clearly the effects of services (Keith, 1984). Additionally, skeptics are quick to note the expense involved with rehabilitation and its team approach; the use of so many professionals and the comparatively long-term stays of rehabilitation clients looks expensive. However, one must not evaluate rehabilitation only by short-term costs, but should look at long-term benefits of clients who are not dependent. Again, the economic case against dependency! Until rehabilitation makes a better case for its services or becomes a stronger voice in the health care community, these services will not be utilized and dependency will continue.

The 1980s and 1990s have seen an increase in the focus on health maintenance, prevention, and independence. Each of these concepts is part of rehabilitation's philosophy. Rehabilitation should be an option for the chronically ill.

Lack of Interest of Professionals in Rehabilitation

Health care has always thrived on acute care, dramatic cures, technology, and caring for a younger population. Unfortunately, the field of rehabilitation generally does not meet any of those criteria. The increased numbers of persons with chronic illnesses have increased the demand for physicians trained in chronic illness and rehabilitation. There remains, however, a lack of qualified physiatrists (physicians with special training in rehabilitation) throughout the country (DeLisa et al., 1988). It has been difficult to get physicians, nurses, and many therapists interested in working with the long-term rehabilitation client. Only one-half of the accredited medical schools in the country have physical medicine and rehabilitation departments within their schools (DeLisa et al., 1988). Even those departments have been allowed very little time to teach rehabilitation concepts (Kottke, Stillwell, & Lehmann, 1982). With little exposure to rehabilitation in medical school curricula, there is less chance of students' becoming interested in it.

Schools of nursing, likewise, emphasize a more acute care approach to the profession. With technology changing so rapidly, a primary goal of these schools is to teach as much acute care knowledge as possible. Care of the chronically ill or rehabilitation client is of less importance, unless, of course, that client is admitted to an acute care setting with acute health problems.

Additionally, health care professionals often see the older client as having a lessened rehabilitation potential. With the increasing numbers of older persons with chronic illness, however, this bias must be eliminated. Rehabilitation potential is not age dependent (Williams, 1984). A "small gain" in an older client may make a major difference and allow that individual the opportunity to live in his or her own home as opposed to a long-term care facility.

Lack of rehabilitation emphasis in medical and nursing curricula is in direct contrast to curricula of the physical, occupational, speech, and recreational therapies. These professions are primarily involved in maximizing client strengths and increasing independence.

The future of rehabilitation for all clients rests with professionals to firmly believe that it is important for the chronically ill client to have access to rehabilitation services.

Inadequate Documentation of Rehabilitation Outcomes

The best measure of the value of medical rehabilitation is client outcome (Kottke et al., 1982). Does the client have better function? Is there increased quality of life? Is the client more independent? Is there better functioning in activities of daily living? These seem to be basic and answerable questions. However, there is inadequate documentation of the effects of rehabilitation.

It is "common knowledge" among rehabilitation professionals that rehabilitation does make a difference and that clients have increased function, independence, and quality of life. But scientific data relating to treatment effectiveness and positive client outcomes are lacking (DeLisa et al., 1988). For rehabilitation to be considered in the cost-conscious health care industry, more stringent documentation must be done to substantiate rehabilitation's claims. Research demands large randomized samples and outcome tools with strong reliability and validity. Rehabilitation has few examples of such research (Haughey, 1989).

Additionally, although it may be difficult to place monetary values on some of the benefits of rehabilitation, examining them through a cost–benefit analysis is important (Conley & Noble, 1988). Continuing economic pressure will force rehabilitation to better define the benefits of its services and document positive client outcomes.

Other Issues

Impact on the Individual and Family   The impact of disability on the chronically ill individual and family is difficult to assess. As each illness produces different deficits and each individual and family have a unique social system, the impact that results is unpredictable. The case study of Judy Johnson reflects how family members,

CASE STUDY

Judy Johnson: Family Reaction to Multiple Sclerosis

Judy Johnson is a 35-year-old female recently diagnosed with multiple sclerosis following a five-year period of unexplained numbness and weakness of her legs, intermittent visual difficulties, and unusual fatigue. Judy had been working on a limited part-time basis as a registered nurse at the local hospital during that time because she had been too ill or fatigued to work regularly.

Judy's husband is on the "fast track" in the corporate world and is having a hard time dealing with Judy's illness. He can't understand why she can't entertain socially as is expected in his company, and he finds himself too busy to learn much about her disease. To his credit, he is doing better since she was given a "real diagnosis." They have two children, ages 10 and 5, and Judy finds she needs help with managing the household so that she can devote her time and energy to the children.

---

in this case the patient and her spouse, view her illness differently.

Looking at the Johnson family, one can ask what emotional impact of the illness this family can expect now and in the future. However, it is expected that the individual will be involved in the grief and mourning process during rehabilitation (see Chapter 11, on coping with fear and grieving). Coming from an acute care setting, there may have been inadequate time to work through the grief associated with loss of function, loss of sensation, changed body image, or other deficits. Within the rehabilitation setting, working with grieving clients is almost expected. Similarly, the family is going through a grieving process, but maybe not at the same speed or in the same manner as the client.

Self-care activities, in general, are taken for granted within society. Independence is a valued commodity, although its importance is not fully realized until it is threatened. Dependence and the inability to perform self-care activities can be devastating for the disabled client. Depression, lack of motivation, and decreased self-esteem often appear because of the inability to deal with dependence. Similarly, this dependence has profound effects on the family system. Role changes are often necessary, and family members take on new responsibilities (see Chapter 12, on family caregivers).

A profound issue for the individual and family concerns the depletion of financial resources (see Chapter 22, on financial impact). Treatment and compliance with the rehabilitation regimen are costly and may produce economic stress on the family. Family members may be required to pursue employment, and even that may not be enough to cope with the medical bills, the lack of income from the disabled person, and the indirect costs of disability.

In general, one thinks of a chronic illness or injury producing a visible disability. Perhaps it is the emphysemic client with noticeable shortness of breath and lack of mobility, or an individual using a wheelchair or walker because of a neuromuscular disease. However, the impact on the individual and family of having an *invisible* disability may be just as devastating (see Chapter 5, on stigma).

An invisible disability refers to a condition that evidences no noticeable outward physical changes. Invisible disabilities may include, but are not limited to, cardiac disease, diabetes mellitus, or a benign type of multiple sclerosis. Although it may seem preferable to have no noticeable signs of disability, the invisible disability may provide the individual, family, and society with unrealistic expectations of the client. This ultimately may affect the psychosocial adjustment of the individual to the chronic illness. The uncertainty of what his or her future health may bring is a heavy burden. The case study of Marion shows how even someone who has long had a disability can react adversely to someone with an invisible problem.

Social isolation and disrupted social relationships for the individual and the family may occur as a result of the illness or disability (see Chap-

CASE STUDY
Marion: Invisibility of Disability

Marion has been confined to a wheelchair for the last few years because of rheumatoid arthritis. She has undergone extensive physical rehabilitation, but still has difficulty functioning physically. One day she could not find a "handicapped" parking space near the grocery store. Her first response was to verify that everyone who was using a handicapped space in the area had appropriate identification on their cars.

When she went into the grocery store, she looked around but didn't notice anyone in a wheelchair or using a walker or cane. She voiced her complaint about "people using handicapped spaces when they weren't really handicapped." What she didn't notice was the shopper who was incapacitated by emphysema. This other shopper has often felt guilty using a handicapped parking place because she has an invisible disability and feels that, perhaps, those parking places should be reserved for the visibly disabled. She feels this way even though her own mobility would be markedly restricted if she could not park in these places.

SOURCE: Adapted from Shanck and Lubkin (1990).

ter 8, on social isolation). The stigma of chronic disease and/or the financial burden of such may cause the individual and family to consciously or unconsciously isolate themselves.

Conversely, friends and family may choose to ignore or separate from the chronically ill individual and family. The amount of energy it takes to be a social support for a chronically ill individual and family may be overwhelming, and the easiest way is to detach from the situation (Strauss et al., 1984).

Additionally, both the individual and family often suffer from loss of control in the rehabilitation process. Although they participate as members of the team, they may feel intimidated by the professional expertise of other team members.

Compliance   Compliance or adherence to a medical regimen is a continuous issue for the rehabilitation client and family. The regimen of the rehabilitation client may consist of a number of activities or therapies to increase independence. If great progress is being made with activities of daily living, there is certainly motivation to continue. However, for some clients, the progress may be slow. At times for those with neurological diseases, stroke, or brain injuries, for example, there is limited, if any, progress. With limited progress, motivation of the client and family may decrease.

For rehabilitation professionals, it may be difficult to understand why regimens are not followed. Strauss and associates (1984) sum up this lack of understanding by health care providers:

> At first blush, regimen management may not seem a problem of such magnitude: regimens are either followed by obedient, sensible patients or ignored at their peril. Indeed, physicians and other health personnel tend to regard patients (or their families) as not only foolish if they do not carry out the prescribed regimens, but downright uncooperative. They talk approvingly or disapprovingly about the adherence or lack of adherence to regimens (p. 34).

However, the issue remains that the rehabilitation client must govern his or her entire life around this very specific, and perhaps complicated, regimen with its attendant set of rules. At times, the regimen may produce more problems than the actual symptomology of the disease or illness.

Phillips (1988) examined issues of compliance and adherence in his book *Patient Compliance*. He identified perhaps 230 to 250 factors that are implicated in noncompliance. Clearly, compliance is a problem with the long-term client and will continue to be a source of frustration for rehabilitation professionals as well.

Substance Abuse Substance abuse occurring after a diagnosis of chronic illness or disability is becoming more frequent, although the true incidence is not known (Falvo, 1991). Some individuals may use alcohol or other substances to combat depression, frustration, boredom, or lack of societal acceptance. Additionally, the social isolation that some persons feel post-diagnosis may increase their susceptibility to abuse or dependence on drugs or alcohol (Falvo, 1991). Also, chronically ill persons often have easy access to prescription medications because of their treatment regimen. Compounding the problem of substance abuse is the fact that individuals with chronic illness often take a variety of medications as part of their regimen, and when combined with alcohol or other nonprescription drugs, these medications may produce unwanted effects in the person.

For some individuals, substance abuse existed prior to the chronic illness or disability and may have contributed to or intensified the chronic condition. One example is the individual who is paralyzed or brain injured as a result of a drunk driving accident and has a history of alcohol abuse.

Greer (1986) states that there is a reason for overlooking the substance abuse of the chronically ill or injured person. Physical or mental disabilities have enough social stigma attached to them without adding the extra stigma of substance abuse.

Rehabilitation professionals speak of the increasing problem with substance abuse, but there is little documentation of its incidence (Greer, 1986). Research in this area is limited as well. Clearly this is an issue for rehabilitation professionals to deal with in the future.

Rehabilitation Potential Health care payors are willing to spend dollars on clients with the most rehabilitation potential. Unfortunately, there is not a clear-cut answer as to who that client is. Perhaps the one standard in accepting a person into a rehabilitation program is, Will the client be able to both physically and psychologically participate in the total rehabilitation program each day? For a number of facilities, this consists of 3 hours of therapy daily.

Each specific disease or condition has its examples of clients who have "better" potential than others. For example, stroke rehabilitation clients have poorer outcomes and prognosis if they have had a previous stroke, are older, have bowel and bladder dysfunction, and visual-spatial deficits (Garrison et al., 1988). Also integral to dealing with the stroke client are the ability to follow instructions, either verbal or gestural, and the extent of memory deficits. With these criteria as a guide, decisions are made by the team as to rehabilitation potential.

Other criteria are used with the multiple sclerosis client. Cobble, Wangaard, Kraft, and Burks (1988) identify that poor rehabilitation outcomes for these clients are associated with poor coordination, cognition and perception deficits, and difficulty training the nonambulatory client to become ambulatory. With these criteria, one would assume that clients with poor coordination and cognitive and perception deficits would not be accepted into a rehabilitation program. However, clients with such deficits do participate in programs.

The issue that makes determining rehabilitation potential so imperfect is that one is dealing with a unique human being. Clients with supposedly poor potential can and do make progress, while those with excellent potential may do poorly.

Solutions

Chronic disease is the number-one health problem in the United States today. It produces changes in the physical, social, emotional, economic, and vocational status of individuals and their families. With the increasing numbers of individuals who are facing such illnesses, different approaches to care must be implemented. The health care system has been successful in intervening in the acute aspects of chronic disease. However, the resulting disabilities that affect many of the chronically ill provide challenges for individuals, families, and society.

How does the health care system care for the chronically ill? It becomes clear that the long-term impact of these conditions affects us all, and as the economic cost of dependency is high, efforts should be made to keep the chronically ill as independent as possible. Rehabilitation is a way of increasing the independence of the chronically ill population. Rehabilitation is an approach to care, a philosophy, and an attitude, as much as it is a set of specialized techniques. In chronic disease, the pathological condition cannot be removed. However, the disability resulting from that pathology may be altered by rehabilitation so that the person can achieve more independence, which in turn increases quality of life.

DeLisa and associates (1988) list six strategies to alter disability in chronic disease. These include (1) prevention or correction of additional disability, (2) enhancement of systems unaffected by the pathological condition, (3) enhancement of functional capacity of affected systems, (4) use of adaptive equipment to promote function, (5) modification of social and vocational environment, and (6) psychological techniques to enhance patient performance and patient education. A comprehensive rehabilitation program employs all of these strategies.

When one is considering rehabilitation for a client, it is often easier to see the short-term costs of providing such services as opposed to the long-term benefits. However, one must look at the advantages of restoring function and meaning to individuals. One needs to ask if the long-term costs of providing dependent care to a chronically ill individual outweigh the short-term costs of rehabilitation and long-term independence.

Certainly, it is not an assumption, or even a goal, that all chronically ill individuals will be independent after rehabilitation. However, the overall goal is to provide services to enhance functioning. Any increase in function benefits both the individual and society by putting less strain on health care resources. With the increasing numbers of the chronically ill, society must examine long-term solutions and view short-term costs in perspective.

Team Approach

When trying to met the physical, social, emotional, economic, and vocational needs of cli-ents, it is ludicrous to imagine that one or two disciplines can accomplish all necessary tasks. Comprehensive rehabilitation of the client with chronic illness relies on the expertise of a number of disciplines. A team approach is seen as a compromise between specialization of disciplines and the need for a comprehensive approach to care (Rothberg, 1981). It is an established practice of rehabilitation to use a "team" approach in caring for clients.

Rehabilitation teams may be either *multidisciplinary* or *interdisciplinary*. Multidisciplinary teams consist of individuals from different disciplines who may or may not coordinate their efforts in the care of a client (Dittmar, 1989). A team of this nature is only a sum of each discipline and does not build on each other's strengths.

Interdisciplinary teams, on the other hand, are based on each discipline communicating on a regular basis and establishing common goals for clients. The interdisciplinary team is synergistic, producing more than each discipline can accomplish individually (DeLisa et al., 1988). Common to such teams is consolidation and validation of knowledge; communication with the client, family, and health care providers; and collaboration of care.

The composition of the interdisciplinary rehabilitation team is influenced by several factors: the specific needs of the clients served, the philosophy of rehabilitation in that facility, financial resources, the availability of personnel, and state and federally mandated policies and requirements (Dittmar, 1989). The client and family are integral members of the rehabilitation team. They *must* be included in the development of a plan of care, and they are expected to be active participants of the team.

In general, team members include the physiatrist, rehabilitation nurse, physical therapist, occupational therapist, speech pathologist, nutritionist, psychologist, and social worker. The team may also include an audiologist, prosthetist, or clergy. Team members may have some overlap in their responsibilities, but this only strengthens the expertise of the team because their common goal is to produce an optimal outcome for the client.

Rehabilitation Settings

Whatever the setting, rehabilitation services have generally been delivered within a service model that is generally designed to deliver rehabilitation care to a mixed diagnosis group of clients (Babicki & Miller-McIntyre, 1992).

Although the interdisciplinary team approach is being used more extensively than the multidisciplinary approach, most facilities provide a general approach to multiple-diagnosis groups of clients as opposed to specific approaches to individual diagnosis groups. Today, some rehabilitation facilities are providing services through the programmatic model, defined as an "integrated delivery care system for a specific diagnostic group of patients using an interdisciplinary team with a central program director" (p. 84).

Rehabilitation services are offered in freestanding rehabilitation facilities, specialized units in acute care hospitals, long-term care facilities, or in the home. In any kind of facility, services may be either inpatient or outpatient, but all are provided through a team approach.

Hospitals and Freestanding Facilities Freestanding and in-hospital rehabilitation facilities are accredited with criteria from two organizations. The oldest is the Joint Commission on the Accreditation of Hospitals (JCOAH), whose original interest was the quality of rehabilitation programs within hospitals, but which has expanded to accrediting freestanding rehabilitation facilities as well (Melvin, 1984).

The Commission of Accreditation of Rehabilitation Facilities (CARF) accredits both inpatient and outpatient rehabilitation facilities of a medical, social, or vocational nature. A major part of CARF review is program evaluation emphasizing client outcomes (Melvin, 1984).

Some freestanding rehabilitation facilities specialize in one or two conditions, primarily spinal cord injury or traumatic brain injury. Others provide care for all types of clients. Rehabilitation units within hospitals generally have a mixed-diagnosis caseload of clients.

Long-Term Care Facilities Skilled nursing facilities may also provide rehabilitation. Although admission to a long-term care facility is often seen as a negative outcome, it may, in fact, be a very appropriate alternative for the elderly client with rehabilitation potential. However, not all skilled nursing facilities provide the same level of rehabilitation services. Services in these facilities are referred to as *restorative*, and consumers of such care need to know the extent of services offered. Skilled nursing settings have some advantages over acute care facilities for the elderly client. The pace is generally slower, lasting months instead of weeks, and the focus is on the individual, with little concern as to how fast progress is made (Osterweil, 1990).

At-Home Rehabilitation A newer approach is providing rehabilitation in the client's home. Usually the cost is considerably less than for inpatient services. With professionals coming to the client, the rationale for in-home rehabilitation is to maintain the client in the lower range of dependency or, at the very least, to maintain the status quo (Keenan, 1990).

Home rehabilitation services may be used to supplement outpatient services. With pressure from Medicare and private insurance, discharge from the acute care setting tends to occur before the client is sufficiently ready to participate, both physically and emotionally, in an inpatient rehabilitation program, causing a need for a modified program. To date, this approach is being used more with the elderly population.

Evaluation of the Client

Primary to viewing rehabilitation as an option for the client is determining his or her rehabilitation potential, an issue for both younger and older clients. Is there a potential to be semi-independent in mobility, or is there a potential to live at home with some assistance? What support is needed and available in the community for the client so that the client can stay at home?

A key in determining rehabilitation potential is the client's motivation to be independent. Internal motivation of the client is essential in completing a program and attaining goals. External motivation may be enough initially, but will not carry the client through the program. Motivation is a factor with all rehabilitation clients (Kemp, 1986).

Evaluation of the client is an ongoing component in the rehabilitation process. As the goal of rehabilitation is to increase functional performance and assist the client to an optimal level, it is essential to measure functional outcomes of the client. Rehabilitation uses the term *functional assessment* to describe such client evaluation. Granger (1984) defines functional assessment as "a method for describing abilities and activities in order to measure an individual's use of the variety of skills included in performing the tasks necessary to daily living, vocational pursuits, social interactions, leisure activities, and other required behaviors" (p. 24). With this definition as a beginning, a comprehensive functional assessment would consist of a number of different tools to measure the multiple variables involved in the rehabilitation client's total being. Therein lies a potential problem—presently there is no tool that inclusive.

Functional assessment tools have a variety of purposes, including (1) the development of a client problem list, (2) evaluation of the client's progress and outcomes, (3) measurement of treatment interventions, (4) cost–benefit effectiveness of care (5) assistance in the rehabilitation program's evaluation and audit, (6) goal setting based on identified strengths and weaknesses of the client, and (7) research.

In general, functional assessment tools are categorized into three groups or scales that provide systematic methods to evaluate client functioning (Hens, 1989). *Global* scales incorporate a multidimensional approach in evaluation of the client. *Categorical* scales limit measurement to a single condition, such as hand function, mental status, or mobility status (Hens, 1989). *Activities of daily living* (ADL) scales concentrate on activities such as eating, bathing, walking, and dressing. An example of an ADL scale is the Barthel index (see Table 24–5). The table presents the items or tasks scored in the Barthel index with the corresponding values for independent performance of the tasks.

When assessing function in the elderly client, however, caution must be used. The above mentioned tools were normed to a general population and may not provide an accurate representation of the elderly (Kane & Kane, 1981). This is particularly true for the client over the age of 75 and for clients who are institutionalized.

Geriatric Rehabilitation

The population over the age of 75 is the fastest growing segment of society (Kemp, Brummel-Smith, & Ramsdell, 1990), and, not surprisingly, their most significant health care problem is chronic disease. However, the elderly client with a chronic disease can live a productive, independent life if given the opportunity to participate in a geriatric rehabilitation program.

Geriatric rehabilitation is a fairly new concept in rehabilitation. Historically, rehabilitation was reserved for younger clients, since it was assumed that the end result of rehabilitation was a vocational outcome. For the elderly client, gainful employment may not be a possibility, but rehabilitation can still be an option. The practice of geriatrics, in general, promotes the functional approach to client care. Thus, it can be argued that rehabilitation, with the strong philosophy of increasing function, is the foundation of geriatric care (Kemp et al., 1990).

The presence of a disabling condition in an older client, as well as in a younger one, does not mean the end of independence. The end point of disability has to be independence. Small gains in independence may enable the older individual to stay at home, with some outside assistance, as compared to living in a long-term care facility. A home health aide assisting the person may then be all that is needed so the client can remain in his or her own home. Geriatric rehabilitation increases function that allows for independence. Rehabilitation for the older client provides long-term solutions for that person. If one looks at the short-term costs of rehabilitation of the older client, they may seem prohibitive. However, the long-term benefits of greater independence outweigh such costs.

According to Brody and Ruff (1986), there are three subgroups of disabled elderly who may benefit from rehabilitation services:

1. The developmentally disabled who are surviving past middle age for the first time

TABLE 24-5. The Barthel index

	"Can Do by Myself"	"Can Do with Help of Someone Else"	"Cannot Do at All"
SELF-CARE SUBSCORE			
1. Drinking from a cup	4	0	0
2. Eating	6	0	0
3. Dressing upper body	5	3	0
4. Dressing lower body	7	4	0
5. Putting on brace or artificial limb	0	−2	0 (N/A)
6. Grooming	5	0	0
7. Washing or bathing	6	0	0
8. Controlling urination	10	5 (accidents)	0 (incontinent)
9. Controlling bowel movements	10	5 (accidents)	0 (incontinent)
MOBILITY SUBSCORE			
10. Getting in and out of chair	15	7	0
11. Getting on and off toilet	6	3	0
12. Getting in and out of tub or shower	1	0	0
13. Walking 50 yards on the level	15	10	0
14. Walking up/down one flight of stairs	10	5	0
15. If not walking: Propelling or pushing wheelchair	5	0	0 (N/A)

Barthel total: Best score is 100; worst score is 0.

Note: Tasks 1–9, the self-care subscore (including control of bladder and bowel sphincters), have a total possible score of 53. Tasks 10–15, the mobility subscore, have a total possible score of 47. The two groups of tasks combined make up the total Barthel index with a total possible score of 100.

SOURCE: From Granger, C., & Gresham, G. (1984). *Functional assessment in rehabilitation medicine* (p. 74). Baltimore: Williams & Wilkins. Used with permission.

2. Adults with long-time traumatic injuries who are surviving longer due to the availability of better medical care
3. The elderly client with a recent disability or chronic disease.

The third group makes up the largest number of potential clients for rehabilitation services. Clearly, services may be appropriate for a number of older clients, but how and where these services are offered differs in every community. The admission criteria for the older client in both inpatient and outpatient rehabilitation facilities may differ from criteria used with the younger client, whom the medical community sees as having a greater number of years to be "productive." However, the increased graying of the population and the number of chronic diseases that this population presents cannot go unnoticed. The health care system has to look beyond the present and believe there is a need to keep the elderly disabled client as independent as possible. Geriatric rehabilitation needs to be seen as a viable option for the chronically ill.

Self-Help Groups

A societal trend has been the shift from seeking help from institutions to self-help (Hymovich & Hagopian, 1992). Increasingly, the chronically ill are taking care of themselves at home or having more family care than institutional care. Part of this self-care trend is the participation in self-help groups.

Self-help groups originally emerged out of needs for mutual support, problem solving, or assisting others in coping (Newton, 1984). It was estimated that in 1986 there were 500,000 mutual aid support groups for individuals to share with others having similar concerns (Parcel, Bartlett, & Bruhn, 1986). The growth of such support groups has been attributed to consumer activism, increased acceptance by health care professionals of patient education, and behavior modification techniques emphasizing self-management (Hymovich & Hagopian, 1992).

Usually these groups are formally organized, have regular meetings that may include a formal presentation, and provide time for group interaction. These groups can provide preventive intervention for the individual with chronic illness. Group membership is usually confined to a specific health problem. For clients with a chronic illness or disability, self-help groups provide long-term support, and further extend the social support system of the individual.

Addressing the Need for Rehabilitation

Although rehabilitation professionals deal with a number of different chronic diseases, the disabilities produced by these diseases are often very similar. For example, rehabilitation services may be provided for a number of mobility-disabled individuals, but each individual's disability may have originated from a very different impairment.

Services for several chronic conditions have addressed the need for, and provided specific rehabilitation guidelines for, clients, including guidelines for cardiac disease, pulmonary disease, and cancer.

Cardiac Rehabilitation   Cardiac rehabilitation was developed from a prevention, wellness perspective. With heart disease the number-one cause of mortality in the United States, there are many potential candidates for such rehabilitation. Cardiac rehabilitation programs are longitudinal, preventive in nature, and demand strong client participation. Cardiac rehabilitation has three phases: Phase I, in-hospital; Phase II, early post-hospitalization; and Phase III, maintenance.

As with all rehabilitation, cardiac rehabilitation addresses the physiological, psychological, social, and vocational aspects of disability (Brammell, 1988).

Pulmonary Rehabilitation   Goals for a pulmonary rehabilitation program include reduction in the average number of hospital days per year and subjective improvement in dyspnea as it relates to function and self-care (Rondinelli & Hill, 1988). As pulmonary disabilities are likely to be permanent and progressive, realistic goals are of utmost importance for the client, family, and interdisciplinary team.

Cancer Rehabilitation   Cancer rehabilitation includes attempts at maximizing both independence and dignity in individuals with cancer (Watson, 1992). The development of cancer rehabilitation began in the 1970s and has moved into the 1990s with more support because of the increased incidence of cancer and the improved survival rates (Watson, 1992).

The goals of cancer rehabilitation include prevention, restoration, support, and palliation (Dietz, 1980). Prevention reduces or prevents the impact of cancer. Restoration strives to return the individual to premorbid status with minimal disability. Support reduces disabilities through rehabilitation interventions. And palliation provides comfort, reduces complications, maintains independence, and provides emotional support.

Rehabilitation Clinical Nurse Specialist

As the provision of health care begins to shift into a cost-benefit, cost-containment model, the clinical nurse specialist will be used more often as a primary or adjunct care provider. Among these nurse specialists is the rehabilitation clinical nurse specialist. The incidence of chronic illness and the accompanying need for nonacute, long-term approaches to care provide a perfect arena for the rehabilitation clinical nurse specialist.

Rehabilitation clinical nurse specialists are prepared at either the master's or doctoral level and are certified in rehabilitation nursing by the

Association of Rehabilitation Nurses (ARN). They provide expertise in the provision of both direct and indirect care of the rehabilitation client. As core members of the interdisciplinary team, these nurses provide expertise in preventing further disability, maintaining function, and restoring lost function. A key component of their role is the emphasis on providing education for the client and family.

Additionally, rehabilitation clinical nurse specialists may provide their expertise and services to private rehabilitation companies and insurance companies as consultants or as case managers. The increased numbers of catastrophic injuries and diseases have shown the need for such expertise, and companies have recognized the importance of the nurse specialist's expertise.

Research

Rehabilitation must develop a stronger research base if it is to survive as a viable option for the chronically ill (DeLisa et al., 1988). Rehabilitation professionals state that rehabilitation makes a difference, client outcomes are successful, and there is increased function and quality of life of disabled clients. But there is no research to validate this contention. If research were available, many would not still question the effectiveness of rehabilitation when compared to the cost. In the past cost–benefit studies of rehabilitation have usually been done from the viewpoint of the institution and not the individual.

Kane (1990) provides an overview of the problems of research in rehabilitation. Rehabilitation professionals attest to the fact that they can recognize a good outcome when they see it, but designing a tight study can be difficult. Randomized studies involving rehabilitation effectiveness are difficult to design. Kane (1990) argues that not providing rehabilitation borders on unethical practice. So one must ask how to set up a tight experimental study with a control group and experimental group.

Another research issue is when the rehabilitation process ends. At what point in time are outcomes measured? Six months? Twelve months? The time factor is important when mea-suring the effectiveness of a program or a specific intervention (Kane, 1990). Additionally, how does one account for the fact that there is a degree of natural recovery in some disease processes, such as a stroke? If the client improves functionally, is it because of rehabilitation or the decreased swelling of the brain?

Rehabilitation must provide more evidence of its worth, and the way to accomplish that is through research. If rehabilitation's existence cannot be justified, in these days of high health care costs, less costly alternatives may be implemented.

Summary

The prevalence of chronic illness will continue, and the health care system needs creative approaches to lessen the impact of chronic illness and its accompanying disabilities. We need to find ways of decreasing dependence and increasing opportunities for the chronically ill. Certainly, the passage of the ADA in 1990 finally allowed the disabled citizens of the United States access to both the private and public sector in regard to employment and public accommodations. This major civil rights legislation will have farreaching effects, some of which are not yet clear.

Rehabilitation is an approach to chronic illness that can decrease the economic cost of dependency. As one looks at cost–benefit ratios of rehabilitation, one needs to look at long-term benefits, not short-term costs. Since rehabilitation services are expensive, social and economic pressure will force the rehabilitation industry to design more cost-effective methods of providing service, such as more outpatient and in-home services. However, maintaining quality of services will be a challenge. Geriatric rehabilitation programs will need to increase, since that population continues to rise and need to be kept independent.

Rehabilitation must develop a stronger research base to validate that it makes a difference in client outcomes and quality of life. It is a true prevention and wellness model of care and can be the basis of future health care in the chronically ill population.

STUDY QUESTIONS

1. Describe impairment, disability, and handicap, and relate those terms to chronic illness.
2. Rehabilitation is a philosophy as much as it is a set of techniques. Name five different components of the philosophy and explain each.
3. Identify three problems in the provision of rehabilitation services to the chronically ill.
4. Describe the different settings where rehabilitation services can be provided.
5. Geriatric rehabilitation is a relatively new concept with special issues of its own. What benefits and problems do you see in this concept?
6. What specific issues of rehabilitation makes doing research difficult?
7. Discuss the three different types of functional assessment tool.

References

Andreoli, K., & Musser, L. (1985). Trends that may affect nursing's future. *Nursing and Health Care, 6*(1), 47–51.

Athelstan, G. (1982). Vocational assessment and management. In F. Kottke, G. Stillwell, & J. Lehmann, (Eds.). *Krusen's handbook of physical medicine and rehabilitation* (3rd ed.) (pp. 163–189). Philadelphia: W. B. Saunders.

Babicki, C., & Miller-McIntyre, K. (1992). A rehabilitation programmatic model: The clinical nurse specialist perspective. *Rehabilitation Nursing, 17*(2), 145–153.

Brammel, H. (1988). Rehabilitation of the cardiac patient. In J. DeLisa (Ed.), *Rehabilitation medicine* (pp. 671–687). Philadelphia: J. B. Lippincott.

Brody, S., & Ruff, G. (Eds.) (1986). *Aging and rehabilitation: Advances in the state of the art.* New York: Springer.

Brummel-Smith, K. (1990). Introduction. In B. Kemp, K. Brummel-Smith, & J. Ramsdell (Eds.), *Geriatric rehabilitation* (pp. 3–21). Boston: Little, Brown.

Cobble, N., Wangaard, C., Kraft, G., & Burks, J. (1988). Rehabilitation of the patient with multiple sclerosis. In J. DeLisa (Ed.), *Rehabilitation medicine* (pp. 612–634). Philadelphia: J. B. Lippincott.

Conley, R., & Noble, J. (1988). Americans with severe disabilities. In J. Goodgold (Ed.), *Rehabilitation medicine* (pp. 924–941). St. Louis: Mosby.

DeLisa, J., Martin, G., & Currie, D. (1988). Rehabilitation medicine: Past, present and future. In J. DeLisa (Ed.), *Rehabilitation medicine* (pp. 3–24). Philadelphia: J. B. Lippincott.

Dietz, J. (1980). Adaptive rehabilitation in cancer. *Postgraduate Medicine, 68,* 145–153.

Dittmar, S. (Ed.) (1989). *Rehabilitation nursing: Practice and application.* St. Louis: Mosby.

Falvo, D. (1991). *Medical and psychosocial aspects of chronic illness and disability.* Gaithersburg, MD: Aspen.

Garrison, S., Rolak, L., Dodaro, R., & O'Callaghan, A. (1988). Rehabilitation of the stroke patient. In J. DeLisa (Ed.), *Rehabilitation medicine* (pp. 565–584). Philadelphia: J. B. Lippincott.

Granger, C. (1984). A conceptual model for functional assessment. In C. Granger & G. Gresham (Eds.), *Functional assessment in rehabilitation medicine* (pp. 14–25). Baltimore: Williams & Wilkins.

Greer, B. (1986). Substance abuse among people with disabilities: A problem of too much accessibility. *Journal of Rehabilitation, 52,* 34–38.

Hanlon, D., & Sharkey, E. (1989). Professional practice of rehabilitation nursing. In S. Dittmar (Ed.), *Rehabilitation nursing: Practice and application* (pp. 73–79). St. Louis: Mosby.

Haughey, B. (1989). Research. In S. Dittmar (Ed.), *Rehabilitation nursing: Practice and application* (pp. 541–567). St. Louis: Mosby

Hens, M. (1989). Functional evaluation. In S. Dittmar (Ed.), *Rehabilitation nursing: Practice and application* (pp. 486–501). St. Louis: Mosby.

Hickey, J. (1992). *The clinical practice of neurological and neurosurgical nursing* (3rd ed.). Philadelphia: W. B. Saunders.

Hymovich, D., & Hagopian, G. (1992). *Chronic illness in children and adults.* Philadelphia: W. B. Saunders.

Kane, R. (1990). Measuring the effectiveness of rehabilitation programs. In B. Kemp, K. Brummel-Smith, & J. Ramsdell (Eds.), *Geriatric rehabilitation* (pp. 429–440). Boston: College-Hill.

Kane, R., & Kane, R. (1981). *Assessing the elderly.* Lexington, MA: Lexington Books.

Keenan, J. (1990). In-home geriatric rehabilitation. In B. Kemp, K. Brummel-Smith, & J. Ramsdell (Eds.), *Geriatric rehabilitation* (pp. 357–369). Boston: Little, Brown.

Keith, R. (1984). Functional assessment in program evaluation for rehabilitation medicine. In

C. Granger & G. Gresham (Eds.), *Functional assessment in rehabilitation medicine* (pp. 122-139). Baltimore: Williams & Wilkins.

Kemp, B. (1986). Psychosocial and mental health issues in rehabilitation of older persons. In S. Brody & G. Ruff (Eds.), *Aging and rehabilitation* (pp. 122-158). New York: Springer.

Kemp, B., Brummel-Smith, K., & Ramsdell, J. (Eds.) (1990). *Geriatric rehabilitation.* Boston: Little, Brown.

Kottke, F., Stillwell, G., & Lehmann, J. (Eds.) (1982). *Krusen's Handbook of physical medicine and rehabilitation* (3rd ed.). Philadelphia: W. B. Saunders.

Mayo, L. (Ed.) (1956). *Guides to action on chronic illness,* New York: National Health Council, Commission on Chronic Illness.

Melvin, J. (1984). The relationship of functional assessment to quality of care review. In C. Granger & G. Gresham (Eds.), *Functional assessment in rehabilitation medicine* (pp. 140-153) Baltimore: Williams & Wilkins.

National Association of Rehabilitation Facilities (NARF) (1991). *NARF issues brief.* Washington, D.C.: NARF.

Newton, G. (1984). Self help groups. *Journal of Psychosocial Nursing, 22*(7), 27-31.

Norton, J. (1990). Compensation and litigation in disabled pain patients. In T. Miller (Ed.), *Chronic pain, volume I* (pp. 147-176). Madison, CT: International Universities Press.

Phillips, E. (1988). *Patient compliance.* Toronto: Hans Huber Publishers.

Rondinelli, R., & Hill, N. (1988). Rehabilitation of the patient with pulmonary disease. In J. DeLisa (Ed.). *Rehabilitation medicine* (pp. 688-707). Philadelphia: J. B. Lippincott.

Ross, B. (1992). The impact of reimbursement issues on rehabilitation nursing practice and patient care. *Rehabilitation Nursing, 17*(5), 236-238.

Rothberg, J. (1981). The rehabilitation team: Future direction. *Archives of Physical Medicine and Rehabilitation, 62*(8), 407-10.

Rusk, H. (1965). Preventive medicine, curative medicine—the rehabilitation. *New Physician, 59*(4), 156-60.

Shanck, A., & Lubkin, I. (1990). Rehabilitation. In I. Lubkin (Ed.), *Chronic illness: Impact and interventions* (2nd ed.) (pp. 403-423). Boston: Jones and Bartlett.

Strauss, A., Corbin, J., Fagerhaugh, S., Glaser, B., Maines, D., Suczek, B., & Wiener, C. (1984). *Chronic illness and the quality of life* (2nd ed.). St. Louis: Mosby.

Stryker, R. (1977). *Rehabilitative aspects of acute and chronic nursing care.* Philadelphia: W. B. Saunders.

Watson, P. (1990). The Americans with Disabilities Act: More rights for people with disabilities. *Rehabilitation Nursing 15*(6), 325-8.

——— (1992). Cancer rehabilitation: An overview. *Seminars in Oncology Nursing, 8*(3), 167-73.

Williams, T. (Ed.) (1984). *Rehabilitation in the aging.* New York: Raven Press.

World Health Organization (WHO). (1980). *International classification of impairments, disabilities and handicaps.* Geneva: WHO.

Bibliography

Berg, R., & Cassells, J. (Eds.) (1990). *The Second fifty years: Promoting health and preventing disability.* Washington, D.C.: National Academy Press.

DeLisa, J. (Ed.) (1988). *Rehabilitation medicine.* Philadelphia: J. B. Lippincott.

Emener, W., Patrick, A., & Hollingsworth, D. (Eds.) (1984). *Critical issues in rehabilitation counseling.* Springfield, IL: Charles C. Thomas.

Krusen, F., Kottke, F., & Ellwood P. (1971), *Handbook of physical medicine and rehabilitation.* Philadelphia: W. B. Saunders.

National Council on Rehabilitation (1944). *Symposium on the processes of rehabilitation.* New York: National Council on Rehabilitation.

Osterweil, D. (1990). Geriatric rehabilitation in the long-term care institutional setting. In B. Kemp, K. Brummel-Smith, & J. Ramsdell (Eds.), *Geriatric rehabilitation* (pp. 347-456). Boston: Little, Brown.

Parcel, G., Bartlett, E., & Bruhn, J. (1986). The role of health education in self-management. In K. A. Holyroyd & T. L. Creer (Eds.), *Self-management of chronic disease* (pp. 3-27). Orlando: Academic Press.

Power, P. (1989). Working with families: An intervention model for rehabilitation nurses. *Rehabilitation Nursing, 14*(2), 73-76.

APPENDIX

Name and Address	Type of Service/Goals/Comments

AGING

American Society on Aging
833 Market Street
San Francisco, CA 94103

To enhance well-being of older individuals, foster unity among those working with the elderly.

Gray Panthers
1424 16th Street, N.W., Suite 602
Washington, D.C. 20036

Consciousness-raising activist group of older adults and young people. Aim: to combat ageism.

Families USA Foundation
1334 G Street, N.W.
Washington, D.C. 20005

Projects and educational activities to help the elderly.

National Council on the Aging
409 3rd Street, S.W.
Washington, D.C. 20024

Cooperates with other organizations to promote concern for older people. National information and consulting center.

National Association of Area Agencies
  on Aging
1112 16th Street, N.W.
Washington, D.C. 20024

Established under provisions of the Older Americans Act. Promotes realistic/reasonable national policy on aging and advocates for needs of older persons at national level.

National Center on Rural Aging
c/o National Council on the Aging
409 3rd Street, N.W.
Washington, D.C. 20024

See National Council on Aging.

SOURCE: From Daniels, P. K., Schwartz, C. A. (Eds.), *Encyclopedia of associations* (28th ed.). Detroit: Gale Research. The organizations selected for the appendix are only a small sample of many thousands listed.

Name and Address	Type of Service/Goals/Comments
National Senior Citizens Law Center 1052 W. 6th Street, Suite 700 Los Angeles, CA 90017	Specializes in legal problems of the elderly; advocates on behalf of the elderly poor in litigation.

AIDS

CDC National AIDS Clearinghouse P.O. Box 6003 Rockville, MD 20849-6003	Primarily for professionals. Provides information on HIV/AIDS. Maintains database.
Gay Men's Health Crisis 129 W. 20th Street New York, NY 10011	Social service agency for treatment of AIDS. Provides support, therapy groups, crisis counselors, preventive programs. Provides legal, financial, health care, and advocacy services.
Pediatric AIDS Coalition 1331 Pennsylvania Avenue, N.W., Suite 721 N Washington, D.C. 20004	Advocates for children with HIV/AIDS and their families. Pediatric task force to meet needs of HIV-infected children.

ALLERGY

Asthma and Allergy Foundation of America 1125 15th Street, N.W., Suite 502 Washington, D.C. 20005	Voluntary health agency focusing on solving health problems posed by allergic diseases.
National Foundation for the Chemically Hypersensitive P.O. Box 222 Aphelia, VA 22530	Disseminates information on symptoms, sources of exposure. Networking. Assistance in handling social security and workers' compensation claims.
National Environmental Health Association 720 S. Colorado Boulevard Suite 970, South Tower Denver, CO 80222	For professionals working with environmental disorders.

CANCER

American Cancer Society 1599 Clifton Road, N.E. Atlanta, GA 30329	Supports education and research. Sponsors Reach for Recovery, Can Surmount, I Can Cope.
Association for Research in Childhood Cancer P.O. Box 251 Buffalo, NY 14225-0251	Funds research in pediatric cancer and provides seed money for pilot projects in cancer research.
Breast Cancer Advisory Center P.O. Box 224 Kensington, MD 20895	Medical service group for breast cancer.
Cancer Cares 1180 Avenue of the Americas New York, NY 10036	Promotes and aids social services to patients and families.

Name and Address	Type of Service/Goals/Comments
Cancer Information Service Office of Cancer Communication NCI/NIH, Building 31, 10A24 9000 Rockville Pike Bethesda, MD 20892	Funded by the National Cancer Institute.
National Alliance of Breast Cancer Organizations 1180 Avenue of the Americas New York, NY 10036	Resource for organizations, programs, individuals. Seeks to influence policy pertaining to breast cancer.
Spirit and Breath Association 8210 Elmwood Avenue, Suite 209 Skokie, IL 60077	Associated with American Cancer Society. Provides support for patients and families. Information exchange.

HEARING OR VISION IMPAIRMENT

American Association of the Deaf-Blind 814 Thayer Avenue, Room 300 Silver Spring, MD 20910	Encourages independent living. Advocates before public bodies. Referral services.
Association for Macular Diseases 210 E. 64th Street New York, NY 10021	Information or resources such as recorded material, low-vision aids. Counseling.
Association of Late-Deafened Adults P.O. Box 641763 Chicago, IL 60664-1763	Information, support, social opportunities via self-help groups. Advocacy. Research. Provides captioning at public meetings.
Better Vision Institute 1800 N. Kent Street, Suite 904 Rosalyn, VA 22209	Advisory council of Vision Council of America. Consultation.
Children of Deaf Adults Box 30715 Santa Barbara, CA 93130	Information for professional organizations and others about families with deaf parents. Support. Clearinghouse for families.
Deafness Research Foundation 9 E. 38th Street, 7th floor New York, NY 10016	Seed grants (1–3 years) for research related to hearing disorders and ear diseases.
National Eye Research Foundation c/o Pamela Baker 910 Skokie Blvd #207A Northbrook, IL 60062	For people in the field of eye care. Sponsors research and education. Public information center.

MENTAL HEALTH
MENTAL RETARDATION/DISABILITY

Anxiety Disorders Association of America[1] 6000 Executive Boulevard Rockville, MD 20852	Research and treatment of anxiety disorders and phobias, panic disorders, obsessive-compulsive behavior.

[1]Formerly the Phobia Society of America.

Name and Address	Type of Service/Goals/Comments
Depression and Related Affective Disorders Association Johns Hopkins Hospital Meyer 3-181 600 N. Wolfe Street Baltimore, MD 21205	Support services. Research. Education programs.
Mental Health Law Project 1101 15th N.W., Suite 1212 Washington, D.C. 20005	To clarify, establish, enforce legal rights of people with mental/developmental disabilities.
Mental Retardation Association of America 211 East 300 South, Suite 212 Salt Lake City, UT 84111	To improve quality of life, promote research for prevention, advocate.
National Association of Developmental Disabilities Councils 1234 Massachusetts Avenue, N.W., Suite 103 Washington, D.C. 20005	Promotes cooperation and communication between government agencies and individual groups.
National Mental Health Association[2] 1021 Prince Street Alexandria, VA 22314-2971	To increase public awareness. Public education. Advocates. Funds research.
Project Overcome 50 Ft. Avenue, Apartment 224 Minneapolis, MN 55406	To eliminate stigma attached to patients with mental illnesses.

NEUROLOGICAL/MUSCULAR DISORDERS

Alzheimer's Association[3] 919 N. Michigan Avenue, Suite 1000 Chicago, IL 60611	For family members. Promotes research, provides education programs, develops family support systems.
American Paralysis Association 500 Morris Avenue Springfield, NJ 07081	Grants for research in spinal cord injuries, head injuries, or stroke.
American Parkinson's Disease Association 60 Bay Street, Suite 401 Staten Island, NY 10301	Information and referral centers. Funds research. Provides counseling services.
Amyotrophic Lateral Sclerosis (ALS) Association 2021 Ventura Boulevard, Suite 321 Woodland Hills, CA 91364	Help and information for ALS patients and families. Funds research.

[2]Formerly the National Association for Mental Health; Mental Health Association.
[3]Formerly the Alzheimer's Disease and Related Disorders Association.

Name and Address	*Type of Service/Goals/Comments*
Children's Attention Deficit Disorders (ADD) 499 N.W. 70th Avenue, Suite 308 Plantation, FL 33317	Support groups. Education. Information resource. Seeks opportunities for good education for ADD children.
Epilepsy Foundation of America 4351 Garden City Drive Landover, MD 20785	Voluntary health agency. Prevention and control, improved lives of those with epilepsy. Education, information, government liaison, research, counseling.
Multiple Sclerosis Foundation 6350 N. Andrews Avenue Ft. Lauderdale, FL 33309	Funds research, education and other services.
National Head Injury Foundation 1776 Massachusetts Avenue, N.W., Suite 100 Washington, D.C. 20036	Improves quality of life. Promotes prevention through education, information, advocacy. Supports research.
National Spinal Cord Injury Association 600 W. Cummings Park, Suite 200 Woburn, MA 01801	Informs and educates professionals and others. Supports research. Assists individuals in reaching personal goals. Provides recreation, advocacy, support groups, peer counseling.
National Stroke Association 300 E. Hampden Avenue, Suite 240 Englewood, CO 80110-2654	To reduce incidence and impact of stroke via research, education. Information clearinghouse. Maintains a hot line.
United Cerebral Palsy Association 1522 K Street, N.W., Suite 1112 Washington, D.C. 20005	Aids persons with cerebral palsy and their families. Supports research and traineeships.

PAIN

American Chronic Pain Association P.O. Box 850 Pocklin, CA 95677	Helps individuals suffering from chronic pain become involved in their own recovery.
American Pain Society 5700 Old Orchard Road, 1st Floor Skokie, IL 60077-1024	For professionals to promote control, management, and understanding.
Chronic Pain Support Group P.O. Box 148 Pennisula, OH 41264	Self-help for patients, family, and friends.
National Headache Foundation 5252 N. Western Avenue Chicago, IL 60625	Disseminates information. Funds studies.
National Chronic Pain Outreach Association 7979 Old Georgetown Road, Suite 100 Bethesda, MD 20814-2429	Disseminates information via clearinghouse. Support groups starter kit. Referrals.

Name and Address	*Type of Service/Goals/Comments*

REHABILITATION
HANDICAPPED/DISABLED

AFTER Rehabilitation and Training Center
  for Limb Deficiencies/Amputations
2559 Fairway Island Drive
Willington, FL

To improve self-image and independence of limb-deficient children.

American Association of Cardiovascular
  and Pulmonary Rehabilitation
7611 Elmwood Avenue, Suite 201
Middleton, WI 53562

To improve clinical practice. Promotes research and education.

American Disability Association
2121 8th Avenue, N., Suite 1623
Birmingham, AL 35203

Support group. Information exchange. Children's services. Education, research, charitable services.

Amputee Shoe and Glove Exchange
P.O. Box 27067
Houston, TX 77227

Information about other amputees to facilitate swaps.

National Rehabilitation Association
633 S. Washington Street
Alexandria, VA 22314

Among other activities, conducts legislative activities, develops accessibility guidelines. Divisions include job placement, National Association of Independent Living, vocational and work adjustment.

SUBSTANCE ABUSE[4]

Alcohol and Drug Problems Association of
  North America
444 N. Capital Street, N.W., Suite 706
Washington, D.C. 20001

Facilitates government and professional activities in field of alcohol and drug abuse via information, promotion of legislation and standards of care.

Alcoholics Anonymous World Services
  (A.A.)
475 Riverside Drive
New York, NY 10613

Self-help support group. Uses 12-step program, which they developed.

Association of Halfway House Alcoholism
  Programs of North America
786 E. 7th Street
St. Paul, MN 55106

Placement, technical assistance, education.

BACCHUS of the United States
National Headquarters
P.O. Box 100430
Denver, CO 80250

Alcohol education to college students.

---

[4]Many other 12-step programs are listed under this heading in the *Encyclopedia of associations,* as are other groups and associations dealing with the problem of substance abuse.

Name and Address	*Type of Service/Goals/Comments*
Drug Anon Focus P.O. Box 20806 New York, NY 10025	Self-help support group for families and friends of people addicted to mood-altering drugs. Follows 12-step method of A.A.
Drugs Anonymous P.O. Box 772 Bronx, NY 10451	Applies A.A. 12-step program to drug-addicted persons.
Women for Sobriety P.O. Box 618 Quakertown, PA 18951	Not a 12-step program. Self-help for women only. Approach recognizes male/female differences in alcohol use and methods for successful recovery.
Rational Recovery Systems P.O. Box 800 Lotus, CA 95651	Not a 12-step program. Self-help group. Based on belief that each individual has power to overcome addiction other than through spiritualism. Provides live-in services.

OTHER ORGANIZATIONS

American Diabetes Association[5] National Center P.O. Box 25757 1660 Duke Street Alexandria, VA 22314	Educates the public. Research in diabetes mellitus prevention and cure.
Burns United Support Groups 441 Colonial Court Grosse Pointe Farms, MI 48236	Support services to burn survivors and their families. Education, children's services.
Crohn's and Colitis Foundation of America[6] 444 Park Avenue, S., 11th floor New York, NY 10016-7374	Research into cause and cure. Education.
National Association for Craniofacially Handicapped P.O. Box 11082 Chatanooga, TN 37401	Financial assistance. Resource file of treatment centers. Support groups. Information.
National Association for Sickle Cell Disease 127 W. 127th, Room 421 New York, NY	Voluntary health agency. Research and education programs. Focus on eradicating sickle cell anemia. Activities mostly in New York.
Phoenix Society for Burn Survivors 11 Rust Hill Road Levittown, PA 19056	Self-help for survivors and their families to ease psychosocial adjustment for severely burned and disfigured persons.

[5]The primary association for diabetes mellitus. There are groups for other metabolic disorders.

[6]Formerly the Foundation for Ileitis and Colitis; National Foundation for Ileitis and Colitis.

INDEX

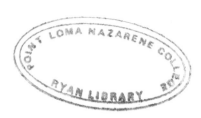